Endometriosis

Tasuku Harada
Editor

Endometriosis

Pathogenesis and Treatment

Springer

Editor
Tasuku Harada
Department of Obstetrics
and Gynecology
Tottori University
Faculty of Medicine
Yonago, Tottori, Japan

ISBN 978-4-431-54420-3 ISBN 978-4-431-54421-0 (eBook)
DOI 10.1007/978-4-431-54421-0
Springer Tokyo Heidelberg New York Dordrecht London

Library of Congress Control Number: 2014942646

Printed on acid-free paper

Springer is part of Springer Science+Business Media (www.springer.com)

Preface

Endometriosis remains an enigmatic disease despite a long history of research into its basic science and clinical aspects. Sampson published his pioneer article in 1927 theorizing that retrograde menstruation may cause peritoneal endometriosis. Since that time, researchers throughout the world have wrestled with the mysteries of the disease. In this book, we bring you a compendium of the present understanding of the pathogenesis of endometriosis as well as how this information may be applied in current therapies. As editor, I invited an international group of distinguished scientists to contribute chapters and was happy that all graciously agreed to do so. In particular, many Asian scientists made significant contributions.

Our hope is that this book will provide useful information and fresh knowledge to all physicians and scientists interested in endometriosis, and that it will stimulate further research and lead to more efficacious treatment modalities.

Yonago, Tottori, Japan

Tasuku Harada

Contents

Part I
Introduction

Chapter 1
Endometriosis: A Mysterious Disease

Tasuku Harada

Abstract Endometriosis is an enigmatic disease, despite a long history of research into its basic science and clinical aspects. Sampson published his pioneer article in 1927, theorizing that retrograde menstruation may cause peritoneal endometriosis. Since that time, researchers throughout the world have wrestled with the mysteries of the disease. In this book, we bring you a compendium of the present understanding of the pathogenesis of endometriosis as well as how this information may be applied in current therapies. As editor, I invited an international group of distinguished scientists to contribute a chapter and was happy that all graciously agreed to do so. Our hope is that this book will provide useful information and fresh knowledge to all doctors and scientists interested in endometriosis, and that it will stimulate further research, and lead to more efficacious treatment modalities.

Keywords Autotransplant • Epigenetics • Eutopic endometrium • Implantation theory • Pathogenesis

1.1 Introduction

Endometriosis is an enigmatic disease, despite a long history of research into its basic science and clinical aspects. Sampson published his pioneer article in 1927, theorizing that retrograde menstruation may cause peritoneal endometriosis [1]. Since that time, researchers throughout the world have wrestled with the mysteries of the disease. In this book, we bring you a compendium of the present understanding of the pathogenesis of endometriosis as well as how this information may be applied in current therapies. As editor, I invited an international group of

T. Harada, M.D., Ph.D., D.M. Sci. (✉)
Department of Obstetrics and Gynecology, Faculty of Medicine,
Tottori University, 36-1 Nishi-cho, Yonago 683-8504, Japan
e-mail: tasuku@med.tottori-u.ac.jp

T. Harada (ed.), *Endometriosis: Pathogenesis and Treatment*,
DOI 10.1007/978-4-431-54421-0_1,

distinguished scientists to contribute a chapter and was happy that all graciously agreed to do so. Our hope is that this book will provide useful information and fresh knowledge to all doctors and scientists interested in endometriosis, and that it will stimulate further research, and lead to more efficacious treatment modalities.

The prevalence of endometriosis in women varies widely: 0.7–11 % in populations presenting for health care, 2–22 % when undergoing surgical sterilization, 17–47 % among infertile women, and 2–74 % in women with chronic pelvic pain [2]. An estimated 2.6 million Japanese women have this disease, extrapolating a prevalence rate of 10 % among reproductive age women. An increase in the incidence of endometriosis is worrisome because the birth rate in Japanese has decreased and age of primiparous is reportedly over 30 years old. The number of newborn babies is decreasing in Japan, while the population over 65 years old is increasing. In such circumstances, infertility due to endometriosis of women is a serious socioeconomical problem in Japan.

The assumption that the incidence of endometriosis is increasing is based on the combination of the implantation theory of retrograde menstruation and the data of well-known studies on epidemiology. Several well-designed epidemiological studies reported that shorter menstrual cycles, longer duration of flow, heavier menstrual flow, and low parity are risk factors for endometriosis [3], indicating an increased number of menstruation and retrograde reflux may increase risk of the disease.

The classic theory on the pathogenesis of endometriosis includes implantation theory, coelomic metaplasia theory, and embryonic Mullerian rests. A recent study found that extrauterine stem cells originating from bone marrow may differentiate into endometriotic tissues [4]. Although many researchers argue that modern technologies of molecular medicine are unveiling the unsolved issues regarding the pathogenesis of endometriosis, Sampson's implantation theory has never been discarded.

Redwine raised a question about an intriguing point in Sampson's theory. His paper entitled "Was Sampson wrong?" proposed that endometriotic tissues may not be autotransplanted tissue. After reviewing more than 200 papers on autotransplants and comparisons of endometriosis and endometrium, Redwine pointed out that a majority of studies found multiple and significant alterations between ectopic endometrium (endometriosis) and original endometrium. He suggested that endometriosis is not a simple autotransplant, indicating that endometriosis is not a displacement (implantation) of normal endometrium. Redwine concluded that Sampson may be wrong [5].

We investigated the expression of inflammatory cytokines and prostaglandins in eutopic endometrium and endometriotic tissues [6–8]. Recently, we obtained interesting data regarding differential expression of inflammatory genes in eutopic endometrium and endometriosis. We obtained endometriotic tissue from ovarian chocolate cysts at the time of laparoscopic surgery, collected the two types of eutopic endometrial tissues, and classified them as follows: (1) the disease-free (F-Em: patients with benign ovarian tumor) and (2) endometriosis with ovarian chocolate cysts (C-Em). Gene expression of interleukin-6 (IL-6), IL-8, and

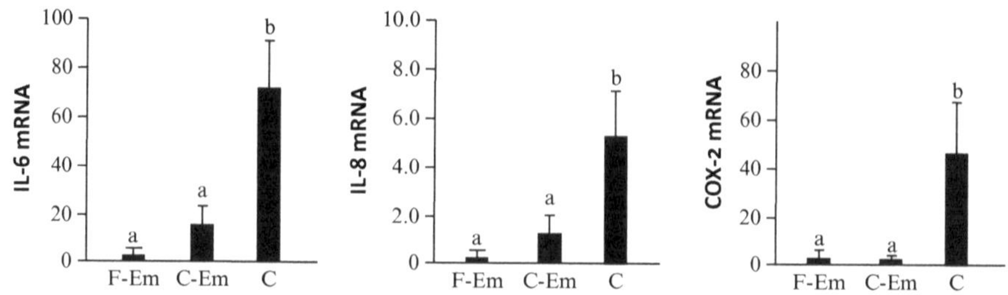

Fig. 1.1 Quantitative analysis of IL-6, IL-8, and COX-2 gene expression in human endometrial and endometriotic tissues. The mRNA levels were evaluated by real-time RT-PCR. The abbreviations of the three types of tissues are as follows: (1) eutopic endometrial tissues of disease-free, F-Em ($n = 15$); (2) eutopic endometrium with ovarian chocolate cyst, C-Em ($n = 15$); and (3) the ovarian chocolate cyst, C ($n = 15$). The mRNA level of F-Em (proliferative phase) set arbitrarily at 1.0. Data are the mean ± SE of three independent experiments. Bars that do not share a letter are significantly different ($P < 0.05$)

cyclooxygenase 2 in endometriotic tissue is enhanced compared with that in both types of eutopic endometrial tissues (Fig. 1.1). With regard to IL-6 and IL-8 mRNA expression, eutopic endometrium in women with endometriosis exhibited greater expression than the disease-free endometrium.

These observations suggest that the biological character of endometriosis tissue regarding inflammatory mediators is quite distinguishable from the eutopic endometrium of disease-free women. Therefore, this implies that endometriosis tissue is not derived from eutopic endometrium as Redwine described. It may also not be an autotransplant disease. On the other hand, we can speculate (1) that eutopic endometrium had already been altered within the uterine cavity before its implantation to the peritoneum or (2) that endometriotic tissues may change their biological character during separation from the uterus, escape from immune clearance, attachment, invasion, establishment of local neurovascularity, and continued growth. In the latter case, however, altered gene expression in the eutopic endometrium of patients with endometriosis cannot be explained. Why modest alterations occur in eutopic endometrium of patients with endometriosis is observed.

Taylor and colleagues published interesting papers, reporting significant changes in multiple markers of endometrial receptivity in the eutopic endometrium after induction of endometriosis in a mouse model [9]. They showed reduction in the Hoxa 10 gene in the eutopic endometrium of the endometriosis model mouse, a similar finding to that observed in women with endometriosis. They also found hypermethylation of the Hoxa 10 gene in the eutopic endometrium of mouse endometriosis model. These data suggest that the presence of endometriotic tissue may induce changes in eutopic endometrial gene expression. The alteration of gene expression is regulated through epigenetic transcriptional repression. In Taylor's subsequent study, cells from endometriotic lesions when induced in the mouse model migrated to the eutopic endometrium [10]. Together with these observations, experimentally induced ectopic endometrium may influence eutopic endometrium through direct movement of cells and influence via epigenetic changes.

Experimental studies in autotransplant animal models used eutopic endometrium in the non-menstrual phase. The transplanted ectopic endometrial tissues gained distinct biological character compared with the eutopic endometrium [11, 12]. These distinct characteristics are observed in human endometriotic tissues, suggesting that biological character of eutopic endometrium can be altered in humans also. Although conclusive data are still not available, we know much more about the details of the nature of transplanted endometrium than our great senior doctors, like Sampson. Endometriosis is still a mysterious disease. The accumulation of research data slowly unveils its character and its application in endometriosis patient care is urgently awaited.

References

1. Sampson JA. Peritoneal endometriosis due to the menstrual dissemination of endometrial tissue into the peritoneal cavity. Am J Obstet Gynecol. 1927;14:422–69.
2. Peterson CM, Johnstone EB, Hammoud AO, Stanford JB, Varner MW, Kennedy A, Chen Z, Sun L, Fujimoto VY, Hediger ML, Buck Louis BM. Risk factors associated with endometriosis: importance of study population for characterizing disease in the ENDO study. Am J Obstet Gynecol. 2013;208:451.
3. Eskenazi B, Warner ML. Epidemiology of endometriosis. Obstet Gynecol Clin North Am. 1997;24:235–58.
4. Sasson IE, Taylor HS. Stem cells and the pathogenesis of endometriosis. Ann N Y Acad Sci. 2008;1127:106–15.
5. Redwine DB. Was Sampson wrong? Fertil Steril. 2002;78:686–93.
6. Harada T, Iwabe T, Terakawa N. Role of cytokines in endometriosis. Fertil Steril. 2001;76:1–10.
7. Iba Y, Harada T, Horie S, Deura I, Iwabe T, Terakawa N. Lipopolysaccharide-promoted proliferation of endometriotic stromal cells via induction of tumor necrosis factor alpha and interleukin-8 expression. Fertil Steril. 2004;82:1036–42.
8. Takenaka Y, Taniguchi F, Miyakoda H, Takai E, Terakawa N, Harada T. Lipopolysaccharide promoted proliferation and invasion of endometriotic stromal cell via induction of cyclooxygehase-2 expression. Fertil Steril. 2010;93:325–7.
9. Lee B, Du H, Taylor HS. Experimental murine endometriosis induces DNA methylation and altered gene expression in eutopic endometrium. Biol Reprod. 2009;80:79–85.
10. Santamaria X, Massasa EE, Taylor HS. Migration of cells from experimental endometriosis to the uterine endometrium. Endocrinology. 2012;153:5566–74.
11. Sharpe KL, Vernon MW. Polypeptides synthesized and released by rat ectopic uterine implants differ from those of the uterus in culture. Biol Reprod. 1993;48:1334–40.
12. Machado DE, Berardo PT, Palmero CY, Nasciutti LE. Higher expression of vascular endothelial growth factor (VEGF) and its receptor VEGFR-2 (Flk-1) and metalloproteinase-9 (MMP-9) in a rat model of peritoneal endometriosis is similar to cancer disease. J Exp Clin Cancer Res. 2010;29:4.

Part II
Basic Science

Chapter 2
Pathological Aspect and Pathogenesis of Endometriosis

Ritsuo Honda and Hidetaka Katabuchi

Abstract Historically, endometriosis was first described in Egyptian scrolls in the sixteenth century BC. The first scientific description of endometriosis was published by Carl Freiherr von Rokitansky in 1860. At this time, the concept of endometriosis as a disease entity was not established and it was assumed to be an enigmatic disease with an unknown pathology. Although extensive basic and clinical research has been carried from the last century until present, the pathogenesis of endometriosis is still controversial. Major theories on the pathogenesis of endometriosis are (1) metastases of endometrial tissues to an ectopic location (transplantation theory), (2) metaplastic development of endometrial tissue on the ectopic site (metaplastic theory), and (3) changes of the embryonic duct remnant epithelium into endometrial epithelium (müllerian remnants theory). A comprehensive understanding of the histopathogenesis of endometriosis is essential to the novel clinical approaches for the enigmatic disease.

Keywords Endometriosis • Pathogenesis • Pathophysiology

2.1 Introduction

Endometriosis is a common gynecological disease of unknown etiology which affects an estimated 10–45 % in infertile females. Endometriosis is defined as the presence of endometrial tissue, consisting of both glandular epithelium and stroma, in ectopic locations. Clinically, it can be associated with many distressing and debilitating symptoms, such as pelvic pain, severe dysmenorrhea, dyspareunia, and infertility, or it may be asymptomatic and incidentally discovered at laparoscopic surgery.

R. Honda, M.D., Ph.D. (✉) • H. Katabuchi
Department of Obstetrics and Gynecology, Faculty of life Sciences, Kumamoto University, 1-1-1 Honjo, Chuo-ku, Kumamoto 860-8556, Japan
e-mail: ritz@kuamoto-u.ac.jp

T. Harada (ed.), *Endometriosis: Pathogenesis and Treatment*,
DOI 10.1007/978-4-431-54421-0_2, © Springer Japan 2014

In 1860, the first histological description of endometriosis was given by von Rokitansky [1]. In 1896, Cullen suggested that adenomyoma, as he called it, resembled the histological features of normal endometrial epithelium and stroma [2]. The term "endometriosis" was first described by Sampson in 1925 [3] and his studies became a pioneering figure of research on the pathogenesis of endometriosis [3–5]. Endometriosis is believed a benign disease, but it has been confirmed that it may lead to recurrence and metastasis and be secondary ovarian cancer from chocolate cysts. Because of the different locations of the disease, its pathogenesis also has been attributed either to transplantation of viable endometrial cell fragments, to coelomic metaplasia, or to embryonic remnants, and several contributing factors are also involved, including retrograde menstruation, disturbances of hormonal conditions, or familial and genetic factors.

2.2 Sites of Endometriosis

Endometriosis is defined as a pathological disease caused by the presence and proliferation of ectopic endometrial tissue in sites other than the endometrial cavity. Endometriosis often develops in the ovary, pouch of Douglas, and uterosacral ligaments and sometimes in the fallopian tubes, uterine cervix, vagina, colon and rectum, vermiform appendix, urinary bladder and tract, and others, that is, mostly in the peritoneum of the pelvic cavity and associated deep tissue [6].

Endometriosis is also occasionally observed in remote organs such as lymph nodes, pudendum, umbilicus, and lung [6]. Cases of endometriosis can occur in tissues beyond the pelvis and have diverse symptoms that depend on the site of development, including pain and/or bleeding, associated with the menstrual cycle. Rarely, endometriosis has been reported in males. However, they were all older men suffering from prostate cancer, who were treated with high doses of estrogens. In these cases, a hypertrophic change of the müllerian remnants was observed in the prostate [7].

2.3 The Theory of Secondary Müllerian System

The term "secondary müllerian system" was first described by Lauchlan in 1972 [8]. He noted the propensity of the peritoneum which covers the surface of the ovary and the peritoneal cavity to müllerian differentiation. The surface mesothelial and the submesothelial stroma of peritoneum exhibit a full spectrum of müllerian differentiation from benign to malignant. Many lesions of secondary müllerian system are described, which are benign, such as endosalpingiosis, of the low grade of malignancy, serous and mucinous and malignant, described as extraovarian peritoneal serous and mucinous carcinomas, and endometriosis is considered as the main lesson of the secondary müllerian system [9]. It is proposed that the development of peritoneal müllerian lesions may be secondary to the proximity of pelvic peritoneum to tubal fimbria and the exposure of the peritoneal surfaces to external agents, such as talc and asbestos, that stimulate the peritoneal müllerian differentiation [10].

2.4 Microscopic Findings of Endometriosis

The focus of endometriosis is basically formed of three components: the endometrial glandular epithelium, an endometrium-specific stroma, and a stroma with fibrosis that forms the lesion in regions of chronic inflammation associated with endometriosis. Findings of fibrosis are associated with infiltration of inflammatory cells such as macrophages, mast cells, monocytes, eosinophil granulocytes, and basophil granulocytes; proliferation of fibroblasts; and smooth muscle metaplasia, angiogenesis, and innervation. Similar to the original endometrium, the ectopic glandular and stromal cells also express estrogen and progesterone receptors. In response to the expression of the sex steroid receptors, stromal cells show a decidual reaction in the pregnant women.

The cell morphology of glandular epithelium may change to that of the epithelium of müllerian ducts; epithelial cells of the fallopian tubes [11], the glandular epithelium of the endocervical canal (Fig. 2.1b), with apocrine-like cells (Fig. 2.1c) and intestinal epithelium (Fig. 2.1d). These changes usually may occur in response to inflammation and others, and it enables epithelial cells to change to their surrounding circumstances to better adapt to their environment [12].

2.5 Theories on the Pathogenesis of Endometriosis

Because of the different locations, possible organs, appearances, and hormone responsiveness, many theories on the pathogenesis of endometriosis have been proposed over about one century. However, no single theory is sufficient to explain the development of this enigmatic disease.

2.5.1 Transplantation

The theory of transplantation implies that the endometrium is replaced from the uterus to another location inside the body. Many different ways of dissemination of endometrial tissue are involved in this concept. Iatrogenic, lymphogenic, and hematogenic spread account for uncommon, extraperitoneal lesion of endometriosis [13, 14]. The most easily understood, scientifically supported, and widely accepted mechanism for the histogenesis of endometriosis is that, at menstruation, some effluent flows retrograde through the lumen of fallopian tubes into the

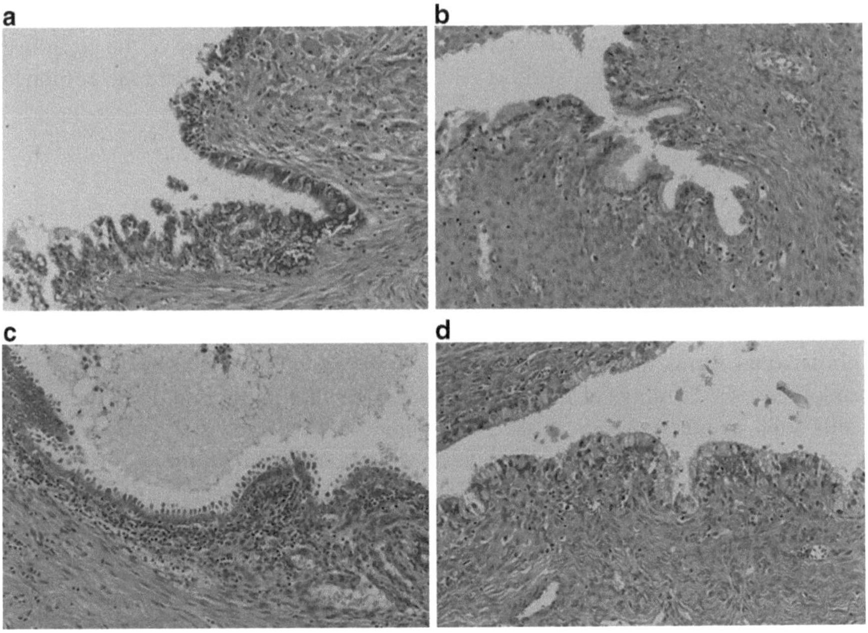

Fig. 2.1 Metaplasia of epithelial cells involved in endometriosis. (**a**) Metaplasia of tubal epithelial cells. (**b**) Metaplasia of endocervical canal glandular cells. (**c**) Apocrine metaplasia. (**d**) Intestinal metaplasia. Hematoxylin–eosin stain, (**a–d**) ×200 (Reprinted from Okamura and Katabuchi [12] with permission of Int Rev Cytol.)

peritoneal cavity (Fig. 2.2). Indeed, the high frequency of this phenomenon is supported by the finding of menstrual blood in the peritoneal fluid of up to 90 % of women with patent fallopian tubes undergoing laparoscopy during the perimenstrual period [16]. Although retrograde menstruation explains the physical displacement of endometrial fragments into the peritoneal cavity, additional steps are necessary for the development of endometriotic implants. Escape from the immune clearance system, during the courses of attachment to the ovarian surface epithelium and peritoneal mesothelium, invasion of the epithelium, establishment of local neurovascularity, and continued growth and survival are necessary if endometriosis is to develop from retrograde passage of the endometrium.

2.5.2 *Coelomic Metaplasia*

The theory of coelomic metaplasia suggests that the mesothelium of the peritoneum including ovarian surface epithelium (OSE) can be transformed into endometrium by metaplasia. The müllerian ducts, which constitute the primordial uterus, are generated through intrusion of the coelomic epithelium in the antenatal stage. For this reason, it has been proposed secondary müllerian system; the organs derived

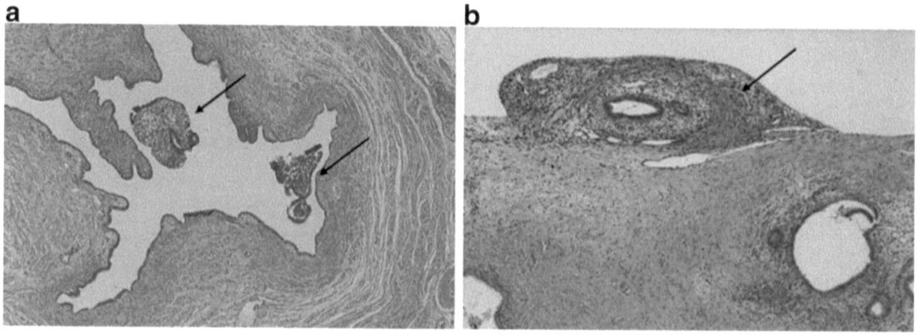

Fig. 2.2 Histogenesis of endometriosis. (**a**) Exfoliated endometrial tissue (*left arrow*) floating in the tubal cavity. (**b**) Endometrial tissue (*left arrow*) adhering to the peritoneum. Hematoxylin–eosin stain, (**a**) ×40, (**b**) ×100 (Reprinted from Katabuchi [15] with permission of J Japan Societ Endo.)

from müllerian duct are generated from the same origin as that of the peritoneal mesothelium and OSE [8, 17]. The peritoneal mesothelium and OSE may undergo metaplasia into the endometrial epithelium and stroma, thereby inducing endometriosis. We rarely come across the histological evidence for this metaplastic progression in the ovarian surface as shown in Fig. 2.3 [17]. Moreover, in the observation of morphological changes in a collagen-embedded culture system of the human OSE [18], the OSE and the coculture of OSE with endometrial stromal cells (ES) showed a luminal structure with estradiol (E_2) supplementary (Fig. 2.4a–c), and, in the OSE/ES coculture, the nuclear position was deviated toward the basal side and the appearance of cilia was observed [19]. The OSE/ES coculture was positive for epithelial membrane antigen (EMA) and cytokeratin, indicating differentiation into glandular cells, while the epithelium of the OSE culture was negative for EMA. These findings suggest that the OSE can differentiate into glandular cells and that E_2 and endometrial stromal cells are involved in this process. Thus, flow of endometrial stromal cells in the menstrual blood back through the fallopian tube may be an important factor in the development of endometriosis [18–20].

2.5.3 Müllerian Ducts Remnants

In the antenatal phase, the coelomic epithelium gives rise to the müllerian ducts, which constitute the fallopian tubes and the uterus and the upper portion of the vagina. During the course of differentiation and migration of the müllerian ducts and fetal organogenesis, some primordial cells might spread in the posterior pelvic floor. This might explain the findings that endometriosis is frequently found in the pouch of Douglas, uterosacral ligaments, and rectovaginal septum and even the presence of endometriosis among young women with Mayer–Rokitansky–Küster–Hauser syndrome.

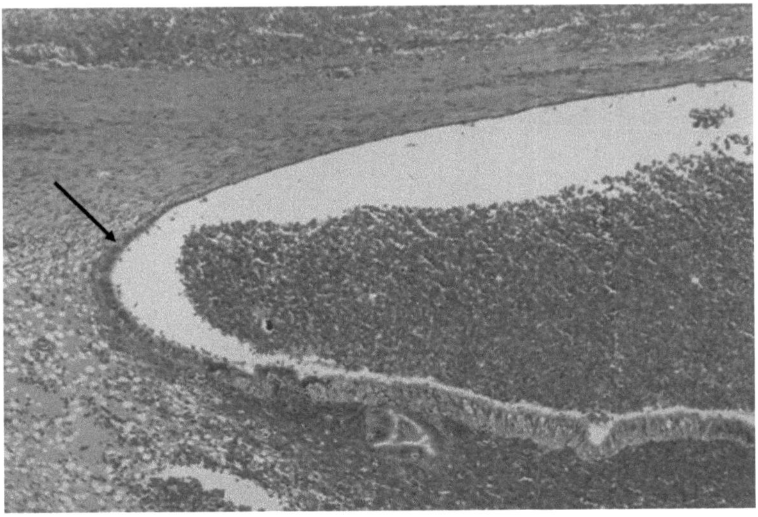

Fig. 2.3 Progression of a cyst enclosed in the ovary to endometriosis. Single layer of the surface epithelium in the cortex of the ovary, which formed the cyst, moved to the glandular epithelium of the endometrium (*right arrow*). Hematoxylin-eosin stain, ×150 (Reprinted from Okamura and Katabuchi [17] with permission of Ital J Anat Embryol.)

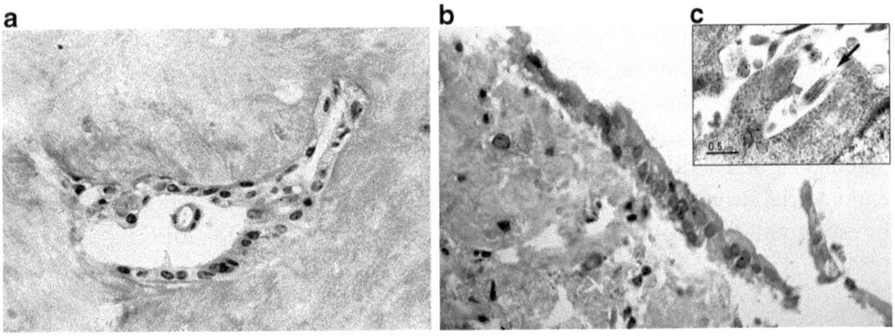

Fig. 2.4 Three-dimensional collagen gel-embedded cultures of the ovarian surface epithelium (OSE). (**a**) In the OSE culture, a cavity formed after addition of estradiol 17β (10 ng/mL). (**b**, **c**) In a coculture of OSE with the endometrial stoma, an epithelium-stoma structure formed, the surface epithelium formed a cavity with a three–dimensional structure, the position of the nucleus was biased toward the basal side, and cilia appeared. Hematoxylin–eosin stain, (**a**) ×200, (**b**) ×400; Uranyl acetate-lead citrate stain, (**c**) ×17,000 (Reprinted from Ohtake et al. [19] with permission of Fertil Steril.)

2.6 The Factors Affecting the Development of Endometriosis

2.6.1 Disturbances of Hormonal Conditions

Hormonal alterations may influence the ability of endometrial cells to proliferate, attach to the mesothelium, and/or evade immune-mediated clearance [11]. Sex steroids including estradiol (E_2) are found intracellularly in patients with endometriosis. Aromatase is specifically expressed in endometrial tissue and converts androstenedione to estrone (E_1), which in turn is converted to E_2 by 17β-hydroxysteroid dehydrogenase (17β-HSD) type 1. 17β-HSD type 2, which converts E_2 to E_1 for regulation of E_2 activity, is found in the normal endometrium, but seems not to be expressed in the tissue of patients with endometriosis, with a consequent increase in the local concentration of E_2 [21]. In addition to estrogen dependence, there is increasing evidence to support a profile of P resistance in the pathophysiology of endometriosis [22]. Endometriotic lesions exhibit an overall reduction in P receptor expression relative to eutopic endometrium and absence of P receptor-B [23]. Additionally, endometrial expression profiling has documented dysregulation of P-responsive genes in the luteal phase [24]. An incomplete transition of endometrium from the proliferative to a secretory phase has significant molecular implantation of refluxed endometrial cells.

2.6.2 Familial and Genetic Factors

The upregulation of the antiapoptotic gene BCL-2 in eutopic and ectopic endometrium from women with endometriosis is reported, and a genetic alteration of endometrial cells influencing their tendency to implant may be hereditary [25]. Linkage analysis has elucidated candidate genes with biological plausibility. The largest of these involved over 1,000 families more than two affected sib pairs and established significance for a susceptibility locus in the regions of chromosome 10q26 and 7p15 [26, 27].

2.6.3 Inflammation

From the studies of macrophages in the female reproductive organ since the 1980s [28, 29], the conceptualization of endometriosis as a pelvic inflammatory condition is established. In patients with endometriosis, the peritoneal fluid is remarkable for an increased number of activated macrophages and important differences in the cytokine/chemokine profile. Macrophages produce and secrete diverse physiologically active substances including cytokines, coagulation factors, fibrinolytic factors, components of complement, plasma proteins, lipids, and enzymes. A proteomics approach identified a unique protein structurally similar to haptoglobin in the peritoneal fluid in patients with endometriosis [30]. This protein was subsequently found to bind to macrophages, reduce their phagocytic activity, and increase their production of IL-6. Other cytokines or chemokines found to be increased in the peritoneal fluid of patients with endometriosis include macrophage migration inhibitory factor, TNF-α, IL-1β, IL-6, and IL-8, regulated on activation normal T expressed and secreted, and monocyte.

2.7 Conclusions

The pathogenesis of endometriosis has been studied among major theories; however, no single theory is sufficient to explain the development of the disease. It has been suggested that peritoneal endometriosis, chocolate cysts of the ovary, and adenomyotic nodules of the rectovaginal septum or deeply infiltrating endometriosis are three different disease entities, each with a different pathogenesis. This concept leads that diverse pathological conditions underlie endometriosis and leads to the proposal of endometriosis as a series of syndromes that develop through different mechanisms depending on the host tissue or organ. Recently, a combination of the metastatic and metaplastic theories has been favored to explain that endometriosis represents a polygenetic disorder, with alterations in multiple biological pathways leading to a metaplastic process under the irritating effect of endometrial tissue shed during retrograde menstrual flow. Thus, endometriosis has a long medical and historical background and is appropriately referred to as an enigmatic disease. Clinical treatment in line with individual pathology is required because of the diverse symptoms and findings. Further assessment of the pathology of endometriosis may open the way for development of new drugs for this disease.

Co-workers in our Department Okamura H, Matsuura K, Ohba T, Tashiro H, Fukumatsu Y, Nakamura M, Ohtake H, Motohara K, Miyamura S.

References

1. von Rokitansky C. Ueber Uterusdrusen-Neubilding in Uterus- und Ovarial – Sarcomen. Ztschr KK Gesellsch Der Aerzte zu Wien. 1860;37:577–81.
2. Cullen TS. Adeno-myoma uteri diffusum benignum. Johns Hopkins Hosp Bull. 1896;6:133–7.
3. Sampson JA. Perforating hemorrhagic cysts of the ovary. Their importance and especially their relation to adenomas of the endometrial type. Arch Surg. 1921;3:245–323.
4. Sampson JA. Inguinal endometriosis. Am J Obstet Gynecol. 1925;10:462–503.

5. Sampson JA. Peritoneal endometriosis due to menstrual dissemination of endometrial tissue into the peritoneal cavity. Am J Obstet Gynecol. 1927;14:422–69.
6. Olive DL, Pritts EA. Treatment of endometriosis. N Engl J Med. 2001;345:266–75.
7. Suginami H. A reappraisal of the coelomic metaplasia theory by reviewing endometriosis occurring in unusual sites and instances. Am J Obstet Gynecol. 1991;165:214–8.
8. Lauchlan SC. The secondary müllerian system. Obstet Gynecol Surv. 1972;27:133–46.
9. Clement PB. Reactive tumor-like lesions of the peritoneum. Am J Clin Pathol. 1995;103:673–6.
10. Lauchlan SC. The secondary Müllerian system revisited. Int J Gynecol Pathol. 1994;13:73–9.
11. Kitawaki J, Kado N, Ishihara H, Koshiba H, Kitaoka Y, Honjo H. Endometriosis: the pathophysiology as an estrogen-dependent disease. J Steroid Biochem Mol Biol. 2002;83:149–55.
12. Okamura H, Katabuchi H. Pathophysiological dynamics of human ovarian surface epithelial cells in epithelial ovarian carcinogenesis. Int Rev Cytol. 2005;242:1–54.
13. Ridley JH. Pathogenesis of endometriosis. A review of facts and fancies. Obstet Gynecol Surv. 1968;23:1–35.
14. Victory R, Diamond MP, Johns DA. Villar's node: a case report and systematic review of endometriosis externa of the umbilicous. J Mnim Invasive Gynecol. 2007;14:23–33.
15. Katabuchi H. J Japan Societ Endo. 2009.
16. Halme J, Hammond MG, Hulka JF, Raj SG, Talbert LM. Retrograde menstruation in healthy women and in patients with endometriosis. Obstet Gynecol. 1984;64:151–4.
17. Okamura H, Katabuchi H. Detailed morphology of human ovarian surface epithelium focusing on its metaplastic and neoplastic capability. Ital J Anat Embryol. 2001;106:263–76.
18. Nakamura M, Katabuchi H, Ohba T, Fukumatsu Y, Okamura H. Isolation, growth and characteristics of human ovarian surface epithelium. Virchows Arch. 1994;424:59–67.
19. Ohtake H, Katabuchi H, Matsuura K, Okamura H. A novel in vitro experimental model for ovarian endometriosis: the three-dimensional culture of human ovarian surface epithelial cells in collagen gels. Fertil Steril. 1999;71:50–5.
20. Okamura H, Katabuchi H, Nitta M, Ohtake H. Structural changes and cell properties of human ovarian surface epithelium in ovarian pathophysiology. Microsc Res Tech. 2006;69:469–81.
21. Zeitoun K, Takayama K, Sasano H, Suzuki T, Moghrabi N, Andersson S, Johns A, Meng L, Putman M, Carr B, Bulun SE. Deficient 17beta-hydroxysteroid dehydrogenase type 2 expression in endometriosis: failure to metabolize 17beta-estradiol. J Clin Endocrinol Metab. 1998;83:4474–80.
22. Bulun SE, Cheng YH, Yin P, Imir G, Utsunomiya H, Attae E, Innes J, Julie KJ. Progesterone resistance in endometriosis: link to failure to metabolize estradiol. Mol Cell Endocrinol. 2006;248:94–103.
23. Attia GR, Zeitoun K, Edward D, Johns A, Carr BR, Bulun SE. Progesterone receptor isoform A but not B is expressed in endometriosis. J Clin Endocrinol Metab. 2000;85:2897–902.
24. Burney RO, Talbi S, Hamilton AE, Vo KC, Nyegaard M, Nezhat CR, Lessey BA, Giudice LC. Gene expression analysis of endometrium reveals progesterone resistance and candidate susceptibility genes in women with endometriosis. Endocrinology. 2007;148:3814–26.
25. Jones RK, Searle RF, Bulmer JN. Apoptosis and bcl-2 expression in normal human endometrium, endometriosis and adenomyosis. Hum Reprod. 1998;13:3496–502.
26. Treloar SA, Wicks J, Nyholt DR, Montgomery GW, Bahlo M, Smith V, Dawson G, Mackay IJ, Weeks DE, Bennett ST, Carey A, Ewen-White KR, Duffy DL, O'Connor DT, Barlow DH, Martin NG, Kennedy SH. Genomewide linkage study in 1,176 affected sister pair families identifies a significant susceptibility locus for endometriosis on chromosome 10q26. Am J Hum Genet. 2005;77:365–76.
27. Painter JN, Anderson CA, Nyholt DR, Macgregor S, Lin J, Lee SH, Lambert A, Zhao ZZ, Roseman F, Guo Q, Gordon SD, Wallace L, Henders AK, Visscher PM, Kraft P, Martin NG, Morris AP, Treloar SA, Kennedy SH, Missmer SA, Montgomery GW, Zondervan KT. Genome-wide association study identifies a locus at 7p15.2 associated with endometriosis. Nat Genet. 2011;43:51–4.

28. Fukumatsu Y, Katabuchi H, Miyamura S, Matsuura K, Okamura H, Naito M, Takahashi K. Activated macrophages in the peritoneal fluid of women with endometriosis: examination of the intracytoplasmic localization of endogenous peroxidase and interleukin-1. Acta Obst Gynaec Jpn. 1992;44:529–36.
29. Okamura H, Katabuchi H, Kanzaki H. Macrophages in reproductive biology. In: Lewis C, Burke B, editors. The Macrophages. London: Oxford University Press; 2002. p. 548–76.
30. Sharpe-Timms KL, Piva M, Ricke EA, Surewicz K, Zhang YL, Zimmmer RL. Endometriotic lesions synthesize and secrete a haptoglobin-like protein. Biol Reprod. 1998;58:988–94.

Chapter 3
Visible and Invisible (Occult) Endometriosis

Khaleque Newaz Khan

Abstract Endometriosis is a chronic disease characterized by endometrial tissue located outside of the uterine cavity and is associated with chronic pelvic pain and infertility. However, an in-depth understanding of the pathophysiology of endometriosis is still elusive. Once generated within pelvis due to retrograde entry of menstrual debris, peritoneal endometriotic lesions time-dependently change their color appearance resulting from certain biochemical change within lesions. A variable pattern of endometriotic lesions within pelvis can be detected by laparoscopy as visible peritoneal endometriosis. It is generally believed that besides ovarian steroid hormones, the growth of endometriosis can be regulated by innate immune system in pelvic microenvironment by their interaction with endometrial cells and immune cells. We conducted a series of studies in perspectives of pelvic inflammation that is triggered primarily by bacterial endotoxin (lipopolysaccharide, LPS) and is mediated by Toll-like receptor 4 (TLR4) and showed their involvement in the growth regulation of visible peritoneal endometriosis. Even with the careful eye of an expert surgeon, we may sometimes miss to detect peritoneal lesion within peritoneal cavity or deep into peritoneum. In such a case, random collection of normal peritoneum may carry the possibility to identify some hidden endometriotic lesions by microscopy and these lesions can be named as invisible endometriosis. Here, we discuss the color appearance of peritoneal lesions, role of innate immune system in visible endometriosis, and finally our recent findings on invisible microscopic endometriosis and their biological and clinical significance.

Keywords Visible endometriosis • Bacterial endotoxin • Innate immunity • TLR4 • Invisible endometriosis

---

K.N. Khan, M.D., Ph.D. (✉)
Department of Obstetrics and Gynecology, Graduate School of Biomedical Sciences, Nagasaki University, 1-7-1 Sakamoto, Nagasaki, 852-8501, Japan
e-mail: nemokhan@nagasaki-u.ac.jp

T. Harada (ed.), *Endometriosis: Pathogenesis and Treatment*,
DOI 10.1007/978-4-431-54421-0_3, © Springer Japan 2014

3.1 Visible Endometriosis: Introduction

Endometriosis, the presence of functional endometrium outside of the uterine cavity, is a common disease, causing abdominal pain, dysmenorrhea, dyspareunia, and infertility in about 10 % of the female population [1]. Besides metaplastic transformation of endometrial and peritoneal mesothelial cells, the transplantation, implantation, and growth of exfoliated menstrual debris on the peritoneal and ovarian surfaces are the widely accepted mechanisms of endometriosis [2, 3]. With the elapse of many decades and publication of abundant number of literatures, exact physiopathology or pathogenesis of endometriosis is still debatable. The potential role of ovarian steroid hormones in the regeneration of endometrium after menstruation and the growth of endometriosis has been demonstrated [4]. However, as a nonself lesion in pelvic environment, the growth or persistence of visible endometriosis can also be regulated by innate immune system. Therefore, we cannot rule out the involvement of an immuno-endocrine crosstalk in the pelvis of women with visible endometriosis.

3.1.1 Pathogenesis and Natural Course of Peritoneal Endometriosis

3.1.1.1 Common Concepts in the Pathogenesis of Endometriosis

In addition to transplantation and implantation theory of Sampson [2] and coelomic metaplasia theory of Meyer [5], immuno-surveillance of the refluxed endometrial cells is another attractive theory for the development of pelvic endometriosis. The immune tolerance or immune defect theory could be responsible for a deficiency in the rejection of the autologous cells derived from the eutopic endometrium in the peritoneal cavity after menstrual reflux. This rejection in the clearance of endometrial cells could be contributed by a dysfunctional immune response in the pelvic cavity [6].

According to the retrograde menstruation theory, endometrial fragments flow back through the patent fallopian tubes, reach the peritoneal cavity, attach on the pelvic mesothelium, invade the peritoneum, and develop into endometriotic lesions [2]. Limited information still exists regarding early endometrial-peritoneal attachment and invasion in the development of endometriosis.

3.1.1.2 Role of Cell Adhesion Molecules in Endometriosis

After overcoming a phase of immune tolerance, a key step in the development of early endometriosis is the ability of endometrial cells to adhere to mesothelium and invade the extracellular matrix. These effects are contributed by a number of intercellular adhesion molecules (ICAMs) and subcellular matrix degrading metalloproteinases (MMPs) [7]. The expressions of these ICAMs such as integrins and E-cadherin and MMPs are already detected in cells derived from menstrual effluent, endometrium, peritoneal fluid, peritoneum, and endometriosis [8].

3.1.1.3 Role of Heme Metabolism in Endometriosis

A potential implication of hemoglobin in the pathogenesis of peritoneal endometriosis has been recently reported [9]. A simple hypothesis is that hemoglobin, being released into the peritoneal cavity after red blood cell lysis, may activate cell adhesion molecules and induce cytokine production, cell proliferation, and the process of neovascularization. Degradation of hemoglobin yields biologically active molecules, heme, and its products of oxidative cleavage by heme oxygenases such as iron, carbon monoxide, biliverdin, and bilirubin. Accumulation of heme in the peritoneal cavity might have a number of deleterious effects including induction of oxidative stress, stimulation of cell adhesion, and cytokine production by macrophages (Mφ). All these biological events are finally involved in the generation of visible peritoneal lesions.

3.1.1.4 Color Changes of Visible Peritoneal Lesions

The lesions of early endometriosis are either transparent or translucent because they still lack formation of vasculatures around them. We named these early lesions as nonopaque lesions [10] because these lesions contain either of watery, serous, or mucinous secretion and there is no collection of blood in the stroma by histology. Once cellular attachment and invasion of endometrial cells are established, the subsequent growth or maintenance of endometriotic lesions is maintained by promotion of mitogenesis and angiogenesis with the continuation of menstrual cycle. The growth-promoting effect of endometriosis is contributed by an orchestrated action of estrogen and other inflammatory or proinflammatory mediators. Over proliferation of microvessels in the growing endometriotic lesions causes oozing of blood in the stroma and appears as blood-filled opaque red lesions by laparoscope [10]. With the progression of time, there is deoxygenation process from hemoglobin to methemoglobin or hemosiderin leading to color changes of these opaque red lesions to black lesion or related lesions. In this stage, collection of blood in the stroma disappears. Black lesion again changes to white lesion due to collection of bilirubin or biliverdin and accumulation of fibrous tissue. In this stage, gland gradually becomes smaller and stroma sometimes disappears due to deposition of fibrous tissue. Finally old lesions disappear and there is new focus of endometriosis due to continuation of menstrual reflux. These sequential events indicate that once exfoliated, the endometrium enters into the pelvic cavity and becomes attached to the mesothelial layer, and then a process of angiogenesis,

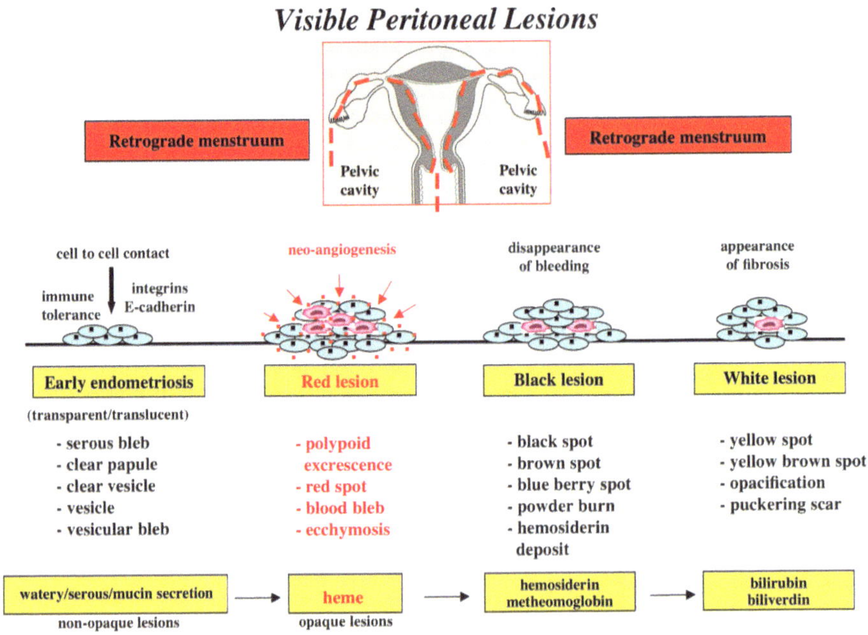

Fig. 3.1 Shows the diagrammatic representation of the natural course of visible peritoneal endometriosis in pelvic cavity. After initial attachment of refluxed endometrial cells with peritoneal cells producing early endometriotic lesions, the consequent events of mitosis, angiogenesis, metabolic degradation of heme, and appearances of fibrosis result in the generation of different morphological appearances of peritoneal endometriosis as shown in this figure

heme metabolism, and fibrosis ensue to maintain the natural course of endometriosis (Fig. 3.1). A panel of nonopaque lesion, blood-filled opaque lesion, blue berry spots, and their corresponding histological pictures is shown in Fig. 3.2.

3.1.2 *Role of Mφ in Pelvic Inflammation and Growth of Visible Endometriosis*

3.1.2.1 Infiltration of Mφ in Eutopic and Ectopic Endometria

As a cell component of innate immune system, peritoneal fluid (PF) and eutopic/ectopic endometria derived from women with endometriosis have been shown to contain higher numbers of activated Mφ than in control women [11, 12]. This results in the secretion of higher concentrations of growth factors and cytokines in the PF as produced by the stimulated Mφ in these patients [11]. Red peritoneal lesions and their adjacent peritoneum had the greatest Mφ infiltration, compared with black/white lesions or chocolate cyst walls. These results indicate that early endometriosis with red peritoneal lesions induces a higher inflammatory response

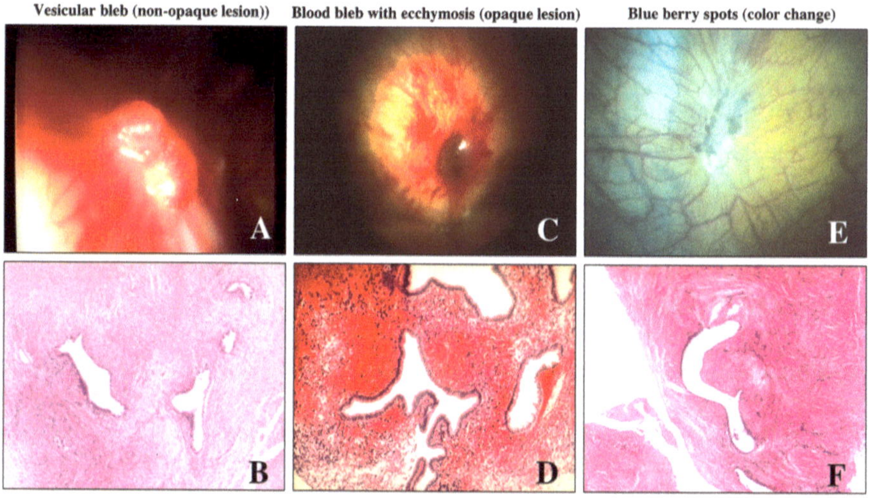

Fig. 3.2 Shows the laparoscopic and corresponding histologic appearance of nonopaque transparent/translucent lesion (**A, B**), blood-filled opaque red lesion (**C, D**), and blue berry spots (**E, F**) in pelvic cavity of women with peritoneal endometriosis. It can be noted here that nonopaque endometriotic lesions such as vesicular bleb (**A**) lack oozing of blood in stroma (**B**) and opaque red lesions such as blood bleb with ecchymosis (**C**) are accompanied by oozing of blood in the stroma of these lesions (**D**). In contrast, black lesions such as blue berry spots (**E**) are manifested by color change and disappearance of blood from the stroma of these lesions (**F**)

in the pelvic cavity than advanced endometriosis [12]. The inflammatory reactions in the eutopic and ectopic endometria suggest that the growth of endometriosis does not depend on the fibrotic extension of disease; rather, it depends on the tissue activity of endometriosis. We presume that extension of disease could be related to pelvic pain, but higher tissue activity of endometriosis associated with abundant recruitment and infiltration of Mφ could be related to infertility.

3.1.2.2 Role of Endotoxin or Lipopolysaccharide (LPS) in Mφ-Mediated Pelvic Inflammation

We examined the ability of peritoneal Mφ to synthesize different macromolecules in basal conditions and after treatment with lipopolysaccharide (LPS), a bacterial endotoxin derived from the cell wall extract of Gram-negative bacteria. We speculated that LPS could be a primary inflammatory mediator of Mφ stimulation in pelvic microenvironment. We found that activated Mφ synthesize and secrete variable amount of different secondary inflammatory mediators such as IL-1, IL-6, IL-10, TNF-α, and other growth factors in response to LPS [13, 14].

3.1.2.3 TLR4-Mediated Cytokine Production and Growth of Endometrial Cells

Bacterial endotoxin (LPS) is recognized by Toll-like receptor 4 (TLR4), a pattern recognition receptor, and transmits NF-κB-mediated cellular signals in association with other accessory molecules [15]. We confirmed gene and protein expression of TLR4 in Mφ, gland cells, and stromal cells derived from the eutopic and ectopic endometria of women with or without endometriosis [16]. In an attempt to examine that the stimulating effect of LPS in the production of cytokines and growth factors is mediated by TLR4, we pretreated peritoneal Mφ and glandular epithelial cells/stromal cells derived from eutopic/ectopic endometria with antibody against TLR4 and then again treated them with LPS. We found that blocking of TLR4 was able to significantly suppress Mφ-mediated production of HGF/VEGF/IL-6/TNF-α as well as growth of endometriotic cells [16]. These results indicate that LPS-mediated inflammatory reaction and growth of endometriotic cells are mediated by TLR4.

3.1.3 Source of Bacterial Endotoxin in Endometriosis

3.1.3.1 Endotoxin Levels in Body Fluids

We measured endotoxin levels in the menstrual fluid (MF) and PF of women with and without endometriosis. We found that the concentration of bacterial endotoxin is two- to fourfold higher in the MF when compared with that in PF. Endotoxin level in MF/PF was also significantly higher in women with endometriosis than in control women [16]. We found the highest endotoxin level during the menstrual phase and persistence of a small amount of endotoxin in the pelvis either in the proliferative phase or in the secretory phase of the menstrual cycle [16]. This indicates that MF of women with endometriosis is highly enriched with bacterial endotoxin followed by the presence of a modest amount in the PF.

3.1.3.2 Source of Endotoxin in Intrauterine and Pelvic Environment

There is a possibility that the lower genital tract of women with or without endometriosis is contaminated with a number of normal bacterial florae including *Escherichia coli* (*E. coli*). Therefore, we speculated that there might be an ascending migration of *E. coli* from the vaginal lumen up into the uterine cavity that causes contamination of menstrual blood and resulting in the subsequent release of endotoxin into menstrual blood and back to the peritoneal fluid. After bacteria culture analysis, we found a significantly higher colony formation (CFU/ml) of *E. coli* in the menstrual blood of women with endometriosis than that in control women [16].

The CFU of *E. coli* was also significantly higher in women containing red peritoneal lesions than in women having only chocolate cyst.

Based on these findings of our serial experiments, we proposed a new "bacterial contamination hypothesis" that may be involved in the growth regulation of visible peritoneal endometriosis via LPS/TLR4 cascade [16]. This *E. coli* contamination of menstrual blood is responsible for higher endotoxin levels in the MF and PF of women with endometriosis. In search of a mechanistic basis of bacterial contamination of menstrual blood, we found that higher concentrations of PGE2 in MF and PF of women with endometriosis were involved in *E. coli* growth by its direct bacterial proliferation effect or indirect immunosuppressive effect [17].

3.1.4 *Inflammation, Stress Reaction, and TLR4 in Endometriosis*

In addition to pelvic inflammation, a wide variety of stressful stimuli, such as heat shock, ultraviolet radiation, viral or bacterial infection, internal physical stress (cell growth, differentiation, invasion), chemical stress (ligand/receptor interaction), oxidative stress, neurogenic stress, pain sensation, and pelvic inflammation, may induce a variable degree tissue stress reaction in pelvis and release stress-induced proteins, such as heat shock proteins (HSPs) [17, 18]. As a danger signal, the effect of HSPs has been reported to be mediated by TLR4 either alone or in combination with LPS.

We demonstrated a variable amount of soluble HSP70 in MF, PF, and in different peritoneal lesions [18, 19]. These body fluid and tissue concentrations of HSP70 were significantly higher in women with endometriosis than in control women. In an in vitro cell culture system, we found that HSP70 was able to induce TLR4-mediated proinflammatory response and growth of endometriotic cells, and a combined effect was observed between HSP70 and LPS in further promoting pelvic inflammation and growth of endometriotic cells [19]. Although polymyxin B, a potent LPS antagonist, or anti-HSP70 antibody, was unable to suppress combined LPS+HSP70-mediated growth of endometriosis, blocking of TLR4 alone significantly suppressed LPS+HSP70-mediated inflammation and growth of endometriosis [19]. Recently it has been demonstrated that in addition to the effects of endogenous danger signals via TLRs, tissue oxidative stress itself may promote NF-κB-mediated or TLR4-mediated growth of endometriosis [20]. In fact, LPS itself has the capacity to produce ROS by Mφ [15]. These findings are consistent with the understanding that LPS, endogenous danger signals, and oxidative stress may promote the onset and progression of visible endometriosis after activation of TLR4 and/or NF-κB signaling.

3.1.5 *Inflammation, Ovarian Steroid, and TLR4 in Endometriosis*

Basically endometriosis is an estrogen-dependent disease and induces an inflammatory reaction in pelvic environment. Irrespective of the phases of the menstrual cycle, a small amount of estrogen is available in the PF of women with and without endometriosis [21]. Therefore, it is important to know the combined effect of estrogen and inflammation in the growth of endometriosis. Based on published reports, gland cells/stromal cells of eutopic/ectopic endometria and Mφ retain ER and PR [18, 21]. Recently, we reported that Mφ-mediated production of HGF/VEGF/IL-6/TNF-α in response to ovarian steroid was further enhanced after treatment with LPS [22]. An additive effect was observed between E_2 and LPS on cytokine production and growth of eutopic/ectopic endometrial stromal cells when compared with their individual treatment. This combined effect of E_2+LPS on pelvic inflammation and cell growth was markedly abrogated after pretreatment of cells with anti-TLR4 antibody and ICI, an ER antagonist [21]. Our findings suggest that a TLR4/ER-mediated immuno-endocrine crosstalk in pelvis may be involved in the growth or progression of endometriosis.

3.2 Invisible (Occult) Endometriosis: Introduction

The detection and visible diagnosis of peritoneal endometriosis is usually performed by laparoscopy, a gold standard modality, and is microscopically confirmed by histopathology. Even with the careful eyes of expert surgeons, there is obvious chance to miss or overlook hidden lesions in visually normal peritoneum. Therefore, immense interest could arise to randomly collect visually normal peritoneum from different anatomical location in pelvis and to investigate the nature of these visually undetectable lesions of endometriosis. The concept of microscopic endometriosis in visually normal peritoneum was first reported by Murphy in 1986 [23] and subsequently confirmed with an incidence rate of 6–13 % [24].

We histologically examined all biopsy specimens derived from visually normal peritoneum of women with and without endometriosis to detect the possible occurrence of invisible (occult) microscopic endometriosis (IME). The designation of visually normal peritoneum was based on modified criteria of Redwine [25]. The question still remains, if hidden endometriosis lesions could be detected in normal peritoneum, are these invisible lesions really inactive as proposed in a previous report [26], or do they truly retain some biological activity? If tissue activity of IME is there, this could be a clinically important issue. To address this question, we recently investigated the expression patterns of some tissue activity markers including ovarian steroid receptors and cell proliferation marker in histologically confirmed IME lesions.

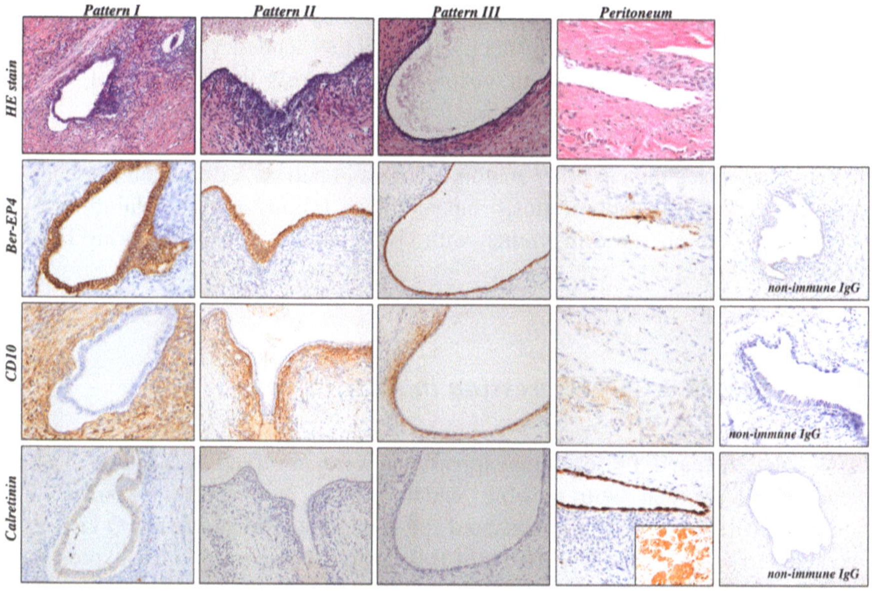

Fig. 3.3 Microscopically detected three patterns of invisible (occult) endometriosis in visually normal peritoneum. Pattern I shows presence of typical gland/stroma; pattern II shows reactive hyperplastic change of endometrioid epithelial cells with surrounding stroma; and pattern III shows single-layered epithelium-lined cystic lesions with surrounding stromal cells (all in HE stain, *upper column*). The identification of glandular epithelial cells, stromal cells, and peritoneal mesothelial cells was confirmed by the immunoreaction to Ber-EP4, CD10, and calretinin, respectively, and are shown against each HE-stained slide. Flat mesothelial cells derived from normal peritoneum and mesothelioma cells as a positive control (*inset*) immunoreactive to calretinin are shown at the *right panel*. The immunoreactions to nonimmune mouse IgG as a negative control are shown on the extreme *right panel*. HE stain, hematoxylin and eosin stain. Magnification of slides (×200)

3.2.1 Pattern of IME in Normal Peritoneum

After careful observation and analysis, we collected 227 visually normal peritoneal samples from 151 women with visible endometriosis and 78 samples from 62 women without any visible peritoneal lesions (control). We detected three patterns of IME: (I) presence of typical gland/stroma, (II) reactive hyperplastic change of endometrioid-like epithelium with surrounding stroma, and (III) single-layered mesothelium- or epithelium-lined cystic lesions with surrounding rim of stromal cells. All these IME lesions were confirmed by their immunoreactivity to Ber-EP4 (marker of gland epithelium), CD10 (marker of stroma), and nonreactivity to calretinin (marker of mesothelial cells) (Fig. 3.3).

We could detect variable patterns of IME in the normal peritoneum derived from 23 women with endometriosis (biopsy samples, $n=27$) and 4 control women (biopsy samples, $n=4$) without visible endometriosis. The detection rate of IME was as follows: for endometriosis, 15.2 % (23/151) and 11.8 % (27/227) and for control women, 6.4 % (4/62) and 5.1 % (4/78) by the number of patients and number of collected samples, respectively. A higher tendency in the incidence of IME was found in women with visible endometriosis than in control women ($p = 0.06$ by patient number and $p = 0.07$ by sample number) [27].

A predominance of IME occurrence was observed in pouch of Douglas and uterovesical space than in other anatomical sites in pelvis. A dominant presence of r-ASRM stages I–II endometriosis and red/black lesions and complaints of dysmenorrhea were observed in women with visible endometriosis harboring IME in their peritoneum [27].

3.2.2 ER/PR/Ki-67 Expression in IME Lesions

A variable ER and PR immunoexpressions were observed in all IME lesions detected in women with visible endometriosis and control women. The immunoreaction of PR as measured by quantitative-histogram (Q-H) score appeared to be higher in all patterns of IME lesions comparing to ER expression.

A stronger immunoreaction of Ki-67 (cell proliferation marker) was found in pattern I/II IME lesions than in pattern III IME lesions detected in women with visible endometriosis. A weak Ki-67 expression was found in pattern I/III IME lesions diagnosed in control women. Ki-67 index (mean percentage of Ki-67-positive nuclei among total cells) was significantly higher in pattern I/II IME lesions than in pattern III IME lesions found in women with visible endometriosis [27].

We are against the argument by Donnez et al. [26] that IME lesions are quiescent and they are nonactive or inactive and that these lesions are clinically irrelevant. Our findings indicate that a proportion of occult lesions are indeed biologically active and a substantial amount of estrogen and different inflammatory mediators in pelvis might be involved in the growth promotion of IME lesions even if it is undetectable by naked eyes. With the influence of both systemic and local estrogen, these IME lesions, even if it is minute in size, may time-dependently increase in size to be recognized by histology. This could be responsible for the subsequent recurrence/occurrence of endometriotic lesions or persistence/recurrence of pain symptoms even after successful excision or ablation of visible peritoneal lesions by laparoscopy. Further studies in human or in primates are necessary to establish this possibility. From the logical point of view, it is difficult to trace these growing lesions on the peritoneal surface by repeated surgical procedures in human.

3.2.3 Origin of IME Lesions

The most alarming questions may arise now, "how can we decide the origin of IME lesions?" Or "is Sampson's theory enough to explain IME lesions?" There is no

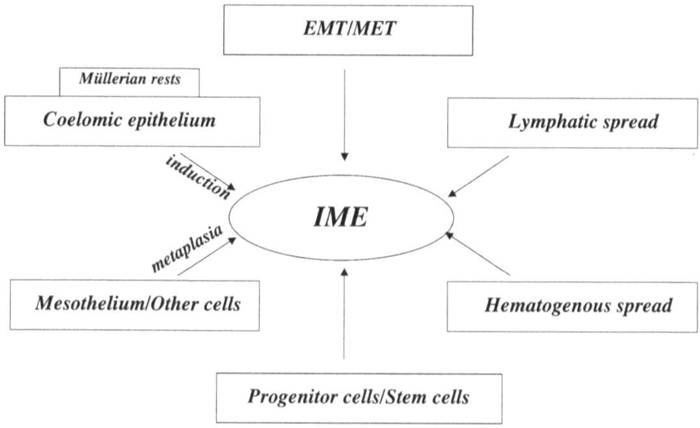

Fig. 3.4 Some hypothetical proposals that may be linked to the possible origin of invisible (occult) microscopic endometriosis (IME) lesions. After initial attachment of menstrual debris to the peritoneum, a sequence of epithelial-mesenchymal transition (EMT) or mesenchymal-epithelial transition (MET) may be involved in the generation of IME. Hematogenous or lymphogenous dissemination of shedding endometrial cells during menstruation could be another mechanism. In addition to possible origin from progenitor cells/stem cells, cellular change of flat mesothelium to cuboidal or columnar cells (metaplasia theory) or activated cells derived from residing coelomic epithelium within peritoneum (müllleriosis, induction theory) in response to pelvic inflammation could be linked to the origin of IME. Cells or tissues derived from müllerian rests in association with peritoneal pockets can be another explanation for the development of IME

definite answer at this moment. But we argue that we can link each and every theory supporting the origin of visible endometriosis [28] to the pathogenesis of IME lesions. If Sampson's theory does not directly support the origin of IME lesions, it can be indirectly explained by lymphatic or hematogenous spread of menstrual debris and subsequent localization deep into peritoneum. We cannot exclude the possibility of genetic factor or metaplastic transformation of peritoneal mesothelial cells (metaplasia theory) in response to estrogen, inflammation, or environmental factors. Despite possible origin of IME as a result of epithelial-mesenchymal transition/mesenchymal-epithelial transition or from stem cells [29, 30], activation of cells derived from coelomic epithelium (müllleriosis, induction theory) within peritoneum may be another possible mechanism to explain the origin of IME [31]. Some hypothetical proposals that might be linked to the possible origin of IME lesions are shown in Fig. 3.4.

3.3 Summary and Perspective

We proposed for the first time a new concept "bacterial contamination hypothesis" in endometriosis. Our results suggest that a substantial amount of endotoxin in peritoneal fluid due to reflux of menstrual blood is involved in pelvic inflammation and may promote TLR4-mediated growth of endometriosis. When there is persistence or recurrence of pain even after successful surgical ablation of visible endometriosis in pelvis, we should keep in mind about its possible link with invisible or occult endometriosis, although emerging evidence supporting this phenomenon is still unknown. In order to avoid confusion in the use of the term "invisible" or "non-visible" microscopic endometriosis among laparoscopists, we can also use the term "occult" microscopic endometriosis (OME) instead of IME to indicate any hidden lesion in visually normal peritoneum (27). Since the growth regulation of endometriosis is difficult to explain uniformly by a single factor, we believe that a mutual orchestration among inflammatory mediator, tissue stress reaction, and estrogen may be involved in the growth, maintenance, or progression of endometriosis once it is generated in the female pelvis. Our ongoing study targeting to find the evidence of a subclinical vaginal infection in women with endometriosis may hold new therapeutic potential in addition to conventional estrogen suppressing agent.

Acknowledgement I gratefully thank Dr. Michio Kitajima of Nagasaki University Hospital and Dr. Akira Fujishita of Saiseikai Nagasaki Hospital for their kind assistance in sample collection; Prof. Masahiro Nakashima of Atomic Bomb Disease Institute, Nagasaki for his experimental advice; and Prof. Hideaki Masuzaki of Nagasaki University Hospital for reading/advice.

References

1. Strathy JH, Molgaard CA, Coulman CB. Endometriosis and infertility: a laparoscopic study of endometriosis among fertile and infertile women. Fertil Steril. 1982;38:667–72.
2. Sampson J. Peritoneal endometriosis due to menstrual dissemination of endometrial tissue into the peritoneal cavity. Am J Obstet Gynecol. 1927;14:422–9.
3. Thomas EJ, Prentice A. The etiology and pathogenesis of endometriosis. Reprod Med Rev. 1992;1:21–36.
4. Nisolle M, Casanas-Rouz F, Donnez J. Immunohistochemical analysis of proliferative activity and steroid receptor expression in peritoneal and ovarian endometriosis. Fertil Steril. 1997;68:912–9.
5. Meyer R. Ueber den Stand der Frage der Adenomyositis und Adenomyom im Allgemeinen und insbesonderes ueber Adenomyositis seroepithelialis und Adeno-myometritis sarcomatosa. Zbl Gynaekol. 1919;36:745–50.
6. Oosterlynck DJ, Cornillie FJ, Waer M, Vandeputte M, Koninckx PR. Women with endometriosis show a defect in natural killer activity resulting in a decreased cytotoxicity to autologous endometrium. Fertil Steril. 1991;56:45–51.
7. Lessey BA, Damjanovich L, Coutifaris C. Integrin adhesion molecules in the human endometrium. Correlation with the normal and abnormal menstrual cycle. J Clin Invest. 1992;90:188–95.
8. van der Linden PJQ, van der Linden EPM, de Goeij AFPM, Ramaekers FC, Dunselman GAJ. Expression of integrins and E-cadherin in cells from menstrual effluent, endometrium, peritoneal fluid, peritoneum, and endometriosis. Fertil Steril. 1994;61:85–90.
9. Langendonckt AV, Casanas-Roux F, Dolmans M-M, Donnez J. Potential involvement of hemoglobin and heme in the pathogenesis of peritoneal endometriosis. Fertil Steril. 2002;77:561–70.

10. Khan KN, Masuzaki H, Fujishita A, Kitajima M, Sekine I, Ishimaru T. Higher activity by opaque endometriotic lesions than non-opaque lesions in women with endometriosis. Acta Obstet Gynecol Scand. 2004;83:375–82.
11. Halme J, Becker S, Haskill S. Altered maturation and function of peritoneal macrophages: possible role in pathogenesis endometriosis. Am J Obstet Gynecol. 1987;156:783–9.
12. Khan KN, Masuzaki H, Fujishita A, Kitajima M, Sekine I, Ishimaru T. Differential macrophage infiltration in early and advanced endometriosis and adjacent peritoneum. Fertil Steril. 2004;81:652–61.
13. Halme J, White C, Kauma S, Estes J, Haskill S. Peritoneal macrophages from patients with endometriosis release growth factor activity in vitro. J Clin Endocrinol Metab. 1988;66:1044–9.
14. Khan KN, Masuzaki H, Fujishita A, Kitajima M, Kohno T, Sekine I, Matsuyama T, Ishimaru T. Regulation of hepatocyte growth factor by basal and stimulated-macrophages in women with endometriosis. Hum Reprod. 2005;20:49–60.
15. Khan KN, Kitajima M, Hiraki H, Fujishita A, Sekine I, Ishimaru T, Masuzaki H. Toll-like receptors in innate immunity: role of bacterial endotoxin and toll-like receptor 4 (TLR4) in endometrium and endometriosis. Gynecol Obstet Invest. 2009;68:40–52.
16. Khan KN, Kitajima M, Hiraki K, Yamaguchi N, Katamine S, Matsuyama T, Fujishita A, Nakashima M, Ishimaru T, Masuzaki H. Escherichia coli contamination of menstrual blood and effect of bacterial endotoxin on endometriosis. Fertil Steril. 2010;94(7):2860–3.e3.
17. Asea A, Rehli M, Kabingu E, Boch JA, Bare O, Auron PE, Stevenson MA, Calderwood SK. Novel signal transduction pathway utilized by extracellular HSP70: role of toll-like receptor (TLR) 2 and TLR4. J Biol Chem. 2002;277:15028–34.
18. Khan KN, Kitajima M, Imamura T, Hiraki K, Fujishita A, Sekine I, Ishimaru T, Masuzaki H. Toll-like receptor 4 (TLR4)-mediated growth of endometriosis by human heat shock protein 70 (Hsp70). Hum Reprod. 2008;23:2210–9.
19. Khan KN, Kitajima M, Inoue T, Tateishi S, Fujishita A, Nakashima M, Masuzaki H. Additive effects of inflammation and stress reaction on Toll-like receptor 4-mediated growth of endometrioid stromal cells. Hum Reprod. 2013;28:2794–803.
20. Kajihara H, Yamada Y, Kanayama S, Furukawa N, Noguchi T, Haruta S, Yoshida S, Sado T, Oi H, Kobayashi H. New insights into the pathophysiology of endometriosis: from chronic inflammation to danger signals. Gynecol Endocrinol. 2011;27(2):73–9.
21. Khan KN, Kitajima M, Hiraki H, Fujishita A, Sekine I, Ishimaru T, Masuzaki H. Immunopathogenesis of pelvic endometriosis: role of hepatocyte growth factor, macrophages and ovarian steroids. Am J Reprod Immunol. 2008;60:383–404.
22. Khan KN, Masuzaki H, Fujishita A, Kitajima M, Sekine I, Matsuyama T, Ishimaru T. Estrogen and progesterone receptor expression in macrophages and regulation of hepatocyte growth factor by ovarian steroids in women with endometriosis. Hum Reprod. 2005;20:2004–13.
23. Murphy AA, Green WR, Bobbie D, dela Cruz ZC, Rock JA. Unsuspected endometriosis documented by scanning electron microscopy in visually normal peritoneum. Fertil Steril. 1986;46:522–4.
24. Nisollle M, Paindaveine B, Bourdone A, Berliere M, Casanas-Rous F, Donnez J. Histologic study of peritoneal endometriosis in infertile women. Fertil Steril. 1990;53:984–8.
25. Redwine DB. 'Invisible' microscopic endometriosis: a review. Gynecol Obstet Invest. 2003;55:63–7.
26. Donnez J, Langendonckt AV. Typical and subtle atypical presentations of endometriosis. Curr Opin Obstet Gynecol. 2004;16:431–7.
27. Khan KN, Fujishita A, Kitajima M, Hiraki K, Nakashima M, Masuzaki H. Occult microscopic endometriosis: an undetectable finding by laparoscopy in normal peritoneum. Hum Reprod. 2014;29(3):462–72.
28. Burney RO, Giudice LC. Pathogenesis and pathophysiology of endometriosis. Fertil Steril. 2012;98(3):511–9.

29. Gaetje R, Kotzian S, Herrmann G, Baumann R, Starzinski-Powitz A. Nonmalignant epithelial cells, potentially invasive in human endometriosis, lack the tumor suppressor molecule E-cadherin. Am J Pathol. 1997;150:461–7.
30. Sasson IE, Taylor HS. Stem cells and the pathogenesis of endometriosis. Ann N Y Acad Sci. 2008;1127:106–15.
31. Redwine DB. Mülleriosis: the single best fit model of origin of endometriosis. J Reprod Med. 1988;33:915–20.

Chapter 4
Role of Stem Cells in the Pathogenesis of Endometriosis

Tetsuo Maruyama

Abstract Endometriosis can be defined as a benign estrogen-dependent disorder in which endometrium-like tissues reside outside of the uterine cavity. Studies now indicate that multiple genetic and epigenetic changes (reminiscent of neoplastic processes) are involved in the pathophysiology of endometriosis. Given the molecular similarities between endometriosis and cancer, it is reasonable to apply the "cancer stem cell model" concept to the pathogenesis of endometriosis. In this article, I review and discuss "the stem cell model for endometriosis" in which endometriosis originates from endometrial stem/progenitor cells within eutopic and ectopic sites.

Keywords Cancer • Endometriosis • Endometrium • Epithelial–mesenchymal transition • Stem cells

4.1 Introduction

Endometriosis can be defined as the presence of endometrium-like tissues outside of the uterine cavity and is frequently associated with dysmenorrhea and dyspareunia [1, 2]. Endometriosis is commonly found associated with the ovaries, pelvic peritoneum, uterine ligaments, and the rectovaginal septum. More rarely, endometriotic sites can include pelvic lymph nodes, the cervix, the intestine, the bladder, and the vagina, and fallopian tubes. More distant sites can include the lungs, skin, kidneys, brain, and spinal column [1–3]. Microscopically, glandular components surrounded by endometrium-like stroma are observed [4]. Smooth muscle cell components (perhaps via smooth muscle metaplasia) can be associated

T. Maruyama (✉)
Department of Obstetrics and Gynecology, School of Medicine, Keio University, 35 Shinanomachi, Shinjuku-ku, Tokyo 160-8582, Japan
e-mail: tetsuo@a5.keio.jp

T. Harada (ed.), *Endometriosis: Pathogenesis and Treatment*,
DOI 10.1007/978-4-431-54421-0_4,

with endometriotic lesions, particularly deeply infiltrating endometriosis [5]. The lesions are often accompanied by angiogenesis and innervation [6, 7]. A number of causes of endometriosis have been proposed. These include retrograde menstruation, iatrogenic direct implantation, coelomic metaplasia, lymphatic and vascular metastasis, embryonic rest, and mesenchymal cell differentiation (induction). Importantly, none of the theories can completely account for all types of endometriotic lesions. Thus, the pathophysiology might be complex, involving several mechanisms.

Current analyses of endometriosis indicate that multiple genetic, epigenetic, environmental, immunological, and/or endocrine processes are involved [8]. Thus far, research has failed to identify one or more specific susceptibility genes. Endometriosis is in fact a benign disorder. However, the underlying molecular mechanisms appear similar to those of cancer [8]. Indeed, evidence indicates that both endometriosis and tumors are monoclonal in origin [9–12]. Furthermore, both endometriotic cells and cancer cells are invasive [13]. To support this interpretation, we point out the enhanced susceptibility to ovarian clear-cell and endometrioid cancers in patients with endometriosis [8]. Given this background, it is reasonable to examine whether the pathophysiology of endometriosis can be explained, at least in part, by the cancer stem cell (CSC) hypothesis. CSCs have the abilities to self-renew and to give rise to differentiated tumor cells. They are also responsible for the overall organization of tumors [14, 15]. Here, I review and discuss an emerging concept and hypothesis, i.e., the "endometriosis stem cell theory" in which endometriosis arises from stem cell(s) originating from bone marrows or eutopic and/or ectopic endometrial stem/progenitor cells [16–18].

4.2 Cancer Stem Cell Theory

Before discussing the stem cell theory for the pathogenesis of endometriosis, I will briefly introduce the current paradigm regarding tissue stem cells (adult stem cells), CSCs, and their roles in cancer formation and metastasis.

4.2.1 Tissue Stem Cells

Tissue-specific stem cells (also termed somatic stem cells or adult stem cells) are found in a quiescent, undifferentiated state throughout the body [19]. They self-renew through symmetric and/or asymmetric cell divisions. Growth is modulated by physiological signals originating from the microenvironment or "stem cell niche." Asymmetric divisions generate lineage-committed cells that differentiate and thereby maintain the tissue of origin. The tissue-specific stem cells and the

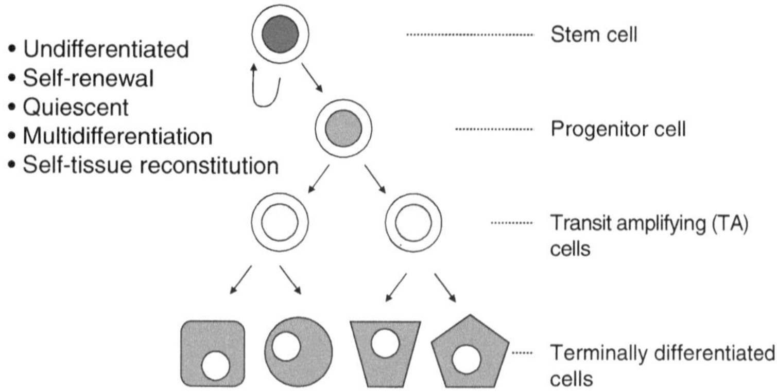

Fig. 4.1 Hierarchy of adult stem cell differentiation. Within its microenvironmental niche, adult stem cells generally remain quiescent. Under the proper conditions, the cells can be stimulated to undergo asymmetric divisions to renew themselves and produce daughter/progenitor cells. The latter cell further divides to produce transit-amplifying (TA) cells. The TA cells promptly proliferate and differentiate into a variety of mature, functional cells

microenvironmental niche work together to keep a balance between the need for cell replacement and the necessity of retaining a pool of primitive cells. In this fashion, the structural and functional requirements of organs and tissues can be met [19]. The hierarchy of tissue stem cells is illustrated in Fig. 4.1.

4.2.2 *CSCs and Primary Tumor Formation*

The "classical" or stochastic model (clonal evolution model) posits that any normal (stem) cell, upon acquiring genetic and/or epigenetic modification(s) giving it selective growth advantage, gives rise to a neoplastic clone of homogenous neoplastic cells [14, 15]. Upon the acquisition of additional genetic and/or epigenetic change(s), it expands as a tumor. In this model, all cells within a tumor have equal tumorigenic potentials [14, 15].

More recently, a hierarchical or CSC model has been developed. This model is based upon the hypothesis that tumors consist of a heterogeneous population of cells, only a small proportion of which are CSCs, also termed tumor-initiating cells [14, 15, 20]. As depicted in Fig. 4.2, a small, self-renewing population of CSCs is responsible for tumor initiation and growth maintenance. Thus, CSCs have been operationally defined by their ability to generate tumors, and tumor-initiating cells are thought to reflect the operational definition of CSCs [20]. The model states that CSCs could originate from tissue stem cells or even differentiated cells that acquired stem cell-like properties (including self-renewal) as a result of genetic and/or epigenetic modifications [14, 15]. In the CSC model, completely mature cells can fully dedifferentiate to become CSCs. In addition to genetic/epigenetic

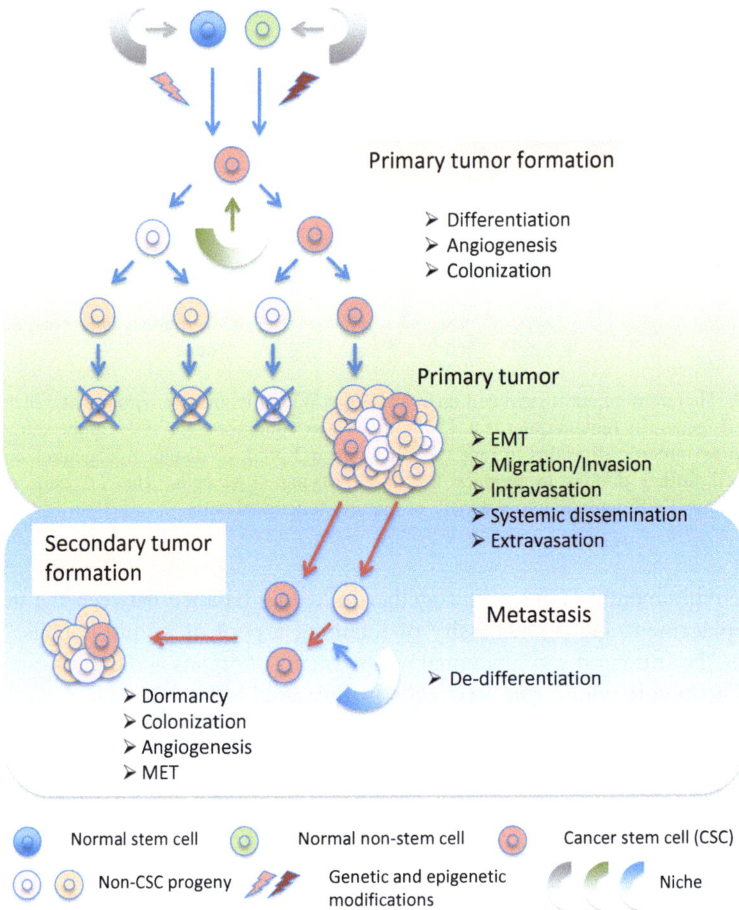

Fig. 4.2 Cancer stem cell (CSC) model for tumor formation and metastasis. Within tumors, a small population of self-renewing CSCs is responsible for initiating tumor growth and maintaining its presence. CSCs might be derived from tissue stem cells or more differentiated cells that gained stem cell properties (including self-renewal) upon genetic and/or epigenetic modifications. Even completely differentiated cells can develop into CSCs through dedifferentiation. The tumor microenvironment (niche) maintains stem cell properties. CSCs that migrate away from the primary site are capable of invasion, intravasation, systemic dissemination, and extravasation. This behavior might be due to the EMT. Upon reaching distant tissues, the cells can reverse the epithelial state by undergoing the MET. This promotes growth and the initiation of angiogenesis. Alternatively, EMT programs per se might lead to the generation of CSCs

modifications, the tumor microenvironment (the CSC niche) is required for the maintenance of stem cell properties. It likely includes many components, such as stromal cells, blood vessels, extracellular matrix (ECM), growth factors, and cytokines in a hypoxic environment. Exposure of non-CSCs to niche factors might result in their acquisition of stem cell properties [14, 15].

4.2.3 Cell Metastasis and Tumor Formation

The metastatic cascade includes tumor cell migration away from the site of the primary tumor. It is now believed by many researchers that this process requires the epithelial–mesenchymal transition (EMT) [20, 21]. The EMT is a biological process in which epithelial cells lose their cell polarity and cell–cell adhesive properties. In exchange, the cells gain migratory and invasive properties and undergo multiple biochemical changes, thereby exhibiting a mesenchymal cell phenotype [22]. The EMT is observed in many processes, including mesoderm and neural tube formation as well as wound healing, tissue regeneration, and organ fibrosis [22]. Our own data indicated that endometrial epithelial cells undergo EMT during embryo implantation [23].

CSCs are likely involved in the formation of metastases [20, 21], as they exhibit invasion, intravasation, systemic dissemination, and extravasation. It is believed that such processes are enhanced by the EMT conversion [20, 21]. Subsequently, CSCs that metastasize to distant tissues show colonization and reversion to an epithelial state through reversal of the EMT, i.e., the mesenchymal–epithelial transition (MET), giving rise to metastatic lesions accompanied by angiogenesis [20]. Alternatively, the activation of EMT programs has been implicated in the generation of CSCs [20, 21]. Furthermore, in addition to CSCs, non-CSC progeny cancer cells might become CSCs through dedifferentiation at the metastatic sites and thereby generate metastatic cancer lesions [20, 21] (Fig. 4.3).

For reference, Fig. 4.2 provides a representative CSC model. However, recent studies have revealed complexities, such as plasticity of stem cell properties and clonal diversity of CSCs in certain tumor types requiring revision of the original CSC model. As a result, more complex models such as the dynamic stemness model and the combinatory CSC and stochastic models have recently emerged [15].

4.3 Endometriosis Stem Cell Theory

Based on the principles of the cancer stem cell model illustrated in Fig. 4.2, I here propose a stem cell model for the pathogenesis of endometriosis as depicted in Fig. 4.3. This model incorporates the implantation theory, which is the most widely accepted version among the many theories in this field. Note, however, that the coelomic metaplasia theory and embryonic rest theory are also compatible with the second part of this model in which some types of mesothelial cells and/or embryonic cell rests of müllerian origin behave as endometriosis-initiating cells (endometriotic stem cells) and thereby give rise to endometriotic lesions at ectopic site(s) [18].

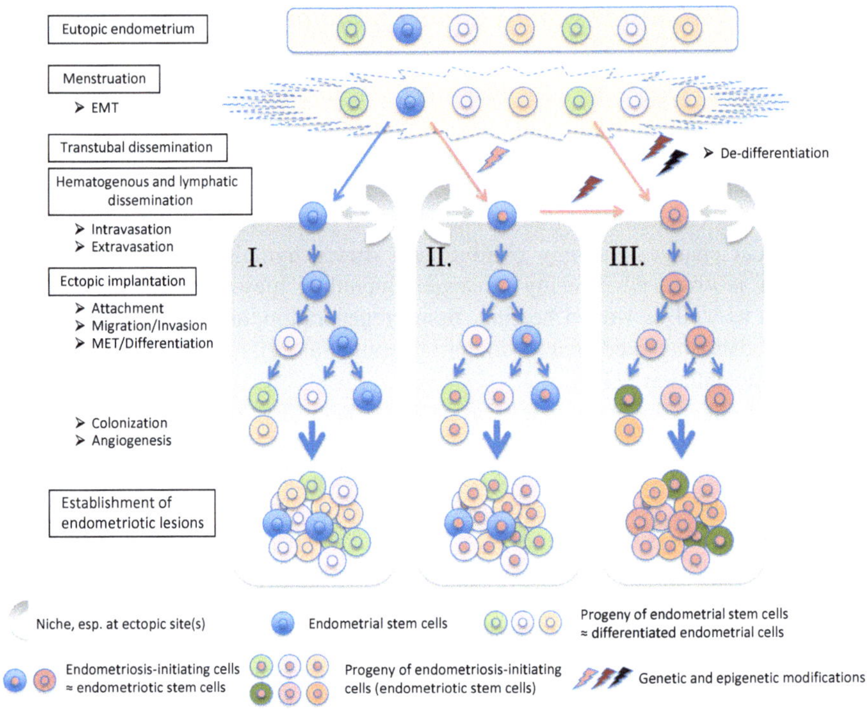

Fig. 4.3 Three proposed stem cell models for the pathogenesis of endometriosis extrapolated from the CSC model. Model I. Endometrial stem cells (EmSCs) are released from eutopic endometrium most likely upon menstruation. EmSCs are transported to ectopic sites via retrograde menstruation, lymphatic and vascular dissemination, direct migration, and invasion or some combination. The EmSCs remain at the ectopic site through attachment, implantation, and/or extravasation followed by invasion. EmSCs initiate self-renewal and/or asymmetric division to generate progenitor cells, transit-amplifying cells, and more differentiated endometrial cells. Because EmSCs and their progeny require a blood supply, angiogenesis is initiated, supporting the expanding colony/endometriotic lesions. Model II. EmSCs undergo genetic and/or epigenetic modifications at the eutopic or ectopic sites and thereafter behave as endometriosis-initiating cells (EmoICs), giving rise to endometriotic lesions as shown in model I. Model III. EmSCs undergo more extensive genetic and/or epigenetic modifications than in model II. Alternatively, terminally differentiated endometrial cells undergo multiple and profound genetic and epigenetic changes and thereby dedifferentiate into EmSC-like cells (not depicted in the schema). In either case, the EmoICs are capable of generating a variety of endometrial cell components in a fashion similar to model I

4.3.1 A Stem Cell Model for the Development of Endometriosis

A stem cell model for endometriosis development is presented below in three variations, i.e., models I, II, and III (Fig. 4.3). In model I, endometrial stem cells are released from eutopic endometrium upon menstruation. The cells could move to ectopic sites via many routes, including lymphatic and vascular dissemination, direct migration and invasion, retrograde menstruation, or some combination thereof. The endometrial stem cells settle ectopically in new sites by attachment, implantation, extravasation, and, finally, invasion. Upon reaching the ectopic site, the endometrial stem cells might undergo self-renewal or divide asymmetrically. In this way, they can self-renew as well as produce progenitor cells, transit-amplifying cells, and more differentiated endometrial cells (Fig. 4.3, model I). This process is based on the behavior of general tissue stem cells (Fig. 4.1). Endometrial stem cells and their proliferating daughter cells require a blood supply to flourish. Therefore, they induce angiogenesis, permitting them to undergo clonal growth. In this fashion, endometriotic lesions are formed.

In model II, endometrial stem cells are subject to genetic (or epigenetic) modifications within the eutopic or ectopic sites. The modifications permit them to act as "endometriosis stem cells," also termed "endometriosis-initiating cells," producing endometriotic lesions. Notably, in this model, they retain the proliferative and differentiative potential of endometrial stem cell-like cells, allowing them to generate components of the endometrium, including glandular, stromal, endothelial, and smooth muscle cells. Like CSCs and tumor-initiating cells as mentioned previously [20], I here operationally define "endometriosis stem cells" by their stem cell-like properties and ability to generate endometriosis with high efficiency, and "endometriosis-initiating cells," therefore, reflect the operational definition of "endometriosis stem cells." Thus, "endometriosis-initiating cells" is used herein as a synonym of "endometriosis stem cells."

In model III, endometrial stem cells undergo additional genetic and/or epigenetic modifications and thereafter behave as "endometriosis-initiating cells," producing endometriotic lesions. Alternatively, terminally differentiated endometrial cells could undergo multiple profound genetic and epigenetic modifications resulting in dedifferentiation into endometrial stem cell-like cells capable of generating a variety of endometrial cell populations, including glandular, stromal, endothelial, and smooth muscle cells. However, it seems likely that such profound modifications would destroy the cells' capability for multipotential differentiation. Hence, this pathway might result in carcinogenesis. Thus, model III might explain endometriosis-originated cancers such as clear-cell carcinoma and endometrioid cancer. In fact, Pten and K-ras double mutations in the mouse give rise to endometrioid adenocarcinoma of the ovary, whereas single mutation of K-ras results in pelvic endometriosis [24].

It is important to note that the processes displayed in models I–III are likely modulated by the microenvironments in which the cells associate themselves. Microenvironmental influences could include menstrual efflux, peritoneal fluids, inflammation, and the ECM of the peritoneum, all of which might regulate molecular/cellular events. Thus, invasion, intravasation, extravasation, colonization, angiogenesis, EMT, and MET could all be affected by the microenvironment. It should be emphasized that EMT and MET could play critical roles in the passage of endometrial stem cells from eutopic sites to ectopic sites and the resultant generation of endometriotic lesions.

4.3.2 Evidence Supporting the Endometriosis Stem Cell Model

The stem cell theory for the pathogenesis of endometriosis is not merely a hypothesis. Rather, a number of studies have emerged that support this model [18, 16]. The supportive evidence is summarized below.

4.3.2.1 EMT and MET Appear to Be Involved in the Pathogenesis of Endometriosis

The metastatic cascades initiated by CSCs and non-CSC cancer cells likely involve the EMT and the MET [20, 21]. In fact, generation of CSCs probably involves the activation of EMT programs [20, 21]. Thus, it is intriguing that EMT- and MET-like processes are also involved in the pathogenesis of endometriosis [25]. For example, menstrual effluent can induce the EMT in mesothelial cells [26]. Consider also "side population" (SP) cells, a population with a high efflux ability of Hoechst 33342 dye defined by flow cytometric techniques [27]. SP cells constitute an undifferentiated population that resides in a number of tissues [28]. SP cells have been isolated from an endometrial cancer cell line, and they represent likely candidates for endometrial CSCs. These cells possess a high capacity to develop into mesenchymal cell lineages, a reflection of EMT activity [29]. These data are consistent with the endometriosis stem cell model. In other words, menstruation might induce EMT pathways in endometrial stem cells and their progeny. In turn, this might induce the cells to migrate away from the eutopic endometrium. Once implanted in an ectopic microenvironment, invasion and establishment of endometriotic lesions could occur through MET at the ectopic site.

4.3.2.2 Expression of Stem Cell Markers in Endometriotic Lesions

In models II and III, Fig. 4.3, primitive endometriosis-initiating cells are thought to express several stem cell markers. Thus, clonal expansion generates endometriotic lesions and the endometriosis-initiating cells retain their original stem cell markers. Experiments have shown that cells present in or adjacent to endometriotic lesions express several stem cell markers including OCT4/POU5F1 and ABCG2 [30–33]. OCT4/POU5F1 is expressed by embryonic stem cells, germ cells, and some types of adult stem cells. This protein plays a crucial role in maintaining stem cell pluripotency [34]. Another stem cell marker is adenosine triphosphate-binding cassette transporter G2 (ABCG2). ABCG2 is highly expressed in a variety of stem cells. It is responsible for removing exogenously added fluorescent dye, Hoechst 33342, and produces the SP phenotype characteristic of stem cells [35]. Thus, the expression of these stem cell markers in endometriotic lesions supports the presence of stem cells and provides indirect evidence for the stem cell model.

4.3.2.3 Tumor Clonality

Most neoplasms are monoclonal in origin. Thus, it is particularly intriguing that endometriotic lesions can also be clonal in nature. The clonality of an endometriotic lesion provides clues to its developmental history. For example, several studies have demonstrated that ovarian endometriomas are in fact monoclonal in origin [9–11]. These molecular findings support the single-cell derivation of endometriomas. However, the developmental history of endometriotic lesions can be more complex. For example, whereas peritoneal endometriotic lesions are polyclonal [12, 36], individual glands of endometriotic lesions are monoclonal [12]. Thus, either single or multiple precursors might give rise to a single peritoneal endometriotic lesion, while the glands arise individually from single stem/progenitor cells [12].

4.3.2.4 Endometriotic Lesions Contain Self-Renewing Mesenchymal Stem Cells

The endometriosis stem cell model predicts that endometriotic lesions should contain a stem cell-like cell population. Chan et al. reported that ovarian endometriomas contain a subset of cells displaying a number of somatic stem cell properties. They include colony-forming activity, self-renewal capacity, and multipotency [37].

4.3.3 The Origin of Stem Cells

Several theories have been proposed to explain both the origin and pathogenesis of endometriosis. These hypotheses include retrograde menstruation (implantation), coelomic metaplasia, and the embryo rest theories [2, 18, 16, 38–40]. Retrograde menstruation (implantation) is the most widely accepted because it is a reasonable explanation for various types of endometriosis, including peritoneal endometriosis [38, 40] and even prepubertal endometriosis when neonatal bleeding is taken into account as a possible cause [41, 42]. In the implantation theory, endometriosis stem cells originate from stem cells that are present in eutopic endometrium and reach ectopic sites via many possible routes as discussed above.

Sasson and Taylor [16] and others proposed that the pathogenesis of endometriosis could be due to endometriosis stem cells that originate from the bone marrow of humans [43, 44], data supported by work in mice [45, 46]. These theories are plausible because a variety of stem/progenitor cells reside in the bone marrow. In this regard, the presence of mesenchymal stem cells is of particular interest. In support of this theory, a murine model of endometriosis was used to demonstrate that bone marrow-derived cells participate in the genesis of epithelial and stromal cells when endometrium was ectopically transplanted into the peritoneum [45].

Theories that propose different stem cell origins do not necessarily contradict one another. It is quite likely that endometrial SP cells include endometrial stem cells [47–51]. Our laboratory showed that endometrial SP cells possess phenotypic properties that are similar to endothelial progenitor cell (EPC)-like cells [49]. Given that EPCs originate from bone marrow [52, 53], it is entirely possible that endometrial SP cells have a similar origin. The fact that bone marrow-derived cells are incorporated into human endometrium at a low level [43, 44] suggests that resident endometrial stem/progenitor cells such as endometrial SP cells are more likely responsible for the cyclic renewal and regeneration of endometrium and also possibly for the establishment of endometriosis than circulating bone marrow-derived cells [54].

4.3.4 Endometrial Stem Cells and Their Relevance to the Pathogenesis of Endometriosis

The best current theory for the pathogenesis of endometriosis posits that stem/progenitor cells in the eutopic endometrium reach ectopic sites through retrograde menstruation or systemic dissemination. At that point, they give rise to endometriotic lesions. Integral to this theory is the presence of EmSCs. Below, the identity and function of EmSCs are discussed.

4.3.4.1 Endometrial Stem Cells

Endometrial stem/progenitor cells and related cells have been isolated and characterized by a number of laboratories [18, 17, 55]. Some of the precursors show "plasticity," i.e., the capacity to differentiate into a variety of endometrial tissue types. For example, endometrial SP cells can differentiate into endothelial, glandular, smooth muscle, and stromal cells, both *in vitro* and *in vivo* [47–51]. Endometrial SP cells have been observed in the functional layer of the human endometrium [49]. Hence, they might contribute to renewal of the endometrium [19]. Intriguingly, when endometrial SP cells are transplanted under the mouse kidney capsule, they migrate into the kidney parenchyma and initiate the formation of blood vessels [49]. Endometrial SP cells can be found in the vascular walls of endometrial small vessels in functional and basal layers, and they have functional properties like EPCs [49]. Endometrial SP cells might initially trigger neovascularization followed by propagation and differentiation into various cellular components of the human endometrium [49].

In addition to endometrial SP cells, endometrial mesenchymal stem cells and endometrial epithelial progenitor cells have been identified and isolated. This was achieved through the use of cell surface markers such as CD146, CD140b/

PDGFR-b, EPCAM, and W5C5 [56–59]. These cell populations are capable of self-renewal and multilineage differentiation, at least in *in vitro* experiments, except for W5C5-positve cells whose stem cell-like properties are verified *in vivo* as well as *in vitro* [59].

Laboratories isolating endometrial SP cells are not in complete agreement with regard to the cells' properties [47–50]. While the endometrial SP cells share some properties, they appear different in regard to their expression of surface markers, clonal efficiency, culture requirements, and location within the normal endometrium. Thus, it is not clear whether there are multiple types of stem cells in the human endometrium or whether these differences are the result of subtle variations in laboratory techniques. In any event, it is an open question whether the endometrium contains populations of precursor cells differing in phenotype and function. If this is indeed the case, it is important to determine their hierarchical relationship.

To better define the nature of endometrial stem cells, our laboratory established a novel *in vivo* endometrial stem cell assay [51]. This approach has a number of advantages, the most important of which is that we could follow multipotential differentiation through use of cell tracking in combination with in vivo model of human endometrial regeneration [51, 60]. We found that the efficiency with which endometrial SP cells reconstituted the endometrium increased when unfractionated endometrial cells were included as support cells. These data clearly showed the importance of the microenvironment in supporting primitive undifferentiated cells [51]. When SP and non-SP cells were labeled with a fluorescent marker by lentiviral labeling, we found that endometrial SP cells had a greater capacity to differentiate into vascular, glandular, and stromal structures *in vivo* compared with non-SP endometrial cells [51]. These experiments verified that endometrial precursors possess a range of differentiation potentials. This newly developed *in vivo* endometrial stem cell assay [51] should prove useful for the identification and analysis of human endometrial stem/progenitor cells.

4.3.4.2 Properties of Endometriosis-Initiating Cells

Based upon the pathogenesis of endometriosis, we can readily predict that endometriosis-initiating cells should possess three sets of properties. In the first case, recall that the functional layer sheds during menstruation and is partially refluxed into the peritoneal cavity through the fallopian tubes. The retrograde menstruation (implantation) theory requires large numbers of endometriosis-initiating cells in the functional layer. In agreement, our data have shown that endometrial SP cells are present in both the basalis and functional layers [49]. However, it has been postulated that stem cells present solely within the basal layer which are not shed during menstruation will then give rise to the new functional layer [61, 62]. There is evidence that fragments of the shed endometrial basalis are found more frequently in the menstrual blood of women with endometriosis than in that of healthy control subjects [63]. Importantly, the expression of stem cell-related markers such as SSEA-1 by endometriotic cells and basal layer cells is similar [64]. The data of the two studies suggest that endometriosis may originate from the basal layer, which, however, does not exclude a possibility that endometrial stem cells such as endometrial SP cells present in the functional layer may also contribute to the cyclic renewal and regeneration of eutopic endometrium and also the establishment of endometriosis.

Second, attachment, migration, and angiogenesis are essential for the implantation and survival of endometriosis-initiating cells at ectopic site(s). These cells, therefore, should have migratory potential and angiogenic capability. Third, to give rise to endometriotic lesion(s) containing glandular structures, endometriosis-initiating cells should demonstrate multi-differentiation potentials to produce a variety of endometrial cell components.

In summary, several groups have shown that endometrial SP cells satisfy most of the predicted properties of endometriosis-initiating cells. That is, endometrial SP cells are present in both the functional and basal layers and have migratory, angiogenic, and stem cell-like properties [49, 50]. These findings strengthen the stem cell theory of endometriosis and support the retrograde menstruation theory.

4.3.5 The Strength and Weakness of the Stem Cell Model

The stem cell theory can account for the weakness of the implantation theory. It can also address the unique characteristics and behavior of endometriosis.

The retrograde menstruation theory has a number of weaknesses. Specifically, it has been extremely difficult to detect the initial pathological steps, i.e., the attachment of endometrial tissue to the peritoneum and its secondary proliferation and invasion [65–67]. A modified version of the stem cell theory explains this shortcoming. This theory posits that endometriosis arises from EmSCs and/or progenitor cells in the implanted endometrial fragments. In other words, EmSCs and/or progenitor cells are both necessary and sufficient for the establishment of endometriosis and can be initiated by a single or very few cells. In this scenario, EmSCs and/or progenitor cells (and not endometrial tissues) implant and give rise to endometriotic lesions. As such, it would be almost impossible to detect the initial attachment and proliferation events of these cells. Thus, endometriotic lesions would only become microscopically detectable after completion of initial events. Note that non-stem/progenitor cells in the endometrium (the bulk of endometrial cells) will not give rise to "persistent" endometriosis even when a large numbers are present ectopically.

We emphasize that endometrial SP cells, the most likely candidate for endometrial stem cells, constitute only ~2 % of the endometrial cell population [49]. Consequently, the chances are low that endometrial stem/progenitor cells will find an ectopic supportive microenvironment and initiate an endometriotic lesion. This might explain the apparent discrepancy between the incidence of endometriosis and the frequent occurrence of retrograde menstruation.

The stem cell theory of endometriosis is weakened by the fact that the characteristics of endometrial and endometriosis stem cells are not universally accepted. Without such consensus, the theory necessarily remains an attractive hypothesis.

4.4 Conclusions

The stem cell theory for the pathogenesis of endometriosis seems to account for many aspects of the pathophysiology of this disease. The theory provides testable hypotheses and suggests new approaches to the development of novel diagnostic tests and treatments. The theory, however, largely depends on determining unequivocally the existence, identity, and function of EmSCs. Such evidence is growing. However, a consensus has not yet been established. Once EmSC populations are defined, significant progress in understanding the pathophysiology of the disease and new clinical approaches can be anticipated.

Acknowledgements I thank Hirotaka Masuda, Masanori Ono, Kaoru Miyazaki, Takashi Kajitani, Hiroshi Uchida, and the other members of my research group for their generous assistance and discussion and Hideyuki Okano and Yumi Matsuzaki for their collaboration with the endometrial and endometriotic stem cell project. We acknowledge the secretarial assistance of Rika Shibata. This work was partly supported by Grant-in-Aid from the Japan Society for the Promotion of Science (to T.M and Y.Y.), Grant-in-Aid from Keio University Sakaguchi-Memorial Medical Science Fund (to T.M.), and Grant-in-Aid from the Japan Medical Association (to T.M.).

References

1. Giudice LC, Kao LC. Endometriosis. Lancet. 2004;364(9447):1789–99.
2. Bulun SE. Endometriosis. N Engl J Med. 2009;360(3):268–79.
3. Jubanyik KJ, Comite F. Extrapelvic endometriosis. Obstet Gynecol Clin North Am. 1997;24 (2):411–40.
4. Robboy SJ, Anderson MC, Russell P. Endometriosis. In: Robboy SJ, Anderson MC, Russell P, editors. Pathology of the female reproductive tract. London: Churchill Livingstone; 2002. p. 445–73.
5. Anaf V, Simon P, Fayt I, Noel J. Smooth muscles are frequent components of endometriotic lesions. Hum Reprod. 2000;15(4):767–71.
6. Taylor RN, Yu J, Torres PB, Schickedanz AC, Park JK, Mueller MD, Sidell N. Mechanistic and therapeutic implications of angiogenesis in endometriosis. Reprod Sci. 2009;16(2):140–6.
7. Medina MG, Lebovic DI. Endometriosis-associated nerve fibers and pain. Acta Obstet Gynecol Scand. 2009;88(9):968–75.
8. Varma R, Rollason T, Gupta JK, Maher ER. Endometriosis and the neoplastic process. Reproduction. 2004;127(3):293–304. doi:10.1530/rep.1.00020.
9. Jimbo H, Hitomi Y, Yoshikawa H, Yano T, Momoeda M, Sakamoto A, Tsutsumi O, Taketani Y, Esumi H. Evidence for monoclonal expansion of epithelial cells in ovarian endometrial cysts. Am J Pathol. 1997;150(4):1173–8.

10. Tamura M, Fukaya T, Murakami T, Uehara S, Yajima A. Analysis of clonality in human endometriotic cysts based on evaluation of X chromosome inactivation in archival formalin-fixed, paraffin-embedded tissue. Lab Invest. 1998;78(2):213–8.
11. Wu Y, Basir Z, Kajdacsy-Balla A, Strawn E, Macias V, Montgomery K, Guo SW. Resolution of clonal origins for endometriotic lesions using laser capture microdissection and the human androgen receptor (HUMARA) assay. Fertil Steril. 2003;79 Suppl 1:710–7.
12. Nabeshima H, Murakami T, Yoshinaga K, Sato K, Terada Y, Okamura K. Analysis of the clonality of ectopic glands in peritoneal endometriosis using laser microdissection. Fertil Steril. 2003;80(5):1144–50.
13. Gaetje R, Kotzian S, Herrmann G, Baumann R, Starzinski-Powitz A. Invasiveness of endometriotic cells in vitro. Lancet. 1995;346(8988):1463–4.
14. Podberezin M, Wen J, Chang CC. Cancer stem cells: a review of potential clinical applications. Arch Pathol Lab Med. 2013;137(8):1111–6. doi:10.5858/arpa.2012-0494-RA.
15. Sugihara E, Saya H. Complexity of cancer stem cells. Int J Cancer. 2013;132(6):1249–59. doi:10.1002/ijc.27961.
16. Sasson IE, Taylor HS. Stem cells and the pathogenesis of endometriosis. Ann N Y Acad Sci. 2008;1127:106–15.
17. Gargett CE, Masuda H. Adult stem cells in the endometrium. Mol Hum Reprod. 2010;16 (11):818–34.
18. Maruyama T, Yoshimura Y. Stem cell theory for the pathogenesis of endometriosis. Front Biosci. 2012;E4:2754–63.
19. Maruyama T, Masuda H, Ono M, Kajitani T, Yoshimura Y. Human uterine stem/progenitor cells: their possible role in uterine physiology and pathology. Reproduction. 2010;140(1):11–22.
20. Scheel C, Weinberg RA. Cancer stem cells and epithelial-mesenchymal transition: concepts and molecular links. Semin Cancer Biol. 2012;22(5–6):396–403. doi:10.1016/j.semcancer.2012.04.001.
21. Shiozawa Y, Nie B, Pienta KJ, Morgan TM, Taichman RS. Cancer stem cells and their role in metastasis. Pharmacol Ther. 2013;138(2):285–93. doi:10.1016/j.pharmthera.2013.01.014.
22. Kalluri R, Weinberg RA. The basics of epithelial-mesenchymal transition. J Clin Invest. 2009;119(6):1420–8. doi:10.1172/JCI39104.
23. Uchida H, Maruyama T, Nishikawa-Uchida S, Oda H, Miyazaki K, Yamasaki A, Yoshimura Y. Studies using an in vitro model show evidence of involvement of epithelial-mesenchymal transition of human endometrial epithelial cells in human embryo implantation. J Biol Chem. 2012;287(7):4441–50. doi:10.1074/jbc.M111.286138.
24. Dinulescu DM, Ince TA, Quade BJ, Shafer SA, Crowley D, Jacks T. Role of K-ras and Pten in the development of mouse models of endometriosis and endometrioid ovarian cancer. Nat Med. 2005;11(1):63–70.
25. Matsuzaki S, Darcha C. Epithelial to mesenchymal transition-like and mesenchymal to epithelial transition-like processes might be involved in the pathogenesis of pelvic endometriosis. Hum Reprod. 2012;27(3):712–21. doi:10.1093/humrep/der442.
26. Demir AY, Demol H, Puype M, de Goeij AF, Dunselman GA, Herrler A, Evers JL, Vandekerckhove J, Groothuis PG. Proteome analysis of human mesothelial cells during epithelial to mesenchymal transitions induced by shed menstrual effluent. Proteomics. 2004;4(9):2608–23. doi:10.1002/pmic.200300827.
27. Goodell MA, Brose K, Paradis G, Conner AS, Mulligan RC. Isolation and functional properties of murine hematopoietic stem cells that are replicating in vivo. J Exp Med. 1996;183 (4):1797–806.
28. Challen GA, Little MH. A side order of stem cells: the SP phenotype. Stem Cells. 2006;24 (1):3–12.
29. Kato K, Takao T, Kuboyama A, Tanaka Y, Ohgami T, Yamaguchi S, Adachi S, Yoneda T, Ueoka Y, Kato K, Hayashi S, Asanoma K, Wake N. Endometrial cancer side-population cells show prominent migration and have a potential to differentiate into the mesenchymal cell lineage. Am J Pathol. 2010;176(1):381–92.

30. Forte A, Schettino MT, Finicelli M, Cipollaro M, Colacurci N, Cobellis L, Galderisi U. Expression pattern of stemness-related genes in human endometrial and endometriotic tissues. Mol Med. 2009;15(11–12):392–401.
31. Chang JH, Au HK, Lee WC, Chi CC, Ling TY, Wang LM, Kao SH, Huang YH, Tzeng CR. Expression of the pluripotent transcription factor OCT4 promotes cell migration in endometriosis. Fertil Steril. 2013;99(5):1332–9.e5.
32. Matsuzaki S, Darcha C. Adenosine triphosphate-binding cassette transporter G2 expression in endometriosis and in endometrium from patients with and without endometriosis. Fertil Steril. 2012;98(6):1512–20.e3.
33. Silveira CG, Abrao MS, Dias Jr JA, Coudry RA, Soares FA, Drigo SA, Domingues MA, Rogatto SR. Common chromosomal imbalances and stemness-related protein expression markers in endometriotic lesions from different anatomical sites: the potential role of stem cells. Hum Reprod. 2012;27(11):3187–97. doi:10.1093/humrep/des282.
34. Sterneckert J, Hoing S, Scholer HR. Concise review: Oct4 and more: the reprogramming expressway. Stem Cells. 2012;30(1):15–21. doi:10.1002/stem.765.
35. Krishnamurthy P, Schuetz JD. Role of ABCG2/BCRP in biology and medicine. Annu Rev Pharmacol Toxicol. 2006;46:381–410. doi:10.1146/annurev.pharmtox.46.120604.141238.
36. Mayr D, Amann G, Siefert C, Diebold J, Anderegg B. Does endometriosis really have premalignant potential? A clonal analysis of laser-microdissected tissue. FASEB J. 2003;17 (6):693–5.
37. Chan RW, Ng EH, Yeung WS. Identification of cells with colony-forming activity, self-renewal capacity, and multipotency in ovarian endometriosis. Am J Pathol. 2011;178 (6):2832–44. doi:10.1016/j.ajpath.2011.02.025.
38. Nisolle M, Donnez J. Peritoneal endometriosis, ovarian endometriosis, and adenomyotic nodules of the rectovaginal septum are three different entities. Fertil Steril. 1997;68(4):585–96.
39. Seli E, Berkkanoglu M, Arici A. Pathogenesis of endometriosis. Obstet Gynecol Clin North Am. 2003;30(1):41–61.
40. Nap AW, Groothuis PG, Demir AY, Evers JL, Dunselman GA. Pathogenesis of endometriosis. Best Pract Res Clin Obstet Gynaecol. 2004;18(2):233–44.
41. Brosens I, Benagiano G. Is neonatal uterine bleeding involved in the pathogenesis of endometriosis as a source of stem cells? Fertil Steril. 2013. doi:10.1016/j.fertnstert.2013.04.046.
42. Brosens I, Puttemans P, Benagiano G. Endometriosis: a life cycle approach? Am J Obstet Gynecol. 2013. doi:10.1016/j.ajog.2013.03.009.
43. Taylor HS. Endometrial cells derived from donor stem cells in bone marrow transplant recipients. JAMA. 2004;292(1):81–5.
44. Ikoma T, Kyo S, Maida Y, Ozaki S, Takakura M, Nakao S, Inoue M. Bone marrow-derived cells from male donors can compose endometrial glands in female transplant recipients. Am J Obstet Gynecol. 2009;201(e601):8.
45. Du H, Taylor HS. Contribution of bone marrow-derived stem cells to endometrium and endometriosis. Stem Cells. 2007;25(8):2082–6.
46. Bratincsak A, Brownstein MJ, Cassiani-Ingoni R, Pastorino S, Szalayova I, Toth ZE, Key S, Nemeth K, Pickel J, Mezey E. CD45-positive blood cells give rise to uterine epithelial cells in mice. Stem Cells. 2007;25(11):2820–6.
47. Kato K, Yoshimoto M, Kato K, Adachi S, Yamayoshi A, Arima T, Asanoma K, Kyo S, Nakahata T, Wake N. Characterization of side-population cells in human normal endometrium. Hum Reprod. 2007;22(5):1214–23.
48. Tsuji S, Yoshimoto M, Takahashi K, Noda Y, Nakahata T, Heike T. Side population cells contribute to the genesis of human endometrium. Fertil Steril. 2008;90(4 Suppl):1528–37.
49. Masuda H, Matsuzaki Y, Hiratsu E, Ono M, Nagashima T, Kajitani T, Arase T, Oda H, Uchida H, Asada H, Ito M, Yoshimura Y, Maruyama T, Okano H. Stem cell-like properties of the endometrial side population: implication in endometrial regeneration. PLoS One. 2010;5 (4):e10387.

50. Cervello I, Gil-Sanchis C, Mas A, Delgado-Rosas F, Martinez-Conejero JA, Galan A, Martinez-Romero A, Martinez S, Navarro I, Ferro J, Horcajadas JA, Esteban FJ, O'Connor JE, Pellicer A, Simon C. Human endometrial side population cells exhibit genotypic, phenotypic and functional features of somatic stem cells. PLoS One. 2010;5(6):e10964.
51. Miyazaki K, Maruyama T, Masuda H, Yamasaki A, Uchida S, Oda H, Uchida H, Yoshimura Y. Stem cell-like differentiation potentials of endometrial side population cells as revealed by a newly developed in vivo endometrial stem cell assay. PLoS One. 2012;7(12):e50749.
52. Urbich C, Dimmeler S. Endothelial progenitor cells: characterization and role in vascular biology. Circ Res. 2004;95(4):343–53.
53. Timmermans F, Plum J, Yoder MC, Ingram DA, Vandekerckhove B, Case J. Endothelial progenitor cells: identity defined? J Cell Mol Med. 2009;13(1):87–102.
54. Deane JA, Gualano RC, Gargett CE. Regenerating endometrium from stem/progenitor cells: is it abnormal in endometriosis, Asherman's syndrome and infertility? Curr Opin Obstet Gynecol. 2013;25(3):193–200. doi:10.1097/GCO.0b013e32836024e7.
55. Cervello I, Mas A, Gil-Sanchis C, Simon C. Somatic stem cells in the human endometrium. Semin Reprod Med. 2013;31(1):69–76. doi:10.1055/s-0032-1331800.
56. Schwab KE, Gargett CE. Co-expression of two perivascular cell markers isolates mesenchymal stem-like cells from human endometrium. Hum Reprod. 2007;22(11):2903–11.
57. Schwab KE, Hutchinson P, Gargett CE. Identification of surface markers for prospective isolation of human endometrial stromal colony-forming cells. Hum Reprod. 2008;23 (4):934–43.
58. Gargett CE, Schwab KE, Zillwood RM, Nguyen HP, Wu D. Isolation and culture of epithelial progenitors and mesenchymal stem cells from human endometrium. Biol Reprod. 2009;80 (6):1136–45.
59. Masuda H, Anwar SS, Buhring HJ, Rao JR, Gargett CE. A novel marker of human endometrial mesenchymal stem-like cells. Cell Transplant. 2012;21(10):2201–14. doi:10.3727/096368911X637362.
60. Masuda H, Maruyama T, Hiratsu E, Yamane J, Iwanami A, Nagashima T, Ono M, Miyoshi H, Okano HJ, Ito M, Tamaoki N, Nomura T, Okano H, Matsuzaki Y, Yoshimura Y. Noninvasive and real-time assessment of reconstructed functional human endometrium in NOD/SCID/γ_c^{null} immunodeficient mice. Proc Natl Acad Sci U S A. 2007;104(6):1925–30.
61. Padykula HA. Regeneration in the primate uterus: the role of stem cells. Ann N Y Acad Sci. 1991;622:47–56.
62. Padykula HA, Coles LG, Okulicz WC, Rapaport SI, McCracken JA, King Jr NW, Longcope C, Kaiserman-Abramof IR. The basalis of the primate endometrium: a bifunctional germinal compartment. Biol Reprod. 1989;40(3):681–90.
63. Leyendecker G, Herbertz M, Kunz G, Mall G. Endometriosis results from the dislocation of basal endometrium. Hum Reprod. 2002;17(10):2725–36.
64. Valentijn AJ, Palial K, Al-Lamee H, Tempest N, Drury J, Von Zglinicki T, Saretzki G, Murray P, Gargett CE, Hapangama DK. SSEA-1 isolates human endometrial basal glandular epithelial cells: phenotypic and functional characterization and implications in the pathogenesis of endometriosis. Hum Reprod. 2013. doi:10.1093/humrep/det285.
65. Redwine DB. Was Sampson wrong? Fertil Steril. 2002;78(4):686–93.
66. Redwine DB. Sampson revisited: a critical review of the development of Sampson's theory of origin of endometriosis. In: Garcia-Velasco JA, Rizk BR, editors. Endometriosis: current management and future trends. New Delhi: Jaypee Brothers Medical Publishers; 2010.
67. Katabuchi H. Endometriosis as an enigmatic pelvic disease [Japanese]. J Jpn Soc Endometriosis. 2008;29:22–31.

Chapter 5
Role of NK Cells in Endometriosis

Nagamasa Maeda

Abstract Impaired natural killer (NK) cell activity in women with endometriosis is thought to promote implantation and the progressive growth of endometrial tissue in accordance with Sampson's hypothesis. However, the mechanisms responsible for decreased NK cell activity and the antigens recognized by NK cells in these women are not clear.

Decreased NK cell activity in the peripheral blood (PB) and peritoneal fluid (PF) of women with endometriosis was first reported by Oosterlynck et al. and subsequent investigators have identified the depression of NK cell function in women with this disorder. Decreased NK cell activity in women with endometriosis is thought to allow the implantation of endometrial tissue in the manner of a graft, but the mechanisms underlying the decline of NK cell activity remain uncertain.

We focused on the expression of HLA-G, a ligand of NK cell receptors, and its changes in eutopic endometrium during the menstrual cycle. HLA-G expression was only identified in eutopic endometrium during the menstrual phase, but not during the proliferative or secretory phases. HLA-G-expressing cells were also detected in peritoneal fluid during the menstrual phase.

Retrograde menstruation may allow HLA-G-expressing endometrial tissue to enter the peritoneal cavity, where it should be scavenged by the immune surveillance system. Because peritoneal NK cells play an important role in this system, impairment of their cytotoxicity via HLA-G could allow the survival and implantation of peritoneal endometrial cells.

In this article, we discuss the pathogenesis of endometriosis from the perspective of intraperitoneal interactions between NK cell receptors and their ligands (antigens) that enter the peritoneal cavity on cells shed from eutopic endometrium via retrograde menstruation.

N. Maeda, M.D. (✉)
Department of Obstetrics and Gynecology, Kochi Medical School,
Kohasu, Oko-cho, Nankoku-city, Kochi 783-8505, Japan
e-mail: maedan@kochi-u.ac.jp

T. Harada (ed.), *Endometriosis: Pathogenesis and Treatment*,
DOI 10.1007/978-4-431-54421-0_5, © Springer Japan 2014

Keywords Endometriosis • Endometrium • HLA-G • KIR • Natural killer cell • NK receptor • Retrograde menstruation • Stress

5.1 Natural Killer (NK) Cells

NK cells are cytotoxic lymphocytes that constitute a major component of the innate immune system. Because these cells can attack target cells without requiring antigen sensitization, they are called "natural killer" cells [1]. NK cells participate in host defenses against infection [2], have antitumor activity [3], and are involved in graft rejection [4]. NK cells can also have an adverse influence on pregnancy [5].

These cells usually express the surface markers CD16 (FcγRIII) [6] and CD56 (neural cell adhesion molecule: NCAM) [7] in humans. In addition to killing target cells, NK cells secrete various cytokines, such as the antiviral cytokine interferon-γ (IFN-γ) [8, 9] and the inflammatory and antitumor cytokine tumor necrosis factor-α (TNF-α) [10].

NK cell activity can be assessed by measuring cytotoxicity for NK-sensitive K562 cells (a chronic myelogenous leukemia cell line) [11, 12]. NK cells do not require activation in order to kill target cells that lack expression of major histocompatibility complex (MHC) class I antigens. Kärre et al. [13, 14] have proposed the "missing self" hypothesis, which states that NK cells act against target cells that do not express MHC determinants characteristic of "self," while toxicity is inhibited when cells express these determinants.

This "missing self" hypothesis has been supported by the identification of killer cell immunoglobulin-like receptors (KIRs) on NK cells that recognize autologous MHC class I antigens [15, 16] and inhibit NK cytotoxicity against target cells bearing these determinants.

5.1.1 Activation of NK Cells

Because of their strong cytotoxicity and the potential for autoreactivity, the activity of NK cells is strictly regulated by several factors. Cytokines play a crucial role in the regulation of NK cells. Cytokines involved in the activation of these cells include interleukin (IL)-2 [8], IL-12 [17], IL-15 [18], IL-18 [19], IL-21 [20], IFN-γ [8], and granulocyte-macrophage colony-stimulating factor (GM-CSF) [21].

NK cells, as well as macrophages and several other cell types, express the Fc receptor (FcγRIII: CD16/Leu-11 antigen), an activating receptor that binds the Fc portion of antibodies and allows NK cells to lyse target cells through antibody-dependent cellular cytotoxicity (ADCC) [22, 23]. Thus, NK cells are fundamentally different from T cells in their lineage and mechanism of nonself recognition.

In addition to the Fc receptor, NK cells express various activating and inhibitory receptors, which maintain the balance of positive and negative signals that controls their cytolytic activity. The KIR family of receptors recognizes and binds both classical and nonclassical MHC class I molecules. Although receptors of this family can have activating or inhibitory cytoplasmic domains, most of these receptors mediate the inhibition of NK cell cytotoxicity. In addition, the nonclassical MHC I molecule HLA-E is recognized by the lectin-like CD94/NKG2 receptor family, which includes both activating and inhibitory receptors [24–26]. Thus, NK cells can simultaneously express both activating and inhibitory receptors.

5.1.2 NK Cells and Endometriosis

In 1991 and 1992, Oosterlynck et al. reported that the NK cell activity against autologous endometrium in PB and PF was reduced in women with endometriosis [27, 28]. Impaired NK cell activity in women with this condition is thought to allow the implantation of endometrial tissue as a graft according to Sampson's hypothesis [29].

The finding of decreased NK cell activity in women with endometriosis and the positive correlation of NK cell activity in both the PB and PF with the severity of this disease has led to consensus about its pathogenesis [30–33].

After removal of endometriotic lesions, decreased NK cell activity and the impaired cytotoxicity of autologous and heterologous lymphocytes against the endometrium are unchanged, and cytotoxicity is still significantly decreased compared with that in women who do not have endometriosis. These findings suggest a primary deficiency of NK cell activity in women with endometriosis, which could explain its frequent relapse after treatment [34].

Survival of endometrial cells in the peritoneal cavity of women with endometriosis [35] is mainly due to decreased NK cell activity, but is also related to resistance of these cells to NK cytotoxicity [36–38].

The "missing self" hypothesis has been supported by the identification of KIRs on NK cells that recognize self-determinants among MHC class I antigens andinhibit NK cell cytotoxicity against target cells bearing these determinants. In women with endometriosis, expression of inhibitory killer immunoglobulin-like receptors on NK cells from PB and PF is significantly upregulated compared with the level of expression in women without endometriosis [39–41], indicating a decrease of NK cell activity and cytotoxicity for endometriotic cells.

5.2 NK Cell Receptors

5.2.1 Killer-Cell Immunoglobulin-Like Receptors (KIRs)

The KIR genes are polymorphic and highly homologous genes that are located in a cluster on chromosome 19q13.4 [25]. The KIR proteins are classified by the number of immunoglobulin (Ig)-like extracellular domain receptors (2 or 3) and by whether they have a long or short cytoplasmic tail. KIR proteins with a long cytoplasmic tail transduce inhibitory signals upon ligand binding via an immunoreceptor tyrosine-based inhibitory motif (ITIM) after binding tyrosine phosphatase SHP1/SHP2, while KIR proteins with a short cytoplasmic tail that lacks the ITIM associate with the tyrosine kinase-binding protein ZAP-70/Syk instead transduce activating signals via an immunoreceptor tyrosine-based activation motif (ITAM) [42–44].

Most KIRs are inhibitory, indicating that recognition of MHC antigens by these receptors suppresses the cytotoxic activity of NK cells, while only a limited number of KIRs have the ability to activate these cells. The ligands for several KIRs are subsets of both classical HLA-Ia antigens (HLA-A, HLA-B, HLA-C) and also nonclassical HLA-Ib antigens (HLA-G) [45, 46].

5.2.1.1 KIR2DL1 and Endometriosis

In women with endometriosis, the decrease of NK cell activity may be related to the inhibitory KIRs expressed by NK cells.

The percentage of cells expressing KIR2DL1 among NK cells in PF and PB was reported to be significantly higher in women with endometriosis than in controls, suggesting that this receptor is probably related to suppression of NK cell activity in endometriosis [39]. The elevated percentage of KIR2DL1$^+$ NK cells in PB from women with endometriosis was not reduced by laparoscopic surgery or by gonadotropin-releasing hormone agonist treatment. Thus, KIR2DL1 overexpression may be a primary event that represents a risk factor for both the development of endometriosis and its recurrence after treatment [40].

5.2.1.2 KIR2DL4 and Endometriosis

KIR2DL4-expressing NK cells have been identified in both the PB and PF [47]. Expression of HLA-G (a ligand for KIR2DL4), ILT-2, and ILT-4 by eutopic endometrium was only detected during the menstrual phase and was not found in either proliferative or secretory endometrium [47]. Because HLA-G-expressing cells were detected in PF during the menstrual phase, retrograde menstruation may allow eutopic endometrial cells bearing HLA-G to enter the peritoneal cavity and react locally with KIR2DL4.

Due to the innate immunological activity of KIR2DL4 targeting HLA-G, KIR2DL4-expressing NK cells in the PF may be cytotoxic for HLA-G-expressing endometrial cells that enter the peritoneal cavity through retrograde menstruation. Mutant (9A)/wild-type (10A) polymorphism would modulate the response of peritoneal NK cells to membrane-bound HLA-G on endometrial cells, and inhibitory ILT-2 and ILT-4 receptors may also influence the local immune response together with KIR2DL4. Thus, impaired cytotoxicity for endometrial cells could allow these cells to survive and result in ectopic implantation that produces peritoneal endometriosis.

5.2.2 *CD94/NKG2A*

CD94/NKG2A is a member of the C-type lectin receptor family composed of a CD94 chain covalently bound with a member of the NKG2 family. The ligand of CD94/NKG2A is HLA-E, a nonclassical HLA-Ib molecule. After binding of CD94 with NKG2A that has the ITIM, the resulting CD94/NKG2A heterodimer forms an inhibitory receptor, whereas association of CD94 with an NKG2 family member lacking the ITIM (NKG2C) may not form an inhibitory receptor.

5.2.2.1 CD94/NKG2A and Endometriosis

Despite its interesting inhibitory function, little has been reported concerning CD94/NKG2A and endometriosis. Women with stage III and stage IV endometriosis were found to have a significantly higher percentage of CD94/NKG2A^{+} peritoneal NK cells than control women [48], and HLA-E (the CD94/NKG2A ligand) has been identified in endometriotic tissues [48]. Because target cells expressing HLA-E show resistance to NK cell-mediated cytotoxicity in a CD94/NKG2A-dependent manner, the increased expression of CD94/NKG2A by peritoneal NK cells may mediate the resistance of endometriotic tissues to NK cell cytotoxicity and thus contribute to the progression of endometriosis [48].

5.2.3 *Immunoglobulin-Like Transcript (ILT)*

The immunoglobulin-like transcript (ILT) gene family has up to 11 members in humans. The extracellular part of each ILT molecule includes at least two and usually four immunoglobulin domains. ILT-2 through ILT-5 are all inhibitory members of this family with different numbers of cytoplasmic ITIM domains. ILT1, ILT7, and ILT8 have a short cytoplasmic tail and a charged amino acid residue in the transmembrane domain, and these family members deliver an activating signal through the cytoplasmic ITAM of the associated common g chain of Fc receptor (FcRg).

5.2.3.1 Immunoglobulin-Like Transcript (ILT) and Endometriosis

ILT-2 and ILT-4 bind to HLA-G with a three- to fourfold higher affinity than that for classical MHC class Ia [49], suggesting that ILT/HLA-G recognition may play a dominant role in regulating the activation of NK cells, T cells, and monocytes. Although ILT is thus thought to have a role in the pathogenesis of endometriosis, surprisingly, there has been no report concerning its interaction with this disease.

5.3 NK Receptor Ligands on Endometrial Cells

5.3.1 HLA Class Ia

In 1990, expression of HLA class I molecules was identified on human endometrial and endocervical epithelial cells [50]. This suggests that KIRs expressed on NK cells can respond to their HLA class I ligands on eutopic endometrium [39–41]. It was also reported that progesterone induces HLA class I mRNA expression by cultured cells from secretory endometrium [51].

In women with endometriosis, HLA class I expression by both glandular cells and stromal cells is significantly elevated compared with that in controls [52]. Furthermore, women with endometriosis show significantly higher expression of HLA class I molecules by eutopic endometrial cells compared with controls [52].

Our investigations have suggested that HLA-C-expressing endometrial cells may enter the peritoneal cavity via retrograde menstruation and react with peritoneal NK cells expressing KIR2DL1 [39–41]. Impaired KIR2DL1 expression by peritoneal NK cells could allow endometrial cells to survive in the peritoneal cavity and undergo ectopic implantation, favoring the onset and progression of endometriosis.

5.3.2 HLA Class Ib

5.3.2.1 HLA-E

HLA-E is one of a family of molecules known as HLA class Ib and it has a very specialized role in the recognition of other cells by NK cells. HLA-E is very highly conserved and presents a small repertoire of peptides of various origins [53]. NK cells recognize the HLA-E/peptide complex via the heterodimeric inhibitory receptor CD94/NKG2A or the activating receptor CD94/NKG2C. When CD94/NKG2A is stimulated, it has an inhibitory effect on NK cell cytotoxic activity and prevents target cell lysis [54].

Expression of HLA-E, the ligand of CD94/NKG2A, has been detected in endometriotic tissues. Target cells bearing HLA-E show resistance to NK cell cytotoxicity in a CD94/NKG2A-dependent manner. Therefore, increased expression of CD94/NKG2A by peritoneal NK cells may mediate the resistance of endometriotic tissue to NK cell cytotoxicity, thus contributing to the progression of endometriosis [48].

5.3.2.2 HLA-G

5.3.2.2.1 Receptors for HLA-G

HLA-G appears to be mainly recognized by ILT-2 and ILT-4 receptors, which are expressed by T and B lymphocytes, as well as NK cells and monocytes, and inhibit the activating signals received by these cells. In addition to ILT, HLA-G can also react with KIR2DL4 expressed on NK cells and T cells. Although the expression of ILT2, ILT3, ILT4, and KIR2DL4 is known to be upregulated by HLA-G in antigen-presenting cells, NK cells, and T cells [55], whether the HLA-G/KIR2DL4 interaction leads to activation or inhibition of NK cells remains a complicated and controversial issue.

5.3.2.2.2 HLA-G and Endometriosis

Hornung et al. reported that HLA-G was not expressed by eutopic endometrium or endometriotic tissue [56] and HLA-G protein was not detectable in peritoneal fluid from endometriosis patients or controls. Moreover, ectopic and normal endometrial tissues and stromal cells did not express HLA-G during the proliferative phase. Accordingly, they concluded that immune cell inhibition in endometriosis is mediated by factors other than HLA-G.

In another study, HLA-G expression was identified in the glandular epithelium of peritoneal endometriotic implants, but not in eutopic endometrium [57]. The authors concluded that differential expression of HLA-G suggests peritoneal inflammation or cellular stress may upregulate mechanisms promoting the survival of ectopic endometrium.

According to our recent findings, KIR2DL4-expressing NK cells can be identified in both the PB and PF. Interestingly, we found that HLA-G (a ligand of KIR2DL4) was only expressed by eutopic endometrium during the menstrual phase and not during the proliferative or secretory phases [47]. In addition, we detected HLA-G-expressing cells in PF during the menstrual phase [47]. This suggests that cells bearing HLA-G may enter the peritoneal cavity through retrograde menstruation, allowing the antigen to react locally with KIR2DL4.

In 2000, Ibrahim et al. reported that stress, including heat shock and arsenite treatment, induces an increase in the expression of various HLA-G alternative transcripts without affecting other MHC class I transcripts (HLA-A, HLA-B, HLA-E, and HLA-F) [58].

A heat shock element (HSE) that binds to heat shock factor 1 (HSF1) trimers under stress conditions has been identified within the HLA-G promoter. When stresses such as heat shock, bacterial infection, and poisons (including arsenite) affect cells, cytoplasmic heat shock factor (HSF)-1, which is usually regulated by HSF-2 and HSF-4, undergoes translocation into the nucleus where it forms trimers and binds with the HSE located in the promoter region of the heat shock protein (Hsp) and HLA-G genes (37), resulting in the induction of hsp70 and HLA-G [58].

We detected HLA-G expression by eutopic endometrial cells during menstruation [47], which presumably reflects the stressful intrauterine environment at this time.

In the normal menstrual cycle, a decrease of the serum progesterone level induces uterine smooth muscle contraction and spiral artery spasm, resulting in menstruation [59]. Transient bacterial invasion and inflammation may also affect the eutopic endometrium during menstruation, and increased expression of Hsp70 and HLA-G by the endometrium may result from such "physiological" stress. Hsp70- and HLA-G-expressing endometrial cells that enter the peritoneal cavity via retrograde menstruation may react with immunocompetent cells such as NK cells in the PF and be eliminated. However, an impaired NK cell response to these antigens could lead to endometrial cell survival in the PF and implantation with subsequent development of endometriosis (Fig. 5.1).

5.4 Conclusions

We demonstrated that HLA-G was expressed in the eutopic endometrium during menstruation, suggesting the existence of physiological stress during the menstrual phase. HLA-G-expressing endometrial cells may enter the peritoneal cavity via retrograde menstruation and react with immunocompetent cells, particularly NK cells. Retrograde menstruation involves the backflow of menstrual discharge from the uterine cavity through the fallopian tubes into the peritoneal cavity. It is a physiological phenomenon that is observed in women with patent tubes.

There is probably a physiological system that removes displaced tissues or debris from the peritoneal cavity and peritoneal NK cells presumably play an important role in this system. Expression of HLA-G by endometrial cells during the menstrual phase and entry of such cells into the peritoneal cavity may induce a local immune response from immunocompetent cells including KIR2DL4-expressing NK cells, while impaired NK cell activity could allow the survival and ectopic implantation of endometrial cells.

Impairment of the physiological immune surveillance system (particularly NK cell function) may favor endometrial cell implantation and thus trigger the onset of endometriosis. Further investigation of the molecular mechanisms leading to

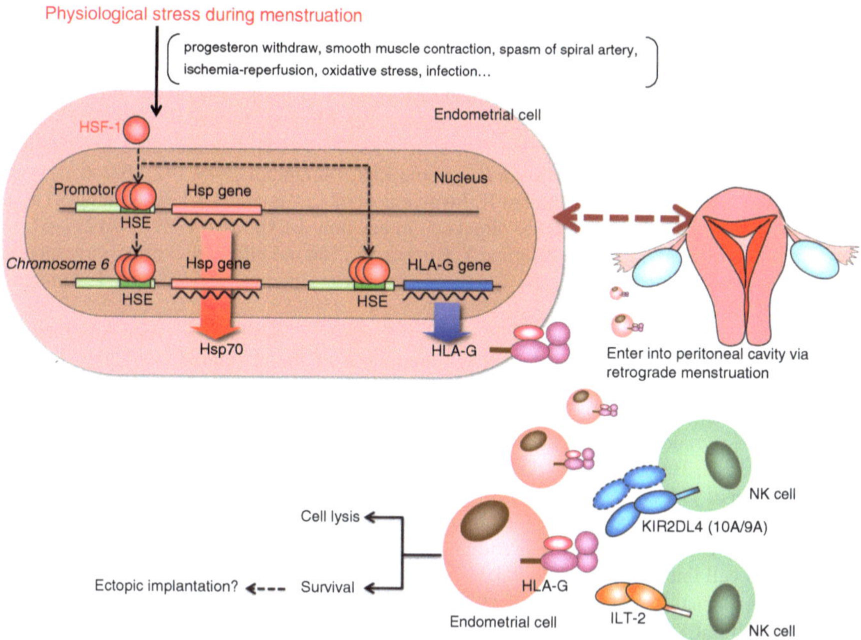

Fig. 5.1 In the usual menstrual cycle, "physiological" stresses such as progesterone withdraw, smooth muscle contraction, spasm of spiral artery, ischemia-reperfusion, oxidative stress, and transient bacterial infection may occur in the uterus. Increased expression of Hsp70 and HLA-G in the endometrium during menstruation may result from such stress pathway. Hsp70- and HLA-G-expressing endometrial cells in the retrograde menstruation may react with immunocompetent cells such as NK cells in PF and finally disappear from peritoneal cavity or survive and develop to endometriosis. *HSF* heat shock factor, *HSE* heat shock element, *HSP* heat shock protein, *KIR* killer immunoglobulin-like receptor, *ILT* immunoglobulin-like transcript

expression of antigens during menstruation and the role of immunocompetent responder cells in the PF may contribute to better understanding of the pathogenesis of endometriosis.

References

1. Klein E, Masucci MG, Masucci G, Vanky F. Natural killer activity of human blood lymphocytes. Mol Immunol. 1982;19:1323–9.
2. Holmberg LA, Ault KA. Characterization of natural killer cells induced in the peritoneal exudates of mice infected with Listeria monocytogenes: a study of their tumor target specificity and their expression of murine differentiation antigens and human NK-associated antigens. Cell Immunol. 1984;89:151–68.
3. Klein E, Vánky F, Vose BM. Natural killer and tumor recognizing lymphocyte activity in tumor patients. Haematologia. 1978;12:107–12.

4. Lefkowitz M, Kornbluth J, Tomaszewski JE, Jorkasky DK. Natural killer-cell activity in cyclosporine-treated renal allograft recipients. J Clin Immunol. 1988;8:121–7.
5. Kwak JY, Beaman KD, Gilman-Sachs A, Ruiz JE, Schewitz D, Beer AE. Up-regulated expression of $CD56^+$, $CD56^+/CD16^+$, and $CD19^+$ cells in peripheral blood lymphocytes in pregnant women with recurrent pregnancy losses. Am J Reprod Immunol. 1995;34:93–9.
6. Werfel T, Uciechowski P, Tetteroo PA, Kurrle R, Deicher H, Schmidt RE. Activation of cloned human natural killer cells via Fc gamma RIII. J Immunol. 1989;142:1102–6.
7. Nitta T, Yagita H, Sato K, Okumura K. Involvement of CD56 (NKH-1/Leu-19 antigen) as an adhesion molecule in natural killer-target cell interaction. J Exp Med. 1989;170:1757–61.
8. Handa K, Suzuki R, Matsui H, Shimizu Y, Kumagai K. Natural killer (NK) cells as a responder to interleukin 2 (IL-2). II. IL-2-induced interferon gamma production. J Immunol. 1983;130:988–92.
9. Hunter CA, Timans J, Pisacane P, Menon S, Cai G, Walker W, Aste-Amezaga M, Chizzonite R, Bazan JF, Kastelein RA. Comparison of the effects of interleukin-1 alpha, interleukin-1 beta and interferon-gamma-inducing factor on the production of interferon-gamma by natural killer. Eur J Immunol. 1997;27:2787–92.
10. Peters PM, Ortaldo JR, Shalaby MR, Svedersky LP, Nedwin GE, Bringman TS, Hass PE, Aggarwal BB, Herberman RB, Goeddel DV, et al. Natural killer-sensitive targets stimulate production of TNF-alpha but not TNF-beta (lymphotoxin) by highly purified human peripheral blood large granular lymphocytes. J Immunol. 1986;137:2592–8.
11. Lozzio BB, Lozzio CB. Properties and usefulness of the original K-562 human myelogenous leukemia cell line. Leuk Res. 1979;3:363–70.
12. Kay HD, Fagnani R, Bonnard GD. Cytotoxicity against the K562 erythroleukemia cell line by human natural killer (NK) cells which do not bear free Fc receptors for IgG. Int J Cancer. 1979;24:141–50.
13. Kärre K. MHC gene control of the natural killer system at the level of the target and the host. Semin Cancer Biol. 1991;2:295–309.
14. Kärre K. Natural killer cell recognition of missing self. Nat Immunol. 2008;9:477–80.
15. Moretta A, Sivori S, Vitale M, Pende D. Existence of both inhibitory (p58) and activatory (p50) receptors for HLA-C molecules in human natural killer cells. J Exp Med. 1995;182:875–84.
16. Moretta A, Bottino C, Vitale M, Pende D, Biassoni R, Mingari MC, Moretta L. Receptors for HLA class-I molecules in human natural killer cells. Annu Rev Immunol. 1996;14:619–48.
17. Hiraki A, Kiura K, Yamane H, Nogami N, Tabata M, Takigawa N, Ueoka H, Tanimoto M, Harada M. Interleukin-12 augments cytolytic activity of peripheral blood mononuclear cells against autologous lung cancer cells in combination with IL-2. Lung Cancer. 2002;35:329–33.
18. Carson WE, Giri JG, Lindemann MJ, Linett ML, Ahdieh M, Paxton R, Anderson D, Eisenmann J, Grabstein K, Caligiuri MA. Interleukin (IL) 15 is a novel cytokine that activates human natural killer cells via components of the IL-2 receptor. J Exp Med. 1994;180:1395–403.
19. Son YI, Dallal RM, Mailliard RB, Egawa S, Jonak ZL, Lotze MT. Interleukin-18 (IL-18) synergizes with IL-2 to enhance cytotoxicity, interferon-gamma production, and expansion of natural killer cells. Cancer Res. 2001;61:884–8.
20. Skak K, Frederiksen KS, Lundsgaard D. Interleukin-21 activates human natural killer cells and modulates their surface receptor expression. Immunology. 2008;123:575–83.
21. Miller JS, Prosper F, McCullar V. Natural killer (NK) cells are functionally abnormal and NK cell progenitors are diminished in granulocyte colony-stimulating factor-mobilized peripheral blood progenitor cell collections. Blood. 1997;90:3098–105.
22. Uciechowski P, Werfel T, Leo R, Gessner JE, Schubert J, Schmidt RE. Analysis of CD16+dim and CD16+bright lymphocytes–comparison of peripheral and clonal non-MHC-restricted T cells and NK cells. Immunobiology. 1992;185:28–40.
23. Uciechowski P, Gessner JE, Schindler R, Schmidt RE. Fc gamma RIII activation is different in $CD16^+$ cytotoxic T lymphocytes and natural killer cells. Eur J Immunol. 1992;22:1635–8.

24. Borrego F, Ulbrecht M, Weiss EH, Coligan JE, Brooks AG. Recognition of human histocompatibility leukocyte antigen (HLA)-E complexed with HLA class I signal sequence-derived peptides by CD94/NKG2 confers protection from natural killer cell-mediated lysis. J Exp Med. 1998;187:813–8.
25. Posch PE, Borrego F, Brooks AG, Coligan JE. HLA-E is the ligand for the natural killer cell CD94/NKG2 receptors. J Biomed Sci. 1998;5:321–31.
26. Braud VM, McMichael AJ. Regulation of NK cell functions through interaction of the CD94/NKG2 receptors with the nonclassical class I molecule HLA-E. Curr Top Microbiol Immunol. 1999;244:85–95.
27. Oosterlynck DJ, Cornillie FJ, Waer M, Vandeputte M, Koninckx PR. Women with endometriosis show a defect in natural killer activity resulting in a decreased cytotoxicity to autologous endometrium. Fertil Steril. 1991;56:45–51.
28. Oosterlynck DJ, Meuleman C, Waer M, Vandeputte M, Koninckx PR. The natural killer activity of peritoneal fluid lymphocytes is decreased in women with endometriosis. Fertil Steril. 1992;58:290–5.
29. Sampson JA. Peritoneal endometriosis due to menstrual dissemination of endometrial tissue into peritoneal cavity. Am J Obstet Gynecol. 1927;14:422–5.
30. Semer D, Reisler K, MacDonald PC, Casey ML. Responsiveness of human endometrial stromal cells to cytokines. Ann N Y Acad Sci. 1991;622:99–102.
31. Gilmore SM, Aksel S, Hoff C, Peterson RD. In vitro lymphocyte activity in women with endometriosis-an altered immune response? Fertil Steril. 1992;58:1148–52.
32. Garzetti GG, Ciavattini A, Provinciali M, Fabris N, Cignitti M, Romanini C. Natural killer cell activity in endometriosis: correlation between serum estradiol levels and cytotoxicity. Obstet Gynecol. 1993;81:665–8.
33. Wilson TJ, Hertzog PJ, Angus D, Munnery L, Wood EC, Kola I. Decreased natural killer cell activity in endometriosis patients: relationship to disease pathogenesis. Fertil Steril. 1994;62:1086–8.
34. Oosterlynck DJ, Meuleman C, Waer M, Koninckx PR. CO2-laser excision of endometriosis does not improve the decreased natural killer activity. Acta Obstet Gynecol Scand. 1994;73:333–7.
35. van der Linden PJ, de Goeij AF, Dunselman GA, van der Linden EP, Ramaekers FC, Evers JL. Expression of integrins and E-cadherin in cells from menstrual effluent, endometrium, peritoneal fluid, peritoneum, and endometriosis. Fertil Steril. 1994;61:85–90.
36. Dmowski WP, Gebel H, Braun DP. Decreased apoptosis and sensitivity to macrophage mediated cytolysis of endometrial cells in endometriosis. Hum Reprod Update. 1998;4:696–701.
37. Gebel HM, Braun DP, Tambur A, Frame D, Rana N, Dmowski WP. Spontaneous apoptosis of endometrial tissue is impaired in women with endometriosis. Fertil Steril. 1998;69:1042–7.
38. Meresman GF, Vighi S, Buquet RA, Contreras-Ortiz O, Tesone M, Rumi LS. Apoptosis and expression of Bcl-2 and Bax in eutopic endometrium from women with endometriosis. Fertil Steril. 2000;74:760–6.
39. Maeda N, Izumiya C, Yamamoto Y, Oguri H, Kusume T, Fukaya T. Increased killer inhibitory receptor KIR2DL1 expression among natural killer cells in women with pelvic endometriosis. Fertil Steril. 2002;77:297–302.
40. Maeda N, Izumiya C, Kusum T, Masumoto T, Yamashita C, Yamamoto Y, Oguri H, Fukaya T. Killer inhibitory receptor CD158a overexpression among natural killer cells in women with endometriosis is undiminished by laparoscopic surgery and gonadotropin releasing hormone agonist treatment. Am J Reprod Immunol. 2004;51:364–72.
41. Matsuoka S, Maeda N, Izumiya C, Yamashita C, Nishimori Y, Fukaya T. Expression of inhibitory-motif killer immunoglobulin-like receptor, KIR2DL1, is increased in natural killer cells from women with pelvic endometriosis. Am J Reprod Immunol. 2005;53:249–54.
42. Lanier LL, Corliss BC, Wu J, Leong C, Phillips JH. Immunoreceptor DAP12 bearing a tyrosine-based activation motif is involved in activating NK cells. Nature. 1998;391:703–7.

43. Bruhns P, Marchetti P, Fridman WH, Vivier E, Daëron M. Differential roles of N- and C-terminal immunoreceptor tyrosine-based inhibition motifs during inhibition of cell activation by killer cell inhibitory receptors. J Immunol. 1999;162:3168–75.
44. Yusa S, Catina TL, Campbell KS. SHP-1- and phosphotyrosine-independent inhibitory signaling by a killer cell Ig-like receptor cytoplasmic domain in human NK cells. J Immunol. 2002;168:5047–57.
45. López-Botet M, Bellón T, Llano M, Navarro F, García P, de Miguel M. Paired inhibitory and triggering NK cell receptors for HLA class I molecules. Hum Immunol. 2000;61:7–17.
46. Borrego F, Kabat J, Kim DK, Lieto L, Maasho K, Peña J, Solana R, Coligan JE. Structure and function of major histocompatibility complex (MHC) class I specific receptors expressed on human natural killer (NK) cells. Mol Immunol. 2002;38:637–60.
47. Kawashima M, Maeda N, Adachi Y, Takeuchi T, Yamamoto Y, Izumiya C, Hayashi K, Furihata M, Udaka K, Fukaya T. Human leukocyte antigen-G, a ligand for the natural killer receptor KIR2DL4, is expressed by eutopic endometrium only in the menstrual phase. Fertil Steril. 2009;91:343–9.
48. Galandrini R, Porpora MG, Stoppacciaro A, Micucci F, Capuano C, Tassi I, Di Felice A. Increased frequency of human leukocyte antigen-E inhibitory receptor. Fertil Steril. 2008;89:1490–6.
49. Shiroishi M, Tsumoto K, Amano K, Shirakihara Y, Colonna M, Braud VM, Allan DS, Makadzange A, Rowland-Jones S, Willcox B, Jones EY, van der Merwe PA, Kumagai I, Maenaka K. Human inhibitory receptors Ig-like transcript 2 (ILT2) and ILT4 compete with CD8 for MHC class I binding and bind preferentially to HLA-G. Proc Natl Acad Sci U S A. 2003;100:8856–61.
50. O'Callaghan CA, Bell JI. Structure and function of the human MHC class Ib molecules HLA-E, HLA-F and HLA-G. Immunol Rev. 1998;163:129–38.
51. Clements CS, Kjer-Nielsen L, McCluskey J, Rossjohn J. Structural studies on HLA-G: implications for ligand and receptor binding. Hum Immunol. 2007;68:220–6.
52. Vernet-Tomás Mdel M, Pérez-Ares CT, Verdú N, Molinero JL, Fernández-Figueras MT, Carreras R. The endometria of patients with endometriosis show higher expression of class I human leukocyte antigen than the endometria of healthy women. Fertil Steril. 2006;85:78–83.
53. Rodgers JR, Cook RG. MHC class Ib molecules bridge innate and acquired immunity. Nat Rev Immunol. 2005;5:459–71.
54. Valés-Gómez M, Reyburn HT, Erskine RA, López-Botet M, Strominger JL. Kinetics and peptide dependency of the binding of the inhibitory NK receptor CD94/NKG2-A and the activating receptor CD94/NKG2-C to HLA-E. EMBO J. 1999;18:4250–60.
55. LeMaoult J, Zafaranloo K, Le Danff C, Carosella ED. HLA-G up-regulates ILT2, ILT3, ILT4, and KIR2DL4 in antigen presenting cells, NK cells, and T cells. FASEB J. 2005;19:662–4.
56. Hornung D, Fujii E, Lim KH, Vigne JL, McMaster MT, Taylor RN. Histocompatibility leukocyte antigen-G is not expressed by endometriosis or endometrial tissue. Fertil Steril. 2001;75:814–7.
57. Barrier BF, Kendall BS, Ryan CE, Sharpe-Timms KL. HLA-G is expressed by the glandular epithelium of peritoneal endometriosis but not in eutopic endometrium. Hum Reprod. 2006;21:864–9.
58. Ibrahim EC, Morange M, Dausset J, Carosella ED, Paul P. Heat shock and arsenite induce expression of the nonclassical class I histocompatibility HLA-G gene in tumor cell lines. Cell Stress Chaperones. 2000;5:207–18.
59. Joseph LM. A healthy menstrual cycle. Clin Nutr Ins. 1997;5:1–7.

Chapter 6
Macrophages in Pathophysiology of Endometriosis

S.F. Ahmad*, N. Michaud*, H. Rakhila*, and A. Akoum

Abstract The mechanisms that sustain endometrial tissues at ectopic sites in patients with endometriosis are poorly understood. It is well established now that endometriosis is associated with changes in population and functions of various leukocytes, including macrophages. Macrophages are the most abundant cells found in the peritoneal fluid and are the consistent feature of endometriotic lesion. They infiltrate endometriotic lesions where they undergo alternative activation as a consequence of signals generated within the invaded tissue. However, instead of clearing endometrial cells from the peritoneal cavity and restoring local homeostasis, macrophages appear to enhance their survival and proliferation by secreting growth, remodelling and inflammatory factors which could contribute to the development of endometriosis as well as to the disease-associated chronic pelvic inflammation and symptoms. Thus, unveiling the molecular mechanisms that underlie macrophage dysfunctions is a critical area of research, which would lead to the development of novel medical treatments for endometriosis. In this chapter, we described how macrophages can play a critical role in the pathophysiology of endometriosis not only via their weakened phagocytic functions but also via other major mechanisms revealed to date.

Keywords Cytokines • Endometriosis • In vivo model • Infertility • Macrophages • Pain • Prostaglandins

*Author contributed equally with all other contributors.

S.F. Ahmad • N. Michaud • H. Rakhila • A. Akoum (✉)
Faculté de Medicine, Endocrinologie de la Reproduction, CHU de Québec, HSFA, Université Laval, Québec, QC, Canada G1L 3L5
e-mail: ali.akoum@crsfa.ulaval.ca

T. Harada (ed.), *Endometriosis: Pathogenesis and Treatment*,
DOI 10.1007/978-4-431-54421-0_6,

Abbreviations

CD	Cluster of differentiation
Cox-2	Cyclooxygenase-2
DCs	Dendritic cells
E2	Oestrogen
FGF	Fibroblast growth factor
ICAM-1	Intercellular adhesion molecule-1
IL	Interleukin
IFN-γ	Interferon gamma
ISO-1	((S,R) 3-(4-hydroxyphenyl)-4,5-dihydro-5-isoxazole acetic methyl ester
LFA-1	Leukocyte function antigen-1
LPS	Lipopolysaccharide
MAPK	Mitogen-activated protein kinase
MCP-1	Monocyte chemotactic protein-1
MIF	Macrophage migration inhibitory factor
MMPs	Matrix metalloproteinases
NF-κB	Nuclear factor kappa B
NGF	Nerve growth factor
NK	Natural killer
PGE2	Prostaglandin-E2
PGF2α	Prostaglandin-F2α
PGs	Prostaglandins
PlGF	Placental growth factor
RANTES	Regulated on activation, normal T cell expressed and secreted
StAR	Steroidogenic acute regulatory protein
TGF	Tumour growth factor
TIMPs	Tissue inhibitors of MMPs
TNF-α	Tumour necrosis factor-alpha
uNK	Uterine natural killer
VEGF	Vascular endothelial growth factor

6.1 Introduction

Endometriosis is associated with changes in the components of the immune system as the peritoneal fluid of women with endometriosis contains increased numbers of immune cells. Dysfunction of the immune system may play an important role in the development of endometriosis since in normal women, menstrual tissue is refluxed into the peritoneal cavity, but it is cleared by immune cells such as macrophages, uterine natural killer (uNK) cells and lymphocytes. However, in women with endometriosis, these subsets of immune cells have been found to be altered in the

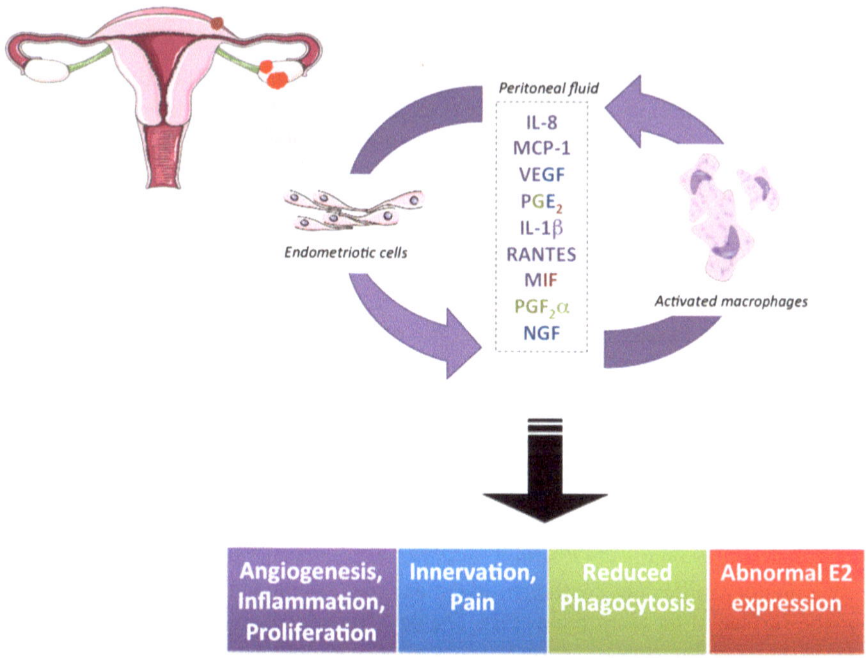

Fig. 6.1 Macrophage in endometriosis: proposed model of positive feedback loops

peritoneal fluid [1]. Macrophages are the most abundant nucleated immune cells found in the peritoneal fluid [2], and their role in endometriosis has been studied for more than three decades. Haney et al. first reported an increase in the number of peritoneal macrophages in women with endometriosis [3]. Several studies confirmed this observation and further reported an increased activation of these cells in women with endometriosis [4–7]. However, activated peritoneal macrophages in women with endometriosis seem to have a reduced capacity to eliminate misplaced endometrial cells. Paradoxically, they rather seem to facilitate endometrial cell survival, invasiveness and growth by secreting growth, angiogenic and tissue remodelling factors and thereby contribute to the development of endometriosis. Interestingly, it was reported that even peripheral blood monocytes enhance eutopic endometrial cell proliferation in women with endometriosis but suppress endometrial cell proliferation in healthy women [8]. Puzzling at first, this phenomenon is being progressively elucidated. It is thus likely that a combination of defects either in macrophages or in the inherent capability of endometrial cells themselves to resist immune suppression and apoptosis in the peritoneal environment is involved. We also believe that activating positive feedback loops and a mutual crosstalk occur within the pelvic cavity of women with endometriosis (where the disease is frequently found) between local immune cells, particularly macrophages, and misplaced or implanted endometriotic cells, which lead to the establishment of a chronic inflammatory process and a local environment that favours ectopic tissue growth (Fig. 6.1).

This chapter provides an overview of the current state of knowledge on macrophages in endometriosis, the functional impairment of these key immune cells and their possible role in the pathophysiology of this disease.

6.2 Physiology of Macrophages

Macrophages are mononuclear phagocytic cells derived from blood monocytes [9]. Monocytes originate from haematopoietic stem cells present in bone marrow, which undergo differentiation. They represent immune effector cells, equipped with chemokine receptors and pathogen recognition receptors that mediate migration from blood to tissues during infection. Extravasation of monocytes from blood to tissue initiates maturation processes leading to mature macrophages or dendritic cells (DCs) [10]. After migration to peripheral tissue, activated monocytes differentiate to inflammatory DCs and macrophages, which are determined by the inflammatory milieu, and pathogen-associated pattern recognition receptors present on the surface of these immune cells. The developmental origin and the function of tissue macrophage subsets, such as microglia (macrophages in the central nervous system), dermal macrophages and splenic marginal zone and metallophilic macrophages, remain insufficiently understood [11]. Resident macrophages in lymphoid and non-lymphoid tissues are the phagocytic cells involved in steady-state tissue homeostasis, and they undergo local activation in response to various inflammatory and immune stimuli. These macrophages are classified as being "elicited", as in the antigen-non-specific response to a foreign body or a sterile inflammatory agent or as being "classically activated" or "alternatively activated" by an antigen-specific immune response. It is difficult to distinguish originally resident macrophages from more recently recruited, elicited or activated macrophages, because cells adapt to a particular microenvironment [12].

6.2.1 Types and Functions

Macrophages are the professional phagocytes expressing numerous membrane adhesion molecules including scavenger receptors such as the cluster of differentiation 36 (CD-36) receptors ensuring targets fixation and endocytosis [9, 13]. Based on membrane-expressed molecules and secretion, macrophages are commonly classified as M1 or M2 phenotype. M1-macrophages are the pro-inflammatory macrophages expressing and secreting cytokines and antimicrobial molecules such as interleukin-1 (IL-1). M2-macrophages are the anti-inflammatory macrophages secreting a majority of growth factors and anti-inflammatory cytokines [14]. It is important to mention that macrophages are dynamic and flexible cells that can change from a phenotype to another depending on their microenvironments [15]. It is a matter of fact that interferon-γ (IFN-γ) and lipopolysaccharide (LPS) generate M1-macrophages, whereas IL-4 and IL-13 activate M2-macrophages [16]. Furthermore, a pallet of phenotype exists between the common M1-macrophages and M2-macrophages activation such as decidual macrophages present in endometrium, which are hybrid M1–M2 phenotype [10, 17, 18]. Scientists finally conclude that the subtle composition of macrophage environment determines their expression profile and thus their role [10].

6.2.2 Macrophages Along the Menstrual Cycle

Macrophages are ubiquitously present as resident cells monitoring tissue environment and ready to react to any discrete change [15]. Actually, oestrogen (E2) has been discovered as a regulator of M2-phenotype and is responsible for decidual macrophages efficiency especially in pregnancy [19]. Indeed, resident macrophages in endometrium are differentially expressed along the menstrual cycle. During proliferative phase, macrophages represent only 1–2 % of all cells and express tumour growth factor (TGF), IL-10, metalloproteinases (MMPs) and tissue inhibitors of MMPs (TIMPs) contributing to endometrial regeneration, enhancing extracellular matrix turnover and fibroblasts recruitment and proliferation [20, 21]. When progesterone level rises, macrophages represent 3–5 % of cells probably due to resident macrophages' proliferation. They express numerous chemoattractant molecules such as macrophage chemotactic protein (MCP)-1, regulated on activation, normal T cell expressed and secreted (RANTES) and IL-8 to allow immune cells infiltration into endometrium where they will prepare for the eventual feto-implantation. Finally, progesterone withdrawal, marking menstrual phase, is characterised by an increase in number of macrophages due to chemoattracted monocyte extravasation [20]. These M1-like macrophages secrete MMP-9, tumour necrosis factor-alpha (TNF)-α and many other pro-inflammatory cytokines and proteolytic enzymes, leading to tissue breakdown and menstruation [21].

In the peritoneal fluid, macrophages are the most abundant cell type. Normally, the peritoneal fluid contains $0.5–20 \times 10^6$ leukocytes/ml, of which 85 % are macrophages [2]. In the absence of pathogens, peritoneal fluid macrophages are present at low level and contribute to tissue homeostasis [22]. Their concentration appears to fluctuate during the menstrual cycle and is maximal during the menses [23]. This is most likely related to the menstrual reflux phenomenon, which is common in almost 90 % of reproductive age women during menstruation. Briefly, a small part of endometrial debris travels through fallopian tubes to the peritoneal compartment instead of being evacuated in vaginal secretions [24, 25], where they are normally phagocytised by peritoneal macrophages [26].

Concisely, macrophages are the phagocytes implicated in an intimate crosstalk between endometrial tissue and the local immune system. Any perturbation in their close environment or intrinsic modifications could trigger profound imbalance in these interactions.

6.3 Pathophysiology of Macrophages in Endometriosis: A Weakened Immune System May Lead to Endometriosis

The discovery that macrophages play a major role in the pathophysiology of endometriosis dates back to 1981 when Dmowski and his group first reported the existence of a deficient cellular immunity in women with endometriosis and a number of functional changes in several immunologic components of the peritoneal fluid [1]. In the same year 1981, other investigators revealed that the number of peritoneal macrophages is increased in infertile women with endometriosis compared with normal women or women with other causes of infertility [3], and an increased phagocytosis of spermatozoa by peritoneal macrophages in patients with endometriosis was then shown [27]. Later on, it was found that endometriosis is associated with an increased influx of macrophages that undergo further maturation and activation and release active substances such as prostaglandins (PGs), which can have adverse effects on the fertility [5, 28]. Data from other studies confirmed these findings and further suggested that peritoneal macrophages in women with endometriosis are in an advanced level of differentiation, which may interfere with gametes and pre-implantation embryos and contribute to endometriosis-associated subfertility [4]. By the end of 1980s, it was well established that concentration, activation and abnormal maturation of peritoneal macrophages may facilitate the onset of endometriosis. A wide array of factors produced by activated macrophages appear to be involved in endometrial cell survival, adhesion, invasion, proliferation and the formation of endometriotic lesions. A key role for macrophages in decreased immunologic surveillance, recognition and destruction of misplaced endometrial cells and possible facilitation of ectopic endometrial tissue growth seems well plausible.

Many aspects of macrophage involvement in endometriosis-related symptoms have also drawn a considerable interest, but the mechanisms by which activated macrophages cause infertility, menstrual disorders and pelvic pain in women with endometriosis remain unclear.

6.3.1 Suppression of Phagocytosis and Apoptosis by Macrophages

Braun et al. have observed a reduction in the number of macrophages in the eutopic endometrium of women with endometriosis [8]. Their results were surprising because an increase in macrophages' number in the peritoneal cavity of these women was well documented [6, 29]. Such a phenomenon would reflect altered chemokine gradients that favour macrophage mobilisation to the ectopic environment due to the presence of cyclical, inflammatory stimuli within that environment. Intrinsic resistance to apoptosis, in conjunction with a physiologic disturbance in macrophage trafficking in the eutopic endometrial environment, would be expected to favour the survival of endometrial cells and lead to their establishment in the ectopic sites. Another study has shown a decrease in the capacity of macrophage-mediated cytolysis of misplaced endometrial cells in the peritoneal locations and an increased resistance of these cells to apoptosis [30].

Taken together, the evidences available to date suggest that defective cytolytic function in macrophages within the peritoneal cavity coupled with the inherent resistance of the endometrial cells to programmed cell death may be fundamental to the pathophysiology of endometriosis.

It is relevant to mention that in women with endometriosis, the ectopic endometrial tissue also seems to escape immune surveillance in the peritoneal cavity. On one hand, several studies have shown that peritoneal macrophages phagocytise and degrade spermatozoids and that peritoneal macrophages isolated from these women have a greater phagocytic ability than those from fertile or infertile women without endometriosis [27, 31]. These results suggest that, if peritoneal macrophages from women with endometriosis enter the reproductive tract via the oviducts, they might adversely influence fertilisation by phagocytising sperm cells [32]. On the other hand, other studies have shown a decreased phagocytic activity against endometrial cells [33, 34]. Thus, instead of eliminating endometrial debris following retrograde menstruation, peritoneal macrophages of patients with endometriosis would favour the development of endometriotic lesions because of the absence of adequate phagocytosis and the large amounts of cytokines and other growth factors released into the peritoneal cavity [35]. It has been suggested that endometrial cells of women with endometriosis contribute to their own survival and escape of immune suppression by secreting various molecules that are capable of interfering with the process of recognition of immune cells [34]. An example of such a phenomenon is the expression of the soluble form of intercellular adhesion molecule (ICAM)-l. ICAM-1 is a co-receptor that interacts with the integrin leukocyte function antigen (LFA)-l present on the surface of leukocytes in order to participate in cell recognition. It has been demonstrated that eutopic endometrial stromal cells of women with endometriosis express a higher concentration of the ICAM-1 soluble form than those of healthy women. In addition, the expression of this form is even higher in ectopic endometrium. Thus, it is possible that the soluble form of ICAM-1 competes with its cellular form to bind to LFA-1, which will disrupt recognition by leukocytes target cells [36].

In most circumstances, macrophages secrete MMP-9 to destroy the extracellular matrix to disperse endometrial tissues into small pieces [37]. In addition, CD-36 receptor is highly expressed on the cell membrane of macrophages to facilitate phagocytosis of these small fragments of endometrial debris. However, in the presence of high concentration of prostaglandin E2 (PGE2), the expression of

MMP-9 and CD-36 is suppressed [38, 39]. This significantly inhibits the phagocytic ability of macrophages and may favour abnormal endometrial tissue growth into the ectopic host sites.

It is worth mentioning here that an apparent inconsistency seems to emerge considering the ability of macrophages to phagocytise sperm cells and their inability to eliminate ectopic endometrial cells. While it is possible that such a difference is at least partly due to inherent properties of endometrial cells of women with endometriosis, the underlying mechanisms remain to be clarified, given their likely impact on the pathogenesis of the disease and the symptoms it causes.

6.3.2 Macrophage Secretions in Endometriosis

Elevated concentrations of cytokines, growth and pro-inflammatory and angiogenic factors have been found in the peritoneal fluid of women with endometriosis. These different factors can originate from a wide variety of sources including endometriotic lesions themselves, macrophages, T cells and follicular fluid after ovulation [40]. IL-1β, IL-8, macrophage migration inhibitory factor (MIF), MCP-1, PGE2 and prostaglandin F2α (PGF2α) are among the main cytokines and eicosanoids that are present at high levels in the peritoneal fluid of women with endometriosis [34, 40–44] and known to be overproduced by activated macrophages. Our previous studies have for the first time detected the existence of endometrial dysfunctions in patients with endometriosis. Thus, endometrial cells are more sensitive to activation by IL-1β, a cytokine that is mainly released by activated monocytes/macrophages and found at high concentrations in the peritoneal fluid of patients with endometriosis [45]. IL-1β, also known as catabolin, can enhance the development of endometriosis by causing the release of factors for blood vessel growth. Other data suggest that IL-1β can also be involved in the up-regulation of MIF expression by ectopic endometrial implants [46].

IL-8, known as an α-chemokine that shows chemotactic activity and acts as a potent angiogenic agent [47], is believed to play a significant role in endometrial physiology and endometriosis. Mainly produced by peripheral macrophages as well [48], IL-8 was detected at higher concentration in the peritoneal fluid of women with endometriosis. In addition to its chemotactic and activating properties for granulocytes, IL-8 was recently found to stimulate proliferation of endometrial cells [49].

MCP-1 is a P-chemokine having a potent chemotactic activity for monocytes, macrophages and lymphocytes [50] and produced by different cell types. In endometriosis, however, MCP-1 was found to be over-expressed in eutopic and ectopic endometrial cells as well as in peritoneal fluid macrophages of women with endometriosis [51, 52], and its peritoneal concentrations appeared to correlate with the stage of the disease [53, 54]. This factor may play a role in the development of endometriotic lesions not only by recruiting and stimulating peritoneal macrophages but also by directly stimulating endometrial cell proliferation [54] and angiogenesis [55, 56]. MCP-1 has potent direct angiogenic effects on endothelial cells [57] and may act indirectly via its ability to stimulate macrophage recruitment and activation and the release of angiogenic factors [52, 58, 59].

RANTES, one of the members of C–C chemokine family that mediate monocyte chemotactic activity, was found to be elevated in peritoneal fluid of women with endometriosis [60]. RANTES peritoneal fluid levels also correlate with advanced endometriosis stage, suggesting that it might contribute to the progression of this disease [60]. Interestingly, our and other studies showed that macrophage-/monocyte-derived pro-inflammatory cytokines such as IL-1β trigger endometriotic cells to produce this monocyte chemoattractant chemokine [61, 62] and point thereby to feedforward amplification loops underlying chronic pelvic inflammation in women with endometriosis.

MIF, originally identified as a protein factor secreted by T cells, inhibits the migration of macrophages in vitro (hence its name: macrophage migration inhibitory factor) [63, 64]. MIF is actually expressed by most immune cells such as monocytes, macrophages or B cells. It has been shown that MIF plays an important role in the cell-mediated immune response by promoting the Th1 response by the production of IL-12 by macrophages [65, 66]. MIF is able to inhibit the immunosuppressive effects of glucocorticoids on the production of pro-inflammatory cytokines such as IL-1β in activated macrophages [66–69]. To illustrate this property, it has been described that MIF induces the expression of cytoplasmic phospholipase A2 which is an important component of the pro-inflammatory cascade and usually blocked by the action of glucocorticoids [70]. Our studies showed that MIF is overproduced by activated peritoneal macrophages in women with endometriosis [52] and further found abundant levels of this factor in peritoneal fluid [43], peripheral blood [44] and eutopic endometrial tissue of endometriosis patients [71]. Furthermore, MIF levels varied according to endometriosis stage and were particularly elevated in women suffering from endometriosis but also complaining from pelvic pain and/or infertility. This, together with the increased peritoneal fluid levels of MIF, was corroborated by other investigators [72, 73]. Our subsequent studies showed that MIF expression is also elevated in the early stage and highly vascularised endometriotic lesions [43] and appeared to act at multiple coordinated levels in the PG biosynthesis cascade, thereby inducing cyclooxygenase-2 (Cox-2) expression in these cells and stimulating PGE2 [74]. From a cellular mechanism point of view, our work suggests the involvement of the transcription factor nuclear factor kappa B (NF-κB) in MIF gene activation in ectopic endometrial cells in response to IL-1β [75]. In addition, our group revealed for the first time the presence of a positive feedback loop by which E2 acts directly on ectopic endometrial cells to up-regulate the expression of MIF, which, in turn, displays the capability of inducing the expression of aromatase, the key and rate-limiting enzyme for E2 synthesis [76]. Our studies also revealed that MIF exerts a potent indirect angiogenic effect by interacting with ectopic endometrial cells and inducing the secretion of major angiogenic factors via CD-44 and CD-74 and mitogen-activated protein kinase (MAPK) signalling pathways [77] and provide evidence for a possible new mechanism underlying endometriosis development and pathophysiology. Angiogenesis or the formation of new blood vessels is essential for the development and the maintenance of endometriotic lesions. Vascular endothelial growth factor (VEGF), one of the major angiogenic factors endowed with the capability of stimulating mitogenesis, migration and differentiation of endothelial cells, is strongly expressed in endometriotic tissue as well as in peritoneal macrophages [78, 79]. Peritoneal-activated macrophages are the major source of VEGF in endometriosis and that this expression is regulated directly by ovarian steroids [80]. Ovarian steroids regulate the production of this growth factor through peritoneal macrophages. E2 acts on various macrophage signalling pathways, influencing in particular those related to sustain the recruitment of inflammatory cells and the remodelling of inflamed tissues, such as MAPK, phosphatidylinositide-3-kinase/protein kinase B and NF-κB. As a consequence, a deregulated response to steroids might influence the survival of ectopic endometrial cells and promote the vascularisation of the lesions [81–85]. It is quite established that hypoxia induces the expression of VEGF [81, 86, 87]. The effects of hypoxia are mainly mediated by hypoxia-inducible factor-1 (HIF-1) protein complex, which is composed of two subunits, HIF-lα, the inducible unit, and HIF-1β, the constitutive unit [88]. In endometriotic tissue, abnormally high levels of complex HIF-lα were found [89], which makes clear that hypoxia is involved in VEGF production in endometriotic lesions and presumably by peritoneal macrophages.

It is of note that peritoneal macrophages strongly express Cox-2 [90], one of the rate-limiting enzyme for PGs secretion. As described in several reports [26, 84, 91, 92], PGE2 and PGF2α themselves induce the over-expression of Cox-2 in macrophages and endometriotic stromal cells, leading to an elevated concentration of their own levels in the peritoneal fluid. On one hand, high levels of PGs act on macrophages to suppress their phagocytic ability by down-regulating MMP-9 and CD-36 [37, 39]. On the other hand, PGs stimulate the steroidogenic capacity of endometriotic stromal cells by up-regulating steroidogenic acute regulatory protein (StAR) and aromatase [93], which induces aberrant biosynthesis of E2. E2 further stimulates the production of mitogens such as fibroblast growth factor-9 (FGF-9), which induces endometriotic cell proliferation [94, 95]. PGE2 can also induce FGF-9 expression by PGE2 receptor 3-dependent transcriptional up-regulation [96, 97]. Other main functions of PGs include the induction of the expression of angiogenic factors such as VEGF and FGF-2 to induce angiogenesis [98, 99]. These effects may play an important role in the survival and proliferation of endometriotic cells. Furthermore, elevated PGs concentrations in endometriosis women is suspected to be involved in pelvic pain and infertility, though more studies will be required to further elucidate the underlying mechanisms [90, 100, 101].

Obviously, macrophages have a rather heterogeneous array of characteristics and dramatically modify their environment not only via the production of cytokines and other pro-inflammatory factors but also via reactive oxygen species (ROS) [102–104]. Production of ROS is known to increase after activation of immune cells, especially macrophages [105] and their production was reported to be increased in serum and peritoneal fluid of patients with endometriosis. In addition, markers of oxidative stress have been found elevated [102–104]. ROS role, as a second messenger of cellular proliferation, has been described. McCubrey et al. found that normal cell proliferation correlated with production of endogenous ROS through the activation of growth-related signalling pathways [106]. Endometriosis is considered a benign disease but shares some features with cancer, such as propensity to invasion, unrestrained growth, neo-angiogenesis, and distant spreading [19, 107]. The known correlation between ROS and proliferation of cancer cells, along with the increased production of ROS in response to chronic inflammation in endometriosis, thus suggests a possible role for ROS in the regulation of endometriotic cell proliferation.

6.4 Deleterious Effects Induced by Macrophages in Endometriosis

The available literature argues in favour of a significant role for macrophages in the growth and development of endometriotic lesions, the generation of pain through interaction with nerve fibres and infertility via the impediment of spermatozoids and/or oocyte functions and endometrial receptivity. It is obvious that little evidence is available as to the existence of a direct cause and effect relationship between endometriosis-associated macrophage dysfunctions and pain or infertility. However, chronic pelvic inflammation in women with endometriosis and many inflammatory and embryotoxic factors involved, abnormally expressed and known for being secreted by activated endometrial and peritoneal macrophages let, in an indirect way, believe in such a role.

6.4.1 Macrophages in Pain Related to Endometriosis

The pathophysiology of pelvic pain associated with endometriosis and macrophages is unclear, especially that there is no correlation between the existence of pain and the extent of damage. Main inflammatory factors, such as PGs (e.g. PGE2 and PGF2α) or cytokines (e.g. MIF), released by macrophages can also irritate tissues, stimulate nerve fibres and cause severe, painful reaction even when very small areas are involved. The eutopic endometrium of women with endometriosis has higher rates of MIF than the eutopic endometrium of normal women; this is correlated with the degree of advancement of the disease. In addition, this increase of the MIF expression is even more obvious in patients with pelvic pain [71]. It is interesting to note that MIF concentration varies during the menstrual cycle. This variation of expression suggests that MIF would be dependent of ovarian hormones [108]. Recent studies have also shown that MIF stimulates Cox-2 expression and PGE2 production in the ectopic endometrial cells [74] leading to chronic inflammation.

The density of nerve fibres in peritoneal endometriotic lesions is much higher than in normal peritoneum. Many inflammatory substances can potentially stimulate the nerve endings of these fibres. Recent studies have demonstrated that VEGF can also act as potent neurotrophic factor in addition to its effects on vessels [109, 110]. But the most important growth factor that plays a role in facilitating development, growth and repair of nerve fibre is the nerve growth factor (NGF). An elevated concentration of PGE2 is thought to stimulate production of NGF [111] which is released from macrophages, as well as endometriotic lesions, and induces smooth muscle metaplasia and innervations. Subsequently, the contraction of smooth muscle cells and hyperalgia of sensory nerve cells, derived from innervations in interstitial lesions, induce endometriotic pain [112].

PGE2 and PGF2α play an important role in inflammation by increasing the vascular permeability, cause of oedema, by generating a fever or by regulating blood flow and are also involved in the sensation of pain [113, 114]. Over their nociceptive properties, PGs seem to be involved in pelvic pain often present in women with endometriosis. Cyclooxygenase inhibitors, such as nonsteroidal anti-inflammatory drugs, are frequently used in the treatment of mild endometriosis and can significantly reduce pain in these patients [90]. The inhibition of certain macrophage activities may have a benefit in the future relief of endometriosis-related pain [22].

In conclusion, several relevant studies provide a plausible link between peritoneal inflammation, increased macrophage number and the development of new nerve fibres throughout the peritoneal cavity, which may be associated with the generation of the pelvic pain sensations in women with endometriosis.

6.4.2 Macrophages in Infertility Related to Endometriosis

It is now well known that macrophages are located into decidua (endometrium of the pregnant uterus) during the implantation window and implicated in the physiological processes of implantation, establishment and maintenance of pregnancy and labour control. Indeed, decidual macrophages (20–25 %) and uNK cells are predominant decidual leukocytes [115, 116]. While other uterine leukocytes are diminished during pregnancy, macrophages proportion remains unchanged. During implantation, macrophages cooperate with developing embryo to insure trophoblast endovascular invasion and anchorage. At this site, only M2-macrophages are found infiltrated into endometrial basalis where they will secrete MMP-7 and MMP-9 degrading extracellular matrix to facilitate trophoblast invasion into myometrium [117]. Moreover, M2-macrophages are able to produce VEGF and placental growth factor (PlGF) implicated in the profound remodelling of uterine vasculature during embryonic growth. Furthermore, those phagocytes participate in maternal cell apoptosis and trophoblast renewal. In fact, maternal decidua cell apoptosis insures trophoblast invasion to remodelling and development of embryo. It is important to notice that phagocytosis of apoptotic bodies are vital to avoid secondary necrosis and so a harmful inflammatory response generating tissue damage [118, 119]. Even more, macrophages are fundamental actors of maternal immune tolerance in pregnancy. Indeed, these immune cells are not only able to secrete molecules such as IL-10, known to inhibit T cell activation, but are also to diminish expression of co-stimulatory molecules (CD-80 and CD-86) and indoleamine 2,3-dioxygenase [116]. They create a microenvironment capable of containing immune response to hemi-allogeneic fetal cells even during infection [120]. Interestingly, macrophages secrete IL-15, an uNK cell chemoattractant, and down-regulate uNK cell cytotoxic capacity [121]. uNK cells are crucial for implantation knowing that they are responsible for trophoblast chemoattraction and invasion by secreting IL-8 and IFNγ-inducible protein-10 that binds to trophoblasts' membrane receptors [122].

Intriguingly, in endometriosis, the number of M2-macrophages is significantly increased in decidua and peritoneal fluid. As explained in the previous section, macrophages are differentially activated in endometriosis overproducing a myriad of pro-inflammatory factors and key processes are crucial for implantation. Decidual macrophages in endometriosis have been shown to secrete elevated concentrations of angiogenic factors (VEGF, MCP-1, IL-8) and to mediate the development of an anarchic vasculature similar to unstructured tumour vasculature [123, 124]. Such an abnormal angiogenic process might disfavours the functional crosstalk between maternal decidua and trophoblasts, which is essential for embryo survival [125]. Acute and controlled inflammation is necessary for pregnancy, but any chronic inflammation leads to spontaneous abortion [126]. As described previously, women with endometriosis are characterised by an exaggerated inflammation that may contribute to infertility in endometriosis [127]. First, disruption of the phagocytic function in endometriosis may promote accumulation of apoptotic bodies and secondary necrosis responsible for inflammation. Second, the cocktail of inflammatory molecules secreted in endometrium generates an acute inflammation, which is deleterious for trophoblastic implantation. In fact, some relate miscarriage to TNF-α increase and normal pregnancy with high concentrations of IL-10 [128]. Chronic inflammation may inhibit trophoblast invasion and immune tolerance [129]. Macrophage phagocytic function is also an issue since sperm phagocytosis has been described in endometriosis patient. Moreover, an activation of specific sperm engulfment surely prevents or disturbs oocyte fertilisation [32]. It seems that endometrial cells express or secrete molecules able to impair phagocytosis in macrophages, but further investigations could provide interesting insights on this phenomenon. In the meantime, endometriosis is also characterised by an oxidant environment inauspicious for pregnancy [130]. Both endometriotic cells and macrophages are responsible for ROS high concentration in peritoneal fluid of women with endometriosis. More precisely, endometriotic lesions activate inducible nitrogen oxide synthase (iNOS) in macrophages leading to an augmentation of NO production [131]. Moreover, the antioxidant machinery (secreting ascorbic acid, GPx, thiol) is down-regulated creating an imbalance in the redox status of peritoneal environment [132–134]. Interestingly, ROS are known to be related to age-related fertility decline, in vitro fertilisation failure and cigarette smoke subfertility [135–137]. In endometriosis, such redox status may affect sperm viability in peritoneal microenvironment, oocyte and embryo quality [130].

Since macrophages are crucial cells in implantation and pregnancy, it is not surprising that their dysfunctions may be a significant possible cause of infertility in endometriosis.

6.4.3 Endometriosis, Macrophages and Cancer

In recent years, a possible link between endometriosis and certain types of cancer, such as ovarian cancer, has been suggested. It is well established that endometriosis shares a number of features with cancer such as abnormal cell proliferation and invasion, the development of new blood vessels [138, 139], the decrease in the number of cells undergoing apoptosis [140] and its stem cell-like activity [141]. Macrophages are important inflammatory mediators and have been implicated in endometriosis through their role in chronic inflammation. As discussed previously in this chapter, macrophages produce a wide range of cytokines which can also induce the progression of tumorigenesis [78]. IL-1 is a potent mediator of inflammation produced by macrophages and it promotes tumorigenesis by stimulating the production of other cytokines and growth factors. Among these, VEGF has been detected in endometriosis-associated ovarian carcinoma [142]. In addition, it has been proposed that VEGF acts as a growth factor for tumours regardless of its role in angiogenesis as there was no correlation observed between VEGF expression and micro-vessel density in ovarian tumours [139].

Taken together, it seems that macrophages might play a role in the development of cancerous transformation at the site of endometriosis by secreting important mediators which are responsible for tumour progression and development. However, further studies are required to ascertain any possible link between endometriosis and cancer.

6.5 Animal Models to Study the Role of Macrophages in Endometriosis

In order to study endometriosis in vivo, an animal model of the disease is required where endometriosis could be induced experimentally by implanting the human endometrial tissue intra-peritoneally. Since endometriosis occurs spontaneously only in humans and some non-human primates, animal models of induced endometriosis have been developed and are of high value for the evaluation of pathophysiological mechanisms underlying the development of this disease. There are two main groups of animal models for endometriosis: rodents and non-human primates. This section of the chapter will summarise the study of macrophages in the animal models for endometriosis.

6.5.1 *Rodents*

Mice and rats are the two established experimental animal models among the rodents. Since rodents do not shed their endometrial tissue and therefore do not develop endometriosis spontaneously, endometriosis can be induced by transplanting endometrial tissue to ectopic sites. These models are classified into two types, homologous and heterologous models. Homologous models have been employed utilising the surgical transplantation of endometrium of the same or syngeneic animals in immunocompetent animals, whereas in heterologous models, human endometrial fragments are transferred either intra-peritoneally or subcutaneously to immunodeficient mice.

Nude and Knockout Mice. As mentioned, animal models represent a useful tool to study in vivo early steps of this disease. The latter approach relies on the transfer of fragments of endometrial tissue harvested from syngeneic donor mice and recapitulates important aspects of the disease [143]. The first experimentally induced endometriosis in mice was reported in 1984 [144], where normal and ectopic human endometrial tissues were successfully transplanted into the peritoneal cavity of athymic nude mice [144]. This study demonstrated that endometrial tissue keeps intact structure and shows the presence of glands and stroma with an infiltration of macrophages. Since then, several groups have used fluorescent markers such as green fluorescent protein [16] or bioluminescent markers such as luciferase expression system to generate endometriosis mouse models [145]. Recent studies on Tie-2 knockout mice demonstrated that alternatively activated macrophages can infiltrate endometriotic lesions and promote angiogenesis [146, 147]. These data indicate that the recruited macrophages have more than one effect. Also, it has been shown that knockdown of annexin A2 inhibited the phagocytic function of macrophages, whereas treatment with annexin A2 recombinant protein enhanced phagocytosis [148]. In addition, we have successfully used the athymic nude mice model to study the role of MIF in the development of endometriosis [149]. As described previously in this chapter, MIF has been a regulator of immune system that promotes the pro-inflammatory functions of immune cells, and its role in angiogenesis, tumorigenesis and autoimmune diseases is well established [74, 150–154]. We have reported previously that expression of MIF is increased in eutopic endometrial tissue of women with endometriosis, which is related to the stage of endometriosis [71]. Furthermore, our research in agreement with others has shown a significant elevation in circulating and local peritoneal levels of MIF [43, 44]. Taking the advantage of athymic nude mice model of experimentally induced endometriosis, we have developed a treatment model of endometriosis. In this study, we have used the in vivo model of experimentally induced endometriosis and challenge MIF in order to discover a possible target for the treatment of endometriosis. We used (S,R) 3-(4-hydroxyphenyl)-4,5-dihydro-5-isoxazole acetic methyl ester (ISO-1), a specific antagonist of MIF [155] where human endometrial tissue was allowed to implant and grow prior to any treatment. Thus our group is the first to report that macrophage migration inhibitory factor can be a suitable target for the treatment of endometriosis as there is no specific targeted treatment available at present [149].

Rat. Among the rodents, rat is another choice as an experimental model for the endometriosis for the researchers. Matsubavashi et al. reported the first study where rats with auto-transplanted endometrium showed the same immunologic changes as humans with endometriosis [156]. In this study the effect of ectopic endometrial lesions on the changes of leukocyte subpopulation in the rat model of endometriosis was reported. This was supported by another independent research where it was reported that the stromal tissue of uterus-attached peritoneum showed proliferation and infiltration of macrophages in rat endometriosis models [157]. Furthermore, it was discovered that an increase in the number of activated macrophages in the endometriotic lesions has a positive correlation with VEGF [158]. Recently, liposomal bisphosphonate [159] and a selective Cox-2 inhibitor [158] have been used as therapeutic drugs targeting macrophages in a rat experimental endometriosis model. These findings have suggested that macrophage depletion effectively inhibits the initiation and growth of endometriotic implants in a rat endometriosis model, and further studies are required to confirm these findings in order to use this approach as a treatment for endometriosis.

6.5.2 Non-human Primates

In the recent past, researchers have started using rhesus macaque (aka rhesus monkey) as an animal model for endometriosis since spontaneous development of the disease requires menstrual shedding. Endometriosis occurs naturally only in some non-human primate species, making development of lesions more comparable to the establishment of disease in humans. Compared with rodents, the non-human primate model of endometriosis is advantageous due to a close recapitulation of human disease and physiology [160]. In a recent study, it has been shown that the activation status of macrophages in endometriosis in the rhesus monkey is more oriented towards the M2 phenotype, in exactly the same way as humans [161].

Concisely, non-human primates have been extensively used for the investigation of endometriosis, but the very high cost of animal handling limits their use. For this reason, the establishment of rodent models for endometriosis via the intra-peritoneal transplantation of pieces of endometrial tissue has been greatly exploited in the recent years.

6.6 Future Research and Perspectives

Altogether, it is evident that impaired functions of macrophages enable endometriotic tissue proliferation and their secretory products are implicated in the pathophysiology of endometriosis and the major symptoms of the disease such as pain and infertility. Presently, there is an urgent need for new approaches to the medical treatment of endometriosis. Since it is obvious that macrophages are closely associated with endometriosis, future treatment strategies may be based on immunological approaches. Currently, treatments are mostly focused on cytokines and growth factors secreted by macrophages which showed abnormal concentrations in the peritoneal fluid and peripheral blood of endometriosis patients. To regulate angiogenesis, the effect of anti-VEGF antibody has been investigated with an endometriosis mouse model. Bevacizumab, first used for cancer chemotherapy, has been shown to decrease VEGF levels in serum and prevent lesion vascularisation and thus trigger endometriotic cell apoptosis [162]. The most promising molecule is metformin, an anti-inflammatory and aromatase inhibitor known as a biguanide insulin sensitiser. Metformin is able to decrease IL-8, IL-6 and VEGF concentration and improve endometriosis symptoms in women with endometriosis [163]. In the same field, statins seem to prevent MCP-1 expression and to reduce the number and size of endometriotic implants in mice [164]. However, there is no treatment available targeting specifically and directly macrophages. An increased understanding of the immune aspects in endometriosis would be beneficial to set up such novel treatment strategies. Inhibiting MIF might be a promising strategy for future therapies targeting endometriosis, and recent in vivo data from our lab using ISO-1, a potent MIF inhibitor, support this hypothesis [149]. Other approaches to MIF inhibition may include anti-MIF or anti-MIF receptor antibodies. Moreover, macrophages can express and secrete various molecules depending on their activation status. Clearly, in endometriosis, peritoneal macrophages show a different secretory and membrane profile. It would be interesting to target macrophage activation and polarisation in order to control the disease. Actually, some strategies already focus on a modulation of macrophage polarisation. For example, in ovarian cancer administration of INF-γ induces macrophage phenotype modifications promoting tumoricidal activity [165, 166]. Similar treatment strategies applied to endometriosis could open new promising avenues for the management of this disease.

In summary, a growing body of evidence indicates that a combination of endometrial and immune cell dysfunctions plays a major role in the pathogenesis of endometriosis and its major symptoms. Macrophages appear to be critically involved via a wide spectrum of secretory products and functional changes that for the most part remain to be elucidated. A better understanding of the role of macrophages and its intriguing and particular interaction with ectopic endometrial cells is crucial for the development of new medical treatments for this serious disease.

During menstruation, endometrial cells reach the peritoneal cavity as a consequence of retrograde menstruation. These cells resist apoptosis and immune suppression, activate the recruitment of immune cells, particularly macrophages, which have a reduced phagocytic ability, and contribute to angiogenesis, pain innervation, abnormal steroid production and ectopic endometrial cell growth. The reciprocal interactions of misplaced endometrial cells and macrophages create deleterious and activating feedback loops that trigger chronic inflammation and other processes involved in endometriosis pathophysiology.

Acknowledgement This study is supported by CIHR grants MOP 93716, 120769 and 123259 to Pr. Ali Akoum, Chercheur National, FRQ-S.

References

1. Dmowski WP, Steele RW, Baker GF. Deficient cellular immunity in endometriosis. Am J Obstet Gynecol. 1981;141(4):377–83.
2. van Furth R, Raeburn JA, van Zwet TL. Characteristics of human mononuclear phagocytes. Blood. 1979;54(2):485–500.
3. Haney AF, Muscato JJ, Weinberg JB. Peritoneal fluid cell populations in infertility patients. Fertil Steril. 1981;35(6):696–8.
4. Dunselman GA, et al. Functional aspects of peritoneal macrophages in endometriosis of women. J Reprod Fertil. 1988;82(2):707–10.
5. Halme J, et al. Increased activation of pelvic macrophages in infertile women with mild endometriosis. Am J Obstet Gynecol. 1983;145(3):333–7.
6. Olive DL, Weinberg JB, Haney AF. Peritoneal macrophages and infertility: the association between cell number and pelvic pathology. Fertil Steril. 1985;44(6):772–7.
7. Zeller JM, et al. Enhancement of human monocyte and peritoneal macrophage chemiluminescence activities in women with endometriosis. Am J Reprod Immunol Microbiol. 1987;13(3):78–82.
8. Braun DP, et al. Monocyte-mediated enhancement of endometrial cell proliferation in women with endometriosis. Fertil Steril. 1994;61(1):78–84.
9. Mantovani B, Rabinovitch M, Nussenzweig V. Phagocytosis of immune complexes by macrophages. Different roles of the macrophage receptor sites for complement (C3) and for immunoglobulin (IgG). J Exp Med. 1972;135(4):780–92.
10. Melin A, et al. Endometriosis and the risk of cancer with special emphasis on ovarian cancer. Hum Reprod. 2006;21(5):1237–42.
11. Geissmann F, et al. Development of monocytes, macrophages, and dendritic cells. Science. 2010;327(5966):656–61.
12. Gordon S. Alternative activation of macrophages. Nat Rev Immunol. 2003;3(1):23–35.
13. Erwig LP. Macrophages and hypoxia in human chronic kidney disease. Kidney Int. 2008;74(4):405–6.
14. Gordon S, Martinez FO. Alternative activation of macrophages: mechanism and functions. Immunity. 2010;32(5):593–604.
15. Murray PJ, Wynn TA. Protective and pathogenic functions of macrophage subsets. Nat Rev Immunol. 2011;11(11):723–37.
16. Hirata T, et al. Development of an experimental model of endometriosis using mice that ubiquitously express green fluorescent protein. Hum Reprod. 2005;20(8):2092–6.
17. Biswas SK, Mantovani A. Macrophage plasticity and interaction with lymphocyte subsets: cancer as a paradigm. Nat Immunol. 2010;11(10):889–96.

18. Houser BL, et al. Two unique human decidual macrophage populations. J Immunol. 2011;186(4):2633–42.
19. Swiersz LM. Role of endometriosis in cancer and tumor development. Ann N Y Acad Sci. 2002;955:281–92. discussion 293–5; 396–406.
20. Thiruchelvam U, et al. The importance of the macrophage within the human endometrium. J Leukoc Biol. 2013;93(2):217–25.
21. Evans J, Salamonsen LA. Inflammation, leukocytes and menstruation. Rev Endocr Metab Disord. 2012;13(4):277–88.
22. Tran LV, et al. Macrophages and nerve fibres in peritoneal endometriosis. Hum Reprod. 2009;24(4):835–41.
23. Oral E, Olive DL, Arici A. The peritoneal environment in endometriosis. Hum Reprod Update. 1996;2(5):385–98.
24. Halme J, et al. Retrograde menstruation in healthy women and in patients with endometriosis. Obstet Gynecol. 1984;64(2):151–4.
25. Sampson JA. Metastatic or embolic endometriosis, due to the menstrual dissemination of endometrial tissue into the venous circulation. Am J Pathol. 1927;3(2):93–110.43.
26. Wu MH, et al. Prostaglandin E2: the master of endometriosis? Exp Biol Med (Maywood). 2010;235(6):668–77.
27. Muscato JJ, Haney AF, Weinberg JB. Sperm phagocytosis by human peritoneal macrophages: a possible cause of infertility in endometriosis. Am J Obstet Gynecol. 1982;144 (5):503–10.
28. Halme J, Becker S, Haskill S. Altered maturation and function of peritoneal macrophages: possible role in pathogenesis of endometriosis. Am J Obstet Gynecol. 1987;156(4):783–9.
29. Braun DP, et al. Relationship between apoptosis and the number of macrophages in eutopic endometrium from women with and without endometriosis. Fertil Steril. 2002;78(4):830–5.
30. Braun DP, et al. Spontaneous and induced synthesis of cytokines by peripheral blood monocytes in patients with endometriosis. Fertil Steril. 1996;65(6):1125–9.
31. Carli C, et al. Direct effect of macrophage migration inhibitory factor on sperm function: possible involvement in endometriosis-associated infertility. Fertil Steril. 2007;88 (4 Suppl):1240–7.
32. Jha P, et al. In vitro sperm phagocytosis by human peritoneal macrophages in endometriosis-associated infertility. Am J Reprod Immunol. 1996;36(4):235–7.
33. Koninckx PR, Kennedy SH, Barlow DH. Endometriotic disease: the role of peritoneal fluid. Hum Reprod Update. 1998;4(5):741–51.
34. Lebovic DI, Mueller MD, Taylor RN. Immunobiology of endometriosis. Fertil Steril. 2001;75(1):1–10.
35. Seli E, Arici A. Endometriosis: interaction of immune and endocrine systems. Semin Reprod Med. 2003;21(2):135–44.
36. Ulukus M, Cakmak H, Arici A. The role of endometrium in endometriosis. J Soc Gynecol Investig. 2006;13(7):467–76.
37. Wu MH, et al. Suppression of matrix metalloproteinase-9 by prostaglandin E(2) in peritoneal macrophage is associated with severity of endometriosis. Am J Pathol. 2005;167(4):1061–9.
38. Chuang PC, et al. Downregulation of CD36 results in reduced phagocytic ability of peritoneal macrophages of women with endometriosis. J Pathol. 2009;219(2):232–41.
39. Chuang PC, et al. Inhibition of CD36-dependent phagocytosis by prostaglandin E2 contributes to the development of endometriosis. Am J Pathol. 2010;176(2):850–60.
40. Giudice LC, Kao LC. Endometriosis. Lancet. 2004;364(9447):1789–99.
41. Akoum A, et al. Secretion of monocyte chemotactic protein-1 by cytokine-stimulated endometrial cells of women with endometriosis. Le groupe d'investigation en gynecologie. Fertil Steril. 1995;63(2):322–8.
42. Akoum A, et al. Secretion of interleukin-6 by human endometriotic cells and regulation by proinflammatory cytokines and sex steroids. Hum Reprod. 1996;11(10):2269–75.

43. Kats R, Metz CN, Akoum A. Macrophage migration inhibitory factor is markedly expressed in active and early-stage endometriotic lesions. J Clin Endocrinol Metab. 2002;87(2):883–9.
44. Morin M, et al. Elevated levels of macrophage migration inhibitory factor in the peripheral blood of women with endometriosis. Fertil Steril. 2005;83(4):865–72.
45. Akoum A, et al. Imbalance in the peritoneal levels of interleukin 1 and its decoy inhibitory receptor type II in endometriosis women with infertility and pelvic pain. Fertil Steril. 2008;89 (6):1618–24.
46. Herrmann Lavoie C, et al. Interleukin-1 stimulates macrophage migration inhibitory factor secretion in ectopic endometrial cells of women with endometriosis. Am J Reprod Immunol. 2007;58(6):505–13.
47. Koch AE, et al. Interleukin-8 as a macrophage-derived mediator of angiogenesis. Science. 1992;258(5089):1798–801.
48. Yoshimura T, et al. Neutrophil chemotactic factor produced by lipopolysaccharide (LPS)-stimulated human blood mononuclear leukocytes: partial characterization and separation from interleukin 1 (IL 1). J Immunol. 1987;139(3):788–93.
49. Arici A, et al. Interleukin-8 induces proliferation of endometrial stromal cells: a potential autocrine growth factor. J Clin Endocrinol Metab. 1998;83(4):1201–5.
50. Velasco G, et al. Cloning and characterization of human MMP-23, a new matrix metalloproteinase predominantly expressed in reproductive tissues and lacking conserved domains in other family members. J Biol Chem. 1999;274(8):4570–6.
51. Jolicoeur C, et al. Increased expression of monocyte chemotactic protein-1 in the endometrium of women with endometriosis. Am J Pathol. 1998;152(1):125–33.
52. Akoum A, et al. Spontaneous and stimulated secretion of monocyte chemotactic protein-1 and macrophage migration inhibitory factor by peritoneal macrophages in women with and without endometriosis. Fertil Steril. 2002;77(5):989–94.
53. Akoum A, et al. Elevated concentration and biologic activity of monocyte chemotactic protein-1 in the peritoneal fluid of patients with endometriosis. Fertil Steril. 1996;66 (1):17–23.
54. Arici A, et al. Monocyte chemotactic protein-1 concentration in peritoneal fluid of women with endometriosis and its modulation of expression in mesothelial cells. Fertil Steril. 1997;67(6):1065–72.
55. Saji H, et al. Significant correlation of monocyte chemoattractant protein-1 expression with neovascularization and progression of breast carcinoma. Cancer. 2001;92(5):1085–91.
56. Soria G, Ben-Baruch A. The inflammatory chemokines CCL2 and CCL5 in breast cancer. Cancer Lett. 2008;267(2):271–85.
57. Salcedo R, et al. Human endothelial cells express CCR2 and respond to MCP-1: direct role of MCP-1 in angiogenesis and tumor progression. Blood. 2000;96(1):34–40.
58. Goede V, et al. Induction of inflammatory angiogenesis by monocyte chemoattractant protein-1. Int J Cancer. 1999;82(5):765–70.
59. Kuroda T, et al. Monocyte chemoattractant protein-1 transfection induces angiogenesis and tumorigenesis of gastric carcinoma in nude mice via macrophage recruitment. Clin Cancer Res. 2005;11(21):7629–36.
60. Hornung D, et al. Chemokine bioactivity of RANTES in endometriotic and normal endometrial stromal cells and peritoneal fluid. Mol Hum Reprod. 2001;7(2):163–8.
61. Lebovic DI, et al. IL-1beta induction of RANTES (regulated upon activation, normal T cell expressed and secreted) chemokine gene expression in endometriotic stromal cells depends on a nuclear factor-kappaB site in the proximal promoter. J Clin Endocrinol Metab. 2001;86 (10):4759–64.
62. Akoum A, Lemay A, Maheux R. Estradiol and interleukin-1beta exert a synergistic stimulatory effect on the expression of the chemokine regulated upon activation, normal T cell expressed, and secreted in endometriotic cells. J Clin Endocrinol Metab. 2002;87 (12):5785–92.

63. Bloom BR, Bennett B. Mechanism of a reaction in vitro associated with delayed-type hypersensitivity. Science. 1966;153(3731):80–2.
64. David JR. Delayed hypersensitivity in vitro: its mediation by cell-free substances formed by lymphoid cell-antigen interaction. Proc Natl Acad Sci U S A. 1966;56(1):72–7.
65. de Jong YP, et al. Development of chronic colitis is dependent on the cytokine MIF. Nat Immunol. 2001;2(11):1061–6.
66. Calandra T, Roger T. Macrophage migration inhibitory factor: a regulator of innate immunity. Nat Rev Immunol. 2003;3(10):791–800.
67. Calandra T, et al. MIF as a glucocorticoid-induced modulator of cytokine production. Nature. 1995;377(6544):68–71.
68. Calandra T, Bucala R. Macrophage migration inhibitory factor (MIF): a glucocorticoid counter-regulator within the immune system. Crit Rev Immunol. 1997;17(1):77–88.
69. Donnelly SC, Bucala R. Macrophage migration inhibitory factor: a regulator of glucocorticoid activity with a critical role in inflammatory disease. Mol Med Today. 1997;3(11):502–7.
70. Bucala R, Donnelly SC. Macrophage migration inhibitory factor: a probable link between inflammation and cancer. Immunity. 2007;26(3):281–5.
71. Akoum A, et al. Macrophage migration inhibitory factor expression in the intrauterine endometrium of women with endometriosis varies with disease stage, infertility status, and pelvic pain. Fertil Steril. 2006;85(5):1379–85.
72. Mahutte NG, et al. Elevations in peritoneal fluid macrophage migration inhibitory factor are independent of the depth of invasion or stage of endometriosis. Fertil Steril. 2004;82 (1):97–101.
73. Lin W, et al. Expression of macrophage migration inhibitory factor in human endometriosis: relation to disease stage, menstrual cycle and infertility. J Obstet Gynaecol Res. 2010;36 (2):344–51.
74. Carli C, et al. Up-regulation of cyclooxygenase-2 expression and prostaglandin E2 production in human endometriotic cells by macrophage migration inhibitory factor: involvement of novel kinase signaling pathways. Endocrinology. 2009;150(7):3128–37.
75. Veillat V, et al. Involvement of nuclear factor-kappaB in macrophage migration inhibitory factor gene transcription up-regulation induced by interleukin-1 beta in ectopic endometrial cells. Fertil Steril. 2009;91(5 Suppl):2148–56.
76. Veillat V, et al. Macrophage migration inhibitory factor is involved in a positive feedback loop increasing aromatase expression in endometriosis. Am J Pathol. 2012;181(3):917–27.
77. Veillat V, et al. Macrophage migration inhibitory factor elicits an angiogenic phenotype in human ectopic endometrial cells and triggers the production of major angiogenic factors via CD44, CD74, and MAPK signaling pathways. J Clin Endocrinol Metab. 2010;95(12): E403–12.
78. Gazvani R, Templeton A. Peritoneal environment, cytokines and angiogenesis in the pathophysiology of endometriosis. Reproduction. 2002;123(2):217–26.
79. Xie K, et al. Constitutive and inducible expression and regulation of vascular endothelial growth factor. Cytokine Growth Factor Rev. 2004;15(5):297–324.
80. McLaren J, et al. Vascular endothelial growth factor is produced by peritoneal fluid macrophages in endometriosis and is regulated by ovarian steroids. J Clin Invest. 1996;98(2):482–9.
81. McLaren J. Vascular endothelial growth factor and endometriotic angiogenesis. Hum Reprod Update. 2000;6(1):45–55.
82. Cakmak H, et al. Immune-endocrine interactions in endometriosis. Front Biosci (Elite Ed). 2009;1:429–43.
83. Gonzalez-Ramos R, et al. Involvement of the nuclear factor-kappaB pathway in the pathogenesis of endometriosis. Fertil Steril. 2010;94(6):1985–94.
84. Langenbach R, et al. Prostaglandin synthase 1 gene disruption in mice reduces arachidonic acid-induced inflammation and indomethacin-induced gastric ulceration. Cell. 1995;83 (3):483–92.

85. Pellegrini C, et al. The expression of estrogen receptors as well as GREB1, c-MYC, and cyclin D1, estrogen-regulated genes implicated in proliferation, is increased in peritoneal endometriosis. Fertil Steril. 2012;98(5):1200–8.
86. Shweiki D, et al. Vascular endothelial growth factor induced by hypoxia may mediate hypoxia-initiated angiogenesis. Nature. 1992;359(6398):843–5.
87. Groothuis PG, et al. Vascular development in endometriosis. Angiogenesis. 2005;8 (2):147–56.
88. Wang GL, et al. Hypoxia-inducible factor 1 is a basic-helix-loop-helix-PAS heterodimer regulated by cellular O2 tension. Proc Natl Acad Sci U S A. 1995;92(12):5510–4.
89. Wu MH, et al. Aberrant expression of leptin in human endometriotic stromal cells is induced by elevated levels of hypoxia inducible factor-1alpha. Am J Pathol. 2007;170(2):590–8.
90. Wu MH, et al. Endometriosis: disease pathophysiology and the role of prostaglandins. Expert Rev Mol Med. 2007;9(2):1–20.
91. Smith WL, Garavito RM, DeWitt DL. Prostaglandin endoperoxide H synthases (cyclooxygenases)-1 and −2. J Biol Chem. 1996;271(52):33157–60.
92. Wu MH, et al. Distinct mechanisms regulate cyclooxygenase-1 and -2 in peritoneal macrophages of women with and without endometriosis. Mol Hum Reprod. 2002;8(12):1103–10.
93. Christenson LK, et al. CCAAT/enhancer-binding proteins regulate expression of the human steroidogenic acute regulatory protein (StAR) gene. J Biol Chem. 1999;274(37):26591–8.
94. Haining RE, et al. Epidermal growth factor in human endometrium: proliferative effects in culture and immunocytochemical localization in normal and endometriotic tissues. Hum Reprod. 1991;6(9):1200–5.
95. Khan IM, Palmer EA, Archer CW. Fibroblast growth factor-2 induced chondrocyte cluster formation in experimentally wounded articular cartilage is blocked by soluble Jagged-1. Osteoarthritis Cartilage. 2010;18(2):208–19.
96. Sun HS, et al. Transactivation of steroidogenic acute regulatory protein in human endometriotic stromal cells is mediated by the prostaglandin EP2 receptor. Endocrinology. 2003;144(9):3934–42.
97. Wing LY, et al. Expression and mitogenic effect of fibroblast growth factor-9 in human endometriotic implant is regulated by aberrant production of estrogen. J Clin Endocrinol Metab. 2003;88(11):5547–54.
98. Jones MK, et al. Inhibition of angiogenesis by nonsteroidal anti-inflammatory drugs: insight into mechanisms and implications for cancer growth and ulcer healing. Nat Med. 1999;5 (12):1418–23.
99. Williams CS, et al. Host cyclooxygenase-2 modulates carcinoma growth. J Clin Invest. 2000;105(11):1589–94.
100. Haney AF. Endometriosis, macrophages, and adhesions. Prog Clin Biol Res. 1993;381:19–44.
101. Burns WN, Schenken RS. Pathophysiology of endometriosis-associated infertility. Clin Obstet Gynecol. 1999;42(3):586–610.
102. Arumugam K, Yip YC. De novo formation of adhesions in endometriosis: the role of iron and free radical reactions. Fertil Steril. 1995;64(1):62–4.
103. Oner-Iyidogan Y, et al. Indices of oxidative stress in eutopic and ectopic endometria of women with endometriosis. Gynecol Obstet Invest. 2004;57(4):214–7.
104. Shanti A, et al. Autoantibodies to markers of oxidative stress are elevated in women with endometriosis. Fertil Steril. 1999;71(6):1115–8.
105. Maathuis JB, Aitken RJ. Protein patterns of human uterine flushings collected at various stages of the menstrual cycle. J Reprod Fertil. 1978;53(2):343–8.
106. McCubrey JA, Franklin RA. Reactive oxygen intermediates and signaling through kinase pathways. Antioxid Redox Signal. 2006;8(9–10):1745–8.
107. Ishikawa H, et al. CCAAT/enhancer binding protein beta regulates aromatase expression via multiple and novel cis-regulatory sequences in uterine leiomyoma. J Clin Endocrinol Metab. 2008;93(3):981–91.

108. Kats R, et al. Cycle-dependent expression of macrophage migration inhibitory factor in the human endometrium. Hum Reprod. 2005;20(12):3518–25.
109. Hashimoto T, et al. VEGF activates divergent intracellular signaling components to regulate retinal progenitor cell proliferation and neuronal differentiation. Development. 2006;133 (11):2201–10.
110. Wittko IM, et al. VEGFR-1 regulates adult olfactory bulb neurogenesis and migration of neural progenitors in the rostral migratory stream in vivo. J Neurosci. 2009;29(27):8704–14.
111. Giudice LC. Clinical practice. Endometriosis. N Engl J Med. 2010;362(25):2389–98.
112. Odagiri K, et al. Smooth muscle metaplasia and innervation in interstitium of endometriotic lesions related to pain. Fertil Steril. 2009;92(5):1525–31.
113. Lee JL, et al. Cyclooxygenases in the skin: pharmacological and toxicological implications. Toxicol Appl Pharmacol. 2003;192(3):294–306.
114. Cabral GA. Lipids as bioeffectors in the immune system. Life Sci. 2005;77(14):1699–710.
115. Koopman LA, et al. Human decidual natural killer cells are a unique NK cell subset with immunomodulatory potential. J Exp Med. 2003;198(8):1201–12.
116. Nagamatsu T, Schust DJ. The contribution of macrophages to normal and pathological pregnancies. Am J Reprod Immunol. 2010;63(6):460–71.
117. Nagamatsu T, Schust DJ. The immunomodulatory roles of macrophages at the maternal-fetal interface. Reprod Sci. 2010;17(3):209–18.
118. Abrahams VM, et al. Macrophages and apoptotic cell clearance during pregnancy. Am J Reprod Immunol. 2004;51(4):275–82.
119. Rico-Rosillo MG, Vega-Robledo GB. Immunological mechanisms involved in pregnancy. Ginecol Obstet Mex. 2012;80(5):332–40.
120. Heikkinen J, et al. Phenotypic characterization of human decidual macrophages. Clin Exp Immunol. 2003;131(3):498–505.
121. Co EC, et al. Maternal decidual macrophages inhibit NK cell killing of invasive cytotrophoblasts during human pregnancy. Biol Reprod. 2013;88(6):155.
122. Hanna J, et al. Decidual NK cells regulate key developmental processes at the human fetal-maternal interface. Nat Med. 2006;12(9):1065–74.
123. Krikun G. Endometriosis, angiogenesis and tissue factor. Scientifica (Cario). 2012;2012:306830.
124. Laschke MW, Giebels C, Menger MD. Vasculogenesis: a new piece of the endometriosis puzzle. Hum Reprod Update. 2011;17(5):628–36.
125. Su MT, Lin SH, Chen YC. Genetic association studies of angiogenesis- and vasoconstriction-related genes in women with recurrent pregnancy loss: a systematic review and meta-analysis. Hum Reprod Update. 2011;17(6):803–12.
126. Romero R, et al. Inflammation in pregnancy: its roles in reproductive physiology, obstetrical complications, and fetal injury. Nutr Rev. 2007;65(12 Pt 2):S194–202.
127. Augoulea A, et al. Pathogenesis of endometriosis: the role of genetics, inflammation and oxidative stress. Arch Gynecol Obstet. 2012;286(1):99–103.
128. Christiansen OB. Reproductive immunology. Mol Immunol. 2013;55(1):8–15.
129. Anton L, et al. Lipopolysaccharide induces cytokine production and decreases extravillous trophoblast invasion through a mitogen-activated protein kinase-mediated pathway: possible mechanisms of first trimester placental dysfunction. Hum Reprod. 2012;27(1):61–72.
130. Agarwal A, et al. The effects of oxidative stress on female reproduction: a review. Reprod Biol Endocrinol. 2012;10:49.
131. Osborn BH, et al. Inducible nitric oxide synthase expression by peritoneal macrophages in endometriosis-associated infertility. Fertil Steril. 2002;77(1):46–51.
132. Lambrinoudaki IV, et al. Measurable serum markers of oxidative stress response in women with endometriosis. Fertil Steril. 2009;91(1):46–50.
133. Mier-Cabrera J, et al. Quantitative and qualitative peritoneal immune profiles, T-cell apoptosis and oxidative stress-associated characteristics in women with minimal and mild endometriosis. BJOG. 2011;118(1):6–16.

134. Szczepanska M, et al. Oxidative stress may be a piece in the endometriosis puzzle. Fertil Steril. 2003;79(6):1288–93.
135. Sobinoff AP, et al. Scrambled and fried: cigarette smoke exposure causes antral follicle destruction and oocyte dysfunction through oxidative stress. Toxicol Appl Pharmacol. 2013;271(2):156–67.
136. Lee TH, et al. The association between microenvironmental reactive oxygen species and embryo development in assisted reproduction technology cycles. Reprod Sci. 2012;19 (7):725–32.
137. Karuputhula NB, et al. Oxidative status in granulosa cells of infertile women undergoing IVF. Syst Biol Reprod Med. 2013;59(2):91–8.
138. Mesiano S, Ferrara N, Jaffe RB. Role of vascular endothelial growth factor in ovarian cancer: inhibition of ascites formation by immunoneutralization. Am J Pathol. 1998;153(4):1249–56.
139. Shen GH, et al. Prognostic significance of vascular endothelial growth factor expression in human ovarian carcinoma. Br J Cancer. 2000;83(2):196–203.
140. Nezhat F, et al. Comparative immunohistochemical studies of bcl-2 and p53 proteins in benign and malignant ovarian endometriotic cysts. Cancer. 2002;94(11):2935–40.
141. Wang Z, et al. Tamoxifen regulates human telomerase reverse transcriptase (hTERT) gene expression differently in breast and endometrial cancer cells. Oncogene. 2002;21 (22):3517–24.
142. Del Carmen MG, et al. Endometriosis-associated ovarian carcinoma: differential expression of vascular endothelial growth factor and estrogen/progesterone receptors. Cancer. 2003;98 (8):1658–63.
143. Somigliana E, et al. Endometrial ability to implant in ectopic sites can be prevented by interleukin-12 in a murine model of endometriosis. Hum Reprod. 1999;14(12):2944–50.
144. Zamah NM, et al. Transplantation of normal and ectopic human endometrial tissue into athymic nude mice. Am J Obstet Gynecol. 1984;149(6):591–7.
145. Becker CM, et al. A novel noninvasive model of endometriosis for monitoring the efficacy of antiangiogenic therapy. Am J Pathol. 2006;168(6):2074–84.
146. Bacci M, et al. Macrophages are alternatively activated in patients with endometriosis and required for growth and vascularization of lesions in a mouse model of disease. Am J Pathol. 2009;175(2):547–56.
147. Capobianco A, et al. Proangiogenic Tie2(+) macrophages infiltrate human and murine endometriotic lesions and dictate their growth in a mouse model of the disease. Am J Pathol. 2011;179(5):2651–9.
148. Wu MH, et al. Suppression of annexin A2 by prostaglandin E(2) impairs phagocytic ability of peritoneal macrophages in women with endometriosis. Hum Reprod. 2013;28(4):1045–53.
149. Khoufache K, et al. Macrophage migration inhibitory factor antagonist blocks the development of endometriosis in vivo. PLoS One. 2012;7(5):e37264.
150. Taylor 3rd JA, et al. Null mutation for macrophage migration inhibitory factor (MIF) is associated with less aggressive bladder cancer in mice. BMC Cancer. 2007;7:135.
151. Nishihira J, et al. Macrophage migration inhibitory factor (MIF): its potential role in tumor growth and tumor-associated angiogenesis. Ann N Y Acad Sci. 2003;995:171–82.
152. Chesney J, et al. An essential role for macrophage migration inhibitory factor (MIF) in angiogenesis and the growth of a murine lymphoma. Mol Med. 1999;5(3):181–91.
153. Bondza PK, Metz CN, Akoum A. Postgestational effects of macrophage migration inhibitory factor on embryonic implantation in mice. Fertil Steril. 2008;90(4 Suppl):1433–43.
154. Bach JP, et al. Role of MIF in inflammation and tumorigenesis. Oncology. 2008;75 (3–4):127–33.
155. Al-Abed Y, et al. ISO-1 binding to the tautomerase active site of MIF inhibits its pro-inflammatory activity and increases survival in severe sepsis. J Biol Chem. 2005;280 (44):36541–4.
156. Matsubayashi H, et al. Leukocyte subpopulation changes in rats with autotransplanted endometrium and the effect of danazol. Am J Reprod Immunol. 1995;33(4):301–14.

157. Uchiide I, Ihara T, Sugamata M. Pathological evaluation of the rat endometriosis model. Fertil Steril. 2002;78(4):782–6.
158. Machado DE, et al. A selective cyclooxygenase-2 inhibitor suppresses the growth of endometriosis with an antiangiogenic effect in a rat model. Fertil Steril. 2010;93(8):2674–9.
159. Haber E, et al. Peritoneal macrophage depletion by liposomal bisphosphonate attenuates endometriosis in the rat model. Hum Reprod. 2009;24(2):398–407.
160. Grummer R. Animal models in endometriosis research. Hum Reprod Update. 2006;12 (5):641–9.
161. Smith KA, et al. Alternative activation of macrophages in rhesus macaques (Macaca mulatta) with endometriosis. Comp Med. 2012;62(4):303–10.
162. Ricci AG, et al. Effect of vascular endothelial growth factor inhibition on endometrial implant development in a murine model of endometriosis. Reprod Sci. 2011;18(7):614–22.
163. Soares SR, et al. Pharmacologic therapies in endometriosis: a systematic review. Fertil Steril. 2012;98(3):529–55.
164. Cakmak H, et al. Statins inhibit monocyte chemotactic protein 1 expression in endometriosis. Reprod Sci. 2012;19(6):572–9.
165. Allavena P, et al. Intraperitoneal recombinant gamma-interferon in patients with recurrent ascitic ovarian carcinoma: modulation of cytotoxicity and cytokine production in tumor-associated effectors and of major histocompatibility antigen expression on tumor cells. Cancer Res. 1990;50(22):7318–23.
166. Duluc D, et al. Interferon-gamma reverses the immunosuppressive and protumoral properties and prevents the generation of human tumor-associated macrophages. Int J Cancer. 2009;125 (2):367–73.

Chapter 7
Inflammation and Cytokines in Endometriosis

Tomio Iwabe and Tasuku Harada

Abstract Endometriosis, a common disease among women of reproductive age, is characterized by the presence and growth of endometrial tissue (glands and stroma) outside the uterus. Dysmenorrhea and infertility common in endometriosis compromise the quality of life of reproductive age women. Despite a long history of clinical experience and experimental research, endometriosis remains an enigma, and its pathogenesis is still controversial. The peritoneal fluid (PF) of women with endometriosis contains an increased number of activated macrophages that secrete a variety of local products, such as growth factors and cytokines. In this chapter, we review the current understanding of the role of cytokines in the pathogenesis of endometriosis.

Keywords Angiogenesis • Cytokine • Peritoneal fluid • Retrograde menstruation • Transcriptional factor

7.1 Introduction

Endometriosis was first acknowledged more than about 100 years ago, and the usual definitions of this disease are based on histology and related to glands, stroma, hemosiderin, and fibromuscular metaplasia [1]. Endometriosis, which occurs in 10 % of reproductive age women, is characterized by the growth of endometrial-like tissue outside the uterus. Dysmenorrhea and infertility, which are common symptoms of endometriosis, compromise the quality of life. This disease is thought to be estrogen dependent. However, the pathogenesis of endometriosis is poorly

T. Iwabe (✉)
Department of Obstetrics and Gynecology, Faculty of Medicine,
Sanin Rosai Hospital, Yonago, Japan
e-mail: iwabe@saninh.rofuku.go.jp

T. Harada
Department of Obstetrics and Gynecology, Faculty of Medicine,
Tottori University, Yonago, Japan

T. Harada (ed.), *Endometriosis: Pathogenesis and Treatment*,
DOI 10.1007/978-4-431-54421-0_7,

understood despite decades of experimental and clinical study. Endometriosis is associated with infertility even among affected women who ovulate and have anatomically patent fallopian tubes. The exact mechanism by which endometriosis interferes with fertility is not known, but data suggest that an aberrant immunological mechanism is involved in its pathophysiology. An important general concept is that of endometriosis as a local pelvic inflammatory process with altered function of immune-related cells in the peritoneal environment. Supporting this concept are recent studies suggesting that the peritoneal fluid (PF) of women with endometriosis contains an increased number of activated macrophages that secrete a variety of local products, such as growth factors and cytokines. Therefore, secreted cytokines in chronic pelvic inflammation is a key factor in the pathogenesis of endometriosis [2].

7.2 Peritoneal Environment

7.2.1 Retrograde Menstruation

Retrograde menstruation, in which fragments of endometrium are refluxed through the fallopian tubes into the peritoneal cavity, occurs only in women and nonhuman primates and in a few exceptional species, such as the elephant and bat. Spontaneous endometriosis, which is clinically confirmed endometriosis in nature, has been reported only in humans and some primates, the rhesus macaque (*Macaca mulatta*), the Japanese macaque (*Macaca fuscata*), the pig-tailed macaque (*Macaca nemestrina*), and the Kenya baboon (*Papio doguera*) [3]. The reproductive organs of women are anatomically similar to that of female baboons; therefore these nonhuman primates are thought to be an adequate animal experimental model. Patients with endometriosis almost always have patent tubes; thus blood and endometrial fragments are able to pass out of the uterus by way of the tubes (Fig. 7.1). Cyclic and retrograde menstruation are common phenomena in both humans and these animals. Several studies suggest that retrograde menstruation strongly relates to endometriosis. Shorter cycles and heavier and longer menstrual flow often occur in women with endometriosis [4]. From the above observation, retrograde menstruation is one of the most important factors in the pathophysiology of endometriosis.

The most widely accepted hypothesis for endometriosis is Sampson's theory of retrograde menstruation [5]. Retrograde menstruation occurs in 76–90 % of investigated women, and endometrial cells have been observed in the peritoneal fluid of 59–79 % of women during menstruation or the early follicular phase; however, endometriosis was diagnosed in only 10 % of this population [6, 7]. Endometriosis was hypothesized to be caused by decreased clearance of peritoneal fluid in endometrial cells due to reduced natural killer (NK) activity and/or decreased macrophage activity [8]. However, the development of endometriosis cannot be explained by this phenomenon. Recently, Khan et al. reported that the menstrual

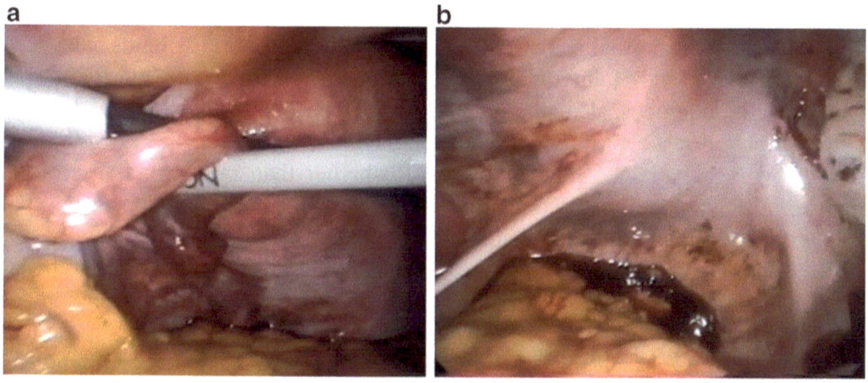

Fig. 7.1 Laparoscopic findings in pelvic cavity during menstrual period. (**a**) Retrograde menstruation from fimbria. (**b**) Cul-de-sac

blood of women with endometriosis is more frequently contaminated with *Escherichia coli* than that of the controls and corresponds to higher levels of endotoxin in the menstrual fluid. Consequently, endotoxin levels are high in the PF due to reflux of menstrual blood into the pelvis. The colony formation of *E. coli* and endotoxin levels in the menstrual fluid was markedly higher in women with red lesion in r-ASRM stage I–II endometriosis patients than in women with endometrioma of stage III–IV endometriosis [9]. We also reported LPS (endotoxin)-promoted proliferation and invasion of endometriotic stromal cells via upregulation of cyclooxygenase 2 (COX2) and prostaglandin E2 (PGE2) [10]. These findings, including that of bacterial contamination, would be a suitable area for future research into the pathophysiology of endometriosis.

7.2.2 Peritoneal Fluid

Peritoneal fluid (PF) containing immune-related cells is often seen in the vesico-uterine cavity or the pouch of Douglas during gynecologic surgery. PF bathes the pelvic cavity, uterus, fallopian tubes, and ovaries and may be a major player controlling the peritoneal microenvironment that influences the development and progression of endometriosis and endometriosis-associated infertility.

The peritoneal cavity is normally empty except for a thin film of fluid that keeps surfaces moist. Peritoneal fluid arises primarily from two sources: plasma transudate and ovarian exudate. Other sources of peritoneal fluid are tubal fluid, retrograde menstruation, and immune cell secretions. Peritoneal fluid depends on follicular activity, corpus luteum vascularity, and hormonal production. The volume of PF within the peritoneal cavity varies during the menstrual cycle, reaching a peak of 20 mL at the time of ovulation [11].

Changes in fluid volume and the presence of various cells, hormones, and other compounds during normal menstrual cycles and in pathologic conditions have been described. Syrop and Halme analyzed PF volume in 426 patients and found that women with endometriosis had a greater PF volume than fertile controls, patients with adhesive disease, or those with unexplained infertility [12]. The PF volume in women with unexplained infertility was also higher than in controls. Therefore, increased PF volume may be commonly associated not only with endometriosis but also with long-lasting, unexplained infertility.

PF contains various free-floating cells, including macrophages, mesothelial cells, lymphocytes, eosinophils, and mast cells. Normally, PF contains leukocytes in concentrations of $0.5–2.0 \times 10^6$ mL^{-1}, of which approximately 85 % are macrophages. Halme et al. postulated that peritoneal macrophage activation might be a central contributor to the pathogenesis of endometriosis [13]. Activated macrophages in the peritoneal cavity of women with endometriosis are potent producers of cytokines. Thus, PF contains a rich cocktail of cytokines. The cytokines are multifunctional proteins whose biological properties suggest a key role in hematopoiesis, immunity, infectious disease, tumorigenesis, homeostasis, tissue repair, and cellular development and growth.

7.3 Cytokines

7.3.1 Cytokines in Peritoneal Fluid

Cytokines, a large family of more than 100 low molecular weight proteins that function as growth and differentiation factors and immune cell modulators, also play a major role in the regulation of immune and inflammatory responses. Immune cell activation results in a burst and cascade of inflammatory cytokines. These cytokines have pleiotropic and redundant activities culminating in the recruitment of numerous cell types to the site of inflammation.

The development of enzyme-linked immunosorbent assay has made it possible to measure a number of cytokines in the PF of women with endometriosis. These include interleukin-1 (IL-1) [14], IL-4 [15], IL-5 [16], IL-6 [17–21], IL-8 [22–24], IL-10 [20, 25, 26], IL-12 [27, 28], IL-13 [29], IL-17 [30], IL-23 [31], IL-33 [32], interferon γ (INFγ) [19], tumor necrosis factor α (TNFα) [14, 21], RANTES [33], monocyte chemotactic protein-1 (MCP-1) [34–36], macrophage colony-stimulating factor (MCSF) [37], transforming growth factor β (TGFβ) [38], and vascular endothelial growth factor (VEGF) [39, 40]. A number of studies report that the level of many cytokines is increased in the PF of women with endometriosis. Cytokines may regulate the actions of leukocytes in the PF or could act directly on the ectopic endometrium, where they may play various roles in the pathogenesis and pathophysiology of endometriosis.

7.3.2 *Source of Cytokines*

Increased levels of cytokines in the PF of women with endometriosis may reflect increased synthesis of cytokines by the peritoneal macrophages, lymphocytes, ectopic endometrial implants, and/or mesothelial cells of the peritoneum, all of which are capable of cytokine production [41, 42]. The main source of cytokines is thought to be the macrophages, which originate in bone marrow, circulate as monocytes, and then migrate to various body cavities.

7.3.2.1 Macrophages

Macrophages are main regulators of the innate response to injured, infected, and neoplastic tissues. The peritoneal macrophages (PMs) are the major resident cells in the peritoneal cavity. They kill cells, such as retrograde endometrial tissues, and their presence is commonly associated with an inflammatory process. Most studies revealed increased cell numbers and activity of PMs in cases of endometriosis, although some studies did not [43, 44]. The increased number of PMs in women with endometriosis may indicate that the presence of endometrial tissue in the peritoneal cavity represents a foreign entity and needs to be removed. Activated PMs might synthesize and secrete different cytokines into the PF including various cytokines and growth factors.

7.3.2.2 T-Lymphocytes

T-lymphocytes are also implicated in the pathogenesis of endometriosis. T-helper cells can be classified into two subsets: type 1 (Th1) and type 2 (Th2). Th1 cells produce IL-2, IL-12, and INFγ, which are potent inducers of cell-mediated immunity. Th2 cells produce mainly IL-4, IL-5, IL-10, and IL-13, which are involved in the suppression of cell-mediated immunity. Hsu et al. investigated the expression of Th1 (IL-2 and INFγ) and Th2 (IL-4 and IL-10) cytokines in the peripheral blood monocytes and PF from patients with endometriosis [15]. They found that cytokine secretion by Th1 and Th2 cells is altered in women with endometriosis. The shift in the balance of Th1/Th2 toward the Th2 arm may contribute to the derangement of an immunologic defense mechanism in endometriosis. Interleukin-10 is well known to be an anti-inflammatory cytokine in regulating inflammatory responses. We also observed that IL-10 expression levels in endometriotic stromal cells were lower than in endometrial stromal cells [26].

7.3.2.3 Others

Recent studies suggest that endometriotic implants also produce cytokines [45, 46]. We demonstrated that endometriotic cells constitutively express IL-6 mRNA and produce IL-6 protein and that adding TNFα stimulated IL-6 gene and protein expression in a dose-dependent manner [47]. When we compared IL-6 production by macrophages and endometriotic stromal cells in patients with endometriosis, similar levels of IL-6 were found to be produced in stromal cells derived from an endometrioma and by macrophages under basal- and TNFα-stimulated conditions.

Numerous leukocytes are harbored in both stromal and intraepithelial parts of normal eutopic endometrium. In women with endometriosis, the member of lymphocytes is increased both in eutopic and ectopic endometria. We postulated that immune cells, such as leukocytes or lymphocytes, and endometriotic tissue interacted via the paracrine mechanism on the source of the cytokines. Therefore, they may contribute to cytokine production in PF and be involved in cellular growth and inflammatory reaction. The findings suggest that endometriotic tissue may be another important source of this cytokine.

7.3.3 Role of Cytokines

The pathogenesis of endometriosis is still a matter of debate, despite extensive research efforts since Sampson's landmark article in 1927 [5]. Sampson's theory of retrograde menstruation, which describes endometrial cells that may attach, implant, and grow, seems plausible because peritoneal lesions are most frequently found in the ovaries and the posterior cul-de-sac where regurgitated menstrual material pools.

One study demonstrated that endometrium can attach to the mesothelial surface of the peritoneum in vitro [48]. The authors described that in all cases of adhesion to intact mesothelium, the endometrium was attached via stromal cells. Another theory, the metaplasia theory, is also attractive since it can explain some rare cases of endometriosis, such as those with the absence of menstruation (Rokitansky–Kuster–Hauser syndrome) [49]. A recent in vitro study supports the metaplasia theory [50]. Unfortunately, neither theory can explain all cases of endometriosis.

7.3.3.1 Implantation of Endometrium

Recent studies demonstrated increased IL-6 production by endometriotic cells in both basal- and cytokine-stimulated conditions compared with their normal counterpart [45]. Tseng et al. examined eutopic endometrium from patients with endometriosis and found an increased basal- and IL-1β-stimulated production of IL-6 compared with patients without endometriosis [46]. This is an important aspect for recent investigation because it suggests that endometrial cells of women who develop endometriosis may function differently from those who do not.

In order to implant and grow, endometrial cells must establish cell–cell or cell–extracellular matrix (ECM) interactions with the peritoneal lining. In these circumstances, cell adhesion molecules are of great importance [51]. A recent report clearly showed that endometrial stromal cells are the critical cells in endometrial attachment to the mesothelial surface of the peritoneum and that endometrial epithelial cells fail to attach to the mesothelium [48]. Most of these interactions between endometrial cells and ECM are mediated by the integrin family of cell surface receptors, which are capable of transducing intracellular signals. It has also been suggested that cellular·adhesion itself stimulates chemokine expression [52].

Garcia-Velasco and Arici showed that increasing the dose of IL-8 stimulates endometrial stromal cells' ability to adhere to an ECM protein, fibronectin [53]. They also showed that the adhesion of endometrial stromal cells to different ECM proteins induces variable levels of IL-8 gene expression and protein secretion and that this event is integrin-mediated [54]. IL-8 may be relevant for the attachment of endometrial implants in the pathogenesis of endometriosis.

According to Sampson's theory of retrograde menstruation, deficient cellular immunity, in particular impaired natural killer (NK) cell function, is one of the etiological factors that could contribute to the survival and implantation of refluxed endometrial cells. Several investigators showed a decrease in NK cell activity in the PF of women with endometriosis compared with women without endometriosis [8, 55, 56]. This observation suggests that the clearing mechanism of retrograde menstruated endometrial cells may be impaired in women with endometriosis because of a defect in the local immune defense system. Oosterlynck et al. found increased TGFβ activity in the PF of women with endometriosis [37]. Transforming growth factor β may be a cytokine that inhibits NK activity in the PF of women with endometriosis.

Intercellular adhesion molecule (ICAM)-1-mediated cell–cell adhesion is essential for various immunological functions, including NK cell-mediated cytotoxicity against endometrium. Recently, Somigliana et al. reported that soluble intercellular adhesion molecules (sICAM)-1 were constitutively shed from the surface of endometrial stromal cells obtained from patients with endometriosis into the culture medium [57]. The enhanced release of sICAM may allow the endometrial stromal cells of patients with endometriosis to escape immunosurveillance and, therefore, to implant in ectopic sites. More interestingly, sICAM-1 production from the macrophages of patients with endometriosis was upregulated by INFγ and IL-6 [58].

Interleukin-12 acts on T and NK cells, inducing cytokine production (primarily INFγ), enhancing NK cell cytotoxic activity, and favoring the generation of T-helper 1 response [59, 60]. Concentrations of IL-12 in the PF are low regardless of the presence or absence of endometriosis, but they are detectable [26]. The administration of IL-12 was recently shown to significantly prevent ectopic endometrial implantation in a murine model of endometriosis [61]. A direct growth inhibitory effect on endometrial cells seems unlikely since endometrial cells do not express receptors for IL-12. A potential explanation for these results is that IL-12 may enhance the growth and augment the cytolytic activity of both NK and T cells. These data support the idea that manipulation of cytokine activity in PF is a novel management approach to controlling the establishment of endometriosis.

7.3.3.2 Angiogenesis

Angiogenesis seldom occurs in adult organs with normal tissues under physiologic conditions. The endometrium represents an exception: the tightly regulated fluctuation of ovarian steroids, estrogen and progesterone concentrations, cyclically triggers the remodeling of the organ vasculature, with angiogenesis and lymphangiogenesis. Angiogenesis, which is the process of generating new capillary blood vessels, occurs in a variety of normal and pathologic processes. It consists of the following steps: dissolution of the basement membrane by the protease derived from vascular endothelial cells, migration and proliferation of the endothelial cells, and formation of the capillary tube [62]. Each step is regulated by various angiogenic factors. Neovascularization is likely to be required for the implant to grow beyond 2–3 mm during tumor growth [63]. An angiogenic mechanism could be involved in the pathogenesis of endometriosis. We can postulate that further outgrowth of these ectopic endometrial implants will depend on new capillary growth according to several studies that indicate that tumors are angiogenesis dependent [64].

Vascular endothelial growth factor (VEGF) is a heparin-binding growth factor of 30–46 KDa, which is active as a disulfide-linked homodimer and is a potent mitogen, morphogen, and chemoattractant for endothelial cells. The angiogenic activity of PF, as well as levels of VEGF in PF, is elevated in women with endometriosis [38, 65]. McLaren et al. demonstrated that PF macrophages are the principal source of the angiogenic growth factor, VEGF, and that the anti-VEGF antibody abolished the enhanced endothelial cell proliferation induced by a conditioned medium from macrophages isolated from the peritoneal cavity of women with endometriosis [39]. McLaren's study suggests that activated macrophages are a major source of VEGF in endometriosis and that estradiol and progesterone directly regulate this expression. Since endometriosis is characterized by pronounced vascularization within and surrounding the ectopic tissue, elevated levels of the potent angiogenic growth factor, VEGF, in the PF and the presence of VEGF-positive macrophages within the ectopic tissue are clinically important in this disease. VEGF-induced angiogenesis may therefore be a critical aspect of the pathophysiology of endometriosis.

IL-8, which is a chemoattractant for neutrophils and an angiogenic agent, induces the proliferation of human melanoma and glioma cells [66, 67]. Arici et al. reported that IL-8 is produced in the human endometrium in vivo, mainly in glandular cells, and that IL-8 induces proliferation of endometrial stromal cell as a potential autocrine growth factor [68, 69]. We demonstrated that IL-8 exerts its growth-promoting actions in endometriotic as well as in normal endometrial cells [24, 70].

TNFα, a secretory product of activated macrophages and a potent inducer of new blood vessel growth, also stimulates proliferation of endometriotic stromal cells. These angiogenic cytokines may play a role in the angiogenesis of endometriosis.

Hypoxia is the stimulus that triggers vessel remodeling in injured and regenerating tissues as well as in tumors. It elicits an adaptive response, which is largely mediated by the hypoxia-inducible transcription factor-1 alpha (HIF1α), under hypoxic conditions. HIF1α translocates to the nucleus where it enhances and accelerates the transcription of genes with appropriate response elements, including angiopoietin 2 (Ang-2), CXCL12, and VEGF [71–73].

In experimental models of endometriosis, early phases of lesion establishment are characterized by a transient hypoxia, which results in the upregulation of HIF1α, with downstream expression of VEGF [74, 75]. Limited ischemia of the endometrium in the early and middle secretory phase occurs: the event is apparently associated with the upregulated expression of VEGF in the late secretory phase of the menstrual cycle in endometriotic women [76]. Interestingly, endometrial fragments from women in which a transient ischemia had been induced by repeated clamping/ unclamping of the uterine artery transplanted onto the chick embryo chorioallantoic membrane demonstrated higher VEGF expression and better survival: this mechanism could facilitate implantation and establishment of the endometrium at ectopic sites [77]. Moreover, response to ischemia is likely to play a role in established lesions of endometriotic patients: the relative expression of HIF1α and VEGF differs at various sites within endometriotic lesions, possibly accounting for some of their heterogeneous histological characteristics [78].

7.3.3.3 Progression and Infiltration

Surrey and Halme demonstrated a direct stimulatory effect of the cell-free fraction of PF samples derived from patients with endometriosis on the proliferation of normal uterine endometrial cells in a short-term culture, indicating that factors in the PF are involved in the progression of endometriosis [79]. Several cytokines, such as IL-8 and TNFα, have growth-promoting effects on endometrial and endometriotic cells [24, 69, 70]. These findings suggest that elevated PF levels of cytokines promote the progression and spread of endometriotic implants in the peritoneal cavity.

We revealed that PF levels of IL-8 significantly enhanced the proliferation of stromal cells derived from ovarian endometriomas [24]. Expression of IL-8 receptor type A (CXCR3A) mRNA was detected in endometriotic stromal cells. These results suggest that IL-8 may promote the progression of endometriosis [70]. We tested the hypothesis that TNFα elevated in PF of patients with endometriosis may contribute to the progression of endometriosis by inducing the production of IL-8. Gene and protein expression of IL-8 in the stromal cells of endometriotic tissues are upregulated by TNFα, and TNFα also stimulated the proliferation of the endometriotic stromal cells. This stimulatory effect of TNFα was abolished by adding either anti-TNFα antibody or anti-IL-8 antibody. Therefore, the action of

TNFα on stromal cells may occur by mediating the proliferative effects of IL-8. The expression of type I and type II receptors for TNFα was observed in endometriotic stromal cells. This evidence suggests that TNFα action mediated by IL-8 may not only be an initiating factor that facilitates adhesion of endometrial cells to the peritoneum, but may also contribute to the development and progression of endometriosis.

We found that the extent of superficial red endometriotic lesions was related to increased levels of IL-6, IL-8, and TNFα in the PF [21]. Red lesions, such as red flame-like lesions, gland-like lesions, and red vesicles, were classified as active lesions of endometriosis because angiogenesis is more pronounced in red lesions than in black or white lesions and because early red lesions invade the ECM. Thus, cytokines may play a role in the early stage of endometriosis.

Hepatocyte growth factor (HGF) was originally characterized as a potent mitogen for adult hepatocytes. HGF is known as a mesenchymal (stromal)-derived pleiotropic growth factor that elicits mitogenic and morphogenic activities on various types of epithelial cells, usually as a paracrine factor [80, 81]. In normal uterine endometrium, stromal-derived HGF promotes proliferation, migration, and lumen formation of endometrial epithelial cells [82]. Overexpression of Met, the receptor for HGF, was observed in several malignant tumors, such as uterine endometrium and ovary [83]. We also showed that the peritoneum and endometriotic stromal cells may be major sources of HGF in peritoneal fluid. Endometrial and endometriotic stromal cells expressed the Met receptor, which was activated by endogenous and exogenous HGF [84]. HGF enhanced stromal cell proliferation and invasion. We also demonstrated that the HGF-stimulated stromal cell invasion was due in part to the induction of urokinase-type plasminogen activator, a member of the extracellular proteolysis system. HGF increased in PF and produced by endometrial stromal cells may induce critical changes in morphology of mesothelial cells and then enhance the endometrial cell attachment and invasion.

7.3.3.4 Infertility

Pelvic endometriosis is frequently associated with infertility even if affected women ovulate and have functional, patent tubes. The exact mechanism by which endometriosis interferes with fertility is not fully understood. A recent study suggests that cytokines are related to infertility in women with endometriosis [2]. Since the ovaries and fallopian tubes are bathed in PF, substances present in PF have the potential to impact greatly on the reproductive function by affecting tubal motility, ovum pickup, or ovulation. It is speculated that a substance or substances from endometriotic tissues enter the PF, interfering with the reproductive process. Interleukin-6, a pleiotropic cytokine produced by a variety of cell types, plays a pivotal role as a mediator of numerous physiologic and pathogenic processes.

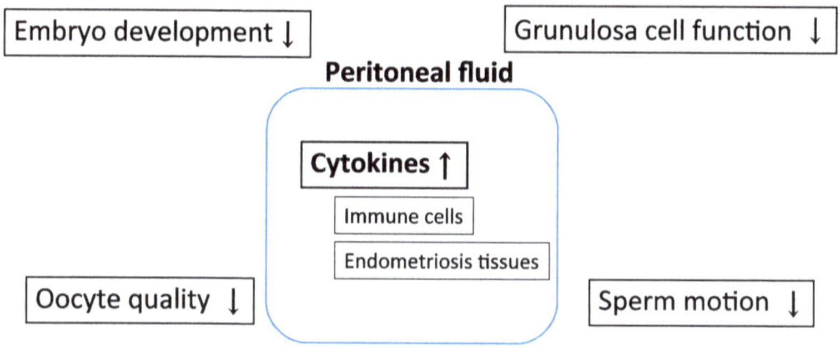

Fig. 7.2 Pathophysiology of endometriosis-associated infertility

It has also been suggested that IL-6 has important functions in reproductive physiology, including the regulation of ovarian steroid production, folliculogenesis, and early events related to implantation [85]. We demonstrated that the addition of human recombinant IL-6 to culture medium suppressed the rate of blastocyst formation of mouse embryos, suggesting that increased IL-6 in the PF of endometriosis patients may contribute to infertility by adversely affecting embryonic development [86]. Recently, Banerjee J et al. showed that IL-6 caused the deterioration in morphology of the microtubule and chromosomal alignment in metaphase-II mouse oocytes [87]. IL-6, generated in the process of oxidative stress, directly affects the quality of the oocyte and may contribute to infertility.

We used a steroidogenic human granulosa-like tumor cell line, KGN cells, as a model for granulosa cells collected during the follicular phase [88]. We demonstrate that IL-6 may reduce aromatase activity and E_2 production via the MAPK signal pathway in human granulosa cells [89]. The results may support the notion that IL-6 is related to impaired estrogen biosynthesis in patients with endometriosis.

Half of the cause of infertility is the male factor. The key predictors of fertilization capability are sperm count and motility. We showed that IL-6 and sIL-6R significantly reduced the percentage of motile and rapidly moving sperm [90]. The inhibition of sperm motility by IL-6 may be involved in the infertility of at least some patients with endometriosis who have highly elevated levels of IL-6 in PF. PF diffusing into the tubal and endometrial environment may affect the sperm and their interaction with the oocyte and embryo development. Many authors have demonstrated that the PF of patients with endometriosis has detrimental effects on several steps of the reproductive process.

These findings suggest that endometriotic implants, which can produce various cytokines, may contribute to reduced fecundity in patients with endometriosis. The role of PF and cytokines in the pathophysiology of endometriosis-associated infertility is summarized in Fig. 7.2. However, data on cytokines and their role in infertility are still incomplete, and future investigation that can reveal the critical roles of cytokines is still needed.

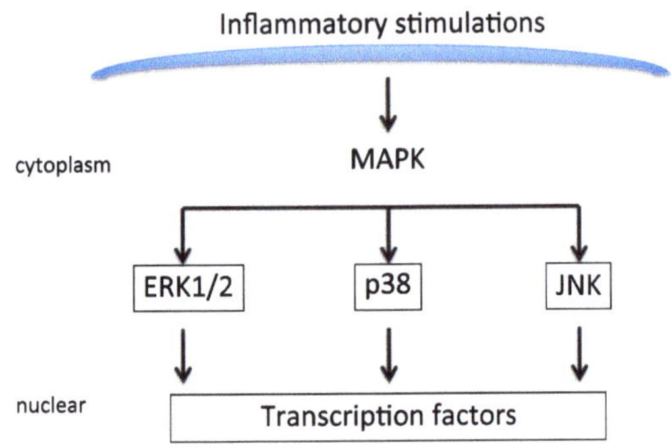

Fig. 7.3 Signal transduction of MAPK pathway

7.3.4 Signal Transduction in Endometriotic Cells

Signal transduction is defined as the response of a cell to the application of an external stimulus. Numerous factors, including cytokines, hormonal factors, genetic predisposition, environmental toxins, and immunological dysfunction, may contribute to the aberrant progression of endometriotic tissue.

7.3.4.1 MAPK Pathway

Many studies have demonstrated that MAPK is involved directly in regulating the pathogenesis of endometriosis [91–93]. MAPK pathways seem to play a pivotal role as intracellular and extracellular signal transducers in endometriotic cells. In the MAPK pathway, the activation of p38, c-jun N-terminal kinase (JNK), and ERK1/2 is important for inflammatory cytokine secretion in endometriotic stromal cells. The most extensively studied mitogen-activated protein kinase (MAPK) pathway is the extracellular signal-regulated kinase (ERK) pathway in which the MAPKKK is Raf, the MAPKK is MEK, and the MAPK is ERK. The activation of the MAPK pathway induced by TNFα through Ras, Raf, MEK, and ERK also affected the activation of AP-1 (Fig. 7.3). We showed that TNFα induced the activation of the signal molecule ERK1/2 of the MAPK cascade in endometriotic cells [94].

Recent studies have shown that p38 mitogen-activated protein kinase (p38 MAPK), an intracellular signal-transducing molecule, plays an important role in the regulation of a variety of inflammatory responses, including expression of proinflammatory cytokines, leukocyte adhesion, and chemotaxis. A number of studies indicated that the p38 MAPK pathway might play an important role in the development and progression of endometriosis [94]. Increased p38 MAPK activation in eutopic and ectopic endometrium indicated that p38 MAPK might be one of the main factors regulating the inflammatory process in endometriosis [95–97]. Yoshino et al. revealed that FR 167653, a p38 mitogen-activated protein kinase inhibitor, inhibits the development of endometriosis, possibly by suppressing peritoneal inflammatory status [98]. Zhou et al. also demonstrated that SB203580, a p38 mitogen-activated protein kinase inhibitor, may suppress the development

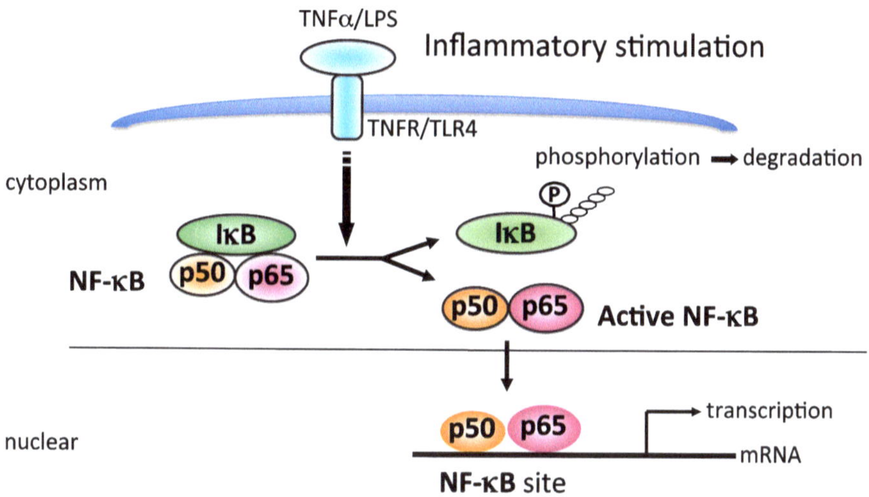

Fig. 7.4 Signal transduction of NF-κB pathway

of EM by inhibiting the expression of proinflammatory cytokines and proteolytic factors. p38 MAPK might play a key role in the progression of endometriosis [99]. These findings suggest that estrogen might to some extent exert its effects on the endometrium through the p38 MAPK pathway.

Many studies have demonstrated that MAPK is involved directly in regulating the pathogenesis of endometriosis. MAPK pathways seem to play a pivotal role as intracellular and extracellular signal transducers in the pathogenesis of endometriosis.

7.3.4.2 NF-kappaB Pathway

Nuclear factor-kappaB (NF-κB) is a family of transcription factors modulating hundreds of genes involved in inflammation, cell proliferation, apoptosis, invasion, angiogenesis, and other cell processes [100]. Therefore, accurate monitoring of NF-κB activation in target cells is crucial to investigating its signal transduction. NF-κB is composed of homo- and heterodimers of five members of the Rel family including p50, p52, p65, RelB, and c-Rel. NF-κB dimers are sequestered in the cytosol of unstimulated cells via noncovalent interactions with a class of inhibitor proteins, called IkBs. NF-κB is normally bound to IκB in cytosol; this binding prevents its movement into the nucleus. Proinflammatory stimuli activate the IκB kinase (IKK) complex and NF-κB essential modulator. Activated IKK phosphorylates IκB, resulting in its polyubiquitination and degradation. The degradation of IκB exposes the nuclear localization signal of NF-κB, resulting in the translocation of the p50/p65 NF-κB dimer to the nucleus in which it can be bound to NF-κB recognition elements in the promoter of proinflammatory cytokines such as TNFα, IL-6, and IL-8 (Fig. 7.4). We demonstrated that NF-κB activation has been involved in the induction of IL-8 in endometriotic tissues [101].

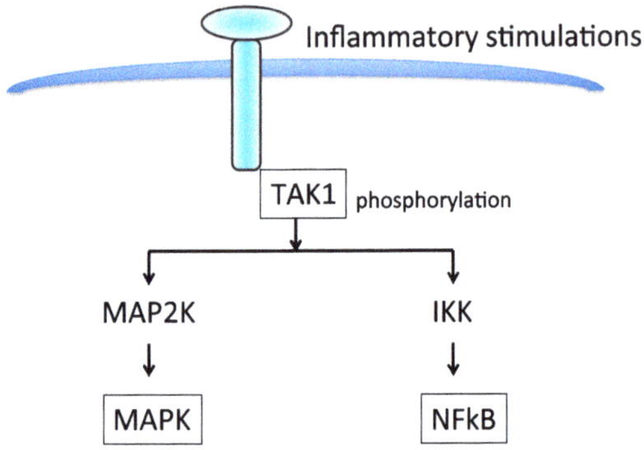

Fig. 7.5 Mechanism of signal transduction by the TAK1 cascade

Multiple publications have strongly suggested participation of the NF-κB pathway in endometriosis pathophysiology. In vitro studies have shown positive regulation of growth factors and proinflammatory and antiapoptotic proteins mediated by NF-κB activation in human endometrial and endometriotic cells [102, 103]. In vivo research in animal models treated with NF-κB inhibitors has revealed reduction of endometriosis development by diminishing inflammation and cell proliferation and inducing apoptosis of endometriotic cells [104, 105]. Constitutive activation of NF-κB was shown to be increased in red endometriotic lesions relative to black endometriotic lesions in women, and iron-mediated NF-κB activation in pelvic macrophages and endometriotic cells has been proposed as a possible mechanism contributing to endometriosis establishment and maintenance [106]. Thus, NF-κB pathways seem to play a pivotal role in the pathophysiology of endometriosis.

TAK1, a serine/threonine kinase, is an essential intracellular signaling component in inflammatory signaling pathways [107]. TAK1 has proven to be a crucial factor in regulating inflammatory responses by controlling production and function of various other cytokines. An accumulation of evidence suggests that TAK1 plays an important role as a second messenger in the activation of NF-κB, p38, and JNK. The activation of TAK1, which works on the TNFα-inducible phosphorylation of both the NF-κB and MAPK pathways, may be indispensable for inflammatory response and progression of endometriosis. TAK1 has been widely accepted as a regulator of the rapid activation of JNK/p38 MAPKs and IκB kinase signaling pathways in response to cellular stimuli (Fig. 7.5).

We showed that TNFα and its downstream TAK1, which are key mediators for NF-κB and MAPK pathways, may be involved in the pathogenesis of endometriosis [108].

7.4 Conclusion

Pathogenesis of endometriosis is very complex, so various factors and directions of studies were needed. Cytokines, which are produced by many cell types in PF, play a diverse role in constructing the peritoneal environment that induces the development and progression of endometriosis. Intense basic research into the specific role of these cells and soluble factors may improve our understanding of endometriosis and result in novel therapeutic modalities for endometriosis.

References

1. Cullen TS. The distribution of adenomyomata containing uterine mucosa. Am J Obstet Gynecol. 1919;80:130–8.
2. Harada T, Iwabe T, Terakawa N. Role of cytokines in endometriosis. Fertil Steril. 2001;76:1–10.
3. D'Hooghe TM, Debrock S. Endometriosis, retrograde menstruation and peritoneal inflammation in women and in baboon. Human Reprod Update. 2002;8:84–8.
4. Eskenazi B, Warner M. Epidemiology of endometriosis. Obstet Gynecol Clin North Am. 1997;24:235–58.
5. Sampson JA. Peritoneal endometriosis due to menstrual dissemination of endometrial tissue into the pelvic cavity. Am J Obstet Gynecol. 1927;14:422–69.
6. Liu D, Hitchcock A. Endometriosis: its association with retrograde menstruation, dysmenorrhoea and tubal pathology. Br J Obstet Gynaecol. 1986;93:859–62.
7. Kruitwagen R, Poels L, Willemsen W, de Ronde IJY, Jap PHK, Rolland R. Endometrial epithelial cells in peritoneal fluid during the early follicular phase. Fertil Steril. 1991;55:297–303.
8. Oosterlynck DJ, Cornillie FJ, Waer M, Vandeputte M, Koninckx PR. Women with endometriosis show a defect in natural killer activity resulting in a decreased cytotoxicity to autologous endometrium. Fertil Steril. 1991;56:45–51.
9. Khan KN, Kitajima M, Hiraki K, Yamaguchi N, Katamine S, Matsuyama T, Nakashima M, Fujishita A, Ishimaru T, Masuzaki H. *Escherichia coli* contamination of menstrual blood and effect of bacterial endotoxin on endometriosis. Fertil Steril. 2010;94:2860–3.
10. Iba Y, Harada T, Horie S, Deura I, Iwabe T, Terakawa N. Lipopolysaccharide-promoted proliferation of endometriotic stromal cells via induction of tumor necrosis factor alpha and interleukin-8 expression. Fertil Steril. 2004;82 Suppl 3:1036–42.
11. Maathuis JB, Van Lock PFA, Michie EA. Changes in volume, total protein and ovarian steroid concentrations of peritoneal fluid throughout the human menstrual cycle. J Endocrinol. 1978;76:123–33.
12. Syrop CH, Halme J. Cyclic changes of peritoneal fluid parameters in normal and infertile patients. Obstet Gynecol. 1987;69:416–8.
13. Syrop CH, Halme J. Peritoneal fluid environment and infertility. Fertil Steril. 1987;48:1–9.
14. Taketani Y, Kuo TM, Mizuno M. Comparison of cytokine levels and embryo toxicity in peritoneal fluid in infertile women with untreated or treated endometriosis. Am J Obstet Gynecol. 1992;167:265–70.
15. Hsu CC, Yang BC, Wu MH, Huang KE. Enhanced interleukin-4 expression in patients with endometriosis. Fertil Steril. 1997;67:1059–64.
16. Koyama N, Matsuura K, Okamura H. Cytokines in the peritoneal fluid of patients with endometriosis. Int J Gynecol Obstet. 1993;43:45–50.
17. Buyalos RP, Funari VA, Azziz R, Watson JM, Martinez-Maza O. Elevated interleukin-6 levels in peritoneal fluid of patients with pelvic pathology. Fertil Steril. 1992;58:302–6.
18. Rier SE, Zarmakoupis PN, Hu X, Becker JL. Dysregulation of interleukin-6 responses in ectopic endometrial stromal cells: correlation with decreased soluble receptor levels in peritoneal fluid of women with endometriosis. J Clin Endocrinol Metab. 1995;80:1431–7.

19. Keenan JA, Chen TT, Chadwell NL, Torry DS, Caudle MR. Interferon-gamma and interleukin-6 in peritoneal fluid and macrophage-conditioned media of women with endometriosis. Am J Reprod Immunol. 1994;32:180–3.
20. Punnonen J, Teisala K, Ranta H, Bennett B, Punonnen R. Increased levels of interleukin-6 and interleukin-10 in the peritoneal fluid of patients with endometriosis. Am J Obstet Gynecol. 1996;174:1522–6.
21. Harada T, Yoshioka H, Yoshida S, Iwabe T, Onohara Y, Tanikawa M, Terakawa N. Increased interleukin-6 levels in peritoneal fluid of infertile patients with active endometriosis. Am J Obstet Gynecol. 1997;176:593–7.
22. Ryan IP, Tseng JF, Schriock ED, Khorram O, Landers DV, Taylor RN. Interleukin-8-concentrations are elevated in peritoneal fluid of women with endometriosis. Fertil Steril. 1995;63:929–32.
23. Arici A, Tazuke SI, Attar E, Kliman HJ, Olive DL. Interleukin-8 concentration in peritoneal fluid of patients with endometriosis and modulation of interleukin-8 expression in human mesothelial cells. Mol Hum Reprod. 1996;2:40–5.
24. Iwabe T, Harada T, Tsudo T, Tanikawa M, Onohara Y, Terakawa N. Pathogenetic significance of increased levels of interleukin-8 in peritoneal fluid of patients with endometriosis. Fertil Steril. 1998;69:924–30.
25. Ho HN, Wu MY, Chao KH, Chen CD, Chen SU, Yang YS. Peritoneal interleukin-10 increases with decrease in activated CD41 T lymphocytes in women with endometriosis. Hum Reprod. 1997;12:2528–33.
26. Tagashira Y, Taniguchi F, Harada T, Ikeda A, Watanabe A, Terakawa N. Interleukin-10 attenuates TNF-alpha-induced interleukin-6 production in endometriotic stromal cells. Fertil Steril. 2009;91(5 Suppl):2185–92.
27. Zeyneloglu HB, Senturk LM, Seli E, Bahtiyar OM, Olive DL, Arici A. The peritoneal fluid levels of interleukin-12 in women with endometriosis. Am J Reprod Immunol. 1998;39:152–6.
28. Mazzeo D, Vigano P, Di Blasio AM, Sinigaglia F, Vignali M, Panina BP. Interleukin-12 and its free p40 subunit regulate immune recognition of endometrial cells: potential role in endometriosis. J Clin Endocrinol Metab. 1998;83:911–6.
29. McLaren J, Dealthy G, Prentice A, Charnock-Jones DS, Smith SK. Decreased levels of the potent regulator of monocyte/macrophage activation, interleukin-13, in the peritoneal fluid of patients with endometriosis. Hum Reprod. 1997;12:1307–10.
30. Zhang X, Xu H, Lin J, Qian Y, Deng L. Peritoneal fluid concentrations of interleukin-17 correlate with the severity of endometriosis and infertility of this disorder. BJOG. 2005;112:1153–5.
31. Antinolo G, Fernandez RM, Noval JA, Garcia-Lozano JC, Borrego S, Marcos I, Molini JL. Evaluation of germline sequence variants within the promoter region of RANTES gene in a cohort of women with endometriosis from Spain. Mol Hum Reprod. 2003;9:491–5.
32. Santulli P, Even M, Chouzenoux S, Millischer AE, de Borghese B, Ziegler D, Batteux F, Chapron C. Profibrotic interleukin-33 is correlated with uterine leiomyoma tumour burden. Hum Reprod. 2013;27:2001–9.
33. Khorram O, Taylor RN, Ryan IP, Schall TJ, Landers DV. Peritoneal fluid concentrations of the cytokine RANTES correlate with the severity of endometriosis. Am J Obstet Gynecol. 1993;169:1545–9.
34. Akoum A, Lemay A, Brunet C, Hebert J. Cytokine-induced secretion of monocyte chemotactic protein-1 by human endometriotic cells in culture. The Groupe d'Investigation en Gynecologie. Am J Obstet Gynecol. 1995;172:594–600.
35. Akoum A, Lemay A, McColl S, Turcot Lemay L, Maheux R. Elevated concentration and biologic activity of monocyte chemotactic protein-1 in the peritoneal fluid of patients with endometriosis. Fertil Steril. 1996;66:17–23.
36. Arici A, Oral E, Attar E, Tazuke SI, Olive DL. Monocyte chemotactic protein-1 concentration in peritoneal fluid of women with endometriosis and its modulation of expression in mesothelial cells. Fertil Steril. 1997;67:1065–72.

37. Fukaya T, Sugawara J, Yoshida H, Yajima A. The role of macrophage colony stimulating factor in the peritoneal fluid in infertile patients with endometriosis. Tohoku J Exp Med. 1994;172:221–6.
38. Oosterlynck D, Meuleman M, Waer M, Koninckx P. Transforming growth factor-b activity is increased in peritoneal fluid from women with endometriosis. Obstet Gynecol. 1994;83:287–92.
39. McLaren J, Prentice A, Charnock-Jones DS, Smith SK. Vascular endothelial growth factor (VEGF) concentrations are elevated in peritoneal fluid of women with endometriosis. Hum Reprod. 1996;11:220–3.
40. McLaren J, Prentice A, Charnock-Jones DS, Millican SA, Muller KH, Sharkey AM, Smith SK. Vascular endothelial growth factor is produced by peritoneal fluid macrophages in endometriosis and is regulated by ovarian steroids. J Clin Invest. 1996;98:482–9.
41. Tabibzadeh S, Santhanam V, Sehgel PB, May LT. Cytokine-induced production of IFN-b2 by freshly explanted human endometrial stromal cells. Modulation by estradiol-17b. J Immunol. 1989;142:3134–9.
42. Betjes MGH, Tuk CW, Struik DG, Kredict RT, Arisz L, Hart M, Beelen RH. Interleukin-8 production by human peritoneal mesothelial cells in response to tumor necrosis factor-a, interleukin-1, and medium conditioned by macrophages co-cultured with Staphylococcus epidermidis. J Infect Dis. 1993;168:1202–10.41.
43. Halme J, Becker S, Wing R. Accentuated cyclic activation of peritoneal macrophages in patients with endometriosis. Am J Obstet Gynecol. 1984;148:85–90.
44. Halme J, Becker S, Haskill S. Altered maturation and function of peritoneal macrophages: possible role in pathogenesis of endometriosis. Am J Obstet Gynecol. 1987;156:783–9.
45. Akoum A, Lemay A, Paradis I, Rheault N, Maheux R. Secretion of interleukin-6 by human endometriotic cells and regulation by proinflammatory cytokines and sex steroids. Hum Reprod. 1996;11:2269–75.
46. Tseng JF, Ryan IP, Milam TD, Murao JT, Schriock ED, Landers DV, et al. Interleukin-6 secretion in vitro is up-regulated in ectopic and eutopic endometrial stromal cells from women with endometriosis. J Clin Endocrinol Metab. 1996;81:1118–22.
47. Tsudo T, Harada T, Iwabe T, Tanikawa M, Nagano Y, Ito M, Terakawa N. Altered gene expression and secretion of interleukin-6 in stromal cells derived from endometriotic tissues. Fertil Steril. 2000;73:205–11.
48. Witz CA, Monotoya-Rodriguez IA, Schenken RS. Whole explants of peritoneum and endometrium: a novel model of the early endometriosis lesion. Fertil Steril. 1999;71:56–60.
49. Rosenfeld DL, Lecher BD. Endometriosis in a patient with Rokitansky- Kuster-Hauser syndrome. Am J Obstet Gynecol. 1981;139:105.
50. Ohtake H, Katabuchi H, Matsuura K, Okamura H. A novel in vitro experimental model for ovarian endometriosis. The three-dimensional culture of human ovarian surface epithelial cells in collagen gels. Fertil Steril. 1999;71:50–5.
51. van der Linden PJ, de Goeij AF, Dunselman GA, van der Linden EP, Ramaekers FL, Evers JL. Expression of integrins and E-cadherin in cells from menstrual effluent, endometrium, peritoneal fluid, peritoneum, and endometriosis. Fertil Steril. 1994;61:85–90.
52. Smith RE, Hogaboam CM, Strieter RM, Lukas NW, Kunkel SL. Cell-to-cell and cell-to-matrix interactions mediate chemokine expression: an important component of the inflammatory lesion. J Leukoc Biol. 1997;62:612–9.
53. Garcia-Velasco JA, Arici A. Interleukin-8 stimulates endometrial stromal cell adhesion to fibronectim. Fertil Steril. 1999;72:336–40.
54. Garcia-Velasco JA, Arici A. Interleukin-8 expression in endometrial stromal cells is regulated by integrin-dependent cell adhesion. Mol Hum Reprod. 1999;5:1135–40.
55. Wilson TJ, Munnery L, Hertzog PJ, Wood EC, Biotech DAM, Kola I. Decreased natural killer cell activity in endometriosis patients: relationship to disease pathogenesis. Fertil Steril. 1994;62:1086–8.

56. Kanzaki H, Wang HS, Kariya M, Mori T. Suppression of natural killer cell activity by sera from patients with endometriosis. Am J Obstet Gynecol. 1992;167:257–61.
57. Somigliana S, Vigano P, Gaffuri B, Guarneri D, Busacca M, Vigbali M. Human endometrial stromal cells as a source of soluble intercellular adhesion molecule (ICAM)-1 molecules. Hum Reprod. 1996;11:1190–4.
58. Fukaya T, Sugawara J, Yoshida H, Murakami T, Yajima A. Intercellular adhesion molecule-1 and hepatocyte growth factor in human endometriosis: original investigation and a review of literature. Gynecol Obstet Invest. 1999;47 Suppl 1:11–7.
59. Kobayashi M, Fitz L, Ryan M, Hewick RM, Clark SC, Chan S, et al. Identification and purification of natural killer cell stimulatory factor (NKSF), a cytokine with multiple biologic effects on human lymphocytes. J Exp Med. 1989;170:827–45.
60. Wysocka M, Kubin M, Vieira LQ, Ozmen L, Garotta G, Scott P, et al. Interleukin-12 is required for IFN- production and lethality in lipopolysaccharide- induced shock in mice. Eur J Immunol. 1995;25:672–6.
61. Somigliana S, Vigano P, Rossi G, Carinelli S, Vignali M, Panina-Bordignon P. Endometrial ability to implant in ectopic sites can be prevented by interleukin-12 in a murine model of endometriosis. Hum Reprod. 1999;14:2944–50.
62. Folkman J, Haudenschild C. Angiogenesis in vitro. Nature. 1980;288:551–6.
63. Folkman J. Clinical applications of research on angiogenesis. N Engl J Med. 1995;333:1757–64.
64. Subik P. Vascularization of tumors: a review. J Cancer Res Clin Oncol. 1982;103:211–26.
65. Oosterlynck DJ, Meuleman H, Sobis M, Vandeputte M, Koninckx PR. Angiogenic activity of peritoneal fluid from women with endometriosis. Fertil Steril. 1993;59:778–82.
66. Schadendorf D, Moller A, Algermissen B, Worm M, Sticherling M, Czarnetzki BM. IL-8 produced by human malignant melanoma cells in vitro in an essential autocrine growth factor. J Immunol. 1993;151:2667–75.
67. Yamanaka R, Tanaka R, Yoshida S, Saitoh T, Fujita K. Growth inhibition of human glioma cells modulated by retrovirus gene transfection with antisense IL-8. J Neurooncol. 1995;25:59–65.
68. Arici A, Seli E, Senturk LM, Gutierrez LS, Oral E, Taylor HS. Interleukin-8 in human endometrium. J Clin Endocrinol Metab. 1998;83:1783–7.
69. Arici A, Seli E, Zeyneloglu HB, Senturk LM, Oral E, Olive DL. Interleukin-8 induces proliferation of endometrial stromal cells: a potential autocrine growth factor. J Clin Endocrinol Metab. 1998;83:1201–5.
70. Iwabe T, Harada T, Tsudo T, Nagano Y, Tanikawa M, Terakawa N. Tumor necrosis factor-a promotes proliferation of the endometriotic stromal cells by inducing interleukin-8 gene and protein expression. J Clin Endocrinol Metab. 2000;85:824–9.
71. Wu MH, Lin SC, Hsiao KY, Tsai SJ. Hypoxia-inhibited dual-specificity phosphatase-2 expression in endometriotic cells regulates cyclooxygenase-2 expression. J Pathol. 2011;225:390–400.
72. Maybin JA, Barcroft J, Thiruchelvam U, Hirani N, Jabbour HN, Critchley HO. The presence and regulation of connective tissue growth factor in the human endometrium. Hum Reprod. 2012;27:1112–21.
73. Henriet P, Gaide Chevronnay HP, Marbaix E. The endocrine and paracrine control of menstruation. Mol Cell Endocrinol. 2012;358:197–207.
74. Becker CM, Beaudry P, Funakoshi T, Benny O, Zaslavsky A, Zurakowski D, Folkman J, D'Amato RJ, Ryeom S. Circulating endothelial progenitor cells are up-regulated in a mouse model of endometriosis. Am J Pathol. 2011;178:1782–91.
75. Lin YJ, Lai MD, Lei HY, Wing LY. Neutrophils and macrophages promote angiogenesis in the early stage of endometriosis in a mouse model. Endocrinology. 2006;147:1278–86.
76. Donnez J, Smoes P, Gillerot S, Casanas-Roux F, Nisolle M. Vascular endothelial growth factor (VEGF) in endometriosis. Hum Reprod. 1998;13:1686–90.

77. Ren QZ, Qian ZH, Jia SH, Xu ZZ. Vascular endothelial growth factor expression up-regulated by endometrial ischemia in secretory phase plays an important role in endometriosis. Fertil Steril. 2011;95:2687–9.
78. Goteri G, Lucarini G, Filosa A, Pierantoni A, Montik N, Biagini G, Fabris G, Ciavattini A. Immunohistochemical analysis of vascular endothelial growth factor cellular expression in ovarian endometriomata. Fertil Steril. 2004;81:1528–33.
79. Surrey ES, Halme J. Effect of peritoneal fluid from endometriosis patients on endometrial stromal cell proliferation in vitro. Obstet Gynecol. 1990;76:792–7.
80. Montesano R, Matsumoto K, Nakamura T, Orci L. Identification of a fibroblast-derived epithelial morphogen as hepatocyte growth factor. Cell. 1991;67:901–8.
81. Barros EJ, Santos OF, Matsumoto K, Makamura T, Nigam SK. Differential tubulogenic and branching morphogenetic activities of growth factors. Proc Natl Acad Sci U S A. 1995;92:4412–6.
82. Sugawara J, Fukaya T, Murakami T, Yoshida H, Yajima A. Hepatocyte growth factor stimulated proliferation, migration, and lumen formation of human endometrial epithelial cells in vitro. Biol Reprod. 1997;57:936–42.
83. Corps AN, Sowter HM, Smith SK. Hepatocyte growth factor stimulates motility, chemotaxis and mitogenesis in ovarian carcinoma cells expressing high levels of c-met. Int J Cancer. 1997;73:151–5.
84. Yoshida S, Harada T, Mitsunari M, Iwabe T, Sakamoto Y, Tsukihara S, Iba Y, Horie S, Terakawa N. Hepatocyte growth factor/Met system promotes endometrial and endometriotic stromal cell invasion via autocrine and paracrine pathways. J Clin Endocrinol Metab. 2004;89:823–32.
85. Tagoh H, Nishimoto N, Ogata A, Yoshizaki K. Multiplicity in the production and the function of IL-6. Clin Immunol. 1989;21:1225–41.
86. Iwabe T, Harada T, Terakawa N. Role of cytokines in endometriosis-associated infertility. Gynecol Obstet Invest. 2002;53 Suppl 1:19–25.
87. Banerjee J, Sharma R, Agarwal A, Maitra D, Diamond MP, Abu-Soud HM. IL-6 and mouse oocyte spindle. PLoS One. 2012;7:e35535.
88. Fujii A, Harada T, Yamauchi N, Iwabe T, Nishi Y, Yanase T, Nawata H, Terakawa N. Interleukin-8 expression is up-regulated by interleukin-1b in steroidogenic human granulosa-like cells. Fertil Steril. 2003;79:151–7.
89. Deura I, Harada T, Taniguchi F, Iwabe T, Izawa M, Terakawa N. Reduction of estrogen production by interleukin-6 in a human granulosa tumor cell line may have implications for endometriosis-associated infertility. Fertil Steril. 2005;83 Suppl 1:1086–92.
90. Yoshida S, Harada T, Iwabe T, Taniguchi F, Mitsunari M, Yamauchi N, Deura I, Horie S, Terakawa N. A combination of interleukin-6 and its soluble receptor impairs sperm motility: implications in infertility associated with endometriosis. Hum Reprod. 2004;19(8):1821–5.
91. Wu Y, Kajdacsy-Balla A, Strawn E, Basir Z, Halverson G, Jailwala P, Wang Y, Wang X, Ghosh S, Guo SW. Transcriptional characterizations of differences between eutopic and ectopic endometrium. Endocrinology. 2006;147:232–46.
92. Velarde MC, Aghajanova L, Nezhat CR, Giudice LC. Increased mitogen-activated protein kinase kinase/extracellularly regulated kinase activity in human endometrial stromal fibroblasts of women with endometriosis reduces 3′,5′-cyclic adenosine 5′-monophosphate inhibition of cyclin D1. Endocrinology. 2009;150:4701–12.
93. Matsuzaki S, Canis M, Vaurs-Barrière C, Pouly JL, Boespflug-Tanguy O, Penault-Llorca F, Dechelotte P, Dastugue B, Okamura K, Mage G. DNA microarray analysis of gene expression profiles in deep endometriosis using laser capture microdissection. Mol Hum Reprod. 2004;10:719–28.
94. Yamauchi N, Harada T, Taniguchi F, Yoshida S, Iwabe T, Terakawa N. Tumor necrosis factor-alpha induced the release of interleukin-6 from endometriotic stromal cells by the nuclear factor-kappaB and mitogen-activated protein kinase pathways. Fertil Steril. 2004;82 Suppl 3:1023–8.

95. Yoshino O, Osuga Y, Hirota Y, Koga K, Hirata T, Harada M, Morimoto C, Yano T, Nishii O, Tsutsumi O, Taketani Y. Possible pathophysiological roles of mitogen-activated protein kinases (MAPKs) in endometriosis. Am J Reprod Immunol. 2004;52:306–11.
96. Grund EM, Kagan D, Tran CA, Zeitvogel A, Starzinski-Powitz A, Nataraja S, Palmer SS. Tumor necrosis factor-alpha regulates inflammatory and mesenchymal responses via mitogen-activated protein kinase kinase, p38, and nuclear factor kappaB in human endometriotic epithelial cells. Mol Pharmacol. 2008;73:1394–404.
97. Lee DH, Kim SC, Joo JK, Kim HG, Na YJ, Kwak JY, Lee KS. Effects of 17β-estradiol on the release of monocyte chemotactic protein-1 and MAPK activity in monocytes stimulated with peritoneal fluid from endometriosis patients. J Obstet Gynaecol Res. 2012;38:516–25.
98. Yoshino O, Osuga Y, Koga K, Hirota Y, Hirata T, Ruimeng X, Na L, Yano T, Tsutsumi O, Taketani Y. FR 167653, a p38 mitogen-activated protein kinase inhibitor, suppresses the development of endometriosis in a murine model. J Reprod Immunol. 2006;72(1–2):85–93.
99. Zhou WD, Yang HM, Wang Q, Su DY, Liu FA, Zhao M, Chen QH, Chen QX. SB203580, a p38 mitogen-activated protein kinase inhibitor, suppresses the development of endometriosis by down-regulating proinflammatory cytokines and proteolytic factors in a mouse model. Hum Reprod. 2010;25:3110–6.
100. González-Ramos R, Defrère S, Devoto L. Nuclear factor-kappaB: a main regulator of inflammation and cell survival in endometriosis pathophysiology. Fertil Steril. 2012;98:520–8.
101. Sakamoto Y, Harada T, Horie S, Iba Y, Taniguchi F, Yoshida S, Iwabe T, Terakawa N. Tumor necrosis factor-alpha-induced interleukin-8 (IL-8) expression in endometriotic stromal cells, probably through nuclear factor-kappa B activation: gonadotropin-releasing hormone agonist treatment reduced IL-8 expression. J Clin Endocrinol Metab. 2003;88:730–5.
102. Ohama Y, Harada T, Iwabe T, Taniguchi F, Takenaka Y, Terakawa N. Peroxisome proliferator-activated receptor-gamma ligand reduced tumor necrosis factor-alpha-induced interleukin-8 production and growth in endometriotic stromal cells. Fertil Steril. 2008;89:311–7.
103. Horie S, Harada T, Mitsunari M, Taniguchi F, Iwabe T, Terakawa N. Progesterone and progestational compounds attenuate tumor necrosis factor alpha-induced interleukin-8 production via nuclear factor kappa B inactivation in endometriotic stromal cells. Fertil Steril. 2005;83:1530–5.
104. González-Ramos R, Van Langendonckt A, Defrère S, Lousse JC, Mettlen M, Guillet A, Donnez J. Agents blocking the nuclear factor-kappaB pathway are effective inhibitors of endometriosis in an in vivo experimental model. Gynecol Obstet Invest. 2008;65:174–86.
105. Takai E, Taniguchi F, Nakamura K, Uegaki T, Iwabe T, Harada T. Parthenolide reduces cell proliferation and prostaglandin E2 synthesis in human endometriotic stromal cells and inhibits development of endometriosis in the murine model. Fertil Steril. 2013;100(4):1170–8.
106. Defrère S, González-Ramos R, Lousse JC, Colette S, Donnez O, Donnez J, Van Langendonckt A. Insights into iron and nuclear factor-kappa B (NF-kappaB) involvement in chronic inflammatory processes in peritoneal endometriosis. Histol Histopathol. 2011;26:1083–92.
107. Ninomiya-Tsuji J, Kishimoto K, Hiyama A, Inoue J, Cao Z, Matsumoto K. The kinase TAK1 can activate the NIK-I kappaB as well as the MAP kinase cascade in the IL-1 signalling pathway. Nature. 1999;398:252–6.
108. Taniguchi F, Harada T, Miyakoda H, Iwabe T, Deura I, Tagashira Y, Miyamoto A, Watanabe A, Suou K, Uegaki T, Terakawa N. TAK1 activation for cytokine synthesis and proliferation of endometriotic cells. Mol Cell Endocrinol. 2009;307(1–2):196–204.

Chapter 8
Epigenetics in Endometriosis

Masao Izawa, Fuminori Taniguchi, and Tasuku Harada

Abstract There is accumulating evidence supporting the concept that endometriosis is a disease associated with an epigenetic disorder. Epigenetics is one of the most expanding fields in the current biomedical research. The word "epigenetics" refers to the study of mitotically and/or meiotically heritable changes in gene expression that occur without changes in the DNA sequence. The disruption of such changes (epigenetic aberration or disorder) underlies a wide variety of pathologies. Epigenetic regulation includes DNA methylation and histone modifications and is responsible for a number of gene transcriptions associated with chromatin modifications that distinguish the states of diseases. As an introduction, we summarize our findings of epigenetic disorder in endometriotic cells and then overview recent studies focused on DNA methylation in endometriosis. We describe our recent challenge and advanced studies from other laboratories using genome-wide (GW) analysis. Finally, we refer to environmental factors as a potential background of epigenetic disorder in endometriosis.

Keywords Aberrant DNA methylation • Aberrant histone modification • Aberrant transcription • Epigenetic disorder

8.1 Why Epigenetics in Endometriosis?

Epigenetics is one of the most promising and expanding fields in the current biomedical research. The word "epigenetics" refers to the study of mitotically and/or meiotically heritable changes in gene expression that occur without changes in the DNA sequence [1]. The disruption of such changes (epigenetic aberration or

M. Izawa, Ph.D. (✉) • F. Taniguchi • T. Harada
Department of Obstetrics and Gynecology, Tottori University Faculty of Medicine,
36-1 Nishi-cho, Yonago 683-8504, Japan
e-mail: 1mizawa@med.tottori-u.a.jp

T. Harada (ed.), *Endometriosis: Pathogenesis and Treatment*,
DOI 10.1007/978-4-431-54421-0_8, © Springer Japan 2014

disorder) underlies a wide variety of pathologies including cancer [2, 3]. Epigenetic regulation includes DNA methylation and histone modifications [4, 5] and is responsible for a number of gene transcriptions associated with chromatin modifications that distinguish the various cell types and the states of diseases. Cancer and many other diseases show aberrant epigenetic regulation [6]. In terms of DNA methylation, cancer cells show genome-wide (GW) hypomethylation and site-specific hypermethylation of promoter CpG islands [2]. This may lead to transcriptional silencing and aberrant transcription from incorrect transcription start sites [4]. In addition, a recent study comparing colorectal cancer tissue with its normal counterpart suggests changes at the CpG island shores [7]. In normal cells, CpG islands and CpG island shores are under the control of physiological methylation, allowing normal gene transcription.

There is accumulating evidence supporting the concept that endometriosis is an epigenetic disease [8]. The concept of aberrant DNA methylation in endometriosis is expanding [9]. Here we describe how the field of epigenetics is reshaping the current thinking about endometriosis. Firstly, we present our study shedding light on aberrant aromatase expression in endometriosis from the viewpoint of epigenetic disorder and then summarize recent advances in endometriosis research using the epigenetic approach. We subsequently describe the advanced technologies of GW methylation analysis and GW association study (GWAS) in endometriosis research. Finally, we refer to environmental factors as a potential background of epigenetic disorder in endometriosis.

8.2 Estrogen Environment in Endometriosis

Endometriotic tissue growth depends on ovarian steroids; thus, medical treatments aim to reduce ovarian steroidogenesis. Continuous exposure to GnRH agonist results in desensitization or downregulation of GnRH receptors leading to reduced serum gonadotropin levels and reduced ovarian hormone production. Treating endometriosis with GnRH agonist reduces both the number of observable endometriotic implants and the frequency and severity of associated pain [10, 11]. Likewise, inhibition of estrogen production by progestins or aromatase inhibitors reduces endometriotic lesions and clinical symptoms [12]. Three major sites for estrogen production are recognized in women with endometriosis: (a) *de novo* synthesis in the ovary, (b) an intrinsic system that depends on aromatase, which converts circulating androstenedione to estradiol (*intracrine*) in the skin and adipose tissue, and (c) a *de novo* system and an *intracrine* system in endometriotic tissues [13, 14]. Among these sites, local estrogen production, which depends on aberrantly expressed aromatase in endometriotic implants, plays an important role in the pathophysiology of endometriosis [15–17]. Local estrogen production by these implants may contribute to the progression of endometriosis even under the hypoestrogenic environment produced by GnRH agonist exposure [17].

8.2.1 Aromatase Upregulation in Endometriosis

Aromatase, an enzyme that catalyzes the conversion of androgens to estrogens, is a key molecule for estrogen production. Aromatase is encoded by a single-copy gene *CYP19* on chromosome 15q21. *CYP19* expression is regulated in a tissue-specific manner, in which alternative usage of multiple promoters with each unique *cis*-acting element has been known [18]. Therefore, identifying the promoter usage becomes the first step in understanding the molecular background of aromatase expression in specific tissues. Bulun et al. previously reported that promoter II is the most potent promoter functioning in endometriotic cells from endometrioma [17]. In addition to promoter II, we recently demonstrated that two proximal promoters, I.3 and I.6, are used additionally in endometriotic cells [14]. At the same time, we observed that aromatase transcription in endometrial cells was at a marginal level depending on the same 3 promoters as those of endometriotic cells [14]. From these observations, we hypothesized that the upregulation of aromatase gene in endometriotic cells may be an epigenetic disorder, since hypermethylation of promoter region in tumor suppressor gene associated with gene silencing has been known.

8.2.2 DNA Demethylation and Aromatase Upregulation in Endometriotic Cells

An epigenetic disorder may lead to the aromatase upregulation in endometriotic cells. We challenged this hypothesis: after treating endometrial cells with 5-aza-deoxycytidine (5-aza-dC, competitive inhibitor for DNA methyltransferase) for 96 h, aromatase transcription was markedly upregulated in the cells (Fig. 8.1). This is the first demonstration that epigenetic modification enhances aromatase mRNA expression [14]. The enhanced aromatase mRNA expression was dependent on the same promoters as those in endometriotic cells (Fig. 8.2). When the effect of trichostatin A (TSA), instead of 5-aza-dC, on aromatase mRNA expression was examined, we observed little effect, suggesting that one of the major factors that suppresses aromatase mRNA expression in endometrial cells is the methylation of aromatase gene and/or its *trans*-acting factor gene. Alternatively, the observation suggests that a disorder of a putative methylation-dependent suppression mechanism may lead to the upregulation of aromatase mRNA expression in endometriotic cells.

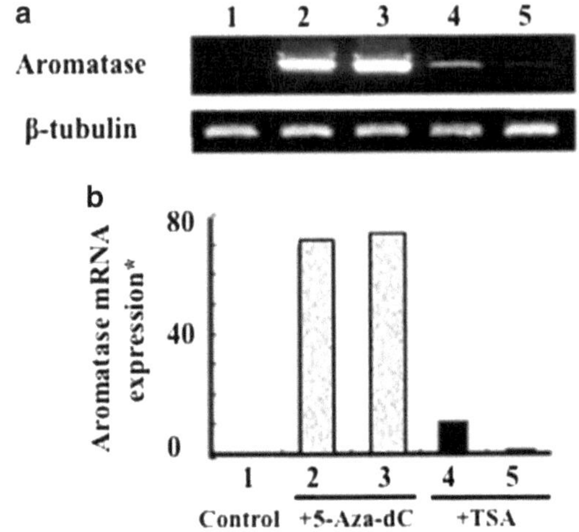

Fig. 8.1 Aromatase mRNA induction in response to 5-aza-dC in endometrial cells. (**a**) RT-PCR: lane 1, untreated control, lanes 2 and 3, treated with 5-aza-dC, and lanes 4 and 5, treated with TSA. (**b**) Semiquantitative analysis

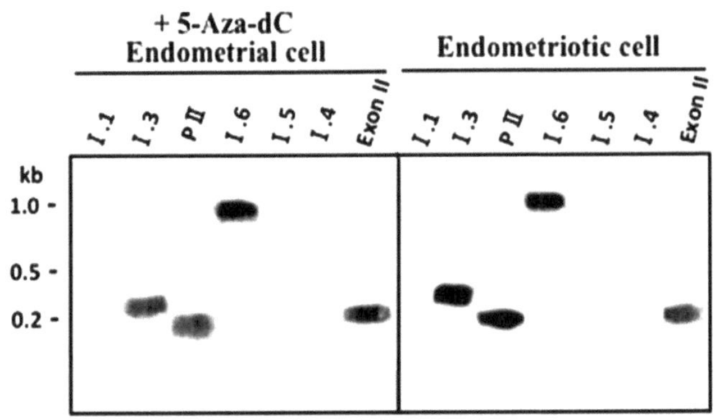

Fig. 8.2 Promoter usage of aromatase mRNA expression. *Left*: 5-aza-dC-treated endometrial cells. *Right*: endometriotic cells

8.2.3 Hypomethylated CpG Island Within the Aromatase Gene in Endometriotic Cells

We searched for the unmethylated CpG locus within the aromatase gene in endometriotic cells [19]. We predicted a CpG island at approximately 20 kb upstream from the end of exon II (Fig. 8.3). In endometriotic cells, the CpG sequence was hypomethylated, while in endometrial cells, the upstream half was hypermethylated and recognized by the methyl-CpG binding proteins, MBD1 and MeCP2 [19]. The downstream half was hypomethylated in both endometrial and endometriotic cells. Because the CpG sequence is located at the promoter-distal region, we speculate that the sequence may act as a *cis*-acting element under the control of methylation.

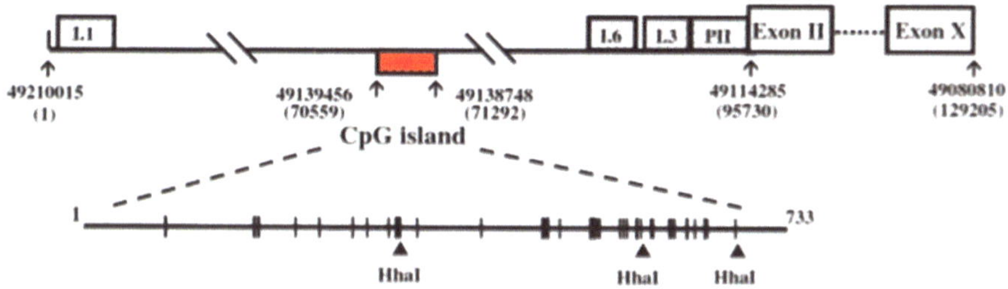

Fig. 8.3 A hypomethylated CpG island at 20 kb upstream from the end of exon II in endometriotic cells

8.3 Nuclear Receptor Genes Under Epigenetic Aberration in Endometriosis

Estrogen receptor (ER) plays pivotal roles in the pathogenesis and progression of endometriosis. Earlier studies have focused on the expression of ERα as well as ERβ in the eutopic endometrium and in endometriotic lesions. Simultaneous expression of ERα and ERβ indicates that the estrogen action might be transmitted in a cooperative manner [20, 21]. In contrast to the high ERα/ERβ expression ratio in the eutopic endometrium, a lower expression of ERα and a markedly higher expression of ERβ in ovarian endometriomas have been reported [22, 23]. The higher ERβ expression in endometriotic tissue may depend on the hypomethylation of the ERβ-promoter region [24]. The increased ERβ expression in endometriotic tissues may suppress ERα expression [25].

8.3.1 ERβ Gene: Hypomethylation and Upregulation

That the development and progression of endometriosis depends on estrogen is well known [26, 27]. ERα and ERβ function as transcription factors and are believed to play key roles in tissue growth of endometrium and endometrioma [22, 23]. Previous studies demonstrated markedly higher levels of ERβ and lower levels of ERα in endometriotic tissues and endometriotic stromal cells [21–23]. Differences in the ERα/ERβ ratio between endometriotic and endometrial stromal cells are suggested to have important functional implications [24]. Recently, Xue et al. [24] demonstrated that the ERβ promoter is hypomethylated in endometriotic cells. Hypomethylation caused the higher expression of ERβ gene in endometriotic cells, while hypermethylation silenced the expression in endometrial cells. Treatment with a demethylating agent significantly increased ERβ mRNA expression in endometrial cells. They proposed that enhanced ERβ transcription in endometriotic cells takes over the ERα promoter activity, thus favoring the suppression of ERα levels [25].

8.3.2 Progesterone Receptor (PR) Gene: Hypermethylation and Downregulation

Progesterone induces differentiation of endometrial stromal cells to decidualized cells and glandular epithelial cells to the secretory phenotype. Representative molecular markers of progesterone action include increased production of epithelial glycodelin and stromal prolactin in the endometrium [28, 29]. Progesterone resistance is known as a feature in some endometriosis and can be attributed to the low level of PR in endometriotic tissue [30–32]. PR-A and PR-B forms are expressed in the stromal and epithelial components of the endometrium [32]. In the endometrium, expressions of PR-A and PR-B are progressively upregulated during the proliferative phase to their highest level immediately before ovulation, and diminish thereafter, suggesting that estradiol stimulates PR expression [25]. PR level may be related to the responsiveness to progesterone in patients [33, 34]. Wu et al. [35] have shown that the promoter region of PR-B is hypermethylated in endometriosis, which may lead to the PR-B downregulation. They recently showed that prolonged stimulation of TNF-α induced partial methylation in the promoter region of PR-B associated with decreased expression of PR-B in an immortalized epithelial-like endometriotic cell line [36]. This seems to provide evidence that phenotypic changes in endometriosis, such as chronic inflammation associated with increased production of proinflammatory cytokines, may cause epigenetic aberrations leading to changes in gene expression [37].

8.4 Other Genes Under Epigenetic Aberration in Endometriosis

8.4.1 Steroidogenic Factor-1 (SF-1) Gene: Hypomethylation and Upregulation

SF-1 is a transcriptional factor essential for the activation of multiple steroidogenic genes for estrogen biosynthesis, such as the genes for steroid acute regulatory (StAR) and aromatase [38–40]. SF-1 is usually undetectable in eutopic endometrial cells [41]. It has been demonstrated that SF-1 mRNA and protein levels in endometriotic cells were significantly higher than those in eutopic endometrial cells [40, 41]. Xue et al. identified a classical CpG island at the promoter region of the SF-1 gene and showed that the SF-1 promoter has increased methylation in eutopic endometrial cells [41]. In endometrial cells, the silencer-type transcription factor MBD2 is recruited to the methylated SF-1 promoter and prevents its interaction with transcriptional activators, resulting in silencing of the SF-1 gene. On the other hand, the SF-1 promoter is hypomethylated in endometriotic cells. Steroidogenic factor-2 (SF-2), a transcription factor highly expressed in endometriotic tissues, binds to the unmethylated SF-1 promoter and activates its transcription in endometriotic cells [42]. The SF-1 expression is under epigenetic control that permits the binding of activator complexes to the SF-1 promoter [41, 42]. SF-1 expression in endometriosis may enhance aromatase expression. Treatment with a demethylating agent has been shown to increase SF-1 mRNA levels in eutopic endometrial cells [26].

8.4.2 E-Cadherin Gene: Hypermethylation and Downregulation

Downregulation of E-cadherin, a known metastasis-suppressor protein in epithelial tumor cells [43], has been shown in endometriotic cells [44]. In two immortalized endometriotic cell lines, the E-cadherin gene was found to be hypermethylated at the promoter region, and treatment with a histone deacetylase inhibitor TSA induced expression [45]. Interestingly, the increased promoter methylation of the E-cadherin gene during aging has been demonstrated [46].

8.4.3 HOXA10 Gene: Hypermethylation and Downregulation

HOXA10 has been expressed in the endometrium, and its expression is under the control of estrogen and progesterone [46–48]. The roles in endometrial development during the menstrual cycle and in establishing uterine receptivity have been suggested [47, 48]. In women with endometriosis, HOXA10 expression is significantly decreased in the eutopic endometrium during the secretory phase, indicating functional defects in uterine receptivity [47, 49]. The promoter region of HOXA10 gene was found to be hypermethylated in the eutopic endometrium from women with endometriosis [50]. As promoter hypermethylation has been suggested as an epigenetic marker of gene silencing, the promoter hypermethylation may be related to the HOXA10 downregulation in the eutopic endometrium of women with endometriosis [47].

8.5 Genome-Wide (GW) Profiling of DNA Methylation and GW Association Study (GWAS) in Endometriosis

Methylation of DNA provides a layer of epigenetic controls that has important implications for diseases including endometriosis. There has been a revolution in DNA methylation analysis technology. Analyses can now be performed on a

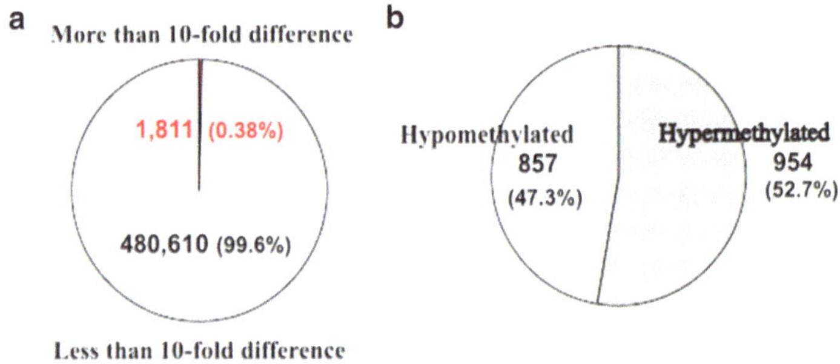

Fig. 8.4 Differentially methylated CpGs in endometriotic cells (**a**) CpGs, which show more than 10-fold difference, were extracted (**b**) the classification

genome-scale and entire methylomes can be characterized at single-base-pair resolution [51]. In endometriosis, a number of aberrant gene expressions have been demonstrated [52, 53]. These aberrations may be related to aberrant DNA methylations. However, it is unknown whether global alterations in DNA methylation patterns occur in endometriosis and to what extent they are involved in its pathogenesis. A whole-genome scanning of CpG methylation status in more than 25,000 promoters has been conducted previously [54]. The results showed highly similar methylation profiles between endometrium and endometriotic lesions. Recently, a new generation of genome-wide DNA methylation BeadChip array including 485,577 CpGs (Infinium HumanMethylation450 BeadChip Array) has been developed [55, 56]. The array covers more than 99 % of human genes and 96 % of CpG islands. Using the array, we recently identified 1,811 CpGs (0.38 %) differentially methylated not only in the promoter region but also in promoter-distal CpGs (Fig. 8.4) [57]. Among them, 954 CpGs (52.7 %) were hypermethylated, while 857 CpGs (47.3 %) were hypomethylated in endometriotic cells. The results indicate that the overall methylation profile in endometriotic cells was highly similar to that in endometrial cells. The observation supports the retrograde menstruation theory by Sampson [58] for the pathogenesis of endometriosis. It is important to note that the CpGs hypomethylated or hypermethylated in endometriotic cells were demonstrated not always in promoter CpG islands. These observations show a facet of epigenetic disorder in endometriosis.

Through a GWAS and a replication study using a total of 1,907 Japanese individuals with endometriosis and 5,292 controls, a significant association of endometriosis with rs10965235 ($P = 5.57 \times 10(-12)$, odds ratio = 1.44), which is located in CDKN2BAS on chromosome 9p21, encoding the cyclin-dependent kinase inhibitor 2B antisense RNA was identified [59]. The findings suggest that these regions are susceptible loci for endometriosis. A GWAS was performed using two case-control cohorts genotyped with the Affymetrix Mapping 500K Array or Genome-Wide Human SNP Array 6.0 in Japanese women with endometriosis [60]. A GWAS in 3,194 individuals with surgically confirmed endometriosis and 7,060 controls from Australia and the UK was conducted [61]. The strongest association signal was reported on 7p15.2 (rs12700667) for endometriosis. rs12700667 is located in an intergenic region upstream of the plausible candidate genes NFE2L3 and HOXA10.

8.6 Epigenetic Aberrations and Environmental Factors in Endometriosis

The known epigenetic modifications are DNA methylation and histone modifications, including methylation, acetylation, ubiquitylation, and phosphorylation [62]. The functional and biological significance of the epigenetic alterations accumulate over a life span. The earliest studies found a pattern of low global DNA methylation levels in aged mammalian tissues [63]. A recent monozygotic (MZ) twin study showed a line of evidence that epigenetic variants accumulate during aging independently of the genetic sequence [64]. The study tested the epigenetic contribution to twin discordance and elucidated the effect of environmental characteristics on gene function. The results revealed that epigenetic difference between siblings is associated with phenotypic discordance, which might be attributed to an unshared environment.

8.6.1 Effect of Environmental Factors on Epigenome

The association between environmental factors and phenotypic discordance within MZ twins has been noticed [64]. However, little is known about the molecular basis by which environmental factors influence gene functions [65]. Typical examples are the abnormal intrauterine environment associated with epigenetic downregulation of genes [66, 67] and the maternal diet associated with the DNA methylation profile of offspring [68–70]. Gene function and chromatin structure can be modulated by environmental factors [71, 72]. In response to a methyl-deficient diet, a significant decrease in repressive dimethyl-H3K9 associated with the upregulation of targeted gene was demonstrated in mice [73]. Environmental factors, including endocrine disrupting chemicals, may affect the epigenome leading to the onset of endometriosis in utero. There might be epigenetic changes during ontogenic development [74, 75].

8.6.2 DNA Methylation, Aging, and Endometriosis

The great fidelity with which DNA methylation patterns in mammals are inherited after each cell division is ensured by the DNA methyltransferases (DNMTs).

However, the aging cell undergoes a DNA methylation drift. Early studies showed that global DNA methylation decreases during aging in many tissue types [63]. The loss of global DNA methylation during aging is probably mainly the result of the passive demethylation of DNA as a consequence of a progressive loss of DNMT activity [76]. Several specific regions of the genomic DNA become hypermethylated during aging [77]. Methylation of promoter CpG islands in nontumorigenic tissues has been reported for several genes, including ER [77]. Interestingly, genes with increased promoter methylation during aging include the E-cadherin gene [46], which is downregulated and hypermethylated in endometriotic cells [65]. Aberrant methylation of CpG islands in 5′ promoters has been suggested to be associated with transcriptional silencing or upregulation in endometriosis [24, 33, 36, 50]. Recent GW methylation studies suggest that tissue- and cell-type-specific methylation is present only in a small percentage of CpG islands in 5′ promoters, while a far greater proportion of CpG island methylation is across gene bodies [78, 79]. In addition, functionally different types of DNA modification, methylation, and hydroxymethylation have been identified [78, 80]. Therefore, methylation of CpG islands in 5′ promoters alone may not be a major player in the aberrant gene expression.

8.6.3 Histone Modification, Aging, and Endometriosis

Histone modifications have a defined profile during aging. For example, the trimethylation of H4-K20, which is enriched in differentiated cells [81], increases with age [82, 83] and decreases in cancer cells [83–87]. A decrease in the histone trimethylation has been observed in the liver after the long-term treatment with the hepatocarcinogen tamoxifen [88]. The loss of trimethylated H4-K20 in cancer can be caused by the loss of expression of the H4-K20-specific methyltransferase Suv4-20h [74]. Although approximately 100 histone methyltransferases and demethylases have been identified in human genome, only a subset of histone methyltransferase inhibitor is in clinical trials for cancer treatment [89].

Acetylation levels of histones are controlled by a balance between histone acetyltransferases and histone deacetylases (HDACs). Histone acetyltransferases transfer acetyl groups from acetyl-CoA to lysine residues on the amino-terminal region of histones and activate gene transcription. Conversely, HDACs restore the positive charge on lysine residues by removing the acetyl groups and prevent transcription. HDACs comprise large multiprotein complexes that target promoter sites through their interaction with sequence-specific transcription sites. HDAC inhibitors (HDACIs) can inhibit cell proliferation, induce cell differentiation and cell cycle arrest, and stimulate apoptosis of various cell types [90]. Hyperacetylation of histones H3 and H4 is often associated with activated transcription, and hypoacetylation of histones H3 and H4 correlates with transcriptional silencing or repression [91]. Kawano et al. [92] recently demonstrated that treatment with HDACIs induced the accumulation of acetylated histones associated with some cell cycle-related gene expressions in endometriotic cells. The advanced human epigenome projects [51, 93] may provide further insight into understanding epigenetic aberrations in endometriosis.

8.7 Conclusion

Epigenetics is one of the most promising and expanding fields in the current biomedical research of diseases including endometriosis. Most important is its translational application. One of the immediate questions to be clarified in endometriosis is which genome is under epigenetic aberration. Here we focused mostly on DNA methylation and reviewed current epigenetics studies in endometriosis.

Epigenetics is currently expanding from DNA methylation to histone modifications (Fig. 8.5) [94]. The development of high-throughput technologies including

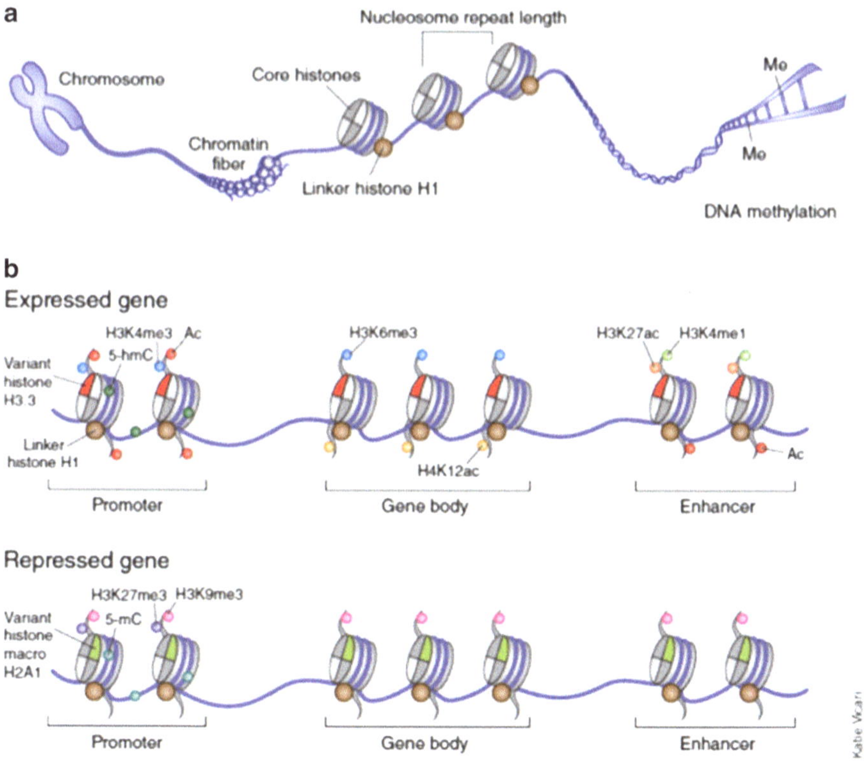

Fig. 8.5 Organization and composition of epigenome. (**a**) A "beads-on-a-string" chromatin fiber includes nucleosome cores connected by linker DNA and linker histone H1. *Me*: methyl group. (**b**) The distribution of DNA methylation and a small subset of histone markings, linker histones, and core histone variants represent a different regulation at active promoters, gene bodies, and enhancers (*top*) as compared to silenced and repressed chromatin (*bottom*)

GW analysis associated with next-generation sequencer is accelerating the study of epigenetic aberration in endometriosis. Using the epigenetic concept as a tool, new diagnostic marker or therapy may be developed to overcome serious problems in patients with endometriosis.

Acknowledgment This work was supported in part by Grants-in-Aid for Scientific Research (C) from Japan Society for the Promotion of Science (Nos. 22591824 and 18591800 to M.I.).

References

1. Berger SL, Kouzarides T, Shiekhattar R, Shilatifard A. An operational definition of epigenetics. Genes Dev. 2009;23:781–3.
2. Esteller M. Epigenetics in cancer. N Engl J Med. 2008;358:1148–59.
3. Jones PA, Baylin BS. The epigenomics of cancer. Cell. 2007;128:683–92.
4. Rodríguez-Paredes M, Esteller M. Cancer epigenetics reaches mainstream oncology. Nat Med. 2011;17:330–9.
5. Li G, Reinberg D. Chromatin higher-order structures and gene regulation. Curr Opin Genet Dev. 2011;21:175–86.
6. Esteller M. Cancer epigenomics: DNA methylomes and histone-modification maps. Nat Rev Genet. 2007;8:286–98.
7. Irizarry RA, Ladd-Acosta C, Wen B, Wu Z, Montano C, Onyango P, Cui H, Gabo K, Rongione M, Webster M, Ji H, Potash JB, Sabunciyan S, Feinberg AP. The human colon cancer methylome shows similar hypo- and hypermethylation at conserved tissue-specific CpG island shores. Nat Genet. 2009;41:178–86.
8. Guo S-W. Epigenetics of endometriosis. Mol Hum Reprod. 2009;15:587–607.
9. Nasu K, Kawano Y, Tsukamoto Y, Takano M, Takai N, Li H, Furukawa Y, Abe W, Moriyama M, Narahara H. Aberrant DNA methylation status of endometriosis: epigenetics as the pathogenesis, biomarker and therapeutic target. J Obstet Gynaecol Res. 2011;37:683–95.
10. Dlugi AM, Miller JD, Knittle J. Lupron depot (leuprolide acetate for depot suspension) in the treatment of endometriosis: a randomized, placebo-controlled, double blind study. Fertil Steril. 1990;54:419–27.
11. Shaw RW. An open randomized comparative study of the effect of goserelin depot and danazol in the treatment of endometriosis. Fertil Steril. 1992;58:265–72.
12. Olive DL, Pritts EA. Treatment of endometriosis. N Engl J Med. 2001;345:266–75.
13. Bulun SE, Imir G, Utsunomiya H, Thung S, Gurates B, Tamura M, Lin Z. Aromatase in endometriosis and leiomyomata. J Steroid Biochem Mol Biol. 2005;95:57–62.
14. Izawa M, Harada T, Ohama Y, Takenaka Y, Taniguchi F, Terakawa N. An epigenetic disorder may cause aberrant expression of aromatase gene in endometriotic stromal cells. Fertil Steril. 2008;89:1390–6.
15. Noble LS, Simpson ER, Johns A, Bulun SE. Aromatase expression in endometriosis. J Clin Endocrinol Metab. 1996;81:174–9.
16. Kitawaki J, Noguchi T, Amatsu T, Maeda K, Tsukamoto K, Yamamoto T, Fushiki S, Osawa Y, Honjo H. Expression of aromatase cytochrome P450 protein and messenger ribonucleic acid in human endometriotic and adenomyotic tissues but not in normal endometrium. Biol Reprod. 1997;57:514–9.
17. Bulun SE, Zeitoun K, Takayama K, Noble L, Michael D, Simpson E, Johns A, Putman M, Sasano H. Estrogen production in endometriosis and use of aromatase inhibitors to treat endometriosis. Endocr Relat Cancer. 1999;6:293–301.

18. Simpson ER, Michael MQ, Agarwal VR, Hinshelwood MM, Bulun SE, Zhao Y. Expression of the CYP19 (aromatase) gene: An unusual case of alternative promoter usage. FASEB J. 1997;11:29–36.
19. Izawa M, Taniguchi F, Uegaki T, Takai E, Iwabe T, Terakawa N, Harada T. Demethylation of a nonpromoter cytosine-phosphate-guanine island in the aromatase gene may cause the aberrant up-regulation in endometriotic tissues. Fertil Steril. 2011;95:33–9.
20. Chang EC, Charn TH, Park S-H, Helferich WG, Komm B, Katzenellenbogen JA, Katzenellenbogen BS. Estrogen Receptors alpha and beta as determinants of gene expression: influence of ligand, dose, and chromatin binding. Mol Endocrinol. 2008;22:1032–43.
21. Charn TH, Liu T-B, Chang EC, Lee YK, Katzenellenbogen JA, Katznellenbogen BS. Genome-wide dynamics of chromatin binding of estrogen receptors α and β:mutual restriction and competitive site selection. Mol Endocrinol. 2010;24:47–59.
22. Fujimoto J, Hirose R, Sakaguchi H, Tamaya T. Expression of oestrogen receptor-alpha and -beta in ovarian endometriomata. Mol Hum Reprod. 1999;5:742–7.
23. Brandenberger AW, Lebovic DI, Tee MK, Ryan IP, Tseng JF, Jaffe RB, Taylor RN. Oestrogen receptor (ER)-alpha and ER-beta isoforms in normal endometrial and endometriosis-derived stromal cells. Mol Hum Reprod. 1999;5:651–5.
24. Xue Q, Lin Z, Cheng YH, Huang CC, Marsh E, Yin P, Milad MP, Confino E, Reierstad S, Innes J, Bulun SE. Promoter methylation regulates estrogen receptor 2 in human endometrium and endometriosis. Biol Reprod. 2007;77:681–7.
25. Trukhacheva E, Lin Z, Reierstad S, Cheng YH, Milad M, Bulun SE. Estrogen receptor (ER) beta regulates ERalpha expression in stromal cells derived from ovarian endometriosis. J Clin Endocrinol Metab. 2009;94:615–22.
26. Bulun SE, Lin Z, Imir G, Amin S, Demura M, Yilmaz B, Martin R, Utsunomiya H, Thung S, Gurates B, Tamura M, Langoi D, Deb S. Regulation of aromatase expression in estrogen-responsive breast and uterine disease: from bench to treatment. Pharmacol Rev. 2005;57:359–83.
27. Attar E, Bulun SE. Aromatase and other steroidogenic genes in endometriosis: Translational aspects. Hum Reprod Update. 2006;12:49–56.
28. Brosens JJ, Hayashi N, White JO. Progesterone receptor regulates decidual prolactin expression in differentiating human endometrial stromal cells. Endocrinology. 1999;140:4809–20.
29. Fazleabas AT, Brudney A, Chai D, Langoi D, Bulun SE. Steroid receptor and aromatase expression in baboon endometriotic lesions. Fertil Steril. 2003;80:820–7.
30. Bulun SE, Cheng YH, Yin P, Imir G, Utsunomiya H, Attar E, Innes J, Kim JJ. P: Progesterone resistance in endometriosis: Link to failure to metabolize estradiol. Mol Cell Endocrinol. 2006;248:94–103.
31. Lessey BA, Metzger DA, Haney AF, McCarty Jr KS. Immunohistochemical analysis of estrogen and progesterone receptors in endometriosis: Comparison with normal endometrium during the menstrual cycle and the effect of medical therapy. Fertil Steril. 1989;51:409–15.
32. Attia GR, Zeitoun K, Edwards D, Johns A, Carr BR, Bulun SE. Progesterone receptor isoform A but not B is expressed in endometriosis. J Clin Endocrinol Metab. 2000;85:2897–902.
33. Lee B, Du H, Taylor HS. Experimental murine endometriosis induces DNA methylation and altered gene expression in eutopic endometrium. Biol Reprod. 2009;80:79–85.
34. Vercellini P, Cortesi I, Crosignani PG. Progestins for symptomatic endometriosis: A critical analysis of the evidence. Fertil Steril. 1997;68:393–401.
35. Wu Y, Strawn E, Basir Z, Halverson G, Guo S-W. Promoter hypermethylation of progesterone receptor isoform B (PR-B) in endometriosis. Epigenetics. 2006;1:106–11.
36. Wu Y, Starzinski-Powitz A, Guo S-W. Prolonged stimulation with tumor necrosis factor-alpha induced partial methylation at PR-B promoter in immortalized epithelial-like endometriotic cells. Fertil Steril. 2008;90:234–7.
37. Wu Y, Shi X, Guo S-W. The knockdown of progesterone receptor isoform B (PR-B) promotes proliferation in immortalized endometrial stromal cells. Fertil Steril. 2008;90:1320–3.

38. Rice DA, Mouw AR, Bogerd AM, Parker KL. A shared promoter element regulates the expression of three steroidogenic enzymes. Mol Endocrinol. 1991;5:1552–61.
39. Morohashi K, Honda S, Inomata Y, Handa H, Omura T. A common trans-acting factor, Ad4-binding protein, to the promoters of steroidogenic P-450 s. J Biol Chem. 1992;267:17913–9.
40. Zeitoun K, Takayama K, Michael MD, Bulun SE. Stimulation of aromatase P450 promoter (II) activity in endometriosis and its inhibition in endometrium are regulated by competitive binding of steroidogenic factor-1 and chicken ovalbumin upstream promoter transcription factor to the same cis-acting element. Mol Endocrinol. 1999;13:239–53.
41. Xue Q, Lin Z, Yin P, Milad MP, Chen YH, Confino E, Reierstad S, Bulun SE. Transcriptional activation of steroidogenic factor-1 by hypomethylation of the 5′ CpG island in endometriosis. J Clin Endocrinol Metab. 2007;92:3261–7.
42. Utsunomiya H, Cheng YH, Lin Z, Reierstad S, Yin P, Attar E, Que Q, Imir G, Thung S, Trukhacheva E, Suzuki T, Sasano H, Kim JJ, Yaegashi N, Bulun SE. Upstream stimulatory factor-2 regulates steroidogenic factor-1 expression in endometriosis. Mol Endocrinol. 2008;22:904–14.
43. Frixen UH, Behrens J, Sachs M, Eberle G, Voss B, Warda A, Löchner D, Birchmeier W. E-cadherin-mediated cell-cell adhesion prevents invasiveness of human carcinoma cells. J Cell Biol. 1991;113:173–85.
44. Starzinski-Powitz A, Gaetje R, Zeitvogel A, Kotzian S, Handrow-Metzmacher H, Herrmann G, Fanning E, Baumann R. Tracing cellular and molecular mechanisms involved in endometriosis. Hum Reprod Update. 1998;4:724–9.
45. Wu Y, Starzinski-Powitz A, Guo S-W. Trichostatin A, a histone deacetylase inhibitor, attenuates invasiveness and reactivates E-cadherin expression in immortalized endometriotic cells. Reprod Sci. 2007;14:374–82.
46. Bornman DM, Mathew S, Alsruhe J, Herman JG, Gabrielson E. Methylation of the E-cadherin gene in bladder neoplasia and in normal urothelial epithelium from elderly individuals. Am J Pathol. 2001;159:831–5.
47. Taylor HS, Bagot C, Kardana A, Olive D, Arici A. HOX gene expression is altered in the endometrium of women with endometriosis. Hum Reprod. 1999;14:1328–31.
48. Taylor HS, Arici A, Olive D, Igarashi P. HOXA10 is expressed in response to sex steroids at the time of implantation in the human endometrium. J Clin Invest. 1998;101:1379–84.
49. Gui Y, Zhang J, Yuan L, Lessey BA. Regulation of HOXA-10 is and its expression in normal and abnormal endometrium. Mol Hum Reprod. 1999;5:866–73.
50. Wu Y, Halverson G, Basir Z, Strawn E, Yan P, Guo S-W. Aberrant methylation at HOXA10 may be responsible for its aberrant expression in the endometrium of patients with endometriosis. Am J Obstet Gynecol. 2005;193:371–80.
51. Laird PW. Principles and challenges of genome-wide DNA methylation analysis. Nat Rev Genet. 2010;11:191–203.
52. Arimoto T, Katagiri T, Oda K, Tsunoda T, Yasugi T, Osuga Y, Yoshikawa H, Nishii O, Yano T, Taketani Y, Nakamura Y. Genome-wide cDNA microarray analysis of gene-expression profiles involved in ovarian endometriosis. Int J Oncol. 2003;22:551–60.
53. Matsuzaki S, Canis M, Vaurs-Barriere C, Pouly JL, Boespflug-Tanguy O, Penault-Llorca F, Dechelotte P, Dastugue B, Okamura K, Mage G. DNA microarray analysis of gene expression profiles in deep endometriosis using laser capture microdissection. Mol Hum Reprod. 2004;10:719–28.
54. Borghese B, Barbaux S, Mondon F, Santulli P, Pierre G, Chapron G, Vaimin D. Genome-wide profiling of methylated promoters in endometriosis reveals a subtelomeric location of hypermethylation. Mol Endocrinol. 2010;24:1872–85.
55. Bibikova M, Barnes B, Tsan C, Ho V, Klotzle B, Le JM, Delano D, Zhang L, Schroth GP, Gunderson KL, Fan JB, Shen R. High density DNA methylation array with single CpG site resolution. Genomics. 2011;98:288–95.

56. Sandoval J, Heyn H, Moran S, Serra-Musach J, Pujana MA, Bibikova M, Esteller M. Validation of a DNA methylation microarray for 450,000 CpG sites in the human genome. Epigenetics. 2011;6(6):692–702.
57. Izawa M, Taniguchi F, Harada T. Genome-wide profiling of DNA methylation in endometriotic cells. J Endometriosis. 2012;4:147.
58. Sampson JA. Peritoneal endometriosis due to menstrual dissemination of endometrial tissue into the peritoneal cavity. Am J Obstet Gynecol. 1927;14:422–69.
59. Uno S, Zembutsu H, Hirasawa A, Takahashi A, Kubo M, Akahane T, Aoki D, Kamatani N, Hirata K, Nakamura Y. A genome-wide association study identifies genetic variants in the CDKN2BAS locus associated with endometriosis in Japanese. Nat Genet. 2010;42:707–10.
60. Adachi S, Tajima A, Quan J, Haino K, Yoshihara K, Masuzaki H, Katabuchi H, Ikuma K, Suginami H, Nishida N, Kuwano R, Okazaki Y, Kawamura Y, Sasaki T, Tokunaga K, Inoue I, Tanaka K. Meta-analysis of genome-wide association scans for genetic susceptibility to endometriosis in Japanese population. J Hum Genet. 2010;55:816–21.
61. Painter JN, Anderson CA, Nyholt DR, Macgregor S, Lin J, Lee SH, Lambert A, Zhao ZZ, Roseman F, Guo Q, Gordon SD, Wallace L, Henders AK, Visscher PM, Kraft P, Martin NG, Morris AP, Treloar SA, Kennedy SH, Missmer SA, Montgomery GW, Zondervan KT. Genome-wide association study identifies a locus at 7p15.2 associated with endometriosis. Nat Genet. 2011;43:51–4.
62. Jenuwein T, Allis CD. Translating the histone code. Science. 2001;293:1074–80.
63. Wilson VL, Jones PA. DNA methylation decreases in aging but not in immortal cells. Science. 1983;220:1055–7.
64. Fraga MF, Ballestar E, Paz MF, Ropero S, Setien F, Ballestar ML, Heine-Suñer D, Cigudosa JC, Urioste M, Benitez J, Boix-Chornet M, Sanchez-Aguilera A, Ling C, Carlsson E, Poulsen P, Vaag Z, Stephan A, Spector TD, Wu YZ, Plass C, Esteller M. Epigenetic differences arise during the lifetime of monozygotic twins. Proc Natl Acad Sci U S A. 2005;102:10604–9.
65. Petronis A. Epigenetics and twins: three variations on the theme. Trends Genet. 2006;22:347–50.
66. Simmons R. Developmental origins of adult metabolic disease: concepts and controversies. Trends Endocrinol Metab. 2005;16:390–4.
67. Gordon L, Joo JH, Andronikos R, Ollikainen M, Wallace EM, Umstad MP, Permezel M, Oshlack A, Morley R, Carlin JB, Saffery R, Smyth GK, Craig JM. Expression discordance of monozygotic twins at birth: effect of intrauterine environment and a possible mechanism for fetal programming. Epigenetics. 2011;6:579–92.
68. Lillycrop KA, Phillips ES, Jackson AA, Hanson MA, Burdge GC. Dietary protein restriction of pregnant rats induces and folic acid supplementation prevents epigenetic modification of hepatic gene expression in the offspring. J Nutr. 2005;135:1382–6.
69. Lillycrop KA. Effect of maternal diet on the epigenome: implications for human metabolic disease. Proc Nutr Soc. 2011;70:64–72.
70. Barnes SK, Ozanne SE. Pathways linking the early environment to long-term health and lifespan. Prog Biophys Mol Biol. 2011;106:323–36.
71. Feil R. Environmental and nutritional effects on the epigenetic regulation of genes. Mutat Res. 2006;600:46–57.
72. Jaenisch R, Bird A. Epigenetic regulation of gene expression: how the genome integrates intrinsic and environmental signals. Nat Genet. 2003;33:245–54.
73. Dobosy JR, Fu VX, Desotelle JA, Srinivasan R, Kenowski ML, Almassi N, Weindruch R, Svaren J, Jarrard DF. A methyl-deficient diet modifies histone methylation and alters Igf2 and H19 repression in the prostate. Prostate. 2008;68:1187–95.
74. Czyz W, Morahan JM, Ebers GC, Ramagopalan SV. Genetic, environmental and stochastic factors in monozygotic twin discordance with a focus on epigenetic differences. BMC Med. 2012;10:93.

75. Cortessis VK, Thomas DC, Levine AJ, Breton CV, Mack TM, Siegmund KD, Haile RW, Laird PW. Environmental epigenetics: prospects for studying epigenetic mediation of exposure-response relationships. Hum Genet. 2012;131:1565–89.
76. Casillas Jr MA, Lopatina N, Andrews LG, Tollefsbol TO. Transcriptional control of the DNA methyltransferases is altered in aging and neoplastically-transformed human fibroblasts. Mol Cell Biochem. 2003;252:33–43.
77. Issa JP. Age-related epigenetic changes and the immune system. Clin Immunol. 2003;109:103–8.
78. Maunakea AK, Nagarajan RP, Bilenky M, Ballinger TJ, D'Souza C, Fouse SD, Johnson BE, Hong C, Nielsen C, Zhao Y, Turecki G, Delaney A, Varhol R, Thiessen N, Shchors K, Heine VM, Rowitch DH, Xing X, Fiore C, Schillebeeckx M, Jones SJM, Haussler D, Marra MA, Hirst M, Wang T, Costello JF. Conserved role of intragenic DNA methylation in regulating alternative promoters. Nature. 2010;466:253–7.
79. Shenker N, Flanagan JM. Intragenic DNA methylation: implication of this epigenetic mechanism for cancer research. Br J Cancer. 2012;106:248–53.
80. Song CX, Szulwach KE, Fu Y, Dai Q, Yi C, Li X, Li Y, Chen CH, Zhang W, Jian X, Wang J, Zhang L, Looney TJ, Zhang B, Godley LA, Hicks LM, Lahn BT, Jin P, He C. Selective chemical labeling reveals the genome-wide distribution of 5-hydroxymethylcytosine. Nat Biotechnol. 2011;29:68–72.
81. Biron VL, McManus KJ, Hu N, Hendzel MJ, Underhill DA. Distinct dynamics and distribution of histone methyl-lysine derivatives in mouse development. Dev Biol. 2004;276:337–51.
82. Prokocimer M, Margalit A, Gruenbaum Y. The nuclear lamina and its proposed roles in tumorigenesis: projection on the hematologic malignancies and future targeted therapy. J Struct Biol. 2006;155:351–60.
83. Sarg B, Koutzamani E, Helliger W, Rundquist I, Lindner HH. Postsynthetic trimethylation of histone H4 at lysine 20 in mammalian tissues is associated with aging. J Biol Chem. 2002;277:39195–201.
84. Olins DE, Olins AL. Granulocyte heterochromatin: defining the epigenome. BMC Cell Biol. 2005;6:39.
85. Fraga MF, Ballestar E, Villar-Garea A, Boix-Chornet M, Espada J, Schotta G, Bonaldi T, Haydon C, Ropero S, Petrie K, Iyer NG, Pérez-Rosado A, Calvo E, Lopez JA, Cano A, Calasanz MJ, Colomer D, Piris MA, Ahn N, Imhof A, Caldas C, Jenuwein T, Esteller M. Loss of acetylation at Lys16 and trimethylation at Lys20 of histone H4 is a common hallmark of human cancer. Nat Genet. 2005;37:391–400.
86. Pogribny IP, Ross SA, Tryndyak VP, Pogribna M, Poirier LA, Karpinets TV. Histone H3 lysine 9 and H4 lysine 20 trimethylation and the expression of Suv4-20 h2 and Suv-39 h1 histone methyltransferases in hepatocarcinogenesis induced by methyl deficiency in rats. Carcinogenesis. 2006;27:1180–6.
87. Tryndyak VP, Kovalchuk Q, Pogribny IP. Loss of DNA methylation and histone H4 lysine 20 trimethylation in human breast cancer cells is associated with aberrant expression of DNA methyltransferase 1, Suv4-20h2 histone methyltransferase and methyl-binding proteins. Cancer Biol Ther. 2006;5:65–70.
88. Tryndyak VP, Muskhelishvili L, Kovalchuk O, Rodriguez-Juarez R, Montgomery B, Churchwell MI, Ross SA, Beland FA, Pogribny IP. Effect of long-term tamoxifen exposure on genotoxic and epigenetic changes in rat liver: implications for tamoxifen-induced hepatocarcinogenesis. Carcinogenesis. 2006;27:1713–20.
89. Peter CJ, Akbarian S. Balancing histone methylation activities in psychiatric disorders. Trends Mol Med. 2011;17:372–9.
90. Takai N, Narahara H. Human endometrial and ovarian cancer cells: histone deacetylase inhibitors exhibit antiproliferative activity, potently induce cell cycle arrest, and stimulate apoptosis. Curr Med Chem. 2007;14:2548–53.
91. Norton VG, Imai BS, Yau P, Bradbury EM. Histone acetylation reduces nucleosome core particle linking number change. Cell. 1989;57(449–457).

92. Kawano Y, Nasu K, Li H, Tsuno A, Abe W, Takai N, Narahara H. Application of the histone deacetylase inhibitors for the treatment of endometriosis: histone modifications as pathogenesis and novel therapeutic target. Hum Reprod. 2011;26:2486–98.
93. Eckhardt F, Lewin J, Cortese R, Rakyan VK, Attwood J, Burger M, Burton J, Cox TV, Davies R, Down TA, Haefliger C, Horton R, Howe K, Jackson DK, Kunde J, Koenig C, Liddle J, Niblett D, Otto T, Pettett R, Seemann S, Thompson C, West T, Rogers J, Olek A, Berlin K, Beck S. DNA methylation profiling of human chromosomes 6, 20 and 22. Nat Genet. 2006;38:1378–85.
94. Jakovcevski M, Akbarian S. Epigenetic mechanisms in neurological disease. Nat Med. 2012;18:1194–204.

Chapter 9
Roles of Prostaglandin E_2 in Endometriosis

Kuei-Yang Hsiao, Meng-Hsing Wu, and Shaw-Jenq Tsai

Abstract Endometriosis is one of the most common gynecological diseases, affecting approximately 10 % of women in reproductive age. It is characterized as the presence of endometrial-like glands and stroma outside the uterus, commonly on the pelvic peritoneum and ovaries. The major symptoms of endometriosis include pelvic pain, dysmenorrhea, dyspareunia, and infertility. During the past decade, intensive investigations on molecular mechanisms responsible for the pathological processes of endometriosis have been conducted. Although many factors have been reported to be involved in these processes, prostaglandin E_2 (PGE_2) no doubt represents as one of the most critical regulators of all. Accumulating data demonstrate that PGE_2 controls many critical functions, such as steroidogenesis, angiogenesis, proliferation, and immune suppression that contribute to the pathogenesis of endometriosis. Herein, we will summarize the most up-to-date information regarding the functional roles of PGE_2 in the development and maintenance of endometriosis.

Keywords Angiogenesis • Hypoxia • Macrophage • Phagocytosis • Proliferation • Prostaglandin • Steroidogenesis • Stromal cells

K.-Y. Hsiao • S.-J. Tsai, Ph.D. (✉)
Department of Physiology, College of Medicine, National Cheng Kung University, 1 University Road, Tainan 70101, Taiwan
e-mail: seantsai@mail.ncku.edu.tw

M.-H. Wu
Department of Obstetrics and Gynecology, College of Medicine, National Cheng Kung University, 1 University Road, Tainan 70101, Taiwan

T. Harada (ed.), *Endometriosis: Pathogenesis and Treatment*,
DOI 10.1007/978-4-431-54421-0_9,

9.1 Introduction

Although the etiology of endometriosis remains unclear, there are several hypotheses proposed including retrograde menstruation theory, embryonic rest theory, coelomic metaplasia theory, and new combined theory [1–5]. Among these, Sampson's retrograde menstruation theory is the most accepted one in which it states that the origin of endometriosis is caused by implanted cast-off endometrial tissues, the retrograde menstruation [3, 4]. Several clinical observations, which described that women with cervical or vaginal obstruction have higher risk of developing endometriosis, are in line with this hypothesis [6–8]. In addition, an animal model of baboon showed that the ligation of cervices increases the incidence of endometriosis [9]. A more convincing evidence is that endometriosis is observed exclusively in species that menstruate [10]. Nevertheless, retrograde menstruation theory is insufficient to explain why only 5–10 % of women with reflux menstruation developed endometriosis when 90 % of women in reproductive age have retrograde menstruation [11]. Furthermore, before the infiltration of vasculature, the retrograded tissues have to escape from the surveillance of immune system, gain the capacity of steroidogenesis (because endometrial cells are highly dependent on estrogen), and establish a self-support system to maintain proliferation to survive in the ectopic sites. Therefore, it is clear that other local or even epigenetic factors must exist to contribute to the pathological processes of this disease. It is obvious that we cannot discuss all the factors involved in endometriosis pathogenesis; therefore, in this review chapter, we will primarily focus on the functional roles of prostaglandin E_2 (PGE_2) and some other factors that are involved in the regulation of PGE_2 biosynthesis.

9.2 Biosynthesis of PGE_2

Prostaglandins, a group of biologically active long-chain fatty acids derived from arachidonic acid, are short-lived eicosanoids that are produced locally in response to numerous stimuli. PGs regulate numerous physiological and pathological processes including but not limited to inflammation, reproduction, respiration, angiogenesis, coagulation, photo-sensing, sleep and awakeness, stem cell generation, and cancer progression [12–16]. In mammals, every cell can synthesize one or more kinds of PGs. The synthesis of PGs involves multiple enzymes and sequential processes. First, it begins with the cleavage of arachidonic acid from diacylglycerol and phospholipids by phospholipase C and A2 (PLC and PLA2), respectively (Fig. 9.1). Then prostaglandin H synthase-1 and synthase-2 (also known as cyclooxygenase-1/cyclooxygenase-2, COX-1/COX-2) convert arachidonic acid to common prostaglandin precursor PGH_2. This enzymatic reaction is the rate-limiting step in the biosynthesis of the 2-series of PGs (PGD_2, PGE_2, $PGF_{2\alpha}$, PGI_2, PGJ_2, and thromboxane A_2). Third, a group of PG synthases, such as microsomal PGE

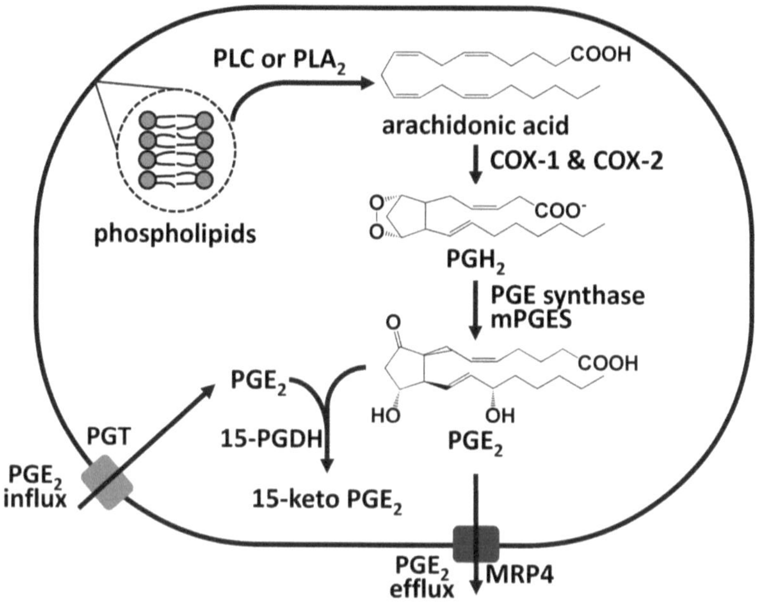

Fig. 9.1 Biosynthesis of prostaglandin E_2. Membrane-bound phospholipids, such as diacylglycerol and phospholipids, are cleaved by phospholipase C and A2 (PLC, PLA2) to yield arachidonic acid, the common precursor of all PGs. Prostaglandin G/H synthase (cyclooxygenase, COX-1/COX-2) then converts arachidonic acid into PGH2, which is further metabolized by microsomal PGE synthase (mPGES) to produce PGE2. PGE transporter (PGT) and multidrug resistance-associated protein 4 (MRP4) are responsible for the uptake and secretion of PGE_2, respectively

synthase (mPGES) and PGF synthases, act on PGH_2 to produce PGE_2 and $PGF_{2\alpha}$, respectively [17–19]. These enzymes coordinate with preferred partners in specific tissue to produce PGs. For example, in the process of PGE_2 synthesis, cytosolic PGES (cPGES) and COX-1 account for constitutive production of PGE_2 [19, 20], while the coupling of mPGES-1 and COX-2 is responsible for inflammation-induced PGE_2 production [17]. As is the rule for locally acting lipid mediators, PGE_2 is not stored but rapidly metabolized once synthesized. The major enzymes responsible for the rapid (within minutes) inactivation of PGE_2 are the cytosolic enzymes 15-ketoprostaglandin Δ13-reductase and 15-hydroxyprostaglandin dehydrogenase (15-PGDH).

9.3 Source of PGE_2 in Endometriosis

Early in the mid-1980s, it was discovered that concentrations of PGE_2 are elevated in the peritoneal fluid collected from women with endometriosis compared to that derived from otherwise healthy women [21]. Later, it became clear that the majority of PGE_2 comes from two cell types—peritoneal macrophages and endometriotic stromal cells [22–25]. Macrophages are the major immune cells recruited to the sites where endometriotic tissues reside within first few hours and it has been found that women with endometriotic lesion have more macrophages [26, 27], especially the activated macrophages [24]. COX-2 was overexpressed in peritoneal macrophages from women with endometriosis while COX-1 was expressed at very low level and elevated COX-1 is only seen in the severe stage of endometriosis. It should be noted that COX-2 levels are undetectable in monocytes (precursor of macrophages) isolated from peripheral blood regardless of their stages [24], indicating that local modulators in the peritoneal cavity promote COX-2 overexpression. Proinflammatory cytokines are commonly elevated in the peritoneal fluid from women with endometriosis [28] and are potentially responsible for COX-2 induction. Indeed, PGE_2, tumor necrosis factor-α (TNF-α), and interlukin-1β (IL-1β) have been demonstrated to promote the expression of COX-2 in peritoneal macrophages [24]. This provides evidence to demonstrate that overproduction of PGE_2 by peritoneal macrophages in women with endometriosis is likely due to the activation of COX-2 by a group of proinflammatory cytokines in the peritoneal fluid.

In parallel to macrophages, ectopic endometriotic stromal cells also produce high levels of PGE_2 [22, 23, 25]. Phospholipase A2 was found to increase in lesion tissues [29, 30], and mPGES was elevated in both epithelial and stromal cells from women with endometriosis [29, 31]. These elevated PLA_2 and mPGES work together with the upregulated COX-2 to increase PGE_2 production.

Aberrant expression of COX-2 in endometriotic stromal cells has been reported by several groups [22, 23, 25]. However, one intriguing phenomenon is that although the ectopic endometriotic tissue consists of the same genetic backgrounds as the eutopic endometrium, it possesses distinct biochemical nature compared to its eutopic counterpart. It has been shown that ectopic stromal cells are at least 100 times more sensitive to IL-1β treatment than eutopic endometrial stromal cells in terms of COX-2 expression. The distinct sensitivity is due to increased transcriptional activity of *COX-2* promoter in ectopic but not eutopic endometrial stromal cells [25]. Because endometriosis is a chronic inflammatory disease and many proinflammatory cytokines, including IL-1β, are elevated in the peritoneal fluid, increased sensitivity enables ectopic endometriotic stromal cells to respond to the level of proinflammatory cytokines that eutopic endometrial stromal cells normally do not respond. This phenomenon may explain why COX-2 and, to some extent, its downstream target genes are consistently overexpressed in ectopic endometriotic tissues.

The underlying molecular mechanism responsible for the increased sensitivity of ectopic stromal cells to stimuli is an area of interest to be investigated because it may provide important information for designing new treatment regimens. Recent studies reveal that predisposition to hypoxic stress may account for the distinct responses of ectopic endometriotic cells. The retrograded tissues encountered hypoxic stress before the formation of new blood vessels in the ectopic site. Typically, cells sense the hypoxia via an oxygen-dependent hydroxylation on hypoxia-inducible factors (HIFs). There are two kinds of HIF members: the α and β subunits, both of which are constitutively transcribed and translated but undergo differential posttranslational modifications. Under normoxic condition, the α subunit undergoes hydroxylation at two proline residues (Pro402 and Pro564), which ultimately results in 26S proteasome-mediated degradation of HIF-α protein [32]. In response to hypoxia, the α subunit accumulates due to the lack of oxygen-induced hydroxylation and degradation. In contrast, the β subunit does not respond to oxygen-dependent degradation and is constitutively expressed. Thus, the level of α subunit determines the gene expression profile of a cell. In endometriotic stromal cells, levels of HIF-1α mRNA and protein were elevated compared to the eutopic endometrial stromal cells [33]. Elevation of HIF-1α protein or treatment with hypoxia causes the downregulation of dual-specificity phosphatase-2 (DUSP2), a downstream inactivator of mitogen-activated protein kinase (MAPK) signaling [34–36]. Downregulation of DUSP2 results in a prolonged activation of ERK and p38 MAPK in ectopic endometriotic stromal cells, which explains the increased sensitivity of COX-2 promoter to IL-1β stimulation because it is mediated by ERK- and p38 MAPK-dependent signaling pathway [25].

In addition to altered COX-2 regulation, PGE_2 transporter/carrier may also play important roles on the PGE_2 production. Up to date, only few transporters/carriers of PGE_2 have been found and are capable of facilitating the uptake or clearance of PGE_2 to regulate pericellular PG levels. The co-expression of prostaglandin transporter, preferentially transporting PGE_2, and 15-PGDH, metabolizing PGE_2 resides in cytoplasm, indeed supporting the idea that uptake of PGE_2 is essential for its metabolism [37]. Multidrug resistance-associated protein 4 (MRP4) is one of the few proteins with high specificity to export PGE_1 and PGE_2 [38]. Interestingly, endometriotic tissue expressed lower 15-PGDH but higher MRP4 mRNA compared to eutopic ones and correlated to higher PGE_2 production/release [29, 39].

9.4 Actions of PGE_2

9.4.1 Control of Steroidogenesis by PGE_2

The development and maintenance of endometriosis are highly dependent on estrogen. This notion was supported by several lines of evidences. First, symptoms of endometriosis usually appear after menarche and regress in menopausal or ovariectomized women [40]. Second, a study using the "monkey" animal model also demonstrated that only the group of animals that received capsules with estrogen or progesterone developed endometriosis [41]. During the menstrual cycle, the level of estrogen reaches its maximum before ovulation and maintains at a certain level in the luteal phase. However, after luteolysis and before the production of estrogen by follicles of the next cycle, the estrogen level drops to a minimal level. This raises the question: what is the source of estrogen supporting

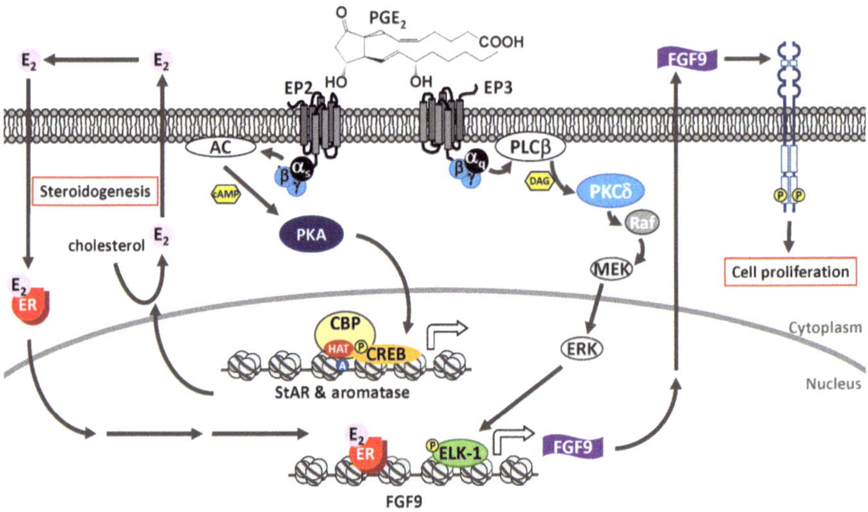

Fig. 9.2 Prostaglandin E_2 promotes cell proliferation by two independent EP receptor-mediated pathways. PGE_2 binds to EP2 receptor and activates adenylyl cyclase (AC) to generate cyclic AMP (cAMP), which then activates protein kinase A (PKA). Activated PKA translocates to the nucleus to phosphorylate cAMP response element-binding protein (CREB), which binds to *StAR* (and aromatase) gene promoter. Phosphorylated CREB recruits CREB-binding protein (CBP), a histone acetyl transferase (HAT), to initiate chromatin remodeling and promote StAR and aromatase gene transcription. Upregulation of StAR and aromatase leads to biogenesis of 17-β estradiol (E_2) that stimulates fibroblast growth factor-9 (FGF9) production in an autocrine manner. On the other hand, PGE_2 binds to EP3 receptor to activate the protein kinase Cδ (PKCδ)-Raf-MEK-ERK signaling pathway that directly results in upregulation of FGF9 transcription. Overexpressed FGF9 then stimulates endometriotic cell proliferation via autocrine and/or paracrine regulations

the survival of endometriotic tissue when the ovarian estrogen is not available? The answers to this question were revealed by multiple studies showing that endometriotic stromal cells actually are capable of producing estrogen. Endometriotic stromal cells not only express proteins/enzymes required for de novo synthesis of estrogen but even express at higher levels compared to its endometrial counterpart. The pro-steroidogenic proteins, including steroidogenic acute regulatory protein (StAR), P450 side chain cleavage enzyme, 3β-hydroxysteroid dehydrogenase, 17α-hydroxylase 17, 20 lyase, aromatase, and 17β-hydroxysteroid dehydrogenase type I, are either aberrantly expressed or elevated in ectopic stromal cells [42–44], whereas the anti-steroidogenic protein, 17β-hydroxysteroid dehydrogenase type II, is suppressed. Among these proteins, StAR and aromatase control two of the most important steps for estrogen production. StAR governs the first step in which hydrophobic cholesterol is carried through the double-membraned mitochondria where the P450 side chain cleavage enzyme resides and aromatase converts androstenedione to estrone.

Expression of StAR in endometriotic stromal cells is induced by PGE_2 (Fig. 9.2). This stimulation is unique to endometriotic stromal cells, but not found in eutopic endometrial stromal cells or epithelial cells [44]. PGE_2-induced StAR expression is mediated via EP2 receptor [45]. Treatment with PKA inhibitor attenuates PGE_2-induced StAR expression, indicating that the EP2 signaling is mediated via typical Gs and PKA/cAMP pathway. In line with this observation, treatment with cell-permeable cAMP also stimulates StAR expression in endometriotic stromal cells. The PKA/cAMP pathway further leads the phosphorylation of cAMP response element-binding protein (CREB), which binds to a CCAAT/enhancer-binding protein (C/EBP) response element in StAR promoter [46]. Phosphorylated CREB recruits CREB-binding protein (CBP), a histone acetyltransferase, causing histone H3 acetylation around StAR promoter and facilitating local nucleosome decondensation, which allows the assembly of transcription complexes [45]. The phosphorylated CREB (15 min), histone H3 acetylation (60 min), and newly transcribed nascent RNA (2 h) were nicely coordinated as the fact that the peak of each molecular event takes place sequentially.

Along with the aberrant expression of StAR in endometriotic stromal cells, expression of aromatase is also regulated by PGE_2 via the EP2 receptor-mediated signaling pathway [47, 48]. Aberrant expression of steroidogenic factor-1 (SF-1) in endometriotic stromal cells alters its sensitivity to PGE_2. It has been found that competition between SF-1 and COUP-TFII on the same DNA-binding site in aromatase promoter may contribute to the change of PGE_2 sensitivity in endometriotic stromal cells [49], whereas in endometrial cells, due to the lack of SF-1, COUP-TFII occupies the aromatase promoter, rendering its transcriptional activity. Since the expression of StAR and aromatase is regulated in a similar and parallel aspect, this mechanism enables PGE_2 to induce de novo estrogen production from the readily available precursor, cholesterol, without depending on the transport of intermediate metabolites from other organs.

9.4.2 *Induction of Peptide Growth Factors by PGE_2*

Although it is clear that endometriosis is an estrogen-dependent disease, estrogen per se is not a mitogen. The mitogenic effect of estrogen usually is mediated by one or more peptide growth factors. Several well-known peptide growth factors, such as insulin-like growth factor-1 (IGF-1), epidermal growth factor (EGF), and fibroblast growth factor-2 (FGF2), have been shown to exert such estrogen-induced growth effect in other cell types [50–53]. However, evidences that link the expression patterns of these growth factors with the pathogenesis of endometriosis are either inconsistent or even controversial. For example, levels of IGF-1 in peritoneal fluid of women with endometriosis were higher [54], not different [55], or even lower [56] as compared with that in peritoneal fluid of women without endometriosis. The levels of EGF and EGF receptor are not different between ectopic endometriotic lesions and eutopic endometrial tissues [57, 58]. Concentrations of FGF-2 in peritoneal fluid and immunoreactive FGF-2 in pelvic endometriotic cells are not different from those of normal or eutopic counterparts [57, 59, 60].

In contrast to the aforementioned peptide growth factors, FGF9 seems to be a promising candidate that carries estrogen's mitogenic effect in endometriotic cells. First, expression of FGF9 is induced by estrogen in normal endometrial stromal cells [61]. Second, FGF-9 is consistently expressed by ectopic endometriotic tissue with greater amounts in early stage compared to that in late stage [62], which correlates with the concentrations of estrogen in the peritoneal fluid of women with endometriosis [44]. Third, expression of FGF9's high-affinity receptors, including FGFR2IIIb, FGFR2IIIc, FGFR3IIIb, and FGFR3IIIc, is detected in ectopic endometriotic stromal cells [61]. Fourth, FGF9 dose-dependently induces endometrial stromal cell proliferation [61, 63]. Taking these four lines of evidence together with the notion that PGE_2 is able to induce estrogen production, it strongly suggests that FGF9 is an estromedin that transmits PGE_2's action in promoting the proliferation of endometriotic cells. Indeed, treatment of endometrial stromal cells with PGE_2 dose-dependently induces FGF9 expression, and PGE_2-preteated conditioned medium is able to induce stromal cell proliferation, an effect that can be blocked by the addition of anti-FGF9 antibody [64]. Interestingly, it was shown that blocking estrogen signaling by estrogen receptor antagonist, ICI182,780, only partially inhibits PGE_2's action [64]. This observation leads to a new discovery that PGE_2 also directly induces FGF9 expression independent of estrogenic effect [64].

How can PGE_2 regulate the same gene expression through two different pathways? To understand this, it is necessary to review the signaling transduction pathways of PGE_2. PGE_2 regulates various physiological and pathological processes by binding to its receptors on the plasma membrane. In mammals, there are four distinct subtypes of PGE_2 receptor, namely EP1, EP2, EP3, and EP4, which are encoded by different genes [65]. All EP receptors are G-protein-coupled receptors. EP2 and EP4 couple to Gs and activate adenylyl cyclase and protein kinase A signaling pathway. Compared to EP2 and EP4, EP1 and EP3 have more complicated pathways. Both EP1 and EP3 have different isoforms generated via alternative splicing varied in their C-terminal cytoplasmic domain, which largely accounts for interaction with G proteins. EP1 has been reported to couple to Gq or Gi/o proteins and promotes the increase of intracellular Ca^{2+} level and/or inhibition of PKA. EP3 couples to Gs, Gq, or Gi proteins and activates the PKA/PKC/MAPK pathway, immobilization of intracellular Ca^{2+}, or inactivation of PKA [65]. Therefore, different signaling pathway(s) can be regulated by PGE_2 dependent on which specific EP was bound [16]. Three EP receptors, EP2, EP3, and EP4, are expressed in human endometrial and endometriotic stromal cells [45].

The effect of PGE_2 on the induction of StAR and aromatase is mediated through binding to the EP2 receptor [45, 47]. In contrast, the induction of FGF9 by PGE_2 is mediated by EP3 receptor and its downstream signaling pathway (Fig. 9.2). Treatment with PGE_2 or selective EP3 agonist, sulprostone, activates PKCδ, which leads to phosphorylation of ERK. Phosphorylated ERK translocates to the nucleus and activates transcription factor ELK-1, which binds to two response elements residing in the promoter of human *FGF9* gene [64]. This direct effect of PGE_2 represents the quick response, which occurs between 8 and 12 h after treatment. On the other hand, the PGE_2-estrogen-FGF9 axis represents a delayed response, which occurs between 24 and 48 h. Taken together, via two different types of receptors, PGE_2 is able to induce the critical survival and proliferating factor, FGF9, to ensure the progression of endometriosis.

9.4.3 Suppression of Phagocytosis by PGE_2

One of the most intriguing questions in the pathogenesis of endometriosis is why the immune system fails to clear the retrogradely transported tissues. Normally, apoptotic tissues such as the shed endometrium will be destroyed and engulfed by immune cells. However, in the case of endometriosis, these tissues obviously have some sort of immune privilege that prevent them from being phagocytosed. During the development of endometriosis, the retrograded endometrial tissues induce local inflammation that recruits immune cells, mainly the macrophage, to the peritoneum [66, 67]. Macrophages represent the first line of defense system that either directly phagocytose these aberrantly present cells or activates other immune cells (such as dendritic cells, natural killer cells, and lymphocytes) to launch the antiproliferation responses [68]. However, peritoneal macrophages isolated from patients with endometriosis have greater ability in producing inflammatory agents and poorer capability in phagocytosis [69, 70]. This phenomenon has puzzled researchers for more than three decades. Recently, through a series of investigations, the mechanism of immune deficiency in endometriotic macrophage becomes more and more clear.

The phagocytosis process begins with secreting proteases by activated macrophages. Matrix metalloproteinases (MMPs) are a group of proteases that participate in extracellular matrix degradation [71]. Macrophages can secrete MMP-2, MMP-7, MMP-9, and MMP-12 to degrade elastin and have been implicated to play an important role in the pathogenesis of emphysema and aortic aneurysm [72–75]. In addition, MMP-9 can facilitate the destruction of the type IV collagen-containing basement membrane which separates the epithelial and stromal compartment [76]. This feature makes MMP-9 becoming the prime candidate secreted by macrophages to destroy the retrogradely transported tissues in the peritoneal cavity.

Another important molecule that also contributes to macrophage's phagocytic function is annexin A2. Annexin A2 has diverse biological functions depending on its cellular localization. When annexin A2 is expressed in membrane-bound form, it promotes the ability of macrophages in remodeling extracellular matrix. Annexin A2 acts as a fibrinolytic receptor that activates plasmin by facilitating the interaction between tissue plasminogen activator and plasminogen [77]. Plasmin serves as a physiological activator which, in turn, converts pro-MMP-9 to active MMP-9. Thus, the activation of membrane annexin A2 will lead to MMP-9 activation. In addition, annexin A2 can be externalized or secreted. Soluble annexin A2 protein activates human monocyte-derived macrophages through toll-like receptor 4 resulting in enhancing phagocytosis [78]. Furthermore, it has been reported that

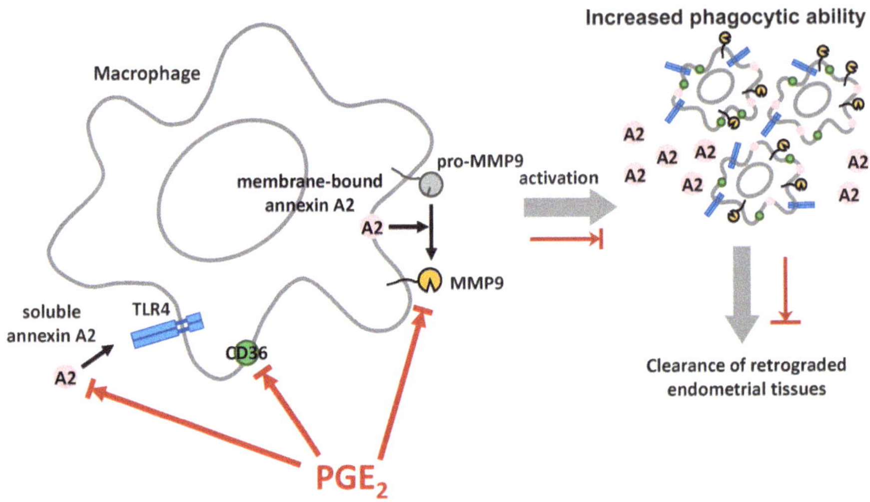

Fig. 9.3 Prostaglandin E_2 inhibits phagocytosis. Under low-PGE_2 condition, macrophages are recruited to the peritoneal cavity due to retrogradely transported endometrial tissue-induced inflammation. Recruited macrophages express high levels of annexin A2 (membrane form and soluble form), MMP9, and CD36 to facilitate phagocytosis. Therefore, the retrograded tissues will be engulfed and removed. However, under high concentrations of PGE_2 (indicated by *red lines*), the expression of annexin A2, MMP9, and CD36 is all suppressed. Thus, macrophages lose their phagocytic ability and retrogradely transported endometrial tissues are able to implant and grow in the peritoneum

membrane externalization of annexin A2 in macrophages mediates apoptotic cell clearance [79].

The third line of phagocytic activity involves expression of scavenger receptors on the macrophages to enhance the uptake and degradation of cell debris [80, 81]. Scavenger receptors are a family of structurally diverse receptors having broad ligand specificity that includes low-density lipoprotein, phosphatidylserine, polyanion, and apoptotic cells [82–84]. The known scavenger receptors that participate in phagocytosis of apoptotic cells by macrophages include class A scavenger receptors (SR-AI, SR-AII, SR-AIII) [83] and class B scavenger receptors (SR-BI, SR-BII, and SR-BIII) [85, 86]. Reduced expression of one of these scavenger receptors may result in loss of phagocytic ability.

By using peritoneal macrophages isolated from individuals with or without endometriosis, we have demonstrated that levels of MMP-9, annexin A2, and SR-BIII (better known as CD36) are all reduced in endometriotic macrophages [87–89] (Fig. 9.3). The decrease in MMP-9, annexin A2, and CD36 is due to exposure to soluble factors in the peritoneal fluid of individuals with endometriosis. Treatment of normal macrophages with peritoneal fluids collected from individuals with endometriosis recaps the phenomenon seen in endometriotic macrophages. In contrast, normal macrophages treated with peritoneal fluids collected from normal individuals are not affected. Interestingly, not only the mRNA and protein levels of

MMP-9 are reduced, the MMP-9 enzymatic activity is also inhibited [89]. This markedly impairs macrophage's ability to digest the basement membrane of retrogradely transported tissues and ultimately contributes to reduced macrophage's phagocytic ability. Since CD36 is one of the first macrophage receptors to be implicated in the recognition of aged or apoptotic cells [90, 91] and annexin A2 participates in both MMP-9 activation and phagocytosis, reduced expression of CD36 and annexin A2 severely impairs the phagocytic ability of macrophages. Indeed, when CD36 or annexin A2 is knocked down from the normal macrophages, the phagocytic ability is reduced. In contrast, when peritoneal macrophages isolated from individuals with endometriosis are transfected with exogenous CD36 or annexin A2, the phagocytic ability is restored [88, 92].

The next question to ask is which factor in the endometriosis peritoneal fluid exerts such inhibitory effect. Because endometriosis is a chronic inflammatory disease and many proinflammatory cytokines are elevated in the peritoneal fluid of endometriosis [24, 93–96], it is likely that reduced phagocytic ability of peritoneal macrophage is mediated by one or some of these proinflammatory cytokines. Through a series of screens, we identified that PGE_2 is the primary factor to inhibit the expression of MMP-9, annexin A2, and CD36 in peritoneal macrophages [88, 89, 92]. PGE_2, via binding to the EP2 and EP4 receptors, activates PKA signaling pathway to suppress the expression of MMP-9, annexin A2, and CD36. As expected, treatment of macrophages with PGE_2 inhibits phagocytic ability, which can be reversed by adding EP2 receptor antagonist [92]. The in vitro results of PGE_2 action in suppressing phagocytosis are further supported by in vivo autologous transplanted mouse model. In this model, uterine endometria from donor mice are peeled off, minced into small pieces, and injected into peritoneal cavity of recipient mice. Recipient mice are treated with or without PGE_2 or selective COX-1/COX-2 inhibitors to blunt the biosynthesis of PGE_2 for 4 weeks. Mice treated with PGE_2 have more endometriotic tissue-like lesions, lower levels of CD36 and annexin A2 in peritoneal macrophages, and reduced phagocytic ability of peritoneal macrophages. In contrast, mice that received selective COX inhibitors develop fewer lesions, express more CD36 and annexin A2 by the peritoneal macrophages, and exert greater phagocytic ability of peritoneal macrophages [88, 92]. Taken altogether, these data reveal that PGE_2 utilizes the same receptor-mediated signaling pathway to target three different molecules involved in phagocytosis. Such a safeguarding system to efficiently inhibit macrophage's phagocytic ability by controlling three target proteins simultaneously is likely due to the evolutional advantage.

9.4.4 *Induction of Angiogenesis by PGE_2*

Establishment of an effective blood supply is a prerequisite for the survival of retrogradely transported endometrial tissues to develop as endometriotic lesions. Newly formed vessels play an indispensible role in the development and progression of endometriosis by providing nutrients, growth factors, and oxygen [97–99]. The newly formed blood vessel can be easily observed on day 4 after the transplantation of mouse endometrium to the peritoneal cavity [27]. Several pro-angiogenic factors that may be involved in blood vessel formation during the development of endometriosis had been reported. Among those, vascular endothelial growth factor (VEGF) and cysteine-rich angiogenic inducer 61 (CYR61) are the most well studied. Concentrations of VEGF in the peritoneal fluid of individuals with endometriosis are greater compared with controls [100]. This VEGF may come from both endometriotic lesions and infiltrated neutrophils and macrophages [27, 97]. Estrogen and COX-2 have been shown to play critical roles in angiogenesis in various tumor models. Both can stimulate VEGF expression and induce endothelial cell proliferation [101–103]. In endometriosis, estrogen has been shown to enhance VEGF production in neutrophils and macrophages [27] while the expression of COX-2 and VEGF is highly correlated in endometriotic lesions [104]. In vitro study reveals that treatment of endometrial epithelial cells with celecoxib, a selective COX-2 inhibitor, inhibits VEGF expression in comparison to that treated with vehicle [105]. In vivo studies also demonstrate inhibitory effects of selective COX-2 inhibitors in the growth of endometriotic lesion and the development of microvascular networks. Treating rats with rofecoxib induced a decrease in the endometriotic lesion size accompanied by a decrease in peritoneal fluid VEGF levels [106]. Ozawa et al. demonstrate that another selective COX-2 inhibitor, NS398, decreases the size of implants in a xenograft model that implants human ovarian endometrioma to peritonea of SCID mice [107]. Laschke et al. report that the expression of proliferating cell nuclear antigen and VEGF as well as the microvessel density within the endometrial grafts is decreased in NS398-treated golden hamster [108]. Machado et al. also report that parecoxib, also a selective COX-2 inhibitor, reduced lesion size, microvessel density, the number of macrophages, and the expression of VEGF in a rat model of peritoneal endometriosis [109].

CYR61, a member of the CCN family of growth regulators, is a pro-angiogenic factor that mediates several distinct functions in cell proliferation, adhesion, migration, differentiation, apoptosis, and extracellular matrix production. Cyr61-deficient mice suffer embryonic death due to vascular defects [110]. Expression of CYR61 mRNA is rapidly induced in an immediate early fashion by a spectrum of stimuli such as growth factors, cytokines, and estrogens [111]. The expression of CYR61 in endometrium is elevated in the proliferative phase and menstrual effluents [112, 113]. Aberrant expression of CYR61 has been found in the ectopic lesions of endometriotic women and baboon [35, 114, 115]. The expression of CYR61 is upregulated by PGE_2 and hypoxia in human endometrial stromal cells and colon cancer cells, respectively [34, 112]. While PGE_2-induced CYR61 is a direct effect, hypoxia-mediated CYR61 may be mediated via downregulation of DUSP2. It has been shown that reduced expression of DUSP2 by hypoxia causes a prolonged phosphorylation of ERK and p38 MAPK, which ultimately leads to upregulation of COX-2 [35, 36]. Therefore, hypoxia-induced CYR61 overexpression is likely also mediated by PGE_2.

Taking together all currently available data, it is clear that COX-2-derived PGE_2 does play a key role in establishing an effective blood supply system either directly or indirectly during the development of endometriosis. Targeting COX-2-derived PGE_2 signaling pathway to blunt new blood vessel formation may be a plausible approach to prevent the development of endometriosis.

9.5 Feed-Forward Loop of PGE_2

The consistent production of self-supporting factors is a sophisticated mechanism that keeps endometriotic cells alive despite of the cyclic rises and falls of estrogen and is also the main reason why there is no effective therapeutic regimen for endometriosis. The central piece of this feed-forward self-supporting system is PGE_2. There are at least three feed-forward loops to maintain PGE_2 at the high concentration in the endometriotic tissues and surrounding local environment (Fig. 9.4). The first positive loop involves estrogen and COX-2. COX-2-derived PGE_2 stimulates StAR and aromatase expression in ectopic stromal cells, which leads to aberrant production of estrogen. Autonomous production of estrogen by ectopic tissues induces several known peptide growth factors such as VEGF and FGFs that serve as autocrine (for endometriotic cell) and paracrine (for endothelial cell) factors to stimulate cell proliferation and angiogenesis. On the other hand, estrogen can induce COX-2 expression and thus PGE_2 production to form the feed-forward auto-amplification loop [116].

The second positive loop requires the cooperation between peritoneal macrophages and endometriotic stromal cells. Peritoneal macrophages secrete proinflammatory cytokines such as IL-1β and PGE_2 to induce COX-2 expression in ectopic endometriotic stromal cells and peritoneal macrophages. As a result, more PGE_2 is produced. The elevated PGE_2 not only induces more COX-2 expression by macrophages but also inhibits phagocytosis. Attenuated phagocytic ability of macrophages enables ectopic endometriotic tissues to grow and produce more PGE_2 upon stimulation by proinflammatory cytokines or estrogen.

The third positive loop, to some extent, may be the most important one to initiate the whole pathological process of endometriosis. It starts with the increase of hypoxic stress due to lack of blood supply to the endometrium right before the onset of menstruation. Increased hypoxic stress causes the accumulation of HIF-1α, which then translocates to the nucleus and dimerizes with HIF-1β to regulate gene expression. Hypoxia-mediated downregulation of DUSP2 causes a prolonged activation of ERK and p38 MAPK, which results in increased sensitivity of *COX-2* gene to proinflammatory cytokine stimulation. As a result, the endometriotic lesions are more vulnerable to exogenous stimulation and produce more PGE_2. Moreover, the activation of ERK enhances nuclear accumulation of HIF-1α [117], which further suppresses DUSP2 and thus enhances ERK activation. This may explain why HIF-1α protein [33] and phosphorylated ERK [118] are elevated in ectopic endometriotic lesions. Because ERK and p38 MAPK signaling controls

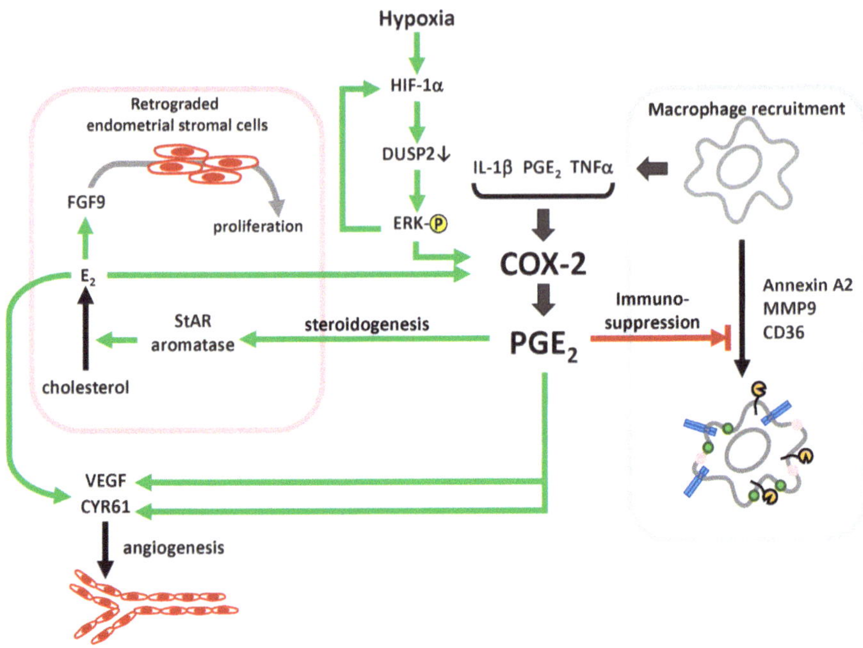

Fig. 9.4 Positive feed-forward loops of PGE_2 actions in endometriosis. Regulation of PGE_2 biosynthesis in ectopic endometriotic stromal cells is regulated by predisposition to hypoxic stress, which inhibits expression of dual-specificity phosphatase-2 (DUSP2) and leads to a prolonged activation of ERK. Phosphorylated ERK stabilizes HIF-1α and, at the same time, enhances proinflammatory cytokine-induced COX-2 expression and PGE_2 production. These proinflammatory cytokines also induce COX-2 expression and PGE_2 production by peritoneal macrophages. Elevated concentration of PGE_2 stimulates steroidogenesis and angiogenesis to promote cell proliferation and inhibits phagocytosis to prevent ectopic endometriotic tissues from destroyed by macrophages. The effects of PGE_2 are augmented by three feed-forward positive regulatory loops: (1) hypoxia-HIF-1α-ERK loop, (2) COX-2-PGE_2-estrogen loop, and (3) COX-2-PGE_2 proinflammatory cytokine loop. See text for details

many endometrial functions such as IL-1β and macrophage migration inhibitory factor-induced COX-2 expression [25, 119, 120], macrophage migration inhibitory factor-stimulated production of angiogenic factors [121], basal endometrial cells survival [122], and estrogen-stimulated cell proliferation [118], downregulation of DUSP2 in ectopic endometriotic cells points out the importance of hypoxia and/or HIF-1α in the pathogenesis of endometriosis.

As we can see in Fig. 9.4, these three positive feed-forward loops are not separated but rather interlinked to form a very complicated auto-amplification gene regulatory network. It involves multiple genes and environmental factors. Thus, how to disrupt these tightly regulated, self-supporting feed-forward loops represents a great challenge in treating endometriosis.

9.6 Targeting PGE_2 Signaling Pathway as a Potential Therapeutic Approach

As reviewed above, PGE_2 exerts multiple pathological functions to regulate the development of endometriosis and minimize or eradicate those effects triggered by PGE_2 and represents a plausible approach to prevent or cure endometriosis. Inhibiting the production of PGE_2 by ectopic endometriotic stromal cells and by peritoneal macrophages might be an option. However, given the short half-life of COX inhibitors and the unfavorable side effects caused by long-term use of NSAIDs, suppressing PGE_2 production to cure endometriosis may not be an ideal choice. An alternative approach is to block the downstream signaling pathways to terminate PGE_2's action. For example, it has been shown recently that blocking EP2/EP4 may prevent PGE_2 to transactivate EGF receptor and induce apoptosis in SV40-immortalized endometriotic stromal and epithelial cells. Similar approach may be applicable to block EP3 receptor on endometriotic stromal cells to inhibit the production of FGF-9 or to target EP2 on macrophages to prevent suppression of phagocytic ability by PGE_2. In addition, inhibition of multiple enzymes to disrupt the positive feedback loops of PGE_2 overproduction may be an alternative. Indeed, dienogest, a synthetic progestin that inhibits COX-2 and aromatase activities, was found to be effective in ameliorating endometriotic symptoms [123–125]. In light of this recent finding, developing effective small molecules to terminate PGE_2-mediated signaling is more likely a promising therapeutic strategy to treat endometriosis.

Acknowledgment This work was supported by grants from National Science Council of Taiwan (NSC-101-2320-B-006-030-MY3 to SJT and NSC-101-2314-B-006-043-MY2 to MHW). KYH wrote the first draft and proof-read the final manuscript. MHW and SJT edited and wrote the final draft. SJT designed and supervised the project. All authors read and approved the final draft.

References

1. Gruenwald P. Origin of endometriosis from the mesenchyme of the coelomic walls. Am J Obstet Gynecol. 1942;44:474.
2. Olive DL, Schwartz LB. Endometriosis. N Engl J Med. 1993;328:1759–69.
3. Sampson JA. Metastatic or embolic endometriosis, due to the menstrual dissemination of endometrial tissue into the venous circulation. Am J Pathol. 1927;3(93–110):43.
4. Sampson JA. Peritoneal endometriosis due to menstrual dissemination of endometrial tissue into the peritoneal cavity. Am J Obstet Gynecol. 1927;14:422–69.
5. von Recklinghausen F. Adenomyomas and cystadenomas of the wall of the uterus and tube: their origin as remnants of the wolffian body. Wien Klin Wochenschr. 1986;8:530.
6. Nunley Jr WC, Kitchin 3rd JD. Congenital atresia of the uterine cervix with pelvic endometriosis. Arch Surg. 1980;115:757–8.
7. Olive DL, Henderson DY. Endometriosis and mullerian anomalies. Obstet Gynecol. 1987;69:412–5.

8. Sanfilippo JS, Wakim NG, Schikler KN, Yussman MA. Endometriosis in association with uterine anomaly. Am J Obstet Gynecol. 1986;154:39–43.
9. D'Hooghe TM. Clinical relevance of the baboon as a model for the study of endometriosis. Fertil Steril. 1997;68:613–25.
10. D'Hooghe TM, Debrock S. Endometriosis, retrograde menstruation and peritoneal inflammation in women and in baboons. Hum Reprod Update. 2002;8:84–8.
11. Halme J, Hammond MG, Hulka JF, Raj SG, Talbert LM. Retrograde menstruation in healthy women and in patients with endometriosis. Obstet Gynecol. 1984;64:151–4.
12. Chen C, Bazan NG. Lipid signaling: sleep, synaptic plasticity, and neuroprotection. Prostaglandins Other Lipid Mediat. 2005;77:65–76.
13. Huang ZL, Sato Y, Mochizuki T, Okada T, Qu WM, Yamatodani A, Urade Y, Hayaishi O. Prostaglandin E2 activates the histaminergic system via the EP4 receptor to induce wakefulness in rats. J Neurosci. 2003;23:5975–83.
14. Kalinski P. Regulation of immune responses by prostaglandin E2. J Immunol. 2012;188:21–8.
15. Pelus LM, Hoggatt J. Pleiotropic effects of prostaglandin E2 in hematopoiesis; prostaglandin E2 and other eicosanoids regulate hematopoietic stem and progenitor cell function. Prostaglandins Other Lipid Mediat. 2011;96:3–9.
16. Sugimoto Y, Narumiya S. Prostaglandin E receptors. J Biol Chem. 2007;282:11613–7.
17. Murakami M, Naraba H, Tanioka T, Semmyo N, Nakatani Y, Kojima F, Ikeda T, Fueki M, Ueno A, Oh S, Kudo I. Regulation of prostaglandin E2 biosynthesis by inducible membrane-associated prostaglandin E2 synthase that acts in concert with cyclooxygenase-2. J Biol Chem. 2000;275:32783–92.
18. Tanikawa N, Ohmiya Y, Ohkubo H, Hashimoto K, Kangawa K, Kojima M, Ito S, Watanabe K. Identification and characterization of a novel type of membrane-associated prostaglandin E synthase. Biochem Biophys Res Commun. 2002;291:884–9.
19. Tanioka T, Nakatani Y, Semmyo N, Murakami M, Kudo I. Molecular identification of cytosolic prostaglandin E2 synthase that is functionally coupled with cyclooxygenase-1 in immediate prostaglandin E2 biosynthesis. J Biol Chem. 2000;275:32775–82.
20. Murakami M, Nakashima K, Kamei D, Masuda S, Ishikawa Y, Ishii T, Ohmiya Y, Watanabe K, Kudo I. Cellular prostaglandin E2 production by membrane-bound prostaglandin E synthase-2 via both cyclooxygenases-1 and −2. J Biol Chem. 2003;278:37937–47.
21. Badawy SZ, Marshall L, Cuenca V. Peritoneal fluid prostaglandins in various stages of the menstrual cycle: role in infertile patients with endometriosis. Int J Fertil. 1985;30:48–52.
22. Chishima F, Hayakawa S, Sugita K, Kinukawa N, Aleemuzzaman S, Nemoto N, Yamamoto T, Honda M. Increased expression of cyclooxygenase-2 in local lesions of endometriosis patients. Am J Reprod Immunol. 2002;48:50–6.
23. Ota H, Igarashi S, Sasaki M, Tanaka T. Distribution of cyclooxygenase-2 in eutopic and ectopic endometrium in endometriosis and adenomyosis. Hum Reprod. 2001;16:561–6.
24. Wu MH, Sun HS, Lin CC, Hsiao KY, Chuang PC, Pan HA, Tsai SJ. Distinct mechanisms regulate cyclooxygenase-1 and −2 in peritoneal macrophages of women with and without endometriosis. Mol Hum Reprod. 2002;8:1103–10.
25. Wu MH, Wang CA, Lin CC, Chen LC, Chang WC, Tsai SJ. Distinct regulation of cyclooxygenase-2 by interleukin-1beta in normal and endometriotic stromal cells. J Clin Endocrinol Metab. 2005;90:286–95.
26. Karck U, Reister F, Schafer W, Zahradnik HP, Breckwoldt M. PGE2 and PGF2 alpha release by human peritoneal macrophages in endometriosis. Prostaglandins. 1996;51:49–60.
27. Lin YJ, Lai MD, Lei HY, Wing LY. Neutrophils and macrophages promote angiogenesis in the early stage of endometriosis in a mouse model. Endocrinology. 2006;147:1278–86.
28. Gupta S, Agarwal A, Sekhon L, Krajcir N, Cocuzza M, Falcone T. Serum and peritoneal abnormalities in endometriosis: potential use as diagnostic markers. Minerva Ginecol. 2006;58:527–51.

29. Lousse JC, Defrere S, Colette S, Van Langendonckt A, Donnez J. Expression of eicosanoid biosynthetic and catabolic enzymes in peritoneal endometriosis. Hum Reprod. 2010;25:734–41.
30. Sano M, Morishita T, Nozaki M, Yokoyama M, Watanabe Y, Nakano H. Elevation of the phospholipase A2 activity in peritoneal fluid cells from women with endometriosis. Fertil Steril. 1994;61:657–62.
31. Chishima F, Hayakawa S, Yamamoto T, Sugitani M, Karasaki-Suzuki M, Sugita K, Nemoto N. Expression of inducible microsomal prostaglandin E synthase in local lesions of endometriosis patients. Am J Reprod Immunol. 2007;57:218–26.
32. Semenza GL. Hypoxia-inducible factor 1 (HIF-1) pathway. Sci STKE. 2007;2007:cm8.
33. Wu MH, Chen KF, Lin SC, Lgu CW, Tsai SJ. Aberrant expression of leptin in human endometriotic stromal cells is induced by elevated levels of hypoxia inducible factor-1alpha. Am J Pathol. 2007;170:590–8.
34. Lin SC, Chien CW, Lee JC, Yeh YC, Hsu KF, Lai YY, Lin SC, Tsai SJ. Suppression of dual-specificity phosphatase-2 by hypoxia increases chemoresistance and malignancy in human cancer cells. J Clin Invest. 2011;121:1905–16.
35. Lin SC, Wang CC, Wu MH, Yang SH, Li YH, Tsai SJ. Hypoxia-induced microRNA-20a expression increases ERK phosphorylation and angiogenic gene expression in endometriotic stromal cells. J Clin Endocrinol Metab. 2012;97:E1515–23.
36. Wu MH, Lin SC, Hsiao KY, Tsai SJ. Hypoxia-inhibited dual-specificity phosphatase-2 expression in endometriotic cells regulates cyclooxygenase-2 expression. J Pathol. 2011;225:390–400.
37. Nomura T, Lu R, Pucci ML, Schuster VL. The two-step model of prostaglandin signal termination: in vitro reconstitution with the prostaglandin transporter and prostaglandin 15 dehydrogenase. Mol Pharmacol. 2004;65:973–8.
38. Reid G, Wielinga P, Zelcer N, van der Heijden I, Kuil A, de Haas M, Wijnholds J, Borst P. The human multidrug resistance protein MRP4 functions as a prostaglandin efflux transporter and is inhibited by nonsteroidal antiinflammatory drugs. Proc Natl Acad Sci U S A. 2003;100:9244–9.
39. Gori I, Rodriguez Y, Pellegrini C, Achtari C, Hornung D, Chardonnens E, Wunder D, Fiche M, Canny GO. Augmented epithelial multidrug resistance-associated protein 4 expression in peritoneal endometriosis: regulation by lipoxin A. Fertil Steril. 2013;99:1965.
40. Missmer SA, Hankinson SE, Spiegelman D, Barbieri RL, Malspeis S, Willett WC, Hunter DJ. Reproductive history and endometriosis among premenopausal women. Obstet Gynecol. 2004;104:965–74.
41. Dizerega GS, Barber DL, Hodgen GD. Endometriosis: role of ovarian steroids in initiation, maintenance, and suppression. Fertil Steril. 1980;33:649–53.
42. Attar E, Tokunaga H, Imir G, Yilmaz MB, Redwine D, Putman M, Gurates B, Attar R, Yaegashi N, Hales DB, Bulun SE. Prostaglandin E2 via steroidogenic factor-1 coordinately regulates transcription of steroidogenic genes necessary for estrogen synthesis in endometriosis. J Clin Endocrinol Metab. 2009;94:623–31.
43. Noble LS, Simpson ER, Johns A, Bulun SE. Aromatase expression in endometriosis. J Clin Endocrinol Metab. 1996;81:174–9.
44. Tsai SJ, Wu MH, Lin CC, Sun HS, Chen SM. Regulation of steroidogenic acute regulatory protein expression and progesterone production in endometriotic stromal cells. J Clin Endocrinol Metab. 2001;86:5765–73.
45. Sun HS, Hsiao KY, Hsu CC, Wu MH, Tsai SJ. Transactivation of steroidogenic acute regulatory protein in human endometriotic stromal cells is mediated by the prostaglandin EP2 receptor. Endocrinology. 2003;144:3934–42.
46. Hsu CC, Lu CW, Huang BM, Wu MH, Tsai SJ. Cyclic adenosine 3′,5′-monophosphate response element-binding protein and CCAAT/enhancer-binding protein mediate prostaglandin E2-induced steroidogenic acute regulatory protein expression in endometriotic stromal cells. Am J Pathol. 2008;173:433–41.

47. Noble LS, Takayama K, Zeitoun KM, Putman JM, Johns DA, Hinshelwood MM, Agarwal VR, Zhao Y, Carr BR, Bulun SE. Prostaglandin E2 stimulates aromatase expression in endometriosis- derived stromal cells. J Clin Endocrinol Metab. 1997;82:600–6.
48. Zeitoun K, Takayama K, Michael MD, Bulun SE. Stimulation of aromatase P450 promoter (II) activity in endometriosis and its inhibition in endometrium are regulated by competitive binding of steroidogenic factor-1 and chicken ovalbumin upstream promoter transcription factor to the same cis-acting element. Mol Endocrinol. 1999;13:239–53.
49. Zeitoun KM, Bulun SE. Aromatase: a key molecule in the pathophysiology of endometriosis and a therapeutic target. Fertil Steril. 1999;72:961–9.
50. Cooke PS, Buchanan DL, Lubahn DB, Cunha GR. Mechanism of estrogen action: Lesions from the estradiol receptor-α knockout mouse. Biol Reprod. 1998;59:470–5.
51. Croze F, Kennedy TG, Schroedter IC, Friesen HG, Murphy LJ. Expression of insulin-like growth factor-I and insulin-like growth factor-binding protein-1 in the rat uterus during decidualization. Endocrinology. 1990;127:1995–2000.
52. Haining RE, Cameron IT, van Papendorp C, Davenport AP, Prentice A, Thomas EJ, Smith SK. Epidermal growth factor in human endometrium: proliferative effects in culture and immunocytochemical localization in normal and endometriotic tissues. Hum Reprod. 1991;6:1200–5.
53. Pierro E, Minici F, Alesiani O, Miceli F, Proto C, Screpanti I, Mancuso S, Lanzone A. Stromal-epithelial interactions modulate estrogen responsiveness in normal human endometrium. Biol Reprod. 2001;64:831–8.
54. Kim JG, Suh CS, Kim SH, Choi YM, Moon SY, Lee JY. Insulin-like growth factors (IGFs), IGF-binding proteins (IGFBPs), and IGFBP-3 protease activity in the peritoneal fluid of patients with and without endometriosis. Fertil Steril. 2000;73:996–1000.
55. Matalliotakis IM, Goumenou AG, Koumantakis GE, Neonaki MA, Koumantakis EE, Dionyssopoulou E, Athanassakis I, Vassiliadis S. Serum concentrations of growth factors in women with and without endometriosis: the action of anti-endometriosis medicines. Int Immunopharmacol. 2003;3:81–9.
56. Sbracia M, Zupi E, Alo P, Manna C, Marconi D, Scarpellini F, Grasso JA, Di Tondo U, Romanini C. Differential expression of IGF-I and IGF-II in eutopic and ectopic endometria of women with endometriosis and in women without endometriosis. Am J Reprod Immunol. 1997;37:326–9.
57. Huang JC, Papasakelariou C, Dawood MY. Epidermal growth factor and basic fibroblast growth factor in peritoneal fluid of women with endometriosis. Fertil Steril. 1996;65:931–4.
58. Huang JC, Yeh J. Quantitative analysis of epidermal growth factor receptor gene expression in endometriosis. J Clin Endocrinol Metab. 1994;79:1097–101.
59. Ferriani RA, Charnock-Jones DS, Prentice A, Thomas EJ, Smith SK. Immunohistochemical localization of acidic and basic fibroblast growth factors in normal human endometrium and endometriosis and the detection of their mRNA by polymerase chain reaction. Hum Reprod. 1993;8:11–6.
60. Seli E, Zeyneloglu HB, Senturk LM, Bahtiyar OM, Olive DL, Arici A. Basic fibroblast growth factor: peritoneal and follicular fluid levels and its effect on early embryonic development. Fertil Steril. 1998;69:1145–8.
61. Tsai SJ, Wu MH, Chen HM, Chuang PC, Wing LY. Fibroblast growth factor-9 is an endometrial stromal growth factor. Endocrinology. 2002;143:2715–21.
62. Wing L-YC, Chuang P-C, Wu M-H, Chen H-M, Tsai S-J. Expression and mitogenic effect of fibroblast growth factor-9 in human endometriotic implant is regulated by aberrant production of estrogen. J Clin Endocrinol Metab. 2003;88:5547–54.
63. Wing LY, Chen HM, Chuang PC, Wu MH, Tsai SJ. The mammalian target of rapamycin-p70 ribosomal S6 kinase but not phosphatidylinositol 3-kinase-Akt signaling is responsible for fibroblast growth factor-9-induced cell proliferation. J Biol Chem. 2005;280:19937–47.

64. Chuang PC, Sun HS, Chen TM, Tsai SJ. Prostaglandin E2 induces fibroblast growth factor 9 via EP3-dependent protein kinase Cdelta and Elk-1 signaling. Mol Cell Biol. 2006;26:8281–92.
65. Breyer RM, Bagdassarian CK, Myers SA, Breyer MD. Prostanoid receptors: subtypes and signaling. Annu Rev Pharmacol Toxicol. 2001;41:661–90.
66. Dunselman GA, Hendrix MG, Bouckaert PX, Evers JL. Functional aspects of peritoneal macrophages in endometriosis of women. J Reprod Fertil. 1988;82:707–10.
67. Haney AF, Muscato JJ, Weinberg JB. Peritoneal fluid cell populations in infertility patients. Fertil Steril. 1981;35:696–8.
68. Dunn GP, Old LJ, Schreiber RD. The immunobiology of cancer immunosurveillance and immunoediting. Immunity. 2004;21:137–48.
69. Dmowski WP, Gebel H, Braun DP. Decreased apoptosis and sensitivity to macrophage mediated cytolysis of endometrial cells in endometriosis. Hum Reprod Update. 1998;4:696–701.
70. Steele RW, Dmowski WP, Marmer DJ. Immunologic aspects of human endometriosis. Am J Reprod Immunol. 1984;6:33–6.
71. Visse R, Nagase H. Matrix metalloproteinases and tissue inhibitors of metalloproteinases: structure, function, and biochemistry. Circ Res. 2003;92:827–39.
72. Campbell EJ, Cury JD, Shapiro SD, Goldberg GI, Welgus HG. Neutral proteinases of human mononuclear phagocytes. Cellular differentiation markedly alters cell phenotype for serine proteinases, metalloproteinases, and tissue inhibitor of metalloproteinases. J Immunol. 1991;146:1286–93.
73. Curci JA, Liao S, Huffman MD, Shapiro SD, Thompson RW. Expression and localization of macrophage elastase (matrix metalloproteinase-12) in abdominal aortic aneurysms. J Clin Invest. 1998;102:1900–10.
74. Dhami R, Gilks B, Xie C, Zay K, Wright JL, Churg A. Acute cigarette smoke-induced connective tissue breakdown is mediated by neutrophils and prevented by alpha1-antitrypsin. Am J Respir Cell Mol Biol. 2000;22:244–52.
75. Welgus HG, Campbell EJ, Cury JD, Eisen AZ, Senior RM, Wilhelm SM, Goldberg GI. Neutral metalloproteinases produced by human mononuclear phagocytes. Enzyme profile, regulation, and expression during cellular development. J Clin Invest. 1990;86:1496–502.
76. McMillan JI, Weeks R, West JW, Bursten S, Rice GC, Lovett DH. Pharmacological inhibition of gelatinase B induction and tumor cell invasion. Int J Cancer. 1996;67:523–31.
77. Brownstein C, Deora AB, Jacovina AT, Weintraub R, Gertler M, Khan KM, Falcone DJ, Hajjar KA. Annexin II mediates plasminogen-dependent matrix invasion by human monocytes: enhanced expression by macrophages. Blood. 2004;103:317–24.
78. Swisher JF, Burton N, Bacot SM, Vogel SN, Feldman GM. Annexin A2 tetramer activates human and murine macrophages through TLR4. Blood. 2010;115:549–58.
79. Fan X, Krahling S, Smith D, Williamson P, Schlegel RA. Macrophage surface expression of annexins I and II in the phagocytosis of apoptotic lymphocytes. Mol Biol Cell. 2004;15:2863–72.
80. Febbraio M, Hajjar DP, Silverstein RL. CD36: a class B scavenger receptor involved in angiogenesis, atherosclerosis, inflammation, and lipid metabolism. J Clin Invest. 2001;108:785–91.
81. Linton MF, Fazio S. Class A scavenger receptors, macrophages, and atherosclerosis. Curr Opin Lipidol. 2001;12:489–95.
82. Krieger M, Herz J. Structures and functions of multiligand lipoprotein receptors: macrophage scavenger receptors and LDL receptor-related protein (LRP). Annu Rev Biochem. 1994;63:601–37.
83. Platt N, da Silva RP, Gordon S. Recognizing death: the phagocytosis of apoptotic cells. Trends Cell Biol. 1998;8:365–72.

84. Rigotti A, Acton SL, Krieger M. The class B scavenger receptors SR-BI and CD36 are receptors for anionic phospholipids. J Biol Chem. 1995;270:16221–4.
85. Savill J, Dransfield I, Hogg N, Haslett C. Vitronectin receptor-mediated phagocytosis of cells undergoing apoptosis. Nature. 1990;343:170–3.
86. Savill J, Hogg N, Ren Y, Haslett C. Thrombospondin cooperates with CD36 and the vitronectin receptor in macrophage recognition of neutrophils undergoing apoptosis. J Clin Invest. 1992;90:1513–22.
87. Chuang PC, Wu MH, Shoji Y, Tsai SJ. Downregulation of CD36 results in reduced phagocytic ability of peritoneal macrophages of women with endometriosis. J Pathol. 2009;219:232–41.
88. Wu MH, Chuang PC, Lin YJ, Tsai SJ. Suppression of annexin A2 by prostaglandin E (2) impairs phagocytic ability of peritoneal macrophages in women with endometriosis. Hum Reprod. 2013;28:1045–53.
89. Wu MH, Shoji Y, Wu MC, Chuang PC, Lin CC, Huang MF, Tsai SJ. Suppression of matrix metalloproteinase-9 by prostaglandin E(2) in peritoneal macrophage is associated with severity of endometriosis. Am J Pathol. 2005;167:1061–9.
90. Navazo MD, Daviet L, Savill J, Ren Y, Leung LL, McGregor JL. Identification of a domain (155–183) on CD36 implicated in the phagocytosis of apoptotic neutrophils. J Biol Chem. 1996;271:15381–5.
91. Trial J, Rice L. Erythropoietin withdrawal leads to the destruction of young red cells at the endothelial-macrophage interface. Curr Pharm Des. 2004;10:183–90.
92. Chuang PC, Lin YJ, Wu MH, Wing LY, Shoji Y, Tsai SJ. Inhibition of CD36-dependent phagocytosis by prostaglandin E2 contributes to the development of endometriosis. Am J Pathol. 2010;176:850–60.
93. Harada T, Yoshioka H, Yoshida S, Iwabe T, Onohara Y, Tanikawa M, Terakawa N. Increased interleukin-6 levels in peritoneal fluid of infertile patients with active endometriosis. Am J Obstet Gynecol. 1997;176:593–7.
94. Iwabe T, Harada T, Tsudo T, Tanikawa M, Onohara Y, Terakawa N. Pathogenetic significance of increased levels of interleukin-8 in the peritoneal fluid of patients with endometriosis. Fertil Steril. 1998;69:924–30.
95. Koyama N, Matsuura K, Okamura H. Cytokines in the peritoneal fluid of patients with endometriosis. Int J Gynaecol Obstet. 1993;43:45–50.
96. Kupker W, Schultze-Mosgau A, Diedrich K. Paracrine changes in the peritoneal environment of women with endometriosis. Hum Reprod Update. 1998;4:719–23.
97. Donnez J, Smoes P, Gillerot S, Casanas-Roux F, Nisolle M. Vascular endothelial growth factor (VEGF) in endometriosis. Hum Reprod. 1998;13:1686–90.
98. Groothuis PG, Nap AW, Winterhager E, Grummer R. Vascular development in endometriosis. Angiogenesis. 2005;8:147–56.
99. Taylor RN, Lebovic DI, Mueller MD. Angiogenic factors in endometriosis. Ann N Y Acad Sci. 2002;955:89–100. discussion 18, 396–406.
100. Mahnke JL, Dawood MY, Huang JC. Vascular endothelial growth factor and interleukin-6 in peritoneal fluid of women with endometriosis. Fertil Steril. 2000;73:166–70.
101. Jones MK, Wang H, Peskar BM, Levin E, Itani RM, Sarfeh IJ, Tarnawski AS. Inhibition of angiogenesis by nonsteroidal anti-inflammatory drugs: insight into mechanisms and implications for cancer growth and ulcer healing. Nat Med. 1999;5:1418–23.
102. Tsujii M, Kawano S, Tsuji S, Sawaoka H, Hori M, DuBois RN. Cyclooxygenase regulates angiogenesis induced by colon cancer cells. Cell. 1998;93:705–16.
103. Williams CS, Tsujii M, Reese J, Dey SK, DuBois RN. Host cyclooxygenase-2 modulates carcinoma growth. J Clin Invest. 2000;105:1589–94.
104. Ceyhan ST, Onguru O, Baser I, Gunhan O. Expression of cyclooxygenase-2 and vascular endothelial growth factor in ovarian endometriotic cysts and their relationship with angiogenesis. Fertil Steril. 2008;90:988–93.

105. Olivares C, Bilotas M, Buquet R, Borghi M, Sueldo C, Tesone M, Meresman G. Effects of a selective cyclooxygenase-2 inhibitor on endometrial epithelial cells from patients with endometriosis. Hum Reprod. 2008;23:2701–8.
106. Dogan E, Saygili U, Posaci C, Tuna B, Caliskan S, Altunyurt S, Saatli B. Regression of endometrial explants in rats treated with the cyclooxygenase-2 inhibitor rofecoxib. Fertil Steril. 2004;82 Suppl 3:1115–20.
107. Ozawa Y, Murakami T, Tamura M, Terada Y, Yaegashi N, Okamura K. A selective cyclooxygenase-2 inhibitor suppresses the growth of endometriosis xenografts via antiangiogenic activity in severe combined immunodeficiency mice. Fertil Steril. 2006;86:1146–51.
108. Laschke MW, Elitzsch A, Scheuer C, Vollmar B, Menger MD. Selective cyclo-oxygenase-2 inhibition induces regression of autologous endometrial grafts by down-regulation of vascular endothelial growth factor-mediated angiogenesis and stimulation of caspase-3-dependent apoptosis. Fertil Steril. 2007;87:163–71.
109. Machado DE, Berardo PT, Landgraf RG, Fernandes PD, Palmero C, Alves LM, Abrao MS, Nasciutti LE. A selective cyclooxygenase-2 inhibitor suppresses the growth of endometriosis with an antiangiogenic effect in a rat model. Fertil Steril. 2010;93:2674–9.
110. Mo FE, Muntean AG, Chen CC, Stolz DB, Watkins SC, Lau LF. CYR61 (CCN1) is essential for placental development and vascular integrity. Mol Cell Biol. 2002;22:8709–20.
111. Chen Y, Du XY. Functional properties and intracellular signaling of CCN1/Cyr61. J Cell Biochem. 2007;100:1337–45.
112. Gashaw I, Stiller S, Boing C, Kimmig R, Winterhager E. Premenstrual regulation of the pro-angiogenic factor CYR61 in human endometrium. Endocrinology. 2008;149:2261–9.
113. MacLaughlan SD, Palomino WA, Mo B, Lewis TD, Lininger RA, Lessey BA. Endometrial expression of Cyr61: a marker of estrogenic activity in normal and abnormal endometrium. Obstet Gynecol. 2007;110:146–54.
114. Absenger Y, Hess-Stumpp H, Kreft B, Kratzschmar J, Haendler B, Schutze N, Regidor PA, Winterhager E. Cyr61, a deregulated gene in endometriosis. Mol Hum Reprod. 2004;10:399–407.
115. Gashaw I, Hastings JM, Jackson KS, Winterhager E, Fazleabas AT. Induced endometriosis in the baboon (Papio anubis) increases the expression of the proangiogenic factor CYR61 (CCN1) in eutopic and ectopic endometria. Biol Reprod. 2006;74:1060–6.
116. Attar E, Bulun SE. Aromatase and other steroidogenic genes in endometriosis: translational aspects. Hum Reprod Update. 2006;12:49–56.
117. Richard DE, Berra E, Gothie E, Roux D, Pouyssegur J. p42/p44 mitogen-activated protein kinases phosphorylate hypoxia-inducible factor 1alpha (HIF-1alpha) and enhance the transcriptional activity of HIF-1. J Biol Chem. 1999;274:32631–7.
118. Murk W, Atabekoglu CS, Cakmak H, Heper A, Ensari A, Kayisli UA, Arici A. Extracellularly signal-regulated kinase activity in the human endometrium: possible roles in the pathogenesis of endometriosis. J Clin Endocrinol Metab. 2008;93:3532–40.
119. Carli C, Metz CN, Al-Abed Y, Naccache PH, Akoum A. Up-regulation of cyclooxygenase-2 expression and prostaglandin E2 production in human endometriotic cells by macrophage migration inhibitory factor: involvement of novel kinase signaling pathways. Endocrinology. 2009;150:3128–37.
120. Tamura M, Sebastian S, Yang S, Gurates B, Fang Z, Bulun SE. Interleukin-1beta elevates cyclooxygenase-2 protein level and enzyme activity via increasing its mRNA stability in human endometrial stromal cells: an effect mediated by extracellularly regulated kinases 1 and 2. J Clin Endocrinol Metab. 2002;87:3263–73.
121. Veillat V, Carli C, Metz CN, Al-Abed Y, Naccache PH, Akoum A. Macrophage migration inhibitory factor elicits an angiogenic phenotype in human ectopic endometrial cells and triggers the production of major angiogenic factors via CD44, CD74, and MAPK signaling pathways. J Clin Endocrinol Metab. 2010;95:E403–12.

122. Ngo C, Nicco C, Leconte M, Chereau C, Arkwright S, Vacher-Lavenu MC, Weill B, Chapron C, Batteux F. Protein kinase inhibitors can control the progression of endometriosis in vitro and in vivo. J Pathol. 2010;222:148–57.
123. Momoeda M, Harada T, Terakawa N, Aso T, Fukunaga M, Hagino H, Taketani Y. Long-term use of dienogest for the treatment of endometriosis. J Obstet Gynaecol Res. 2009;35:1069–76.
124. Shimizu Y, Mita S, Takeuchi T, Notsu T, Mizuguchi K, Kyo S. Dienogest, a synthetic progestin, inhibits prostaglandin E2 production and aromatase expression by human endometrial epithelial cells in a spheroid culture system. Steroids. 2010;76:60–7.
125. Yamanaka K, Xu B, Suganuma I, Kusuki I, Mita S, Shimizu Y, Mizuguchi K, Kitawaki J. Dienogest inhibits aromatase and cyclooxygenase-2 expression and prostaglandin E(2) production in human endometriotic stromal cells in spheroid culture. Fertil Steril. 2012;97:477–82.

Chapter 10
Sex Steroids and Endometriosis

Jo Kitawaki

Abstract Endometriosis develops mostly in women of reproductive age and regresses after menopause, suggesting that the growth of lesions is estrogen dependent. Estrogen metabolism differs considerably in women with a normal endometrium compared to those with estrogen-dependent uterine diseases, including endometriosis, adenomyosis, or fibromas. Altered expression patterns of estrogen receptor (ER)-α/ER-β, progesterone receptor (PR)-A/PR-B, and 17-β-hydroxysteroid dehydrogenase type 1 (HSD17B1)/type 2 (HSD17B2) in endometriotic tissue may upregulate aromatase and increase local estrogenic activity. Polymorphisms in *ESR1*, *ESR2*, *PR*, *HSD17B1*, 17α-hydroxylase (*CYP17A1*), and aromatase (*CYP19*) genes have been investigated putative associations with endometriosis susceptibility.

Keywords Endometriosis • Endometrium • Estrogen • Polymorphism • Steroid receptors

10.1 Introduction

Endometriosis, a common gynecological disorder in women of reproductive age, is characterized by the presence of endometrium-like lesions outside the uterine cavity. The main symptoms are pelvic pain, including dysmenorrhea, chronic pelvic pain and deep dyspareunia, and infertility [1]. Endometriosis develops in approximately 10 % of women of reproductive age and regresses after menopause or ovariectomy. The occurrence of endometriosis before menarche has not been reported. The suppression of estrogen levels using a gonadotropin-releasing

J. Kitawaki (✉)
Department of Obstetrics and Gynecology, Kyoto Prefectural University of Medicine,
Graduate School of Medical Science, Kyoto 602-8566, Japan
e-mail: kitawaki@koto.kpu-m.ac.jp

T. Harada (ed.), *Endometriosis: Pathogenesis and Treatment*,
DOI 10.1007/978-4-431-54421-0_10, © Springer Japan 2014

hormone agonist causes regression of the lesions. The recovery of estrogen levels after discontinuing therapy causes a relapse. Endometriosis may relapse in postmenopausal women who have been treated with estrogen-replacement therapy, suggesting that endometriosis progresses and regresses in an estrogen-dependent fashion.

10.2 Mechanisms of Estrogen-Dependent Growth

Breast cancer, endometrial cancer, endometriosis, adenomyosis, and fibromas are diseases that progress in an estrogen-dependent fashion. These lesions commonly contain ER, PR, and androgen receptors. Interestingly, all of the estrogen-dependent diseases of the breast and uterus contain not only ER but also aromatase, an enzyme that catalyzes the conversion of androgens to estrogens. Together with the circulating estrogen, local estrogen production increases the estrogen concentration and stimulates the growth of tissue mediated by the ER. Immunohistochemical studies have shown that ER and PR are localized to the nucleus of both glandular and stromal cells [2–9], whereas aromatase is exclusively localized to the cytoplasm of epithelial glandular cells [9].

Expression patterns of steroid-related molecules, including steroid receptors and enzymes involved in estrogen metabolism, differ between endometriotic tissues and eutopic endometria. Electron microscopic analysis has shown that one-third of endometriotic implants are out of phase with the menstrual cycle [10], and a light microscopic study showed that only 13 % of endometriotic implants were synchronous with the corresponding eutopic endometria [11].

10.2.1 Steroid Receptors

ER-β levels are higher and ER-α levels are lower in women with endometriosis than in those with a normal endometrium. Higher ER-β levels are caused by hypomethylation of a CpG island at the promoter region of this gene. In endometriotic cells, the excess expression of ER-β is responsible for the estrogen-dependent responses, and this expression inhibits ER-α action [12].

The single PR gene is translated into one of two isoforms (PR-A or PR-B) by activating the corresponding promoters. PR-A is a truncated form of PR-B that lacks the N-terminal 164 amino acids; PR-A acts as a repressor of PR-B function. In endometriotic tissue, PR-B is undetectable [13] due to hypermethylation of the *PR* gene and PR-A is markedly reduced [14]. Furthermore, excess ER-β occupies the estrogen responsive element at PR promoter region and blocks transcription of PR that is normally activated by ER-α [15].

10.2.2 *Estrogen Metabolism*

10.2.2.1 Aromatase

Steroidogenic factor 1 (SF1), an orphan nuclear receptor, is expressed at a 12,000 times higher concentration in women with endometriosis than in those with a normal endometrium. SF1 is involved in the prostaglandin E_2 (PGE_2)-stimulated increase in aromatase expression [15]. In endometrial cells, a CpG island at the SF1 promoter is highly methylated and binds to a silencer-type transcription factor, whereas in endometriotic cells, SF1 promoter is unmethylated and binds to a coactivator.

A positive feedback cycle indicates that aromatase and cyclooxygenase-2 (COX-2), a PGE_2 synthase, are responsible for the continuous local formation of estrogen and PGE_2 in endometriotic stromal cells [16]. PGE_2 is a major mediator of endometriosis-associated pain. Aromatase expression might be induced by PGE_2 in endometriotic cells. Aromatase produces estradiol, which consequently promotes PGE_2 production by inducing COX-2 expression [17]. Danazol and dienogest, a fourth-generation progestin, which is used for relieving endometriosis-associated pelvic pain, downregulate expression of aromatase and COX-2 in endometriotic cells [18].

In the normal endometrium of women, aromatase is not expressed, but it is expressed in the endometrium of women with estrogen-dependent uterine diseases such as endometriosis, adenomyosis, or fibromas [9, 19, 20]. In endometriotic cells, the increased expression of SF1 activates aromatase transcription [21]. Immunohistochemical detection of aromatase P450 protein in endometrial biopsies can be used as a screening test for endometriosis [22]. However, detection of aromatase mRNA is less specific for screening of endometriosis [23].

10.2.2.2 17β-Hydroxysteroid Dehydrogenase Type 1 and Type 2

In endometriotic tissues, HSD17B1, an enzyme that converts estrone to the more potent estradiol, predominates, whereas expression of HSD17B2, an enzyme responsible for weakening the activity of estradiol and converting it into less active estrone, is undetectable [24] or at a lower level than HSD17B1 [20, 25]. This is partially responsible for raising the local estrogen activity level.

In contrast in the endometrium, an oxidative reaction that weakens the activity of estradiol to estrone by HSD17B2 predominates and the expression of HSD17B1 is undetectable [26] or extremely low [25]. During the proliferative phase, the expression level and activity of HSD17B2 are comparable in endometria of women with estrogen-dependent diseases and women without disease. However, during the secretory phase, while the expression and activity of HSD17B2 increase four- to sixfold in diseased endometria, there is no cyclical change in normal endometrium [20, 27]. Although it is not possible to distinguish histologically between normal and diseased endometria, estrogen metabolism is different between the two states. Furthermore, in endometriotic tissues, progesterone does not stimulate HSD17B2 because there is no PR-B [13], whereas endometrium of women with endometriosis acquires ability to stimulate HSD17B2 by progesterone.

10.3 Polymorphisms in Genes Involved in Steroid Metabolism

Both environmental and genetic factors have been implicated in the pathogenesis of endometriosis. Family and twin studies have indicated that there is a two- to ninefold increase in the risk of developing endometriosis in first-degree relatives of women with endometriosis, suggesting it is a genetic disorder with polygenic or multifactorial inheritance [28–30]. Studies have revealed associations between the polymorphisms of many genes, including the genes involved in steroid metabolism and endometriosis susceptibility.

10.3.1 ESR1

Polymorphisms in the gene coding for ER-α (*ESR1*) have been investigated in European and Asian women. Single-nucleotide polymorphisms in intron 1 of the *ESR1* gene have been assessed in *Pvu*II (−398 T/C) and *Xba*I (−351A/G) restriction fragment length polymorphisms. Several studies found statistically significant differences between the cases and controls in the distribution of *Pvu*II alleles [31–34], but other studies found no association with *Pvu*II polymorphisms [35–38]. One study found an association with an *Xba*I polymorphism [34], and three studies found an association with the TA dinucleotide repeat polymorphism [31, 36, 39, 40].

10.3.2 ESR2

One study in Japanese women showed association with the gene coding for *ER*-β (*ESR2*) *Alu*I polymorphism [35], but other studies found no association [33, 41]. One study showed that shorter CA dinucleotide repeats in the *ESR2* gene were linked to endometriosis in women without infertility [40].

10.3.3 PR

Several studies in Austria, Italy, and Brazil showed association between the 306-bp insertion polymorphism in intron G of the *PR* gene (PROGINS) and the risk of endometriosis risk [42–44].

10.3.4 HSD17B1

Several studies showed that, in an A/G polymorphism of the *HSD17B1* gene, the A allele was found to be associated with a significantly increased risk of endometriosis [40, 45].

10.3.5 CYP17

One study showed a possible association of endometriosis in Taiwanese women with a *Msp*A1 (T/C) polymorphism in the *CYP17A1* gene [39], whereas other studies found no association between any *CYP17A1* gene polymorphisms and endometriosis risk [46–48].

10.3.6 CYP19

In intron 4 of the *CYP19* gene, there is a TTTA repeat microsatellite polymorphism, and 50-bp upstream of the TTTA polymorphism, a 3-base pair (CTT) insertion/deletion polymorphism. A study in Japanese women showed an association between this 3-base pair insertion/deletion polymorphism and endometriosis risk [46]. The TTTA repeat polymorphism was found to increase endometriosis risk in Greek women [49]. A study in Italian women showed a significant association of AA and CC genotypes in Val80 and C1558T polymorphisms with endometriosis risk [50]. However, two other studies showed no association between *CYP19* gene polymorphisms and endometriosis susceptibility [40, 45].

10.4 Conclusions

Altered expression patterns of a range of receptors and enzymes involved in steroid metabolism (ER-α/ER-β, PR-A/PR-B, and HSD17B1/HSD17B2) in endometriotic tissue may upregulate aromatase and increase local estrogenic activity, thus stimulating the growth of lesions. Substantial differences in estrogen metabolism exist between normal endometrium and the endometrium in women with uterine diseases, including endometriosis, adenomyosis, or fibromas. Polymorphisms in *ESR1*, *ESR2*, *PR*, *HSD17B1*, *CYP17A1*, and *CYP19* genes have all been investigated with varying success. Further investigations to distinguish pathologic from normal endometria and genetic polymorphism associations will contribute to a better understanding of endometriosis and help develop novel therapeutic strategies for this disease.

References

1. Vercellini P, Somigliana E, Viganò P, Abbiati A, Barbara G, Fedele L. Chronic pelvic pain in women: etiology, pathogenesis and diagnostic approach. Gynecol Endocrinol. 2009;25:149–58.
2. Lessey BA, Metzger DA, Haney AF, McCarty Jr KS. Immunohistochemical analysis of estrogen and progesterone receptors in endometriosis: comparison with normal endometrium during the menstrual cycle and the effect of medical therapy. Fertil Steril. 1989;51:409–15.
3. Prentice A, Randall BJ, Weddell A, McGill A, Henry L, Horne CH, Thomas EJ. Ovarian steroid receptor expression in endometriosis and in two potential parent epithelia: endometrium and peritoneal mesothelium. Hum Reprod. 1992;7:1318–25.
4. Bergqvist A, Ljungberg O, Skoog L. Immunohistochemical analysis of oestrogen and progesterone receptors in endometriotic tissue and endometrium. Hum Reprod. 1993;8:1915–22.
5. Jones RK, Bulmer JN, Searle RF. Immunohistochemical characterization of proliferation, oestrogen receptor and progesterone receptor expression in endometriosis: comparison of eutopic and ectopic endometrium with normal cycling endometrium. Hum Reprod. 1995;10:3272–9.
6. Howell RJ, Dowsett M, Edmonds DK. Oestrogen and progesterone receptors in endometriosis: heterogeneity of different sites. Hum Reprod. 1994;9:1752–8.
7. Nisolle M, Casanas-Roux F, Wyns C, de Menten Y, Mathieu PE, Donnez J. Immunohistochemical analysis of estrogen and progesterone receptors in endometrium and peritoneal endometriosis: a new quantitative method. Fertil Steril. 1994;62:751–9.
8. Fujishita A, Nakane PK, Koji T, Masuzaki H, Chavez RO, Yamabe T, Ishimaru T. Expression of estrogen and progesterone receptors in endometrium and peritoneal endometriosis: an immunohistochemical and in situ hybridization study. Fertil Steril. 1997;67:856–64.
9. Kitawaki J, Noguchi T, Amatsu T, Maeda K, Tsukamoto K, Yamamoto T, Fushiki S, Osawa Y, Honjo H. Expression of aromatase cytochrome P450 protein and messenger ribonucleic acid in human endometriotic and adenomyotic tissues but not in normal endometrium. Biol Reprod. 1997;57:514–9.
10. Schweppe KW, Wynn RM. Ultrastructural changes in endometriotic implants during the menstrual cycle. Obstet Gynecol. 1981;58:465–73.
11. Metzger DA, Olive DL, Haney AF. Limited hormonal responsiveness of ectopic endometrium: histologic correlation with intrauterine endometrium. Hum Pathol. 1988;19:1417–24.
12. Xue Q, Lin Z, Cheng YH, Huang CC, Marsh E, Yin P, Milad MP, Confino E, Reierstad S, Innes J, Bulun SE. Promoter methylation regulates estrogen receptor 2 in human endometrium and endometriosis. Biol Reprod. 2007;77:681–7.
13. Attia GR, Zeitoun K, Edwards D, Johns A, Carr BR, Bulun SE. Progesterone receptor isoform A but not B is expressed in endometriosis. J Clin Endocrinol Metab. 2000;85:2897–902.
14. Wu Y, Strawn E, Basir Z, Halverson G, Guo SW. Promoter hypermethylation of progesterone receptor isoform B (PR-B) in endometriosis. Epigenetics. 2006;1:106–11.

15. Xue Q, Lin Z, Yin P, Milad MP, Cheng YH, Confino E, Reierstad S, Bulun SE. Transcriptional activation of steroidogenic factor-1 by hypomethylation of the 5′ CpG island in endometriosis. J Clin Endocrinol Metab. 2007;92:3261–7.
16. Bulun SE. Endometriosis. N Engl J Med. 2009;360:268–79.
17. Bulun SE, Zeitoun K, Takayama K, Noble L, Michael D, Simpson E, Johns A, Putman M, Sasano H. Estrogen production in endometriosis and use of aromatase inhibitors to treat endometriosis. Endocr Relat Cancer. 1999;6:293–301.
18. Yamanaka K, Xu B, Suganuma I, Kusuki I, Mita S, Shimizu Y, Mizuguchi K, Kitawaki J. Dienogest inhibits aromatase and cyclooxygenase-2 expression and prostaglandin E_2 production in human endometriotic stromal cells in spheroid culture. Fertil Steril. 2012;97:477–82.
19. Noble LS, Simpson ER, Johns A, Bulun SE. Aromatase expression in endometriosis. J Clin Endocrinol Metab. 1996;81:174–9.
20. Matsuzaki S, Canis M, Pouly JL, Déchelotte PJ, Mage G. Analysis of aromatase and 17-β-hydroxysteroid dehydrogenase type 2 messenger ribonucleic acid expression in deep endometriosis and eutopic endometrium using laser capture microdissection. Fertil Steril. 2006;85:308–13.
21. Zeitoun K, Takayama K, Michael MD, Bulun SE. Stimulation of aromatase P450 promoter (II) activity in endometriosis and its inhibition in endometrium are regulated by competitive binding of steroidogenic factor-1 and chicken ovalbumin upstream promoter transcription factor to the same *cis*-acting element. Mol Endocrinol. 1999;13:239–53.
22. Kitawaki J, Kusuki I, Koshiba H, Tsukamoto K, Fushiki S, Honjo H. Detection of aromatase cytochrome P-450 in endometrial biopsy specimens as a diagnostic test for endometriosis. Fertil Steril. 1999;72:1100–6.
23. Dheenadayalu K, Mak I, Gordts S, Campo R, Higham J, Puttemans P, White J, Christian M, Fusi L, Brosens J. Aromatase P450 messenger RNA expression in eutopic endometrium is not a specific marker for pelvic endometriosis. Fertil Steril. 2002;78:825–9.
24. Zeitoun K, Takayama K, Sasano H, Suzuki T, Moghrabi N, Andersson S, Johns A, Meng L, Putman M, Carr B, Bulun SE. Deficient 17β-hydroxysteroid dehydrogenase type 2 expression in endometriosis: failure to metabolize 17β-estradiol. J Clin Endocrinol Metab. 1998;83:4474–80.
25. Dassen H, Punyadeera C, Kamps R, Delvoux B, Van Langendonckt A, Donnez J, Husen B, Thole H, Dunselman G, Groothuis P. Estrogen metabolizing enzymes in endometrium and endometriosis. Hum Reprod. 2007;22:3148–58.
26. Utsunomiya H, Suzuki T, Kaneko C, Takeyama J, Nakamura J, Kimura K, Yoshihama M, Harada N, Ito K, Konno R, Sato S, Okamura K, Sasano H. The analyses of 17β-hydroxysteroid dehydrogenase isozymes in human endometrial hyperplasia and carcinoma. J Clin Endocrinol Metab. 2001;86:3436–43.
27. Kitawaki J, Koshiba H, Ishihara H, Kusuki I, Tsukamoto K, Honjo H. Progesterone induction of 17β-hydroxysteroid dehydrogenase type 2 during the secretory phase occurs in the endometrium of estrogen-dependent benign diseases but not in normal endometrium. J Clin Endocrinol Metab. 2000;85:3292–6.
28. Moen MH, Magnus P. The familial risk of endometriosis. Acta Obstet Gynecol Scand. 1993;72:560–4.
29. Kennedy S, Mardon H, Barlow D. Familial endometriosis. J Assist Reprod Genet. 1995;12:32–4.
30. Treloar SA, O'Connor DT, O'Connor VM, Martin NG. Genetic influences on endometriosis in an Australian twin sample. Fertil Steril. 1999;71:701–10.
31. Georgiou I, Syrrou M, Bouba I, Dalkalitsis N, Paschopoulos M, Navrozoglou I, Lolis D. Association of estrogen receptor gene polymorphisms with endometriosis. Fertil Steril. 1999;72:164–6.
32. Kitawaki J, Obayashi H, Ishihara H, Koshiba H, Kusuki I, Kado N, Tsukamoto K, Hasegawa G, Nakamura N, Honjo H. Oestrogen receptor-α gene polymorphism is associated with endometriosis, adenomyosis and leiomyomata. Hum Reprod. 2001;16:51–5.

33. Luisi S, Galleri L, Marini F, Ambrosini G, Brandi ML, Petraglia F. Estrogen receptor gene polymorphisms are associated with recurrence of endometriosis. Fertil Steril. 2006;85:764–6.
34. Hsieh YY, Wang YK, Chang CC, Lin CS. Estrogen receptor α-351 XbaI*G and −397 PvuII*C-related genotypes and alleles are associated with higher susceptibilities of endometriosis and leiomyoma. Mol Hum Reprod. 2007;13:117–22.
35. Wang Z, Yoshida S, Negoro K, Kennedy S, Barlow D, Maruo T. Polymorphisms in the estrogen receptor β gene but not estrogen receptor α gene affect the risk of developing endometriosis in a Japanese population. Fertil Steril. 2004;81:1650–6.
36. Kim SH, Choi YM, Jun JK, Kim SH, Kim JG, Moon SY. Estrogen receptor dinucleotide repeat polymorphism is associated with minimal or mild endometriosis. Fertil Steril. 2005;84:774–7.
37. Renner SP, Strick R, Oppelt P, Fasching PA, Engel S, Baumann R, Beckmann MW, Strissel PL. Evaluation of clinical parameters and estrogen receptor α gene polymorphisms for patients with endometriosis. Reproduction. 2006;131:153–61.
38. Xie J, Wang S, He B, Pan Y, Li Y, Zeng Q, Jiang H, Chen J. Association of estrogen receptor α and interleukin-10 gene polymorphisms with endometriosis in a Chinese population. Fertil Steril. 2009;92:54–60.
39. Hsieh YY, Chang CC, Tsai FJ, Lin CC, Tsai CH. Estrogen receptor α dinucleotide repeat and cytochrome P450c17α gene polymorphisms are associated with susceptibility to endometriosis. Fertil Steril. 2005;83:567–72.
40. Lamp M, Peters M, Reinmaa E, Haller-Kikkatalo K, Kaart T, Kadastik U, Karro H, Metspalu A, Salumets A. Polymorphisms in ESR1, ESR2 and HSD17B1 genes are associated with fertility status in endometriosis. Gynecol Endocrinol. 2011;27:425–33.
41. Lee GH, Kim SH, Choi YM, Suh CS, Kim JG, Moon SY. Estrogen receptor β gene +1730 G/A polymorphism in women with endometriosis. Fertil Steril. 2007;88:785–8.
42. Wieser F, Schneeberger C, Tong D, Tempfer C, Huber JC, Wenzl R. PROGINS receptor gene polymorphism is associated with endometriosis. Fertil Steril. 2002;77:309–12.
43. Lattuada D, Somigliana E, Vigano P, Candiani M, Pardi G, Di Blasio AM. Genetics of endometriosis: a role for the progesterone receptor gene polymorphism PROGINS? Clin Endocrinol. 2004;61:190–4.
44. De Carvalho CV, Nogueira-De-Souza NC, Costa AM, Baracat EC, Girão MJ, D'Amora P, Schor E, da Silva ID. Genetic polymorphisms of cytochrome P450c17α (CYP17) and progesterone receptor genes (PROGINS) in the assessment of endometriosis risk. Gynecol Endocrinol. 2007;23:29–33.
45. Tsuchiya M, Nakao H, Katoh T, Sasaki H, Hiroshima M, Tanaka T, Matsunaga T, Hanaoka T, Tsugane S, Ikenoue T. Association between endometriosis and genetic polymorphisms of the estradiol-synthesizing enzyme genes HSD17B1 and CYP19. Hum Reprod. 2005;20:974–8.
46. Kado N, Kitawaki J, Obayashi H, Ishihara H, Koshiba H, Kusuki I, Tsukamoto K, Hasegawa G, Nakamura N, Yoshikawa T, Honjo H. Association of the *CYP17* gene and *CYP19* gene polymorphisms with risk of endometriosis in Japanese women. Hum Reprod. 2002;17:897–902.
47. Asghar T, Yoshida S, Nakago S, Morizane M, Ohara N, Motoyama S, Kennedy S, Barlow D, Maruo T. Lack of association between endometriosis and the CYP17 MspA1 polymorphism in UK and Japanese populations. Gynecol Endocrinol. 2005;20:59–63.
48. Juo SH, Wang TN, Lee JN, Wu MT, Long CY, Tsai EM. CYP17, CYP1A1 and COMT polymorphisms and the risk of adenomyosis and endometriosis in Taiwanese women. Hum Reprod. 2006;21:1498–502.
49. Arvanitis DA, Koumantakis GE, Goumenou AG, Matalliotakis IM, Koumantakis EE, Spandidos DA. CYP1A1, CYP19, and GSTM1 polymorphisms increase the risk of endometriosis. Fertil Steril. 2003;79 Suppl 1:702–9.
50. Vietri MT, Cioffi M, Sessa M, Simeone S, Bontempo P, Trabucco E, Ardovino M, Colacurci N, Molinari AM, Cobellis L. CYP17 and CYP19 gene polymorphisms in women affected with endometriosis. Fertil Steril. 2009;92:1532–5.

Chapter 11
Aromatase Expression in Endometriosis and Its Significance

Hiroshi Ishikawa and Makio Shozu

Abstract Endometriosis is a chronic inflammatory disease frequently observed in the ovary, pelvic peritoneum, and rectovaginal septum. The growth and progression of an endometriotic lesion depends on a sex steroid, estrogen. Aromatase, a key enzyme in estrogen biosynthesis, is highly expressed in the endometriotic tissue, resulting in in situ production of estrogen that, in addition to endocrine estrogen from the ovary, may contribute to the etiology and progression of endometriosis. The aberrant expression of aromatase together with the elevated expression of 17β-hydroxysteroid dehydrogenase type 1 and the absence of 17β-hydroxysteroid dehydrogenase type 2 observed in the endometriotic tissue would contribute to an increase in the tissue concentration of estrogen. Aromatase expression is regulated at multiple levels, from the transcription of *CYP19A1* and epigenetic codes to posttranslational modification and degradation of the protein. Among the multiple promoters of *CYP19A1*, the most proximal promoter PII is the most active in endometriosis and is regulated by cAMP, prostaglandin E2, steroidogenic factor-1, and possibly the end product estrogen. Hypomethylation of CpG islands on *CYP19A1* observed in the endometriotic tissue may contribute to the upregulation of aromatase expression.

Similar to spontaneous menopause, inhibition of in situ estrogen biosynthesis may regress endometriosis. The use of aromatase inhibitors (AIs), which selectively inhibit aromatase activity in human tissues, is a possible treatment for inhibiting local estrogen biosynthesis in endometriosis. AIs have been used as monotherapy or in combination therapies with progestins, oral contraceptive pills, and gonadotropin-releasing hormone agonists to reduce endometriosis-related pain in premenopausal women.

Keywords Aromatase • Aromatase inhibitor • Estrogen • Letrozole

H. Ishikawa, M.D., Ph.D. • M. Shozu, M.D., Ph.D. (✉)
Department of Reproductive Medicine, Graduate School of Medicine, Chiba University, 1-8-1 Inohana, Chuo-ku, Chiba 260-8670, Japan
e-mail: shozu@faculty.chiba-u.jp

T. Harada (ed.), *Endometriosis: Pathogenesis and Treatment*,
DOI 10.1007/978-4-431-54421-0_11, © Springer Japan 2014

11.1 Introduction

Endometriosis is defined as the proliferation of the endometrial gland-like epithelium and surrounding stroma outside the uterus. It is frequently observed in the pelvic peritoneum, ovary, and rectovaginal septum. In total, 6–10 % of women of reproductive age are suffering from endometriosis-related pain, i.e., menorrhagia, dyspareunia, and chronic pelvic pain. Moreover, endometriosis may cause infertility. Although considerably rare, ovarian endometrioma can transform and give rise to ovarian cancer during long-term management of the disease.

Endometriosis becomes symptomatic in the reproductive age and is self-limited after spontaneous menopause. Similar to spontaneous menopause, long-term inhibition of ovulation using progestins, oral contraceptive pills (OCPs), and gonadotropin-releasing hormone (GnRH) agonists alleviates the symptoms. On the other hand, estrogen use in postmenopausal women induces symptomatic regrowth of endometrial lesions. These findings suggest that the progression of endometriosis is closely associated with estrogen as well as ovulation.

The ovary synthesizes estrogens de novo from cholesterol and supplies most of the circulating estrogens in women of reproductive age. In addition to the ovary, a small amount of estrogens can be synthesized in situ at peripheral fat, bones, the skin, the brain, and vessels, which are unable to synthesize estrogen from cholesterol de novo but are able to convert circulating androgens to estrogens [1, 2].

There are 2 rate-limiting steps in estrogen biosynthesis. The first step is the mobilization of cholesterol across the mitochondrial membrane into the mitochondria. This step is mediated by the steroidogenic acute regulatory protein (StAR) expressed in the mitochondria. The second step is the enzymatic reaction converting androgens to estrogens by aromatase. Aromatase is a member of the cytochrome P450 superfamily and is expressed in the endoplasmic reticulum. Aromatase is a unique enzyme that can catalyze aromatization. The rate of estrogen synthesis depends on these 2 steps in the ovary, where estrogen is synthesized de novo. On the other hand, the synthesis depends only on the second step in peripheral organs. In these peripheral organs, expression levels of aromatase determine the production rate of estrogen as long as circulating androgen is supplied [3].

Estrogen plays essential roles in reproduction, bone development, and epiphyseal closure in puberty, bone mineral metabolism, and possibly cognitive function. In addition to the physiological roles, recent studies have focused on the pathological roles and revealed that the overproduction of estrogen in situ causes diseases. Breast cancer tissues express a high level of aromatase, and the resulting in situ estrogen promotes cancer cell growth in postmenopausal women. Endometriosis is another example in which the aberrant expression of aromatase is involved in disease pathogenesis. The inhibition of in situ estrogen synthesis using an aromatase inhibitor (AI) is therefore a potential choice of treatment, similar to that seen in the case of breast cancer.

Here, we review the aromatase expression in endometriotic tissues and the mechanisms underlying the aberrant expression. Following this, we discuss the pathophysiological significance of in situ estrogen in endometriotic tissues and of aromatase as a molecular target treatment for refractory endometriosis.

11.2 Aromatase Genes and Their Expression in Endometriotic Tissues

11.2.1 Genomic Structure of CYP19A1

Aromatase is a unique enzyme responsible for the conversion of androgens to estrogens in humans. Aromatase is encoded by *CYP19A1* on chromosome 15q22, which spans approximately 132 kb and is composed of at least 9 alternative first exons and their 9 downstream coding exons (exons 2–10). Each first exon contains a unique 5′-untranslated sequence and a unique upstream promoter sequence. Each promoter possesses multiple transcriptional regulatory element-binding sites, which enable tissue-specific and promoter-specific regulation of aromatase expression.

The transcription of aromatase begins from 1 of the 9 first exons, is extended to exon 10, and ends at 1 of the 2 poly A signals located at the end of the 3′-untranslated region of exon 10. The resulting primary transcripts give rise to mRNA by splicing all introns. Because there are 9 different first exons, at least 9 different mRNAs are formed; however, all of these encode the same aromatase protein because the protein coding sequence is located in the shared exon 2 and its downstream.

11.2.2 Regulation of Aromatase Expression

11.2.2.1 Expression of Aromatase and In Situ Estrogen

Aromatase is highly expressed in ovarian granulosa cells of Graafian follicles and in placental cytotrophoblasts. Aromatase is also expressed in Sertoli cells, neurons, adipose stromal cells, vascular smooth muscle cells, skin fibroblasts, bone osteoblasts and osteoclasts, hepatocytes, and uterine myometrium. More recently, aromatase expression has been reported in the stomach, lung, colon, and macrophages, albeit at a low level [4–7]. Almost all estrogen receptor (ER)-positive cells express aromatase, although the expression levels vary.

In addition to normal tissues, aromatase is expressed in some pathological conditions such as breast cancer, endometriosis, uterine fibroids, and endometrial cancer. Estrogens synthesized in situ within these peripheral organs can bind to ERs of their own cells or those of neighboring cells and stimulate proliferation, thereby playing a role in disease pathogenesis. The biological actions of this in situ estrogen are more potent than those expected from a comparable amount of endocrine estrogen, possibly because in situ estrogen directly acts on neighboring cells with neither dilution into the circulating volume nor binding to proteins that interfere with the hormonal action.

11.2.2.2 Tissue-Specific Regulation of Aromatase

As described above, aromatase expression is regulated in a tissue-specific manner in multiple tissues by the alternate use of multiple promoters. For example, aromatase transcription is driven in the ovary by the most proximal promoter PII, which is regulated by cAMP downstream of a gonadotropin, follicle-stimulating hormone (FSH). The transcription in the brain is driven by promoter 1f. A further upstream promoter, I.4, drives the transcription in adipose tissues. In these promoters, specific steroid hormones are essential for expression: testosterone and glucocorticoid for promoters 1f and I.4, respectively. Local factors such as growth factors and cytokines also play regulatory roles in these promoters. For the placenta, promoter I.1 is a predominant promoter, while all other promoters are transcribed at very low levels. Promoter I.1 is quite different from other promoters in terms of its structure and function: it does not have a nuclear half site for binding of the NR5A (SF1) and permits constitutive expression, while others strictly downregulate basal expression.

The promoter-specific regulation is realized by relatively short upstream segments of promoters (less than approximately 500 bp), where tissue-specific enhancers and regulatory *cis*-elements possibly exist. Thus, a part of genomic DNA containing these short sequences mimics the physiological regulation by factors such as FSH, steroid hormones, cytokines, and prostaglandins. Using transgenic mice, it has been shown that these short sequences are capable of tissue-specific expression in the ovary and placenta [8]. However, the absolute level of expression of these transgenes (promoter constructs) is generally lower than that observed in vivo, suggesting that undiscovered enhancers exist outside the promoter region. Another explanation has recently been reported for the low level of in vitro expression compared with that of in vivo expression. Estrogen as a product of aromatase binds to the *TSPYL5* promoter and induces the expression of TSPYL5, which in turn is integrated into the transcriptional machinery of aromatase and efficiently enhances its expression [9]. This explains the reason why expression levels of aromatase demonstrated by promoter constructs that lack estrogen synthesizing activity are generally low.

11.2.2.3 Promoter Switching

Physiological expression of aromatase in human tissues, except for the placenta, is basically downregulated, and upregulation occurs only when appropriate stimuli exist. In comparison, it has been known that high levels of aromatase are constitutively expressed in pathological conditions of the breast. For example, aromatase is highly expressed in adipose tissues surrounding breast tumors in postmenopausal women [10]. Similarly, aberrant expression of aromatase has been confirmed in other pathological conditions such as endometriosis, uterine fibroids, endometrial cancer, and lung cancer [3, 11–13].

Promoter switching is a possible event underlying the aberrant expression of aromatase in pathological conditions. This was initially described in breast adipose tissues of women with or without breast cancer [14]. The normal breast adipose tissue of cancer-free women expresses low levels of aromatase by the predominant use of promoter I.4, whereas the adipose tissue surrounding breast tumors expresses high levels of aromatase by the predominant use of promoters PII and I.3. A possible explanation for "promoter switching" is that cancer-derived or cancer-prone local factors drive aromatase expression. Consistent with this, local factors drive aromatase expression. A promoter construct composed of tandem sequences of mini-promoters of *CYP19A1* mimics promoter switching in the breast [15].

11.2.3 CYP19A1 *Polymorphisms and Risk of Endometriosis*

Endometriosis is 6–7 times more frequent among first-degree relatives and is presumed to have a multifactorial inheritance. Several studies have reported polymorphisms of *CYP19A1* in endometriosis, including dysequilibrium for both breast cancer and endometrial cancer. As shown in Table 11.1, the polymorphisms of *CYP19A1* have been associated with the risk of endometriosis; however, the results are controversial [16–24].

Recent genome-wide association studies (GWAS) identified genetic variants in multiple loci that have been associated with endometriosis. These single-nucleotide polymorphisms (SNPs) have never been identified by traditional candidate gene strategies for specific diseases. GWAS-identified endometriosis-associated SNPs have ethnic differences [25]. No SNPs on chromosome 15q22, where *CYP19A1* maps, have been identified by GWAS.

11.2.4 Epigenetic Regulation of Aromatase

An epigenetic change is defined as heritable changes in gene expression that do not represent changes in the DNA sequence. DNA methylation and histone modification are the most often explored epigenetic mechanisms. Transcriptional regulation by noncoding RNAs, particularly micro RNAs (miRNAs), is another distinct epigenetic mechanism.

Table 11.1 Association between CYP19A1 gene polymorphisms and the risk of endometriosis

Nucleotide polymorphisms	Location	Author	Cases	Range of age (mean ± SD)	Control	Range of age (mean ± SD)	Staging of cases (number of subjects)[a]	Results
rs 10046 C1558T	3′ untranslated region of Exon 10	Szczepanska et al.	115	20–39	197	19–39	I (59), II (56)	No association[b]
		Lamp et al.	150	18–45 (32.1 ± 6.1)	199	30–50 (39.8 ± 5.3)	I (53), II (39), III (36), IV (22)	No association
		Vietri et al.	104	22–45 (36.8 ± 6.7)	86	18–48 (37.8 ± 5.1)	Undescribed	Genotype CC was overpresented in cases (48.1 % vs. 30.2 %)
		Hur et al.	224	Undescribed	188	Undescribed	III to IV (224)	No association
		Huber et al.	32	(52.3 ± 5.4)	790	(34.6 ± 7.0)	I (0), II (21), III (10), IV (1)	No association
rs700519 C > T, Arg264Cys	Exon7	Wang et al.	300	(34.3 ± 6.9)	337	(52.2 ± 4.2)	I (7), II (52), III (165), IV (76)	No association
		Tsuchiya et al.	79	20–45	59	20–45	I (21), II (10), III (23), IV (25)	No association
		Huber et al.	32	(52.3 ± 5.4)	790	(34.6 ± 7.0)	I (0), II (21), III (10), IV (1)	No association
rs2236722 T > C, Trp39Arg	Exon2	Wang et al.	300	(34.3 ± 6.9)	337	(52.2 ± 4.2)	I (7), II (52), III (165), IV (76)	No association
		Hur et al.	224	Undescribed	188	Undescribed	III to IV (224)	No association
240 A > G, Val80	At codon80 in exon3	Vietri et al.	104	22–45 (36.8 ± 6.7)	86	18–48 (37.8 ± 5.1)	Undescribed	Genotype AA was overpresented in cases (50.0 % vs. 32.6 %)
		Hur et al.	224	Undescribed	188	Undescribed	III to IV (224)	No association

3 bp insertion/deletion	50 bp upstream from the (TTTA)n tract in intron4	Lamp et al.	150	18–45 (32.1 ± 6.1)	199	30–50 (39.8 ± 5.3)	I (53), II (39), III (36), IV (22)	No association
		Kado et al.	140	24–48 (36.3 ± 8.1)	177	(63.8 ± 6.1)	I to II (32), III to IV (108)	Del/Del was frequently observed in cases
rs1004982	Intron	Trabert et al.	256	18–49	567	Matched to cases	Undescribed	Increased risk of endometriosis
rs18700479	Intron							Increased risk of endometriosis
rs936307	Intron							Increased risk of endometriosis
(TTTA) repeat number	Intron4	Lamp et al.	150	18–45 (32.1 ± 6.1)	199	30–50 (39.8 ± 5.3)	I (53), II (39), III (36), IV (22)	No significant association between [TTTA] repeat <7 and [TTTA] repeat 8–13
		Hur et al.	224	Undescribed	188	Undescribed	III to IV (224)	No significant association between [TTTA] repeat <7 and [TTTA] repeat 8–13
		Kado et al.	140	24–48 (36.3 ± 8.1)	177	(63.8 ± 6.1)	I to II (32), III to IV (108)	No significant association between [TTTA] repeat <7 and [TTTA] repeat 8–13
		Arvanitis et al.	275	21–37 (27.2 ± 3.2)	346	26–53 (34.5 ± 7.4)	Undescribed	[TTTA] 10 allele increased risk by 4.99 times for endometriosis

[a] The staging was assessed by the revised American Society for Reproductive Medicine score
[b] No statistically significant association was observed among different genotypes

11.2.4.1 DNA Methylation of *CYP19A1*

Changes in the methylation status of CpG islands of *CYP19A1* have been reported in endometriosis [26]. A CpG island located approximately 70 kb downstream from exon 1.1 of *CYP19A1* is hypomethylated in endometriosis (stromal cells obtained from ovarian chocolate cysts) but hypermethylated in the eutopic endometrium (stromal cells obtained from disease-free women). The methyl-CpG-binding proteins MBD1 and MeCP2, which contain an amino-terminal methyl-CpG-binding domain and a carboxy-terminal transcriptional repression domain, bind to the hypermethylated region of the CpG island in eutopic tissues, which in turn may suppress aromatase expression in the eutopic endometrium [27].

The treatment of endometrial stromal cells with 5-aza-deoxycytidine (an irreversible inhibitor of DNA methyltransferase1, which is essential for maintaining the methylation status of genomic DNA) induces aromatase expression in endometrial stromal cells obtained from disease-free women. The demethylation of the CpG islands in *CYP19A1* may be relevant to the upregulation of aromatase [28], although other explanations are possible because 5-aza-deoxycytidine alters the expression level of a broad spectrum of genes that may indirectly or directly affect aromatase expression.

11.2.4.2 Histone Modification

Histone modifications affect the chromatin structure and the subsequent interaction of transcription factors with their response elements in the promoters. The acetylation of histone H3 and histone H4 activates transcription by loosening the chromatin structure and allowing the recruitment of transcription factors to their response elements. In contrast, trimethylation of lysine at sites 9 and 27 on histone H3 inactivates transcription by causing the chromatin to become more condensed. Histone modifications affect *Cyp19a1* mRNA expression in rat granulosa cells [29]. We found that the acetylation of H3 and H4 at the promoter I.4 region occurs during the induction of aromatase expression by dexamethasone in breast cancer cell lines. No histone modification has been reported for aromatase regulation in endometriosis till date.

11.2.4.3 Regulation of Aromatase by miRNA

miRNAs are short noncoding RNAs that act by targeting partially complementary sequences within mRNAs. They consist of 19–25 nucleotides and commonly exist in the 3′-untranslated region of the target genes. Traditionally, miRNAs negatively regulate the transcription of their target genes. A single miRNA may target many genes, and each of them may in turn be regulated by different miRNAs [30].

The transcriptional repression of aromatase mRNA by miRNAs has been reported in mammalian ovarian tissues (miR-503 and miR-378 directly inhibit aromatase, miR-224 and miR-383 indirectly inhibit aromatase), trophoblast differentiation (miR-19b and miR-106a downregulate aromatase), and endometrial cancer (miR98 represses aromatase) [31–33]. There has been no report on miRNA regulation of aromatase mRNA in endometriosis.

11.2.5 Posttranslational Regulation of Aromatase

In addition to the mRNA level, aromatase activity is regulated at the protein level. It has been reported that phosphorylation and dephosphorylation of amino acids in the aromatase protein alter the enzymatic activity [34, 35].

Recently we found a novel mechanism underlying posttranslational regulation by autophagy [36]. Insulin-like growth factor-1 enhances aromatase activity over 50 % as early as 1 h in THP-1 myeloid leukemia cells through the inhibition of autophagy. A part of the newly synthesized aromatase protein is continuously transported to the lysosome and is degraded when aromatase protein synthesis is increased.

Another mechanism underlying posttranslational regulation has been proposed. A series of transfection experiments revealed that mRNA stability and protein translation efficiency vary among the 5′-noncoding sequence of exon 1 of aromatase [37]. The 5′-noncoding sequence of exons I.3 and I.4 contains the *cis*-acting elements responsible for the modulation of aromatase levels.

No study has reported the posttranslational regulation of aromatase in endometriosis where aromatase is highly expressed and translated.

11.3 Aromatase Expression in Endometriosis

11.3.1 Aberrant Biosynthesis of Estrogen in Endometriosis

There is unequivocal clinical evidence that the development and progression of endometriosis depends on ovarian estrogen. In addition to endocrine estrogen, numerous studies have shed light on the role of estrogen synthesized by endometriotic cells in situ. Although there have been no reports on direct measurements of the concentration of estrogen in the endometriotic tissues, comprehensive accumulated data have indicated the overproduction of estrogen in situ and its role in the pathogenesis in endometriotic tissues.

The endometriotic tissue expresses higher levels of aromatase than the eutopic endometrium, and it efficiently converts androstenedione to estrogen [38–42]. Moreover, endometriotic tissues do not inactivate estradiol by conversion to estrone because of the reduced expression of 17β-hydroxysteroid dehydrogenase (17β-HSD) type 2, whereas the eutopic endometrial epithelium does [43, 44]. Thus, endometriosis has more available estrogen, which possibly stimulates disease progression. Interestingly, the eutopic endometrium of women with endometriosis overexpresses aromatase before actual implantation to the abdominal cavity. This supports the notion that the overexpression of aromatase in the endometrium is a pathogenic factor that causes ectopic implantation and growth of endometrial tissues in regurgitating menstrual blood [45]. This remains to be determined in future.

The diagnostic use of the aberrant expression of aromatase has been examined. A Japanese group collected endometrial biopsy specimens from patients and immunostained the specimens for aromatase. Receiver operating characteristic curve analysis revealed a cut value of 20 H-scores with 91 % sensitivity, 100 % specificity, 100 % positive predictive value, and 72 % negative predictive value to distinguish the eutopic endometrium from women with or without endometriosis [46].

In addition to a high aromatase activity and reduced expression of 17β-HSD type 2, the expression of 17β-HSD type 1 is higher in the endometriotic tissues than in the eutopic endometrium. 17β-HSD type 1 converts estrone, a primary estrogen synthesized from androstenedione, to estradiol, an active form of estrogen, thereby enhancing the action of estrogen as a product. Compared with the eutopic endometrium, the aberrant expression of aromatase, the elevated expression of 17β-HSD type 1, and the reduced expression of 17β-HSD type 2 in the endometriotic tissue collectively give rise to elevated local levels of estradiol [47]. Another study reported that compared with the normal endometrium, aromatase, 17β-HSD types 1 and 7 (but not type2), sulfatase, and ERβ were statistically significantly upregulated, while ERα was significantly downregulated in ovarian endometrioma. There were no significant differences in 17β-HSD type 2, sulfotransferase, and progesterone receptors A and B gene expression [48]. Aromatase and 17β-HSD type1 mRNA levels were extremely low in the normal human endometrium, while mRNAs for 17β-HSD types 2 and 4, expressed sequence tags, and sequence-tagged sites were readily detectable [49].

Endometriotic tissues express a complete set of steroidogenic enzymes to synthesize estrogen: cholesterol side-chain cleavage enzyme (P450scc), 3-β-hydroxysteroid dehydrogenase 2 (HSD3B2), 17-hydroxylase/17,20-lyase (P450c17), and aromatase. The rate-limiting steps in estrogen synthesis are cholesterol mobilization into the side-chain cleavage enzyme (the initial step) and aromatization (the last step). Both these steps are enhanced in endometriotic tissues: StAR, which facilitates the entry of cytosolic cholesterol into the mitochondria, is overexpressed in endometriotic tissues compared with the normal endometrium. A master transcription regulator for steroidogenesis, steroidogenic factor 1 (SF1 or Ad4BP), also called NR5A1, is expressed at a higher level in endometriotic tissues than in endometrial tissues [39]. This explains the overexpression of a series of, if not all, steroidogenic enzymes in endometriotic tissues.

Prostaglandin E2 (PGE2) is another gateway regulator of the aberrant expression of steroidogenic enzymes in endometriotic tissues. Inflammatory endometriotic tissues express a high level of cyclooxygenase-2 (COX-2) and synthesize substantial amounts of PGE2, which in turn induces a series of steroidogenic enzymes, resulting in the production of progesterone, estrone, and estradiol. Estrogen in turn enhances the expression of COX-2. Thus, PGE2 and estrogen form a different cycle along with their synthesizing enzymes [50, 51]. Increased PGE2 and estrogens synergistically stimulate the progression of endometriosis [39].

Compared with the normal and eutopic endometrium, the expression of ERα and ERβ is increased in endometriotic tissues [52]. Predominant expression of ERα mRNA compared with that of ERβ mRNA has been reported [53]. In addition, the downregulation of ERα and upregulation of ERβ in ovarian endometrioma compared with those in the normal endometrium have been reported [54]. A role of ERβ in the regulation of ERα in endometriotic stromal cells has been elucidated. ERβ knockdown significantly increased ERα mRNA and protein levels in endometriotic stromal cells, whereas ERβ overexpression decreased ERα mRNA and protein levels. High levels of ERβ suppress ERα expression and the response to estradiol in both endometrial and endometriotic stromal cells via binding to classic and nonclassic DNA motifs in alternatively used ERα promoters [55]. Estrogen is believed to have a strong effect on endometriotic tissues through binding of ERα and ERβ.

11.3.2 Regulation of Aromatase In Situ in Endometriosis

The overexpression of aromatase mRNA has been confirmed in endometriotic tissues and endometriotic stromal cells isolated and cultured from ovarian endometrioma. The level of the transcript correlates with the 17β-estradiol-producing activity in vitro in endometriotic stromal cells [3, 39, 41]. The aromatase activity of endometriotic stromal cells is stimulated by the peritoneal fluid, tumor necrotizing factor-α, and interleukin-6 [56].

Macrophage migration inhibitory factor (MIF), a major pro-inflammatory and growth-promoting factor expressed in active endometriotic lesions, enhances the aromatase activity of endometriotic cells by posttranscriptional mRNA stabilization of aromatase. The resulting aromatase increases in situ estrogen, which in turn upregulates MIF expression. Accordingly, MIF and aromatase produce a positive feedback loop to enhance their mutual expression and promote endometriosis. Whether miRNA-mediated regulation is involved in this reciprocal enhancement between MIF and aromatase remains unclear. The inhibition of endogenous MIF may be a therapeutic candidate for endometriosis [57].

As described earlier, COX-2 is another regulator of aromatase expression for reciprocal enhancement in endometriotic tissues. Compared with the eutopic endometrium, COX-2 is overexpressed in endometriotic tissues of healthy women, enhancing PGE2 production in situ. PGE2 induces aromatase, and the resulting estrogen in turn stimulates COX-2 expression. This may prove to be another mechanism underlying the transcriptional enhancement of aromatase [39].

SF1 is a master transcription factor of steroidogenic enzymes, as explained earlier. SF1 induces the transcription of StAR, an essential protein in the initiation of steroidogenesis via cholesterol translocation into the mitochondria. SF1 binds to nuclear half sites of promoter PII of *CYP19A1* and induces aromatase expression in endometriotic tissues. SF1 efficiently induces the transcription from promoter PII in cooperation with the transcriptional cAMP response element-binding protein [42]. In comparison, the chicken ovalbumin upstream promoter transcription factor (COUP-TF) alternatively binds to the nuclear half sites of promoter PII in the eutopic endometrium. This may explain why aromatase is constitutively suppressed in the eutopic endometrium, particularly in healthy women.

Why does the transcription factor switch from COUP-TF to SF1 in endometriotic tissues? A CpG island located upstream of *SF1* promoter is highly methylated in the normal eutopic endometrium but unmethylated in endometriotic tissues. Thus, cancelation of silencing by genomic methylation seems to be a major mechanism underlying the reactivation of SF1 in endometriotic tissues, resulting in an overexpression of aromatase [58].

Many factors that may contribute to the induction and subsequent maintenance of aromatase expression in endometriosis have been reported. Some of these interact with each other and reciprocally increase expression. The contribution of each gene to the pathogenesis of endometriosis remains to be determined.

11.4 Aromatase Inhibitor (AIs)

11.4.1 AIs

AIs were originally developed for the treatment of breast cancer. By the 1990s, it had been revealed that breast cancer tissues synthesize estrogen in situ, which promotes breast cancer cell growth. After the molecular cloning of aromatase in the late 1990s, the aberrant expression of aromatase was identified as a cause of the overproduction of estrogen in situ. AIs were then developed as a new endocrine treatment of breast cancer. Initial trials showed that AIs reduced the level of estrogen in situ and suppressed the progression of cancer in postmenopausal women [59, 60]. Subsequent large-scale studies confirmed the therapeutic advantages over tamoxifen and reported the reduction of cancer development in the contralateral breast, suggesting a cancer preventive effect [61]. The role of in situ estrogen in pathology was first exemplified in breast cancer, and this established aromatase as a molecular target for endocrine therapy.

AIs are now widely used for the treatment of ER-positive breast cancer in postmenopausal women. The use of AIs shows a survival benefit compared with that of other endocrine therapies in women with advanced breast cancer [62].

Table 11.2 Three generations of aromatase inhibitors

	Aromatase inhibitor	
Generation	Nonsteroidal	Steroidal
First	Aminoglutethimide	
Second	Fadrozole	Formestane
Third	Letrozole anastrozole	Exemestane

11.4.2 Pharmacology

The functional aromatase enzyme complex is composed of 2 polypeptides: aromatase cytochrome P450 and NADPH-cytochrome P450 reductase. The former is a product of *CYP19A1*, a single gene on chromosome 15q22, which binds to androgens and hydroxylates them twice at the C19 position located between the A and B rings, resulting in aromatization of the A ring. The latter is a flavoprotein, ubiquitously distributed in most cells. NADPH-cytochrome P450 reductase confers an electron from NADP to aromatase for the enzymatic reaction.

AIs are classified into three generations according to the history of development (Table 11.2). The first-generation inhibitor aminoglutethimide is not selective to aromatase and causes a "medical adrenalectomy," leading to lethargy, skin rashes, and nausea. The second-generation inhibitors include fadrozole and formestane, which are more selective than aminoglutethimide. A risk of glucocorticoid suppression is reduced but still exists. The third-generation AIs include letrozole, anastrozole, and exemestane (6-methylenandrost-1, 4-diene-3, 17-dione). These are more selective and potent; thus, they are excellent for use in clinical practice [63, 64]. The former two are nonsteroidal, while the latter is steroidal. Both types bind to a substrate-binding site of aromatase as a false substrate. The next step in the binding differs between the 2 types of compounds. A steroidal compound forms an unbreakable complex with the aromatase protein, and the enzymatic activity of the aromatase is thus permanently blocked once the binding occurs. This may lead to accelerated degradation of the aromatase protein [65]. Thus, enzymatic activity does not recover even if all unattached inhibitors are removed, and the enzymatic activity can only be restored by new enzyme synthesis [66]. In contrast, nonsteroidal compounds can dissociate from aromatase, resulting in recovery of the enzymatic activity. The difference in inhibitory mechanisms between steroidal and nonsteroidal AIs is expected to provide rationale for alternate treatments for patients with breast cancer who are resistant or refractory to other types of AIs [67].

The third-generation AIs can decrease the local concentration of estradiol by 97–99 %. The therapeutic dose of AIs for breast cancer significantly reduces circulating estrogen levels in postmenopausal women. In comparison, the inhibition of estradiol synthesis in premenopausal women is not sufficient, with only a 20–30 % reduction in circulating estrogen levels [68, 69]. This less effective suppression in premenopausal women is because of androgen availability for nonsteroidal inhibitors: androgen as a substrate is present at micromolar concentrations in the ovary (follicle), while circulating androgen at nanomolar concentrations is the only source of androgen for extraglandular (peripheral) estrogen synthesis. Competitive binding is insufficient in androgen-rich follicles, resulting in insufficient inhibition.

Another mechanism underlying the insufficient suppression observed in premenopausal women is the compensatory increase in FSH. The suppression of estrogen synthesis causes an increase in FSH secretion, which stimulates follicular development and aromatase expression and eventually restores estradiol secretion to some extent [70].

11.4.3 Side Effects of AIs

AIs cause undesired health issues related to the presence or absence of estrogen suppression. Bone loss and fracture are the most important issues, particularly in postmenopausal women who use AIs for more than 6 months. Concomitant use of bisphosphonate is recommended for women who have additional risk factors for fracture [71]. Compared with the use of tamoxifen, long-term use of AIs increases the odds of cardiovascular disease [72]. Other side effects associated with the use of AIs are hot flushes, headache, joint stiffness or pain, leg cramps, arthralgia, nausea, and diarrhea. All of them are generally mild and are therefore tolerable.

It has been reported that AIs + norethindrone acetate or other OCs prescribed for the treatment of endometriosis cause bone mineral loss, as seen in the case of breast cancer. The change is significant but not symptomatic. This is partly because of the shorter duration of therapy compared with that for patients with breast cancer and partly because of the bone protective action of concomitantly used sex steroids [64].

11.4.4 AIs for the Treatment of Endometriosis

In most cases, the progression of endometriotic lesions and endometriosis-related symptoms can be controlled by the use of various types of medications, surgery, or a combination of both. Thus, trials of AIs are limited to patients with severe pain, including deep pareunia and chronic pain, who are refractory to established treatment options. The use of AIs in endometriosis was initially reported for postmenopausal women with refractory endometriosis of the rectovaginal space [73]. The therapeutic effect is now tested in premenopausal women suffering from refractory alleviation of endometriosis-related pain.

As described earlier, the application of AIs to premenopausal women leads to an elevation in FSH levels and subsequent follicular development, which increases estradiol, thereby potentially nullifying the therapeutic effect. Thus, additional agents to control ovarian activation are required. To this end, progesterone or progestins, OCs, and GnRH agonists have been tested. All of these are used in the conventional therapy for endometriosis.

11.4.4.1 AI Monotherapy

A few reports have provided evidence of the efficacy of AI monotherapy for the treatment of endometriosis-related pain in premenopausal women. In these studies, vaginally administered anastrozole (0.25 mg/day) combined with oral elemental calcium (1.2 g/day) and cholecalciferol (800 IU/day) for 6 months improved rectovaginal endometriosis-related dysmenorrhea [74].

A prospective randomized clinical trial has been conducted to compare the effect of short-term letrozole and a GnRH agonist (triptorelin) versus case control on the pregnancy rate and recurrence of endometriosis after laparoscopic surgery [75]. The overall pregnancy and recurrence rate of the letrozole group (2.5 mg/day for 2 months) were similar to those of the triptorelin group. The pregnancy and recurrence rate among the 3 groups were as follows: 23.4 and 6.4 % in the letrozole group, 27.5 and 5 % in the triptorelin group, and 28.1 and 5.3 % in the control group, respectively.

Another case report has revealed the efficacy and side effects of AIs in the treatment of premenopausal patients with endometriosis-related chronic pelvic pain refractory to conventional treatment. Four premenopausal patients were treated with either anastrozole (1 mg/day) combined with alendronate (10 mg/day) or letrozole (2.5 mg/day) combined with calcium (1.5 g/day) and vitamin D (800 U/day) for 6 months, and marked improvement of pelvic pain was observed in all the patients without significant hormonal change and bone mineral loss [76]. The most common side effect was irregular bleeding with anastrozole and joint pains with letrozole.

Thus, AI monotherapy for endometriosis-related pain is tolerable for a short duration, if the prevention of bone mineral loss is adequate.

11.4.4.2 Combination of AIs with Progesterone or Progestins

A prospective noncomparative study on the efficacy of letrozole + norethindrone acetate for endometriosis-related chronic pelvic pain has been conducted [77]. This study included 10 women who were refractory to conventional medication for endometriosis-related pain. The diagnosis of endometriosis was confirmed by laparoscopic biopsy. The combined use of letrozole (2.5 mg/day), norethindrone acetate (2.5 mg/day), calcium citrate (1,250 mg/day), and vitamin D (800 IU/day) for 6 months relieved the pain in 9 of 10 women. The authors concluded that letrozole is a candidate for the medical management of refractory endometriosis-related pain.

Two refractory cases with severe pain were treated with the cyclic administration of anastrozole combined with progesterone. One treatment course consisted of 21 days of treatment with anastrozole (1 mg/day), progesterone (200 mg/day), and calcitriol (1,25-dihydroxyvitamin D3; 0.5 μg/day), followed by 7 days without treatment. In addition, rofecoxib (a selective COX-2 inhibitor; 12.5–50 mg/day) was continuously administered. A six-course treatment resulted in a rapid, progressive reduction in pain, and the remission lasted over 24 months after treatment [78].

Another large-scale, prospective, open-label, nonrandomized trial including 82 women with pain caused by rectovaginal endometriosis has been conducted. Patients received either norethisterone acetate (2.5 mg/day) alone or a combination of letrozole (2.5 mg/day), norethisterone acetate (2.5 mg/day), elemental calcium (1,000 mg/day), and vitamin D3 (880 IU/day) for 6 months. Both regimens were similarly effective for dysmenorrhea; however, the efficacy differed between the 2 regimens with respect to chronic pelvic pain and deep dyspareunia. The reduction rate of the intensity of the pain scale in the combination therapy was 1.4–1.5-fold larger than that in therapy with norethisterone acetate alone [79]. A carryover effect was not observed in both regimens in terms of pain relief. Side effects, including joint pain ($n = 5$) and myalgia ($n = 5$), hair loss ($n = 1$), and decreased libido ($n = 1$), were only reported for the combination therapy ($n = 41$). However, withdrawal due to side effects was not statistically different between the combination group ($n = 4$) and the norethisterone acetate group ($n = 3$).

Overall, the use of AIs enhances the therapeutic efficacy of progesterone/progestins with regard to pelvic pain and deep dyspareunia that are refractory to established treatments. However, the improvement in the pain relapses soon after the completion of treatment, and the side effects, albeit minor, are increased. For extended treatment, great caution is required regarding side effects related to long-term use of AIs, such as bone loss and arthritis, as reported in case of long-term AI monotherapy for breast cancer.

11.4.4.3 Combination of AIs with OCPs

The efficacy of AIs for refractory endometriosis has been also examined in combination with OCPs. A phase 2 prospective open-label trial was conducted on 15 premenopausal women with documented refractory endometriosis and chronic pelvic pain [80]. The use of anastrozole (1 mg/day) and 1 tablet of ethinyl estradiol (20 μg/day)/levonorgestrel (0.1 mg/day) daily for 6 months significantly relieved the pain. Side effects were mild, and no adverse effects on major organs were observed.

The efficacy of AIs + OCPs for premenopausal patients with ovarian endometriomas and chronic pelvic pain, who were previously treated with surgery and medication with an unsatisfactory result, has been reported. Five women received letrozole (2.5 mg/day), desogestrel (0.15 mg/day), ethinyl estradiol (0.03 mg/day), calcium (1,200 mg/day), and vitamin D (800 IU/day) daily for 6 months. Ovarian endometriomas disappeared and the pain was relieved in all 5 women. Loss of bone mineral density was not observed [81]. This result is excellent; however, interpretation is limited because of the small number of patients and the fact that the study was nonrandomized and did not include controls. In addition, the primary target of the treatment was ovarian endometrioma and not rectovaginal endometriosis.

Further randomized trials are necessary to elucidate the benefits of a combination of AIs with OCPs.

11.4.4.4 Combination of AIs with GnRH Agonists

One prospective randomized trial examined whether the addition of anastrozole to goserelin is superior to goserelin alone in terms of adjuvant therapy after conservative surgery [82]. Forty women with stage IV (the revised American Society for Reproductive Medicine score > 40) severe endometriosis received either goserelin (3.6 mg/4 weeks) alone or goserelin + anastrozole (1 mg/day). Compared with goserelin alone, 6 months of treatment with goserelin + anastrozole significantly increased the pain-free interval (1.7 months versus >2.4 months) and decreased symptom recurrence rates until 2 years (35 % versus 7.5 %). The postmenopausal quality of life and bone mineral density at 2 years after medical therapy remained unaffected.

These studies were designed to evaluate the efficacy of AIs combined with progestins or GnRH agonists and actually suggested that the addition of AIs is beneficial for pain relief but may cause unfavorable side effects. Therefore, which is better for combination with AIs in terms of risk and benefit: progestins or GnRH agonists? A randomized prospective study was designed to compare the efficacy and tolerability of AIs combined with either progestin or a GnRH agonist [83]. Women with rectovaginal endometriosis were treated with letrozole (2.5 mg/day) for 6 months and were randomized to also receive either oral norethisterone acetate (2.5 mg/day) or triptorelin (11.25 mg every 3 months). The reduction in the intensity of nonmenstrual pelvic pain and deep dyspareunia did not differ between the 2 medications, whereas the interruption of treatment and bone mineral loss were more frequent and severe and patient satisfaction was therefore lower in the triptorelin group. AIs possibly enhance the efficacy of conventional medicines for endometriosis in premenopausal women; however, they may cause intolerable side effects.

11.4.5 AIs for the Treatment of Infertility in Women with Endometriosis

In 2001, a new application of letrozole for ovulation induction in clomiphene citrate (CC)-resistant anovulatory women was reported [84]. The administration of letrozole in the early follicular phase would release the pituitary/hypothalamic axis from estrogenic negative feedback and increase FSH, somewhat similar to the mechanisms of CC.

The clinical features of AIs as ovulation-inducing medicines differ from those of CC. CC causes thinning of the endometrium during the therapeutic cycle and decreases the cervical mucus, whereas AIs do not. This negative effect on the endometrium explains the reason why the pregnancy rate of CC-treated women is somewhat lower than that expected from the ovulation rate. AIs do not have the negative effects on the endometrium. A reason for the difference is the half-life of the medicine: CC, particularly an isomer of CC existing in the medicine, lasts longer in the body and exerts an antiestrogenic action for a longer period than letrozole: the half-lives are 5–7 days and 45 h for CC and letrozole, respectively. In addition, CC increases circulating estrogen, which binds to ER and accelerates its degradation. Thus, it takes time to recover estrogen responsibility through de novo synthesis of ER after CC is eliminated from the blood. In comparison, AIs do not induce ER degradation and are rapidly eliminated from the body after the cessation of administration. Thus, the endometrium maintains its sensitivity to estrogen and quickly recovers to the level of untreated cycles after the cessation of medication, whereas estrogen levels are decreased to half to one-third of the levels observed in natural cycles. This supports the absence of any direct antiestrogenic effects of letrozole on the endometrium [85].

Despite the lack of a negative effect on the endometrium, meta-analysis does not support that AIs achieve higher pregnancy rates than CC for women with polycystic ovary syndrome. Meta-analyses of 6 randomized controlled trials comparing letrozole with CC demonstrated that letrozole improved the ovulation rate per patient, without a statistically significant difference in the ovulation rate per cycle or pregnancy, live birth, multiple pregnancy, or miscarriage rates [86]. Treatment with letrozole for unexplained infertility is almost equally effective to that with CC; however, it may have some advantages in terms of low serum estradiol levels, the pregnancy rate per cycle, and the abortion rate [70, 87, 88]. There is a report on the efficacy of AIs for infertility in women with endometriosis: the pregnancy rate with letrozole was the same as that with CC alone in an intrauterine insemination program for women with minimal to mild endometriosis who did not achieve pregnancy after 6–12 months following laparoscopic treatment [89].

The use of AIs for ovulation induction is an off-label use and the safety has not been established. A concern about teratogenicity was reported in an abstract in 2005; however, there have been no additional studies published since then. In contrast, a large multicenter retrospective study showed that compared with CC, AIs do not increase congenital cardiac anomalies [90].

11.4.6 AIs for the Treatment of Endometriosis in Postmenopausal Women

Endometriosis spontaneously resolves after menopause; however, endometriosis may progress and cause symptoms, albeit rare. Such patients have been treated with surgery, including hysterectomy, at earlier ages and experience recurrent endometriosis-related pain. AIs have been reported to be successful in the treatment of postmenopausal women with endometriosis [91, 92]. As expected, no additional medication is required to prevent FSH increases during AIs use.

11.5 Conclusions

Endometriotic tissues overexpress aromatase and synthesize estrogen in situ, which may play roles in pathogenesis and progression by enhancing auto-implantation, proliferation, and angiogenesis. Researchers propose several mechanisms underlying this overexpression, namely switching of the transcriptional regulators from COUP-TF to SF1; overexpression of COX-2, MIF, and cytokines; and changes in the methylation status of CpG islands in *CYP19A1*.

Clinical trials of AIs have been conducted and have revealed that AIs reduce endometriosis-related pain, particularly in recurrent cases. The effectiveness supports the notion that locally synthesized estrogen plays a role in the progression of endometriosis, unlike anticipated. Short-term use of AIs (less than 6 months) either as monotherapy or in combination with other medications for ovulation inhibition reduced endometriosis-related pain without significant severe side effects. Future studies will be required to confirm these conclusions.

References

1. Simpson ER. Sources of estrogen and their importance. J Steroid Biochem Mol Biol. 2003;86 (3–5):225–30.
2. Bulun SE, Sebastian S, Takayama K, Suzuki T, Sasano H, Shozu M. The human CYP19 (aromatase P450) gene: update on physiologic roles and genomic organization of promoters. J Steroid Biochem Mol Biol. 2003;86(3–5):219–24.
3. Bulun SE, Lin Z, Imir G, Amin S, Demura M, Yilmaz B, Martin R, Utsunomiya H, Thung S, Gurates B, Tamura M, Langoi D, Deb S. Regulation of aromatase expression in estrogen-responsive breast and uterine disease: from bench to treatment. Pharmacol Rev. 2005;57 (3):359–83.
4. Izawa M, Inoue M, Osaki M, Ito H, Harada T, Terakawa N, Ikeguchi M. Cytochrome P450 aromatase gene (CYP19) expression in gastric cancer. Gastric Cancer. 2008;11(2):103–10.
5. Demura M, Demura Y, Ameshima S, Ishizaki T, Sasaki M, Miyamori I, Yamagishi M, Takeda Y, Bulun SE. Changes in aromatase (CYP19) gene promoter usage in non-small cell lung cancer. Lung Cancer. 2011;73(3):289–93.
6. Sato R, Suzuki T, Katayose Y, Miura K, Shiiba K, Miki Y, Kamogawa Y, Yamamoto K, Takayuki 2nd, Egawa S, Unno M, Sasano H. Aromatase in colon carcinoma. Anticancer Res. 2012;32(8):3069–75.
7. Mor G, Yue W, Santen RJ, Gutierrez L, Eliza M, Berstein LM, Harada N, Wang J, Lysiak J, Diano S, Naftolin F. Macrophages, estrogen and the microenvironment of breast cancer. J Steroid Biochem Mol Biol. 1998;67(5–6):403–11.
8. Kamat A, Hinshelwood MM, Murry BA, Mendelson CR. Mechanisms in tissue-specific regulation of estrogen biosynthesis in humans. Trends Endocrinol Metab. 2002;13(3):122–8.
9. Liu M, Ingle JN, Fridley BL, Buzdar AU, Robson ME, Kubo M, Wang L, Batzler A, Jenkins GD, Pietrzak TL, Carlson EE, Goetz MP, Northfelt DW, Perez EA, Williard CV, Schaid DJ, Nakamura Y, Weinshilboum RM. TSPYL5 SNPs: association with plasma estradiol concentrations and aromatase expression. Mol Endocrinol. 2013;27(4):657–70.
10. Simpson ER, Dowsett M. Aromatase and its inhibitors: significance for breast cancer therapy. Recent Prog Horm Res. 2002;57:317–38.

11. Ishikawa H, Reierstad S, Demura M, Rademaker AW, Kasai T, Inoue M, Usui H, Shozu M, Bulun SE. High aromatase expression in uterine leiomyoma tissues of African-American women. J Clin Endocrinol Metab. 2009;94(5):1752–6.
12. Verma MK, Miki Y, Sasano H. Aromatase in human lung carcinoma. Steroids. 2011;76 (8):759–64.
13. Segawa T, Shozu M, Murakami K, Kasai T, Shinohara K, Nomura K, Ohno S, Inoue M. Aromatase expression in stromal cells of endometrioid endometrial cancer correlates with poor survival. Clin Cancer Res. 2005;11(6):2188–94.
14. Agarwal VR, Bulun SE, Leitch M, Rohrich R, Simpson ER. Use of alternative promoters to express the aromatase cytochrome P450 (CYP19) gene in breast adipose tissues of cancer-free and breast cancer patients. J Clin Endocrinol Metab. 1996;81(11):3843–9.
15. Harada N, Matsumoto T, Yoshimura N, Sakamoto H, Honda S. Analysis of transcriptional regulation of human breast aromatase by in vitro and in vivo studies. J Steroid Biochem Mol Biol. 2001;79(1–5):151–6.
16. Szczepanska M, Wirstlein P, Skrzypczak J, Jagodzinski PP. Polymorphic variants of CYP17 and CYP19A and risk of infertility in endometriosis. Acta Obstet Gynecol Scand. 2013;92:1188–93.
17. Lamp M, Peters M, Reinmaa E, Haller-Kikkatalo K, Kaart T, Kadastik U, Karro H, Metspalu A, Salumets A. Polymorphisms in ESR1, ESR2 and HSD17B1 genes are associated with fertility status in endometriosis. Gynecol Endocrinol. 2011;27(6):425–33.
18. Vietri MT, Cioffi M, Sessa M, Simeone S, Bontempo P, Trabucco E, Ardovino M, Colacurci N, Molinari AM, Cobellis L. CYP17 and CYP19 gene polymorphisms in women affected with endometriosis. Fertil Steril. 2009;92(5):1532–5.
19. Hur SE, Lee S, Lee JY, Moon HS, Kim HL, Chung HW. Polymorphisms and haplotypes of the gene encoding the estrogen-metabolizing CYP19 gene in Korean women: no association with advanced-stage endometriosis. J Hum Genet. 2007;52(9):703–11.
20. Huber A, Keck CC, Hefler LA, Schneeberger C, Huber JC, Bentz EK, Tempfer CB. Ten estrogen-related polymorphisms and endometriosis: a study of multiple gene-gene interactions. Obstet Gynecol. 2005;106(5):1025–31.
21. Wang HS, Wu HM, Cheng BH, Yen CF, Chang PY, Chao A, Lee YS, Huang HD, Wang TH. Functional analyses of endometriosis-related polymorphisms in the estrogen synthesis and metabolism-related genes. PLoS One. 2012;7(11):e47374.
22. Tsuchiya M, Nakao H, Katoh T, Sasaki H, Hiroshima M, Tanaka T, Matsunaga T, Hanaoka T, Tsugane S, Ikenoue T. Association between endometriosis and genetic polymorphisms of the estradiol-synthesizing enzyme genes HSD17B1 and CYP19. Hum Reprod. 2005;20(4):974–8.
23. Trabert B, Schwartz SM, Peters U, De Roos AJ, Chen C, Scholes D, Holt VL. Genetic variation in the sex hormone metabolic pathway and endometriosis risk: an evaluation of candidate genes. Fertil Steril. 2011;96(6):1401–6.e3.
24. Arvanitis DA, Koumantakis GE, Goumenou AG, Matalliotakis IM, Koumantakis EE, Spandidos DA. CYP1A1, CYP19, and GSTM1 polymorphisms increase the risk of endometriosis. Fertil Steril. 2003;79 Suppl 1:702–9.
25. Zhao H, Chen ZJ. Genetic association studies in female reproduction: from candidate-gene approaches to genome-wide mapping. Mol Hum Reprod. 2013;19(10):644–54.
26. Izawa M, Taniguchi F, Uegaki T, Takai E, Iwabe T, Terakawa N, Harada T. Demethylation of a nonpromoter cytosine-phosphate-guanine island in the aromatase gene may cause the aberrant up-regulation in endometriotic tissues. Fertil Steril. 2011;95(1):33–9.
27. van Kaam KJ, Delvoux B, Romano A, D'Hooghe T, Dunselman GA, Groothuis PG. Deoxyribonucleic acid methyltransferases and methyl-CpG-binding domain proteins in human endometrium and endometriosis. Fertil Steril. 2011;95(4):1421–7.
28. Izawa M, Harada T, Taniguchi F, Ohama Y, Takenaka Y, Terakawa N. An epigenetic disorder may cause aberrant expression of aromatase gene in endometriotic stromal cells. Fertil Steril. 2008;89(5 Suppl):1390–6.

29. Lee L, Asada H, Kizuka F, Tamura I, Maekawa R, Taketani T, Sato S, Yamagata Y, Tamura H, Sugino N. Changes in histone modification and DNA methylation of the StAR and Cyp19a1 promoter regions in granulosa cells undergoing luteinization during ovulation in rats. Endocrinology. 2013;154(1):458–70.
30. Kong YW, Ferland-McCollough D, Jackson TJ, Bushell M. MicroRNAs in cancer management. Lancet Oncol. 2012;13(6):e249–58.
31. Donadeu FX, Schauer SN, Sontakke SD. Involvement of miRNAs in ovarian follicular and luteal development. J Endocrinol. 2012;215(3):323–34.
32. Kumar P, Luo Y, Tudela C, Alexander JM, Mendelson CR. The c-Myc-regulated microRNA-17~92 (miR-17~92) and miR-106a ~ 363 clusters target hCYP19A1 and hGCM1 to inhibit human trophoblast differentiation. Mol Cell Biol. 2013;33(9):1782–96.
33. Panda H, Chuang TD, Luo X, Chegini N. Endometrial miR-181a and miR-98 expression is altered during transition from normal into cancerous state and target PGR, PGRMC1, CYP19A1, DDX3X, and TIMP3. J Clin Endocrinol Metab. 2012;97(7):E1316–26.
34. Shozu M, Sumitani H, Murakami K, Segawa T, Yang HJ, Inoue M. Regulation of aromatase activity in bone-derived cells: possible role of mitogen-activated protein kinase. J Steroid Biochem Mol Biol. 2001;79(1–5):61–5.
35. Charlier TD, Harada N, Balthazart J, Cornil CA. Human and quail aromatase activity is rapidly and reversibly inhibited by phosphorylating conditions. Endocrinology. 2011;152 (11):4199–210.
36. Zhang B, Shozu M, Okada M, Ishikawa H, Kasai T, Murakami K, Nomura K, Harada N, Inoue M. Insulin-like growth factor I enhances the expression of aromatase P450 by inhibiting autophagy. Endocrinology. 2010;151(10):4949–58.
37. Wang H, Li R, Hu Y. The alternative noncoding exons 1 of aromatase (Cyp19) gene modulate gene expression in a posttranscriptional manner. Endocrinology. 2009;150(7):3301–7.
38. Noble LS, Takayama K, Zeitoun KM, Putman JM, Johns DA, Hinshelwood MM, Agarwal VR, Zhao Y, Carr BR, Bulun SE. Prostaglandin E2 stimulates aromatase expression in endometriosis-derived stromal cells. J Clin Endocrinol Metab. 1997;82(2):600–6.
39. Attar E, Tokunaga H, Imir G, Yilmaz MB, Redwine D, Putman M, Gurates B, Attar R, Yaegashi N, Hales DB, Bulun SE. Prostaglandin E2 via steroidogenic factor-1 coordinately regulates transcription of steroidogenic genes necessary for estrogen synthesis in endometriosis. J Clin Endocrinol Metab. 2009;94(2):623–31.
40. Bukulmez O, Hardy DB, Carr BR, Auchus RJ, Toloubeydokhti T, Word RA, Mendelson CR. Androstenedione up-regulation of endometrial aromatase expression via local conversion to estrogen: potential relevance to the pathogenesis of endometriosis. J Clin Endocrinol Metab. 2008;93(9):3471–7.
41. Velasco I, Rueda J, Acien P. Aromatase expression in endometriotic tissues and cell cultures of patients with endometriosis. Mol Hum Reprod. 2006;12(6):377–81.
42. Zeitoun KM, Bulun SE. Aromatase: a key molecule in the pathophysiology of endometriosis and a therapeutic target. Fertil Steril. 1999;72(6):961–9.
43. Zeitoun K, Takayama K, Sasano H, Suzuki T, Moghrabi N, Andersson S, Johns A, Meng L, Putman M, Carr B, Bulun SE. Deficient 17beta-hydroxysteroid dehydrogenase type 2 expression in endometriosis: failure to metabolize 17beta-estradiol. J Clin Endocrinol Metab. 1998;83(12):4474–80.
44. Delvoux B, Groothuis P, D'Hooghe T, Kyama C, Dunselman G, Romano A. Increased production of 17beta-estradiol in endometriosis lesions is the result of impaired metabolism. J Clin Endocrinol Metab. 2009;94(3):876–83.
45. Bulun SE. Endometriosis. N Engl J Med. 2009;360(3):268–79.
46. Kitawaki J, Kado N, Ishihara H, Koshiba H, Kitaoka Y, Honjo H. Endometriosis: the pathophysiology as an estrogen-dependent disease. J Steroid Biochem Mol Biol. 2002;83(1–5):149–55.
47. Bulun SE, Zeitoun KM, Takayama K, Sasano H. Estrogen biosynthesis in endometriosis: molecular basis and clinical relevance. J Mol Endocrinol. 2000;25(1):35–42.

48. Smuc T, Pucelj MR, Sinkovec J, Husen B, Thole H, Lanisnik Rizner T. Expression analysis of the genes involved in estradiol and progesterone action in human ovarian endometriosis. Gynecol Endocrinol. 2007;23(2):105–11.
49. Dassen H, Punyadeera C, Kamps R, Delvoux B, Van Langendonckt A, Donnez J, Husen B, Thole H, Dunselman G, Groothuis P. Estrogen metabolizing enzymes in endometrium and endometriosis. Hum Reprod. 2007;22(12):3148–58.
50. Lu B, Jiang YJ, Choy PC. 17-Beta estradiol enhances prostaglandin E2 production in human U937-derived macrophages. Mol Cell Biochem. 2004;262(1–2):101–10.
51. Tamura M, Deb S, Sebastian S, Okamura K, Bulun SE. Estrogen up-regulates cyclooxygenase-2 via estrogen receptor in human uterine microvascular endothelial cells. Fertil Steril. 2004;81 (5):1351–6.
52. Pellegrini C, Gori I, Achtari C, Hornung D, Chardonnens E, Wunder D, Fiche M, Canny GO. The expression of estrogen receptors as well as GREB1, c-MYC, and cyclin D1, estrogen-regulated genes implicated in proliferation, is increased in peritoneal endometriosis. Fertil Steril. 2012;98(5):1200–8.
53. Matsuzaki S, Murakami T, Uehara S, Canis M, Sasano H, Okamura K. Expression of estrogen receptor alpha and beta in peritoneal and ovarian endometriosis. Fertil Steril. 2001;75 (6):1198–205.
54. Smuc T, Hevir N, Ribic-Pucelj M, Husen B, Thole H, Rizner TL. Disturbed estrogen and progesterone action in ovarian endometriosis. Mol Cell Endocrinol. 2009;301(1–2):59–64.
55. Trukhacheva E, Lin Z, Reierstad S, Cheng YH, Milad M, Bulun SE. Estrogen receptor (ER) beta regulates ERalpha expression in stromal cells derived from ovarian endometriosis. J Clin Endocrinol Metab. 2009;94(2):615–22.
56. Velasco I, Acien P, Campos A, Acien MI, Ruiz-Macia E. Interleukin-6 and other soluble factors in peritoneal fluid and endometriomas and their relation to pain and aromatase expression. J Reprod Immunol. 2010;84(2):199–205.
57. Veillat V, Sengers V, Metz CN, Roger T, Leboeuf M, Mailloux J, Akoum A. Macrophage migration inhibitory factor is involved in a positive feedback loop increasing aromatase expression in endometriosis. Am J Pathol. 2012;181(3):917–27.
58. Xue Q, Lin Z, Yin P, Milad MP, Cheng YH, Confino E, Reierstad S, Bulun SE. Transcriptional activation of steroidogenic factor-1 by hypomethylation of the 5' CpG island in endometriosis. J Clin Endocrinol Metab. 2007;92(8):3261–7.
59. Santen RJ, Harvey HA. Use of aromatase inhibitors in breast carcinoma. Endocr Relat Cancer. 1999;6(1):75–92.
60. Miller WR, Stuart M, Sahmoud T, Dixon JM. Anastrozole ('Arimidex') blocks oestrogen synthesis both peripherally and within the breast in postmenopausal women with large operable breast cancer. Br J Cancer. 2002;87(9):950–5.
61. Petit T, Dufour P, Tannock I. A critical evaluation of the role of aromatase inhibitors as adjuvant therapy for postmenopausal women with breast cancer. Endocr Relat Cancer. 2011;18(3):R79–89.
62. Gibson L, Lawrence D, Dawson C, Bliss J. Aromatase inhibitors for treatment of advanced breast cancer in postmenopausal women. Cochrane Database Syst Rev. 2009;4:CD003370.
63. Turkistani A, Marsh S. Pharmacogenomics of third-generation aromatase inhibitors. Expert Opin Pharmacother. 2012;13(9):1299–307.
64. Pavone ME, Bulun SE. Aromatase inhibitors for the treatment of endometriosis. Fertil Steril. 2012;98(6):1370–9.
65. Lintermans A, Neven P, Paridaens R. Drug safety evaluation of exemestane. Expert Opin Drug Saf. 2011;10(3):473–87.
66. Buzdar AU. Pharmacology and pharmacokinetics of the newer generation aromatase inhibitors. Clin Cancer Res. 2003;9(1 Pt 2):468S–72472.
67. Gluck S. Exemestane as first-line therapy in postmenopausal women with recurrent or metastatic breast cancer. Am J Clin Oncol. 2010;33(3):314–9.

68. Lonning PE. Oestrogen suppression–lessons from clinical studies. Best Pract Res Clin Endocrinol Metab. 2004;18(1):33–45.
69. Puhalla S, Brufsky A, Davidson N. Adjuvant endocrine therapy for premenopausal women with breast cancer. Breast. 2009;18 Suppl 3:S122–30.
70. Badawy A, Elnashar A, Totongy M. Clomiphene citrate or aromatase inhibitors for superovulation in women with unexplained infertility undergoing intrauterine insemination: a prospective randomized trial. Fertil Steril. 2009;92(4):1355–9.
71. Bundred NJ. Aromatase inhibitors and bone health. Curr Opin Obstet Gynecol. 2009;21 (1):60–7.
72. Amir E, Seruga B, Niraula S, Carlsson L, Ocana A. Toxicity of adjuvant endocrine therapy in postmenopausal breast cancer patients: a systematic review and meta-analysis. J Natl Cancer Inst. 2011;103(17):1299–309.
73. Takayama K, Zeitoun K, Gunby RT, Sasano H, Carr BR, Bulun SE. Treatment of severe postmenopausal endometriosis with an aromatase inhibitor. Fertil Steril. 1998;69(4):709–13.
74. Hefler LA, Grimm C, van Trotsenburg M, Nagele F. Role of the vaginally administered aromatase inhibitor anastrozole in women with rectovaginal endometriosis: a pilot study. Fertil Steril. 2005;84(4):1033–6.
75. Alborzi S, Hamedi B, Omidvar A, Dehbashi S, Alborzi M. A comparison of the effect of short-term aromatase inhibitor (letrozole) and GnRH agonist (triptorelin) versus case control on pregnancy rate and symptom and sign recurrence after laparoscopic treatment of endometriosis. Arch Gynecol Obstet. 2011;284(1):105–10.
76. Verma A, Konje JC. Successful treatment of refractory endometriosis-related chronic pelvic pain with aromatase inhibitors in premenopausal patients. Eur J Obstet Gynecol Reprod Biol. 2009;143(2):112–5.
77. Ailawadi RK, Jobanputra S, Kataria M, Gurates B, Bulun SE. Treatment of endometriosis and chronic pelvic pain with letrozole and norethindrone acetate: a pilot study. Fertil Steril. 2004;81(2):290–6. doi:10.1016/j.fertnstert.2003.09.029.
78. Shippen ER, West Jr WJ. Successful treatment of severe endometriosis in two premenopausal women with an aromatase inhibitor. Fertil Steril. 2004;81(5):1395–8.
79. Ferrero S, Camerini G, Seracchioli R, Ragni N, Venturini PL, Remorgida V. Letrozole combined with norethisterone acetate compared with norethisterone acetate alone in the treatment of pain symptoms caused by endometriosis. Hum Reprod. 2009;24(12):3033–41.
80. Amsterdam LL, Gentry W, Jobanputra S, Wolf M, Rubin SD, Bulun SE. Anastrozole and oral contraceptives: a novel treatment for endometriosis. Fertil Steril. 2005;84(2):300–4.
81. Lall Seal S, Kamilya G, Mukherji J, De A, Ghosh D, Majhi AK. Aromatase inhibitors in recurrent ovarian endometriomas: report of five cases with literature review. Fertil Steril. 2011;95(1):291.e15–8.
82. Soysal S, Soysal ME, Ozer S, Gul N, Gezgin T. The effects of post-surgical administration of goserelin plus anastrozole compared to goserelin alone in patients with severe endometriosis: a prospective randomized trial. Hum Reprod. 2004;19(1):160–7.
83. Ferrero S, Venturini PL, Gillott DJ, Remorgida V. Letrozole and norethisterone acetate versus letrozole and triptorelin in the treatment of endometriosis related pain symptoms: a randomized controlled trial. Reprod Biol Endocrinol. 2011;9:88.
84. Mitwally MF, Casper RF. Use of an aromatase inhibitor for induction of ovulation in patients with an inadequate response to clomiphene citrate. Fertil Steril. 2001;75(2):305–9.
85. Pavone ME, Bulun SE. Clinical review: the use of aromatase inhibitors for ovulation induction and superovulation. J Clin Endocrinol Metab. 2013;98(5):1838–44.
86. He D, Jiang F. Meta-analysis of letrozole versus clomiphene citrate in polycystic ovary syndrome. Reprod Biomed Online. 2011;23(1):91–6.
87. Samani FG, Farzadi L, Nezami N, Tarzamni MK, Soleimani F. Endometrial and follicular development following letrozole intervention in unexplained infertile patients failed to get pregnant with clomiphene citrate. Arch Gynecol Obstet. 2009;280(2):201–5.

88. Fouda UM, Sayed AM. Extended letrozole regimen versus clomiphene citrate for superovulation in patients with unexplained infertility undergoing intrauterine insemination: a randomized controlled trial. Reprod Biol Endocrinol. 2011;9:84.
89. Abu Hashim H, El Rakhawy M, Abd Elaal I. Randomized comparison of superovulation with letrozole vs. clomiphene citrate in an IUI program for women with recently surgically treated minimal to mild endometriosis. Acta Obstet Gynecol Scand. 2012;91(3):338–45.
90. Tulandi T, Martin J, Al-Fadhli R, Kabli N, Forman R, Hitkari J, Librach C, Greenblatt E, Casper RF. Congenital malformations among 911 newborns conceived after infertility treatment with letrozole or clomiphene citrate. Fertil Steril. 2006;85(6):1761–5.
91. Sasson IE, Taylor HS. Aromatase inhibitor for treatment of a recurrent abdominal wall endometrioma in a postmenopausal woman. Fertil Steril. 2009;92(3):1170.e1–4.
92. Oxholm D, Knudsen UB, Kryger-Baggesen N, Ravn P. Postmenopausal endometriosis. Acta Obstet Gynecol Scand. 2007;86(10):1158–64.

Chapter 12
Apoptosis in Endometriosis

Apostolos Kaponis, Georgia Kollia, Fuminori Taniguchi, Tasuku Harada, and George Decavalas

Abstract Endometriosis is an inflammatory, estrogen-dependent disease characterized by the growth of endometrial tissues outside the uterus. The eutopic endometrium from women with endometriosis has some fundamental differences compared with the normal endometrium of women without endometriosis. The differences could contribute to the survival of regurgitating endometrial cells into the peritoneal cavity and the development of endometriosis. One mechanism that gained a lot of interests is the finding that apoptosis appeared in eutopic and ectopic endometrium of patients with endometriosis. A common characteristic of endometriotic cells is their ability to evade the apoptotic machinery. Endometriosis could result from increased cellular proliferation or decreased apoptosis in response to appropriate stimuli. This chapter focused on the physiological role of apoptosis in normal endometrium and the alterations in regulation of apoptosis in eutopic and ectopic endometrium from women with endometriosis. Finally, the role of apoptosis in the treatment of endometriosis is reviewed to link the basic research findings into clinical applications.

Keywords Apoptosis • Bcl-2 • Endometriosis • Fas/FasL • Medical treatment

---

A. Kaponis, M.D., Ph.D. (✉) • G. Kollia • G. Decavalas
Department of Obstetrics and Gynecology, Patra University School of Medicine, Rio, 26441, Peloponnisos, Patra, Greece
e-mail: kaponisapostolos@hotmail.com

F. Taniguchi • T. Harada
Department of Obstetrics and Gynecology, Tottori University Faculty of Medicine, Yonago, Japan

T. Harada (ed.), *Endometriosis: Pathogenesis and Treatment*,
DOI 10.1007/978-4-431-54421-0_12,

12.1 Introduction

Endometriosis is a common and enigmatic disease characterized by the presence of endometrium-like glandular tissue and stroma outside the uterus. The pathophysiology of the disease remains a mystery. Nearly all women of reproductive age exhibit some degree of reflux of endometrial debris [1]. Menstrual effluents, retrogradely shed into the peritoneal cavity, were observed to contain viable endometrial cells [2]. These mechanisms are necessary but insufficient to explain why only some patients develop the disease. The fact that the *eutopic endometrium* of women with endometriosis shares changes with ectopic tissue and that these changes are not found in the eutopic endometrium of disease-free women has advanced the view that the primary defect in endometriosis is to be found in the eutopic endometrium [3]. Cells and tissue elements, derived from such an altered eutopic endometrium and shed into the peritoneal cavity, have been proposed to have a higher potential for implantation and growth on peritoneal surfaces and development into endometriosis [4]. Many differences are observed between eutopic endometrium of disease-free women and ectopic tissue of a patient with endometriosis. These differences can be explained as the direct influence of the different environment of peritoneal fluid (PF) [5]. One of the endometrial alterations appearing in eutopic and ectopic endometrium from women with endometriosis refers to the regulation of apoptosis. In particular, decreased susceptibility of endometrial tissue to apoptosis may contribute to the pathogenesis of endometriosis.

12.2 Apoptosis in Pathophysiology of Endometriosis

Endometrial cells from women with and without endometriosis have fundamental differences. Endometrial cells from women with endometriosis has enhanced proliferation and increased ability to implant and survive in ectopic locations. Impaired sensitivity of endometrial tissue to apoptosis contributes to abnormal implantation and growth of endometrium at ectopic sites. The inability of endometrial cells to transmit a "death" signal or their ability to avoid cell death is associated with increased expression of *antiapoptotic factors* (e.g., Bcl-2) and decreased expression of *proapoptotic factors* (e.g., BAX) [6]. It is unclear whether the abnormal apoptosis in the eutopic endometrium from patients with endometriosis is primary in origin or secondary after establishment of pelvic endometriosis process. This could be attributed to the fact that at the time of clinical presentation and diagnosis most women have already established disease and therefore, it is very difficult to investigate the early developmental stages of the endometriosis.

Reflux of endometrial fragments during menstruation into the peritoneal cavity is a common phenomenon. Under normal conditions, cells that do not adhere to their extracellular matrix enter apoptosis as they receive different signals from their adhesion receptors [7]. In endometriosis, these cells have the ability to adhere to mesothelial cells of peritoneum, to proliferate, and to produce neoangiogenesis resulting in the development of active endometriosis. The effect of MMPs on apoptotic factors and their regulation by steroid hormones may provide a link between endometrial turnover and the invasive process necessary for the development of endometriosis. Immunoglobulin-like cell adhesion molecules (nectins and Necls) involved in apoptosis and cell proliferation have also stronger expression in eutopic and ectopic endometrium of women with endometriosis [8]. High levels of *VEGF* and IL-1β have been found in the PF of patients with endometriosis. VEGF and IL-1β reduce apoptosis and decrease *Bax* expression in endometrial epithelial cells from patients with endometriosis. VEGF and IL-1β may protect endometriotic cells from undergoing apoptosis favoring the establishment and progression of endometriotic lesions by promoting the formation of new blood vessels and by protecting endometriotic cells from undergoing cell death [9].

Intrinsic abnormalities in transplanted eutopic endometrium are contributed to the pathogenesis of endometriosis. Abnormal signaling pathways in the eutopic endometrium of women with endometriosis have been recently reported. Two different groups demonstrated increased activity of the protein kinase A and B pathways regulating the function of many cellular proteins involved in apoptosis and proliferation [10, 11]. It was suggested that increased Akt phosphorylation may be related to the altered apoptosis/proliferation harmony in endometriosis. Another pathway whose activation confers a resistant to apoptosis phenotype in endometriotic cell is the NF-κB [12]. In vivo, *NF-κB* inhibition in early-stage endometriotic lesions induced in nude mice was found to decrease the proliferation of endometriotic cells and stimulate their apoptosis [13].

cDNA microarray analysis has provided an interesting insight for altered gene expression profiles in patients with endometriosis. Arimoto et al. found 97 upregulated and 337 downregulated genes in women with endometriosis [14]. Genes related to apoptosis (GADD34, GADD45A, GADD45B, PIG11) and the tumor suppressor TP53 gene were downregulated in endometriotic tissues. These findings are inconsistent with the decreased spontaneous apoptosis observed in eutopic endometrium from women with endometriosis.

Survivin is a member of the inhibitors of apoptosis family (IAP). IAP proteins directly inhibit the terminal effector caspases 3 and 7 and thus protect cells from apoptosis. Endometriotic cells express more survivin genes than normal endometrial cells without endometriosis [15]. Survivin plays a critical role in susceptibility of endometriotic stromal cells to apoptosis and survivin inhibitors may be effective as treatment for endometriosis [16]. Increased survivin expression was present in eutopic and ectopic epithelial cells, but only ectopic epithelial cells lost the cyclic variation of survivin expression during menstrual cycles.

Recently, aberrant *miRNA* expression has been shown to play an important role in the pathogenesis of endometriosis as a part of epigenetic mechanisms. A global miRNA microarray technique used to evaluate the expression of miRNAs in endometriotic cyst stromal cells [17]. In normal endometrial stromal cells miR-196b targets c-myc and Bcl-2 expression, inhibits proliferation, and induces apoptosis. In contrast, in endometriotic cells, the expression of miR-196b was repressed by DNA hypermethylation of the miR-196b gene and this repression may be involved in the development of proliferative and antiapoptotic characteristics of endometriosis [17].

Steroid hormones are able to modulate the apoptotic machinery in endometriotic cells. Estradiol has proinflammatory and antiapoptotic effects in endometrial cells, and these effects appear to exacerbate in women with endometriosis. In these women, physiological estradiol concentrations are able to induce an enhanced inflammatory response mediated by local chemokine production and to reinforce mechanisms of cell survival mediated by extracellular signal-regulated kinases and Bcl-2 [18]. On the other hand, the main effect of progesterone is to inhibit interleukin-8 (IL-8) and other chemokines in stromal cells from both eutopic and ectopic endometrium. Progesterone is effective to induce apoptosis through the inhibition of Bcl-2 and NF-κB [18].

12.3 Apoptosis in the Normal Endometrium

Apoptosis helps to maintain cellular homeostasis during the menstrual cycle by eliminating senescent cells from the functional layer of the uterine endometrium [19]. In normal endometrium, apoptotic cells were identified in the glandular epithelium of late secretory and menstruating endometrium due to progesterone withdrawal, while very little apoptosis was detected during the proliferative phase or at the beginning of the secretory phase [20]. The pattern of apoptosis negatively correlates to serum estradiol concentrations in the proliferative phase [20]. Considering the cyclical nature of apoptosis in normal endometrium, it seems likely that estrogen and progesterone can regulate the signals that result in apoptosis in this tissue.

Bcl-2 has been considered to inhibit apoptosis in the endometrium during the proliferative phase. Bcl-2 cyclically expressed in endometrial glandular and stromal cells peaks during the late proliferative phase, while it decreases dramatically in the early and mid-secretory phase to reappear in the late secretory phase. In contrast, myometrial smooth muscle cells showed consistent Bcl-2 immunoreactivity throughout the menstrual cycle [21]. Higher expression of Bcl-2 was observed in the basal layer, whereas death receptor Fas and caspase-3 were higher in the functional layer of the endometrium [22]. These results fit well with the functional biology of endometrium. Since the basal layer remains relatively constant throughout the menstrual cycle, apoptosis is less common in this layer. The functional layer that undergoes cyclical growth, differentiation, and shedding appears with increased level of apoptosis.

Susceptibility of any given cells to a potential apoptotic stimulus may be determined by the ratio of pro- and antiapoptotic Bcl-2 family members presented in the cell at that time [23]. *Bax* and *Bak* are Bcl-2 family members promoting cell death susceptibility, possibly by countering the effect of Bcl-2 on cellular survival through heterodimer interaction. BAX and BAK were upregulated in the glandular epithelial cells during the secretory phase of the normal menstrual cycle [24, 25]. These data imply the existence of a dynamic interplay among many members of the Bcl-2 family in triggering apoptosis.

The *Fas ligand* (*FasL*) belongs to the tumor necrosis factor superfamily. The Fas/FasL interaction is essential in inducing apoptosis. Fas expression seems to be unchanged in the different phases of the menstrual cycle [26]. FasL exhibits peak expression during the secretory and menstrual phases [27]. Taken together, Bcl-2 is expressed in human endometrial glandular cells during the proliferative phase but not during the late secretory phase. In contrast, both Fas and FasL are expressed throughout the cycle in weak or moderate amount, except relatively higher expression of FasL in the late secretory phase. It is generally accepted that Bcl-2 blocks apoptosis via the mitochondrial pathway and not the death receptor pathway induced by the Fas/FasL system. Therefore, in the normal human endometrium, caspase-8 is initially activated by the Fas/FasL signal, resulting in the caspase cascade. Activated caspase-8 can switch on both the death receptor pathway and the *mitochondrial pathway* via Bid degradation [28]. It is possible that both the mitochondrial and the death receptor pathways are involved in apoptosis of human endometrial cells.

12.4 Apoptosis in Endometriosis

The percentage of apoptosis in sloughed endometrial cells is greatly reduced among women with endometriosis implying that the number of surviving cells that enter the peritoneal cavity is greater in women who develop endometriosis. The apoptosis indices in the eutopic endometrium of women with endometriosis were lower compared to women without endometriosis [29]. This difference caused primarily by a significant decrease in apoptosis during the late secretory/menstrual and early proliferative phases in women with endometriosis. The cyclic variability of apoptosis may be lost in these women.

12.4.1 Bcl-2 Family in Endometriosis

The expression of Bcl-2 in endometrial glandular cells has a cyclic pattern in eutopic endometrium in patients with endometriosis, but that cyclic changes were not apparent in peritoneal and ovarian endometriotic tissues [21]. Jones et al. did not detect apoptosis in stromal cells from peritoneal endometriotic tissues [30]. In accordance with these findings, Bcl-2 is expressed to a greater extent in stromal cells from ectopic tissues. This overexpression may be directly correlated to the increase in the number of estrogen receptors expressed by ectopic stroma [31]. ncreased expression of Bcl-2 protein was found in proliferative eutopic endometrium from women with endometriosis when compared with normal endometrium from healthy women [32]. BAX expression was absent in proliferative endometrium, whereas there was an increase in its expression in secretory endometrium from women with endometriosis and healthy women. The *Bcl-xL/Bcl-xS* ratio (antiapoptotic/proapoptotic) was substantially higher in eutopic endometrium from women with endometriosis compared to endometria from women without endometriosis [33]. Altered expression of Bcl-2 family members in eutopic endometrium of women with endometriosis resulted to a decreased number of apoptotic cells and consequently to their abnormal survival in the ectopic locations.

Increased *prostaglandin* E_2 (PGE_2) signaling was observed in ectopic endometriotic tissues compared with eutopic endometrium tissues during the menstrual cycle [34]. The ability of endometriotic cells to circumvent apoptotic signals can be the result of increased PGE_2 signaling, which is associated with abundant expression of the antiapoptotic Bcl-2 and Bcl-$_{XL}$ proteins, low expression of proapoptotic Bax protein, phosphorylation/inactivation of proapoptotic Bad protein, and activation of multiple cell survival signaling pathways (ERK1/2, Akt, nuclear factor-κB, β-catenin) [35].

12.4.2 Fas/FasL System in Endometriosis

Few studies have been published on the expression of *Fas* in endometriotic tissues. Harada et al. found that Fas is expressed randomly in both eutopic and ectopic glandular endometrial cells [36]. Fas expression was constant in both tissues throughout the menstrual cycle. Abundant expression of Fas antigen was found in NKcells of PF of women with early stages of endometriosis [37]. The activated PF NK-cells can be intensively eliminated via the Fas/FasL apoptosis, thus providing conditions for the survival of ectopic endometrium cells and the development of the disease at the initial stages of endometriosis.

In contrast with Fas, many studies indicated that higher expression of FasL by endometriotic cells contributes to their survival and the development of endometriosis. The levels of soluble/active FasL are higher in serum and PF in women with moderate to severe endometriosis than in women with early-stage disease or in disease-free women [38]. Higher levels of *soluble FasL* in the PF of women with endometriosis may contribute to increased apoptosis of Fas-bearing immune cells in the peritoneal cavity, leading to their decreased scavenger activity [31]. This may result in prolonged survival of endometrial cells into the peritoneal cavity.

The sources of the elevated levels of soluble FasL in the peritoneal cavity were endometriotic lesions and PF leukocytes. Endometrial glandular and stromal cells presented with increased FasL expression. *Peritoneal macrophages* in endometriosis might stimulate a Fas-mediated apoptosis of immune cells [38]. FasL expression in the endometriotic cells may protect them from attack by T lymphocytes. Consequently, ectopic endometrium cells escaping from immune surveillance in the peritoneal cavity may contribute to the maintenance of the disease. It is, therefore, possible that many endometriotic cells not only become resistant to Fas-mediated apoptosis, but additionally they have acquired the ability to utilize this pathway to their advantage by launching a "Fas counterattack" against the host's immune system.

Upregulation of FasL expression by endometriotic cells could be induced after the adhesion of these cells to the extracellular matrix proteins laminin, fibronectin, and collagen IV [39]. MMPs have been implicated in the conversion of FasL to active/soluble forms, suggesting that these molecules can activate or release factors involved in the apoptotic process [40]. FasL expression that occurs when endometrial stromal cells attach to the extracellular matrix may be one of the critical events in the development of endometriosis.

Interleukin-8 (IL-8), a chemokine for neutrophils and a potent angiogenic agent, is elevated in the PF of women with endometriosis [41]. IL-8 promotes proliferation of stromal cells derived from endometriotic tissues [42], suggesting that it may facilitate growth of endometriotic implants. Selam et al. demonstrated a concentration-dependent increase in IL-8-induced FasL expression in endometrial stromal cells. Elevated IL-8 levels in PF, via stimulation of FasL, induce apoptosis in activated T lymphocytes and contribute to an immune-privileged environment around the endometriosis implants supporting their survival [43]. On the other hand, IL-8 exerts a chemotactic activity primarily on neutrophils and inhibits their apoptosis even in the presence of Fas engagement. IL-8 is one of the neutrophil survival factors in the PF of endometriosis patients. IL-8 exerts the antiapoptotic effects by activating the PTEN/Akt pathway and mediating the expression of survivin and Bcl-2 [44]. IL-2 also enhanced survival and invasiveness of endometrial stromal cells in an autocrine manner by activating Akt and MAPK/Erk1/2 signal pathway [45]. The impaired clearance of cells responsible for innate immunity in the PF of patients with endometriosis may be associated with the development of the disease.

12.4.3 Apoptosis and Treatment of Endometriosis

Endometriosis is an estrogen-dependent disease. Current therapeutic alternatives consist of various hormone treatments aimed at decreasing circulating estrogen to postmenopausal levels. Incubation with *GnRH agonists* increased the apoptotic rate in eutopic and ectopic endometrium cells from women with endometriosis [46]. Treatment with GnRH-a affects the expression of a diverse range of genes, including those that encode apoptotic factors. GnRH-a significantly induced apoptosis, as was shown from the increased expression of activated caspase-3, in eutopic endometrium cells and lesions from women with endometriosis [47]. GnRH-a inhibit cell proliferation and increase the apoptotic rate in eutopic endometrium cell cultures, an effect that appears to be mediated by an increase in the expression of the proapoptotic proteins Bax and FasL and a decrease in the expression of the antiapoptotic protein Bcl-2[48]. GnRH-a treatment attenuated IL-8 expression by reducing TNF-α-induced NF-κB activation [49]. *Inhibitors of NF-κB activity* (BAY 11-7085, apigenin, pyrrolidine dithiocarbamate) were used to examine the potential application for the treatment of endometriosis. It has been shown that NF-κB inhibitors significantly inhibited the cell proliferation and induced apoptosis [50–52].

Mutants of estrogen receptor genes delivered to endometriotic cells via an adenovirus vector decreased cell proliferation, induced apoptosis, and decreased cytokine production, suggesting that adenovirus-mediated gene therapy may represent a potential therapy for endometriosis in the future [53]. *Aromatase* overexpression is observed in endometriotic tissues. Aromatase inhibitors, letrozole and anastrozole, produced significant and positive effects on apoptosis of epithelial endometrial cells from patients with endometriosis [54]. Combined *oral contraceptives* (OC) can be administered to women with endometriosis in order to reduce pain symptoms and to prevent progression or recurrence of the disease [55]. OC can enhance programmed cell death (decreased Bcl-2/BAX expression ratio) in the eutopic endometrium of women with endometriosis [56]. Progestogens exert inhibitory effects on endometrial proliferation and enhance apoptosis in the endometrium [27]. Levonorgestrel increased Fas expression and enhanced apoptotic index in eutopic and ectopic endometrium of patients with endometriosis [57].

Several new compounds have been investigated as new treatment modalities for endometriosis in in vitro or in animal models (*bufalin, beta-hydroxyisovalerylshikonin, raloxifene, fasudil*). These compounds act as apoptosis-induced agents in endometriotic cells [58–61]. Histone deacetylase inhibitors have been shown also to induce apoptosis in endometriotic cells [62]. Selective *inhibition of cyclooxygenase-2* prevented survival, migration, and invasion of human endometriotic epithelial and stromal cells, which was due to decreased PGE_2 production [63]. Modulation of apoptotic factors may result in the effective treatment of endometriosis.

Apoptosis has an important role in the development of endometriosis. Manipulation of cell death processes could be used to treat endometriosis. However, it is important to remember that no biochemical pathway stands on its own. Apoptosis represents the final execution step that defines the fate of a cell. However, the decision for the survival or the death of a cell has been taken earlier through various and complicated gene regulations. Advances in molecular biology and genetics will help us to understand these issues and may yield prevention and treatment modalities for endometriosis in the near future.

References

1. Halme J, Hammond MG, Hulka JF, Raj S, Talbert LM. Retrograde menstruation in healthy women and in patients with endometriosis. Obstet Gynecol. 1984;64:151–4.
2. Arumugam K, Lim JM. Menstrual characteristics associated with endometriosis. Br J Obstet Gynecol. 1997;104:948–50.

3. Kruitwagen RFPM, Poels LG, Willemsen WNP, de Ronde IJ, Jap PH, Rolland R. Endometrial epithelial cells in peritoneal fluid during the early follicular phase. Fertil Steril. 1991;55:297–303.
4. Sharpe Timms KL. Endometrial anomalies in women with endometriosis. Ann N Y Acad Sci. 2001;943:131–47.
5. Leyendecker G, Kunz G, Noe M, Herbertz M, Mall G. Endometriosis: a dysfunction and disease of the archimetra. Hum Reprod Update. 1998;4:752–62.
6. Meresman GF, Vighi S, Buquet RA, Contreras-Ortiz O, Tesone M, Rumi LS. Apoptosis and expression of Bcl-2, Bax in eutopic endometrium from women with endometriosis. Fertil Steril. 2000;74:760–6.
7. Aplin AE, Howe A, Alahari SK, Juliano RL. Signal transduction and signal modulation by cell adhesion receptors: the role of integrins, cadherins, immunoglobulin-cell adhesion molecules, and selectins. Pharmacol Rev. 1998;50:197–263.
8. Ballester M, Gonin J, Rodenas A, Bernaudin JF, Rouzier R, Coutant C, Darai E. Eutopic endometrium and peritoneal, ovarian and colorectal endometriotic tissues express a different profile of nectin-1, -3, -4 and nectin-like molecule 2. Hum Reprod. 2012;27:3179–86.
9. Bilotas M, Meresman G, Buquet R, Sueldo C, Baranao RI. Effect of vascular growth factor and interleukin-1β on apoptosis in endometrial cell cultures from patients with endometriosis and controls. J Reprod Immunol. 2010;84:193–8.
10. Cinar O, Seval Y, Uz YH, Cakmak H, Ulukus M, Kayisli UA, Arici A. Differential regulation of Akt phosphorylation in endometriosis. Reprod Biomed Online. 2009;19:864–71.
11. Aghajanova L, Horcajadas JA, Weeks JL, Esteban FJ, Nezhat CN, Conti M, Giudice LC. The protein kinase A pathway-regulated transcriptome of endometrial stromal fibroblasts reveals compromised differentiation and persistent proliferative potential in endometriosis. Endocrinology. 2010;151:1341–55.
12. Kaponis A, Iwabe T, Taniguchi F, Ito M, Deura I, Decavalas G, Terakawa N, Harada T. The role of NF-kappaB in endometriosis. Front Biosci. 2012;4:1213–34.
13. Gonzalez-Ramos R, Van Langendonckt A, Defrere S, Lousse JC, Mettelen M, Guillet A, Donnez J. Agents blocking the nuclear factor-kappaB (NF-κB) pathway are effective inhibitors of endometriosis in an in vivo experimental model. Gynecol Obstet Invest. 2008;65:174–86.
14. Arimoto T, Katagiri T, Oda K, Tsunoda T, Yasugi T, Osuga Y, Yoshikawa H, Nishii O, Yano T, Taketani Y, Nakamura Y. Genome-wide cDNA microarray analysis of gene-expression profiles involved in ovarian endometriosis. Int J Oncol. 2003;22:551–60.
15. Ueda M, Yamashita Y, Takehara M, Terai Y, Kumagai K, Ueki K, Kanda K, Yamaguchi H, Akise D, Hung YC, Ueki M. Survivin gene expression in endometriosis. J Clin Endocrinol Metab. 2002;87:3452–9.
16. Watanabe A, Taniguchi F, Izawa M, Suou K, Uegaki T, Takai E, Terakawa N, Harada T. The role of surviving in the resistance of endometriotic stromal cells to drug-induced apoptosis. Hum Reprod. 2009;24:3172–9.
17. Abe W, Nasu K, Nakada C, Kawano Y, Moriyama M, Narahara H. miR-196b targets c-myc and Bcl-2 expression, inhibits proliferation and induces apoptosis in endometriotic stromal cells. Hum Reprod. 2013;28:750–61.
18. Reis FM, Petraglia F, Taylor RN. Endometriosis: hormone regulation and clinical consequences of chemotaxis and apoptosis. Hum Reprod Update. 2013;19:406–18.
19. Kokawa K, Shikone T, Nakano R. Apoptosis in the human uterine endometrium during the menstrual cycle. J Clin Endocrinol Metabol. 1996;81:4144–7.
20. Vaskivuo TE, Stenback F, Karhumaa P, Risteli J, Dunkel L, Tapanainen JS. Apoptosis and apoptosis-related proteins in human endometrium. Mol Cell Endocrinol. 2000;165:75–83.
21. Watanabe H, Kanzaki H, Narukawa S, Inoue T, Katsuragawa H, Kaneko Y, Mori T. Bcl-2 and Fas expression in eutopic and ectopic human endometrium during the menstrual cycle in relation to endometrial cell apoptosis. Am J Obstet Gynecol. 1997;176:360–8.

22. Rogers PA, Lederman F, Plunkett D, Affandi B. Bcl-2, Fas, and caspase-3 expression in endometrium from levonorgestrel implant users with and without breakthrough bleeding. Hum Reprod. 2000;15:152–61.
23. Chittenden T, Harrington EA, O'Connor R, Flemington C, Lutz RJ, Evan GI, Guild BC. Induction of apoptosis by the Bcl-2 homologue Bak. Nature. 1995;374:731–3.
24. Narkar M, Kholkute S, Chitlange S, Nandedkar T. Expression of steroid hormone receptors, proliferation and apoptotic markers in primate endometrium. Mol Cell Endocrinol. 2006;246:107–13.
25. Tao XJ, Sayegh RA, Tilly JT, Isaacson KB. Elevated expression of the proapoptotic BCL-2 family member, BAK, in the human endometrium coincident with apoptosis during the secretory phase of the cycle. Fertil Steril. 1998;70:338–43.
26. Bilotas M, Baranao RI, Buquet R, Sueldo C, Tesone M, Meresman G. Effects of GnRH analogues on apoptosis and expression of Bcl-2, Bax, Fas, and FasL proteins in endometrial epithelial cell cultures from patients with endometriosis and controls. Hum Reprod. 2007;22:644–53.
27. Peng X, Maruo T, Matsuo H, Takekida S, Deguchi J. Serum deprivation-induced apoptosis in cultures porcine granulosa cells is characterized by increased expression of p53 protein, Fas antigen and Fas ligand and by decreased expression of PCNA. Endocr J. 1998;45:247–53.
28. Abe H, Shibata MA, Otsuki Y. Caspase of Fas-mediated apoptosis in human normal endometrium and endometrial carcinoma cells. Mol Hum Reprod. 2006;12:535–41.
29. Gebel HM, Braun DP, Tambur A, Frame D, Rana N, Dmowski DP. Spontaneous apoptosis of endometrial tissue is impaired in women with endometriosis. Fertil Steril. 1998;9:1042–7.
30. Jones RK, Searle RF, Bulmer JN. Apoptosis and bcl-2 expression in normal human endometrium, endometriosis and adenomyosis. Hum Reprod. 1998;13:3496–502.
31. Fujishita A, Chavez RO, Nakane PK, Yamabe T, Koji T, Ishimau T, Masuzaki H. Expression of estrogen and progesterone receptors in endometrium and peritoneal endometriosis: an immunohistochemical and in situ hybridization study. Fertil Steril. 1997;67:856–64.
32. McLaren J, Prentice A, Charnock-Jones DS, Sharkey AM, Smith SA. Immunocolonization of the apoptosis regulating proteins Bcl-2 and Bax in human endometrium and isolated peritoneal fluid macrophages in endometriosis. Hum Reprod. 1997;12:146–52.
33. Braun DP, Ding J, Shaheen F, Willey JC, Rana N, Dmowski WP. Quantitative expression of apoptosis-regulating genes in endometrium from women with and without endometriosis. Fertil Steril. 2006;87:263–8.
34. Banu SK, Lee JH, Speights VO, Starzinski-Powitz A, Arosh JA. Selective Inhibition of Prostaglandin E2 Receptors EP2 and EP4 Induces Apoptosis of Human Endometriotic Cells through suppression of ERK1/2, Akt, NF_B, and β-Catenin Pathways and activation of intrinsic apoptotic mechanisms. Mol Endocrinol. 2009;23:1291–305.
35. Harada M, Suganuma N, Furuhashi M, Nagasaka T, Nakashima N, Kikkawa F, Tomoda Y, Furui K. Detection of apoptosis in human endometriotic tissues. Mol Hum Reprod. 1996;2:307–15.
36. Eidukaite A, Siaurys A, Tamosiunas V. Aberrant expression of CD95 and CD69 molecules among CD56+ cells in women with endometriosis. Am J Reprod Immunol. 2006;55:276–81.
37. Garcia Velasco JA, Mulayim N, Kayisli UA, Arici A. Elevated soluble Fas ligand levels may suggest a role for apoptosis in women with endometriosis. Fertil Steril. 2002;78:855–9.
38. Garcia Velasco J, Arici A, Zreick T, Naftolin F, Mor G. Macrophage-derived growth factors regulate FasL expression in endometrial stromal cells: a role in endometriosis. Mol Hum Reprod. 1999;5:642–50.
39. Selam B, Kayisli UA, Garcia Velasco JA, Arici A. Extracellular matrix-dependent regulation of Fas ligand expression in human endometrial stromal cells. Biol Reprod. 2002;66:1–5.
40. Kayagaki N, Kawasaki A, Ebata T, Ohmoto H, Ikeda S, Inoue S, Yoshino K, Okumura K, Yagita H. Metalloproteinase-mediated release of human Fas ligand. J Exp Med. 1995;182:1777–83.

41. Harada T, Iwabe T, Terakawa N. Role of cytokines in endometriosis. Fertil Steril. 2001;76:1–10.
42. Iwabe T, Harada T, Tsudo T, Nagano Y, Yoshida S, Tanikawa M, Terakawa N. Tumor necrosis factor-alpha promotes proliferation of endometriotic stromal cells by inducing interleukin-8 gene and protein expression. J Clin Endocrinol Metab. 2000;85:824–9.
43. Selam B, Kayisli UA, Garcia Velasco JA, Akbas GE, Arici A. Regulation of Fas ligand expression by IL-8 in human endometrium. J Clin Endocrinol Metabol. 2002;8:3921–7.
44. Li MQ, Luo XZ, Meng YH, Mei J, Zhu XY, Jin LP, Li DJ. CXCL8 enhances proliferation and growth and reduces apoptosis in endometrial stromal cells in an autocrine manner via a CXCR-triggered PTEN/AKT signal pathway. Hum Reprod. 2012;27:2107–16.
45. Li MQ, Li HP, Meng YH, Wang XQ, Zhu XY, Mei J, Li DJ. Chemokine CCL2 enhances survival and invasiveness of endometrial stromal cells in an autocrine manner by activating Akt and MAPK/Erk1/2 signal pathway. Fertil Steril. 2012;97:919–29.
46. Meresman GF, Bilotas MA, Buquet RA, Baranao R, Sueldo C, Tesone M. Gonadotropin-releasing hormone agonist induces apoptosis and reduces cell proliferation in eutopic endometrial cultures from women with endometriosis. Fertil Steril. 2003;80:702–7.
47. Khan KN, Kitajima M, Hiraki K, Fujishita A, Sekine I, Ishimaru T, Masuzaki H. Changes in tissue inflammation, angiogenesis and apoptosis in endometriosis, adenomyosis and uterine myoma after GnRH agonist therapy. Hum Reprod. 2010;25:642–53.
48. Tesone M, Bilotas M, Barañao RI, Meresman G. The role of GnRH analogues in endometriosis-associated apoptosis and angiogenesis. Gynecol Obstet Invest. 2008;66 Suppl 1:10–8.
49. Sakamoto Y, Harada T, Horie S, Iba Y, Taniguchi F, Yoshida S, Iwabe T, Terakawa N. Tumor necrosis factor-a-induced interleukin-8 (IL-8) expression in endometriotic stromal cells, probably through nuclear factor-kappaB activation: gonadotropin-releasing hormone agonist treatment reduced IL-8 expression. J Clin Endocrinol Metabol. 2003;88:730–5.
50. Nasu K, Nishida M, Ueda T, Yuge A, Takai N, Narahara H. Application of the nuclear factor-kappaB inhibitor, BAY 11-7085, for the treatment of endometriosis: an in vitro study. Am J Physiol Endocrinol Metab. 2007;293:E16–23.
51. Suou K, Taniguchi F, Tagashira Y, Kiyama T, Terakawa N, Harada T. Apigenin inhibits tumor necrosis factor α-induced cell proliferation and prostaglandin E2 synthesis by inactivating NFκB in endometriotic stromal cells. Fertil Steril. 2011;95:1518–21.
52. Zhang JJ, Xu ZM, Zhang CM, Dai HY, Ji XQ, Wang XF, Li C. Pyrrolidine dithiocarbamate inhibits nuclear factor-κB pathway activation, and regulates adhesion, migration, invasion and apoptosis of endometriotic stromal cells. Mol Hum Reprod. 2011;17:175–81.
53. Othman EE, Salama S, Ismail N, Al-Hendy A. Toward gene therapy of endometriosis: adenovirus-mediated delivery of dominant negative estrogen receptor genes inhibits cell proliferation, reduces cytokine production, and induces apoptosis of endometriotic cells. Fertil Steril. 2007;88:462–71.
54. Meresman GF, Bilotas M, Abello V, Buquet R, Tesone M, Sueldo C. Effects of aromatase inhibitors on proliferation and apoptosis in eutopic endometrial cell cultures from patients with endometriosis. Fertil Steril. 2005;84:459–63.
55. Harada T, Momoeda M, Taketani Y, Hoshiai H, Terakawa N. Low-dose oral contraceptive pill for dysmenorrhea associated with endometriosis: a placebo-controlled, double-blind, randomized trial. Fertil Steril. 2008;90:1583–8.
56. Meresman GF, Auge L, Baranao RI, Lombardi E, Tesone M, Sueldo C. Oral contraceptives suppress cell proliferation and enhance apoptosis of eutopic endometrial tissue from patients with endometriosis. Fertil Steril. 2002;77:1141–7.
57. Yuan P, Huang Y, Wu H, Teng Z, Zhang J, Xin X. Induction of a local pseudo-pregnancy via levonorgestrel-loaded microspheres for the treatment of endometriosis in a rabbit model. Hum Reprod. 2010;25:462–9.

58. Nasu K, Nishida M, Ueda T, Takai N, Bing S, Narahara H, Miyakawa I. Bufalin induces apoptosis and G0/G1 cell cycle arrest of endometriotic stromal cells a promising agent for treatment of endometriosis. Mol Hum Reprod. 2005;11:817–23.
59. Nishida M, Nasu K, Ueda T, Yuge A, Takai N, Narahara H. Beta-hydroxyisovalerylshikonin induces apoptosis and G0/G1 cell cycle arrest of endometriotic stromal cells preliminary in vitro study. Hum Reprod. 2006;21:2850–6.
60. Altintas D, Kokcu A, Kandemir B, Tosun M, Cetinkaya MB. Comparison of the effects of raloxifene and anastrozole on experimental endometriosis. Eur J Obstet Gynecol Reprod Biol. 2010;150:84–7.
61. Tsuno A, Nasu K, Kawano Y, Yuge A, Li H, Abe W, Narahara H. Fasudil inhibits the proliferation and contractility and induces cell cycle arrest and apoptosis of human endometriotic stromal cells: a promising agent for the treatment of endometriosis. J Clin Endocrinol Metab. 2011;96:E1944–52.
62. Kawano Y, Nasu K, Li H, Tsuno A, Abe W, Takai N, Narahara H. Application of the histone deacetylase inhibitors for the treatment of endometriosis: histone modifications as pathogenesis and novel therapeutic target. Hum Reprod. 2011;26:2486–98.
63. Banu SK, Lee J, Speights Jr VO, Starzinski-Powitz A, Arosh JA. Cyclooxygenase-2 regulates survival, migration and invasion of human endometriotic cells through multiple mechanisms. Endocrinology. 2008;149:1180–9.

Chapter 13
Role of Nerve Fibres in Endometriosis

Natsuko Tokushige

Abstract Endometriosis is an oestrogen-dependent inflammatory disease. Endometriosis is often associated with pain symptoms such as dysmenorrhoea, dyspareunia, dyschezia, dysuria and low back pain. Although increased immune cells in peritoneal fluid, adhesions, retrograde menstruation and prostaglandins are considered to be causes of pain symptoms in endometriosis, the underlying mechanisms by which pain is generated still remain unknown. Recently numerous studies have focused on nerve fibres and neurotrophins in eutopic endometrium and endometriotic lesions from women with endometriosis as well as in animal models as a source of pain generation. Nerve fibres in eutopic and ectopic endometrium may be activated and/or sensitised by many inflammatory mediators to cause pain and tenderness. Neurotrophins are known to regulate the survival, development and function of nerve fibres. However, many other molecules may act as a neurotrophic factor in endometriosis. Increased numbers of nerve fibres, increased amount of neurotrophins and different types of nerve fibres in endometriosis may explain why women with endometriosis experience pain.

Keywords Endometriosis • Nerve fibres • Pain

13.1 Different Types of Nerve Fibres

Nerve fibres in the body arise from cell bodies in dorsal root ganglia (DRG) and nerve fibres in the head arise from cell bodies in trigeminal ganglion. Nerve fibres are categorised into six groups, namely Aα, Aβ, Aγ, Aδ, B and C fibres. Cell bodies with the largest diameters give rise to myelinated Aα, Aβ and Aγ fibres, and cell bodies with small and medium diameter give rise to thinly myelinated Aδ and B and

N. Tokushige (✉)
Department of Obstetrics and Gynaecology, University of Tottori, Tottori, Japan
e-mail: natsuko_tokushige31@yahoo.co.jp

T. Harada (ed.), *Endometriosis: Pathogenesis and Treatment*,
DOI 10.1007/978-4-431-54421-0_13, © Springer Japan 2014

unmyelinated C fibres. Aα, Aβ and Aγ fibres are large (5–15 μm in diameter) with myelin sheaths around them and they conduct at a rapid rate (20–100 m/s). Aα, Aβ and Aγ fibres carry the sensation of light pressure to deep muscle and soft touch to skin and do not produce pain. Pain impulses originate at nociceptors, which are sensory neurons that respond to potentially damaging stimuli. When receptors receive pain stimuli, the stimuli are transmitted to the central nervous system (CNS) by either Aδ fibres or C fibres via DRG [1]. Aδ fibres are smaller fibres with myelin sheaths and they conduct at a slower rate (10–25 m/s) than Aα or Aβ fibres due to their size (1–5 μm in diameter). C fibres are small unmyelinated fibres (0.3–1 μm in diameter) and they conduct at a rate of 0.5–2 m/s. Aδ fibres mediate rapid, acute and sharp pain (first pain), and C fibres mediate dull and diffuse pain (second pain) to the CNS [2].

13.2 Nociceptors and Pain Transmission

There are two types of nociceptors, namely high threshold mechanoreceptors and polymodal nociceptors. High threshold mechanoreceptors respond to mechanical damage such as cutting, crushing or pinching, and polymodal nociceptors respond to all kinds of damaging stimuli, such as irritating chemicals released from injured tissue. Information from high threshold mechanoreceptors are rapidly transmitted to the brain mainly by Aδ fibres, and the location of pain can be recognised. However, information from polymodal nociceptors is transmitted to the brain slowly and the location of pain is usually unrecognised.

Nociceptors can be further divided into peptidergic which contains peptides, such as substance P (SP) and calcitonin gene-related peptide (CGRP), and non-peptidergic which binds isolectin B4 (IB4) [3]. Aδ and C fibres express many of the molecules that have been implicated in the pain activation and sensitisation. These molecules include numerous ion channels and receptors for chemical mediators in their sensory endings. Most nociceptors express only part of the receptors, but prolonged inflammation can lead to an up-regulation of receptors for excitatory compounds. It is likely that the expression of some receptors for chemical mediators may be increased in endometriosis.

The pain from the periphery enters the spinal cord via DRG and it is passed to the nociceptive second-order neurons in the dorsal horn of the grey matter. Second-order neurons are divided into two groups, namely nociceptive-specific (NS) neurons and wide dynamic range (WDR) neurons [4]. Neurotransmitters such as glutamic acid and SP are released from the nerve terminals and they can activate DL-α-amino-3-hydroxy-5-methylisoxazole-4-propionic acid receptor (AMPA) and N-methyl-D-aspartic acid (NMDA) receptors on the second-order neurons. The pain goes to the thalamus and then enters the cerebral cortex or cerebral limbic system. Not all neurotransmitters activate AMPA or NMDA, and some neurotransmitters such as gamma-aminobutyric acid (GABA) and serotonin suppress pain sensation. Neurotransmitters can actually control pain transmission in the brain and spinal cord.

13.3 Pain-Producing Substances

The sensitisation and activation of nociceptors after inflammation result from the release of a variety of chemicals by damaged cells and tissues in the vicinity of the injury. These substances include bradykinin, histamine, prostaglandins (PGs), serotonin and nerve growth factor (NGF). They sensitise (lower the threshold) or activate the terminals of the nociceptor by interacting with cell-surface receptors expressed by these neurons. Primary sensory neurons have been shown to contain bioactive peptides that can cause local inflammation. These peptides include SP, CGRP, neuropeptide Y and vasoactive intestinal polypeptide (VIP). Inflammatory mediators activate the non-selective cation channel transient receptor potential vanilloid 1 (TRPV1) which leads to an influx of calcium. Tryptase released from degranulated mast cells cleaves PAR-2 at the plasma membrane of sensory nerve endings. Increased calcium causes depolarisation of the nerve and activated PAR-2 stimulates the release of bioactive peptides including SP and CGRP from sensory nerve endings.

SP and CGRP can contribute to the inflammatory response by causing vasodilation, plasma extravasation (leakage of proteins and fluid from postcapillary venules) and cellular infiltration by interacting with endothelial cells, arterioles, mast cells, neutrophils and immune cells [5]. SP acts on mast cells in the vicinity of sensory nerve endings to evoke degranulation and the release of histamine, which further induces a release of SP and NGF. SP also acts on platelets to release serotonin, providing a positive feedback [6]. CGRP inhibits SP degradation by a specific endopeptidase (SPE) [7] and enhances SP release, amplifying the effects [6]. VIP induces vasodilation and histamine release from mast cells. Histamine and serotonin levels rise in the extracellular space, secondarily sensitising nearby nociceptors. This leads to a gradual spread of hyperalgesia and/or tenderness.

13.4 Research on Nerve Fibres in the Uterus

Research on nerve fibres in the human uterus began about 1680 [8]. Kilian [9] was one of the first researchers to investigate nerve fibres in the human endometrium [9]. Frankenhauser [10] reported unmyelinated nerve fibres to the smooth muscle of the myometrium with branches to the stroma and the lining epithelium of the human endometrium [10]. Patenko [11], Kostlin [12] and Clivio [13] also demonstrated a fine plexus of unmyelinated nerve fibres in the submucosa from which fine fibrils extended to the epithelium of the human endometrium. Von Gawronsky [14] showed large nerve bundles extending parallel to the endometrial-myometrial junction, with fine branches into the human endometrial stroma [14]. Labhardt [15] and Mabuchi [16] were unable to demonstrate nerve fibres in the human endometrium; however, Dahl [17] described numerous fine nonmodulated nerve fibres in the human endometrium, ending in small treelike branches in the stroma and as straight fibres between the cells of the epithelium. Stöhr [18] reported nerve fibres in the mucosa of the human uterus, even fine fibres to the epithelium. Davis [19] did not find nerve fibres beneath the mucosa of the body of the human uterus. Brown and Hirsch [20] reported nerve fibres in the basal layer of the endometrium in the infantile uterus but were unable to demonstrate the mode of termination in those tissues. These investigators used the silver reduction methods to stain nerve fibres in the human uterus. There is a discrepancy between these studies and it is considered that the silver staining method did not clearly differentiate the nerves and reveal the nerve fibres in the uterus compared with immunohistochemistry.

State and Hirsch [21] used Goldner's modification of Masson's trichrome stain to demonstrate nerve fibres in human uteri with no obvious pathologic changes. Some nerve fibres were present in the lower third of the basal layer of the endometrium that have branches terminating in the stroma, in the basolar arterioles and at the origin of the spiral arterioles. No nerve fibres were detected beyond the basal layer of the endometrium. They also demonstrated some nerve fibres in the myometrium and at the endometrial-myometrial junction. In this study, the nerve fibres in the endometrium were found to be unmyelinated. Koppen [22], Stöhr [23], Krantz [24] and Witt [25] reported that branches of nerve fibres accompanying arteries had been clearly revealed only in the basal layer of the endometrium and there were no nerve fibres in the outer two-thirds of the endometrium by Goldner's modification of Masson's trichrome stain.

Lerner et al. [26] reported abnormal innervation in the myometrium from women with chronic pelvic pain and dysmenorrhoea. There was a marked proliferation of unmyelinated nerve bundles in the myometrium, but nerve fibres in the endometrium were not mentioned in this study. Quinn and Kirk [27] investigated uterine innervation in normal and some clinical conditions such as adenomyosis and chronic pelvic pain. They performed immunohistostaining using an antibody against protein gene product (PGP9.5). They demonstrated nerve bundles at the endometrial-myometrial interface and throughout the myometrium in nulliparous and parous subjects with no histologic abnormality. There was nerve fibre proliferation throughout the myometrium with small-diameter nerve fibres eccentric courses throughout the myometrial stoma in some subjects with chronic pelvic pain.

Some researchers have identified types of nerve fibres in the human uterus. SP- and CGRP-immunoreactive nerve fibres were present in the human myometrium [28]. Heinrich et al. [29] demonstrated neuropeptide (NPY), SP, neurotensin (NT) and VIP-immunoreactive nerve fibres in the basal layer of the endometrium and myometrium in nonpregnant women. Lynch et al. [30] and Helm et al. [31] also detected VIP-immunoreactive nerve fibres in the endometrium and myometrium in women with no pathologic abnormality.

Nerve fibres in the endometrium in animals have also been investigated by some researchers. A number of tyrosine hydroxylase (TH), dopamine β-hydroxylase (DβH), NPY and VIP-immunoreactive nerve bundles and fibres were present in equine endometrium [32], and CGRP-immunoreactive nerve fibres were in equine and rat endometrium [32, 33], secretoneurin (SN)-immunoreactive nerve fibres were in rat endometrium [34], VIP-immunoreactive nerve fibres were in rat and porcine endometrium [35, 36], adrenergic and acetylcholine (ACh)-immunoreactive nerve fibres were in sheep endometrium [37], and AChE- and NPY-immunoreactive nerve fibres were in rat endometrium [38].

TH-immunoreactive nerve fibres are considered to regulate uterine contractility, uterine blood flow and endometrial secretion as those nerve fibres are often associated with blood vessels, endometrial glands and myometrial smooth muscle. SP and CGRP are co-expressed in a subpopulation of nerve fibres (sensory Aδ and C). SP induces contraction in the human uterus [28] and controls blood flow [39]. In contrast, CGRP is a potent vasodilator [40] and inhibitor of spontaneous contractile activity in the human uterus [28]. Also CGRP inhibits uterine contractility caused by SP in rat uterus [41], regulates sensory transmission and glandular secretion [42, 43] and has a proliferative effect on human endothelial cells [43]. NPY is known to co-exist with noradrenaline and considered to regulate vascular tone and exert inhibitory effect on myometrial contractility [28]. VIP is a potent vasodilator of the uterine artery and involves in smooth muscle relaxation, blood flow increase and secretion [36]. ACh is associated with myometrial and vascular smooth muscle [44] and evokes contraction of the myometrium [45]. VIP co-exists with ACh [46] and promotes relaxation of the myometrium through inhibition of the excitatory action of ACh [47]. CGRP also inhibits ACh-stimulated uterine contraction and this is dose dependent [33]. SN is contained in sensory C fibres and parasympathetic neurons [34] and co-exists with SP and CGRP [48]. SN may regulate vascular control and smooth muscle contraction and play a role in the process of neurogenic inflammation that involves the activation of sensory C fibres, which release SP, neurokinin A, CGRP and nitric oxide from their peripheral terminals to increase vascular permeability, protein extravasation, tissue oedema, vasodilation and activation and recruitment of inflammatory immune cells. TH and DβH are present in adrenergic nerve fibres and they are associated with vascular and nonvascular smooth muscle and participate in the regulation of myometrial contractions and blood flow [49]. It would be interesting to see how these nerve fibres are correlated with variation in pain symptoms and response to hormone treatment.

13.5 Nerve Fibres and Neurotrophins in the Uterus from Women with Endometriosis

Quinn and Kirk [27] reported that there was widespread nerve fibre proliferation (small-diameter nerve fibres) in the uterine isthmus suggesting nerve fibre damage in the uterine isthmus in women complaining of chronic pelvic pain. Few of these women had endometriosis, but they did report widespread nerve fibre proliferation in the uterus and cervix in one woman with advanced endometriosis and with painful periods and intercourse. These nerve fibres were prominently seen around arteries and veins throughout the uterine isthmus. Quinn and Armstrong [50] reported widespread nerve fibre proliferation with extensive perivascular nerve fibre proliferation around both arteries and veins in the myometrium in an endometriosis patient with dysmenorrhoea and dyspareunia. In another study, increased numbers of nerve fibres were seen in the myometrium from women with advanced endometriosis compared with women without endometriosis [51]. These studies demonstrated the proliferation of nerve fibres; however, types of nerve fibres in the endometrium and myometrium from women with endometriosis were not investigated in these studies. It has been demonstrated that no nerve fibres were detected in the functional layer of the endometrium from women without endometriosis; however, there were several small nerve fibres present in the functional layer of the endometrium from women with endometriosis (the mean density of nerve fibres: 13.4 mm^2) [52]. There were more nerve fibres in the basal layer of the endometrium and myometrium from women with endometriosis than women without endometriosis. Several thick nerve trunks were seen in the basal layer of the endometrium or at the endometrial-myometrial interface in women with endometriosis, but these nerve fibres were not seen in women without endometriosis. Many small nerve fibres were also present throughout the basal layer of the endometrium, but only a few nerve fibres were seen in women without endometriosis. Many more nerve fibres and nerve trunks were seen in the myometrium in women with endometriosis than in women without endometriosis. In women with endometriosis, nerve fibres in the functional layer of the endometrium were sensory C fibres; sensory C, sensory Aδ and adrenergic fibres in the basal layer; and sensory C, sensory Aδ, adrenergic and cholinergic fibres in the myometrium [53]. These results indicate that abnormal innervation in the uterus may be associated with pain generation in women with endometriosis who suffer from chronic pelvic pain.

Progestogens and combined oral contraceptives are often used to treat women with endometriosis-associated pain. Progestogens and combined oral contraceptives significantly reduced the nerve fibre density in the functional and the basal layers of the endometrium and myometrium from women with hormonally treated endometriosis compared with that from women with untreated endometriosis [54]. Hormonal treatments may reduce pain symptoms by decreasing nerve fibres in the endometrium and myometrium in women with endometriosis.

13.6 Conscious Pain Mapping

Several groups have studied conscious pain mapping since it has been assumed that endometriotic lesions are the source of localised pain and tenderness, and conscious pain mapping may help to identify potential areas causing pelvic pain. Palter and Olive [55] first described conscious pain mapping to identify a focal source of pain and generalised visceral hypersensitivity in a majority of women with chronic pelvic pain (CPP). They found that deep infiltrating sclerotic endometriosis of the rectum, active peritoneal endometriosis and an adhesion of small bowel were apparent sources of cause of pain. Demco [56] found that most women localised or mapped their pain to their endometriotic lesions and the surrounding peritoneum. In this study, pain extended beyond the lesions to normal-looking peritoneum. Almeida and Val-Gallas [57] found 48 positive findings in 50 women with conscious pain mapping and Howard et al. [58] also reported that conscious pain mapping successfully identified tender lesion in 70 % of women. It seems that most endometriotic lesions themselves appear to be capable of generating pain stimuli, and conscious pain mapping can be useful in detecting a source of pain. However, not all endometriotic lesions produce pain and it is likely that there may be other sources of pain generation in women with endometriosis.

13.7 Nerve Fibres in Endometriotic Lesions

Tamburro et al. [59] demonstrated the expression of transforming growth factor β1 (TGFβ1) in nerve fibres in endometriotic lesions from women with dysmenorrhoea associated with endometriosis. There was a significant correlation between the dysmenorrhoea and maximal intensity of staining of TGFβ1 and a relationship between the colour of the lesions and maximal intensity of staining of TGFβ1. Greater maximal intensity of staining of TGFβ1 was seen in red, deep lesions than in black and normal peritoneum. TGFβ1 is increased in the peritoneal fluid of women with endometriosis [60] and can increase cyclooxygenase-2 (COX-2) activity to produce more PGs [59]. Since there were no morphologic differences in the nerve fibres between endometriotic peritoneal lesions and normal peritoneum, substances that are present in the nerve fibres appear to be associated with causing pelvic pain in women with endometriosis. Tulandi et al. [61] demonstrated nerve fibres in endometriotic lesions in women with endometriosis by using an antibody against neurofilament (NF). They reported that the distance between endometrial glands and nerve fibres in endometriotic lesions from women with pain was closer than in women with no pain. Quinn and Kirk [62] reported widespread nerve fibre proliferation (small-diameter nerve fibres) in endometriotic lesions from a woman with pelvic pain. Berkley et al. [63] demonstrated nerve fibres in endometriotic lesions in a rat model and these nerve fibres were protein gene product 9.5 (PGP9.5), CGRP, SP and vesicular monoamine transporter (VMAT) immunoreactive. SP and CGRP are present in myelinated and unmyelinated sensory nerve fibres (Aδ fibres and C fibres), and VMAT is present in sympathetic fibres.

In peritoneal endometriotic lesion from endometriosis patients who presented pain symptoms, nerve fibres were innervated by sensory C, sensory Aδ, cholinergic and adrenergic fibres, and the mean density of nerve fibres was 16 mm^2. Progestogens and combined oral contraceptives significantly reduced nerve fibre density in peritoneal endometriotic lesions from hormone-treated women with endometriosis (the mean density of nerve fibres: 10.6 mm^2) compared with peritoneal endometriotic lesions from untreated women with endometriosis (the mean density of nerve fibres: 16.3 mm^2) [65]. Nerve fibres expressing growth-associated protein 43, which is a marker of neuronal development and sprouting in peritoneal endometriotic lesion as well as SP, have also been reported by another group [66]. The same group has shown the relationship between the severity of pain symptoms and the density of nerve fibres in peritoneal endometriotic lesions [67]. There were more nerve fibres stained with PGP 9.5 and NF in endometriosis patients whose pain score was at least 3 or more than those whose pain score was 2 or less. This study has shown that there is a correlation between the density of nerve fibres and pain severity in peritoneal endometriotic lesions in women with endometriosis. Alvarez et al. have developed peritoneal endometriotic lesions in a rat model by implanting with autologous uterus in the gastrocnemius muscle [68]. Those lesions showed peptidergic nerve fibres (CGRP-positive), non-peptidergic nerve fibres (IB4-positive) as well as GAP43-positive nerve fibres. Since no studies have demonstrated IB4-positive nerve fibres in endometriotic lesions from women with endometriosis, it would be interesting to investigate the presence of IB4-positive nerve fibres and to find out the roles of these nerve fibres in endometriosis.

Deep infiltrating endometriosis (DIE) is often associated with severe pain and is defined as endometriotic lesions penetrating into the retroperitoneal space or the wall of the pelvic organs for a distance of 5 mm or more [69]. Patients with deep pelvic infiltrating endometriosis usually have much stronger pain than those with other types of endometriosis [69–71]. Anaf et al. [70] have demonstrated that endometriosis patients with DIE had significantly higher preoperative pain scores than patients with peritoneal or ovarian endometriosis. In their study, mast cells located <25 μm from nerve fibres were significantly more abundant in DIE than in peritoneal and ovarian endometriosis. Wang et al. have reported that there were more nerve fibres in DIE (the mean density of nerve fibres: 68 mm^2) than in peritoneal endometriosis (the mean density of nerve fibres: 16 mm^2) [72]. Those nerve fibres were sensory C, sensory Aδ, cholinergic and adrenergic fibres. When compared with the locations of DIE, more nerve fibres were detected in DIE in the sigmoid colon, appendix and rectum (the mean density of nerve fibres: 172 mm^2) than in the uterosacral ligament, cul-de-sac or peritoneal sidewall (the mean density of nerve fibres: 68 mm^2).

There are many substances secreted from endometriotic lesions including PGs [73], tumour necrosis factor-α (TNF-α) [74] and NGF [75]. These substances could sensitise and/or activate sensory and sympathetic nerve fibres that are present in endometriotic lesions. TRPV1, a key molecule in nociception, has been identified in the human cervix uteri in the nonpregnant state [76]. The levels of TRPV1 can be increased in painful inflammatory diseases, and TRPV1 can trigger the release of SP and CGRP from peripheral nerve terminals during inflammation [77]. It would be interesting to see whether TRPVI may be present in ectopic endometrium in women with endometriosis.

Most women with endometriosis present some kind of pain symptoms such as dysmenorrhoea or dyspareunia. However, a few endometriosis patients do not show any pain symptoms. When peritoneal endometriotic lesions from women with endometriosis who did not have any pain symptoms were stained with PGP 9.5, some nerve fibres were still detected. Therefore, not only the presence of nerve fibres but also types of nerve fibres or molecules in endometriotic lesions may be associated with pain generation in women with endometriosis. There may be some molecules which can desensitise nerve fibres in those who do not experience pain symptoms. Further studies will be required as to nerve fibres and substances secreted from endometriotic lesions from endometriosis patients who do not have any pain symptoms.

13.8 Neurotrophins (NGF, BDNF, NT-3, NT-4/5) in Eutopic and Ectopic Endometrium

NGF belongs to the neurotrophin family, together with brain-derived neurotrophic factor (BDNF) [78], neurotrophins-3 (NT-3) [79] and neurotrophins-4/5 (NT-4/5) [80]. NGF exerts its effects by binding to a tyrosine kinase A receptor (TrkA), and BDNF and NT-4/5 bind TrkB, and NT-3 binds TrkC instead [81]. p75, a low-affinity glycoprotein, also binds all neurotrophins [82].

NGF was strongly expressed near endometriotic glands in peritoneal and ovarian endometriosis [64, 75], and neurotrophin-3 (NT-3) expression was also observed in peritoneal endometriosis [66]. In ovarian endometriosis, NGF, BDNF, NT-3, NT-4/5 and NTRK2 mRNA expressions were detected by quantitative reverse transcriptase-polymerase chain reaction (RT-PCR) [83]. Browne et al. have demonstrated that NT-4/5 and BDNF mRNAs concentrations in eutopic endometrium detected on the antibody microarrays and reverse transcriptase-polymerase chain reaction were much higher in endometriosis patients than in women without endometriosis [84]. However, another study has reported that there was no difference in amounts of NGF, BDNF, NT-3, TrkA and NGFRp75 in eutopic endometrium between women with and without endometriosis using immunofluorescence staining, Western blot and a neuronal growth assay [85]. The discrepancy may be due to different kinds of pain symptoms, severity of pain or the density of nerve fibres among those patients. Much more detailed studies will be needed to determine the expression of these neurotrophins.

NGF has several effects through a variety of mechanisms. NGF stimulates the development, growth and survival of neurons, particularly of sensory neurons [86]. NGF increases synthesis and release of neuropeptides such as SP and CGRP from sensory nerve endings [87] and stimulates degranulation of mast cells. Recent evidence has implicated NGF as a key mediator of inflammation and pain. NGF is up-regulated in nerve fibres associated with the inflamed area during inflammation. NGF can increase the sensitivity and excitability of peripheral neurons to cause pain by directly or indirectly sensitising sensory nerve fibres [88]. NGF in turn activates mast cells and neutrophils which can release additional inflammatory mediators such as histamine, serotonin and bradykinin to cause hypersensitivity [89]. NGF has also been reported to promote angiogenesis [90]. NGF induces proliferation of endothelial cells [91] and of vascular smooth muscle cells [92] and stimulates the production of vascular endothelial growth factor (VEGF) [93]. NGF is expressed in vascular endothelial cells [94] and a variety of cell types such as T and B lymphocytes [95], mast cells [96], eosinophils [97], monocytes/macrophages [98], neutrophils and basophils [99]. Increased angiogenesis in eutopic endometrium in women with endometriosis demonstrated by several studies [100, 101] and increased numbers of immune cells may lead to further production of NGF, promoting further nerve fibre outgrowth and pain sensation.

13.9 Effects of Oestrogen on Nerve Fibres

It is well established that oestrogen has multiple effects on the female reproductive system and peripheral nervous system including pain sensitivity and neural regulation of vascular function. Endometriosis is oestrogen dependent for continued growth and proliferation, and it usually becomes less active with menopause as the oestrogen level decreases. However, oestrogen replacement therapy can reactivate the disease. Oophorectomy significantly decreased NGF and BDNF levels while oestrogen treatment increased these levels [102, 103], and oestrogen also up-regulated NGF and BDNF expressions in the endometrium [104–106]. Several studies have shown that neuroprotective effects of oestrogen were blocked by ER antagonists [107–109]. Ovariectomy caused a significant decrease in NGF protein content in the uterus, and short-term treatment of ovariectomised mice with oestrogen and/or progesterone increased uterine NGF mRNA and restored NGF protein to concentrations similar to intact control mice [110].

In animals, stronger immunostaining of NGF and TrkA was observed in luminal epithelial cells and glandular cells in the estrous period and early pregnancy as compared to the non-breeding period in the uterus of the wild ground squirrels [111]. p75 was immunolocalised only in luminal epithelial and glandular cells during the estrous period, early pregnancy and non-breeding period. The mean mRNA levels of NGF and TrkA and p75 were significantly higher in the estrous period and early pregnancy as compared to the non-breeding period.

Strong immunostaining of NGF and its receptors NTRK1 and TNFRSF1B was observed in uteri of golden hamsters on the day of proestrus as compared to the other stages of the estrous cycle [112]. There was a positive correlation between uterine NGF expression and plasma concentrations of estradiol-17beta, and estradiol-17beta stimulated expression of NGF and its two receptors in the uterus.

Neutral endopeptidase (NEP) is the enzyme responsible for degradation of SP and oestrogen treatment of ovariectomised rats resulted in a four-fold decrease in uterine NEP relative to control ovariectomised rats, resulting in increased SP levels [113].

Angiotensin-converting enzyme (ACE) is an enzyme responsible for degradation of bradykinin and treatment of postmenopausal women with oestrogen caused an increase in bradykinin and a decrease in ACE [114]. Steroidal hormones may induce further production of neuropeptides and neurotransmitters by altering enzyme expressions to sensitise sensory nerve terminals to cause prolonged pain sensation.

Oestrogen receptor-alpha (ER-alpha) and ER-beta are expressed in sensory neurons of the dorsal root ganglia (DRG) [115], so oestrogen could directly act on sensory nerve fibres to enhance axon outgrowth. Receptors for other steroidal hormones such as progesterone may be expressed in nerve fibres and they may also have direct effects on nerve fibres.

13.10 Prostaglandins and Neurotrophins

The correlation between prostaglandins and endometriosis-associated pain is well established. PGE_2 is present in sensory and sympathetic nerve fibres and can sensitise and activate sensory nerve fibre terminals to induce pain [116]. Prostaglandins may act neuroprotectively to induce the production and release of neurotrophins to promote the survival and outgrowth of nerve fibres. Toyomoto et al. [117] reported that PGE_2 induced and stimulated the secretion and synthesis of NGF and BDNF, and Kanda et al. [118] also demonstrated that PGE_2 enhanced the production of neurotrophin-4 (NT-4) via EP3 receptor.

COX-2 is an enzyme which catalyses the synthesis of prostaglandins from arachidonic acid and COX-2 may have a key function with respect to inflammation and pain. Previous studies have shown that COX-2 is expressed in neurons and COX-2 expression in eutopic endometrium in women with endometriosis was higher than in those without endometriosis [119]. Also, increased COX-2 expression in endometriotic lesions of different anatomical sites (ovarian, peritoneal and deep infiltrating endometriosis) has been reported [120–122], resulting in further modification of the production of prostaglandins in different sites.

13.11 Molecules That May Be Associated with Nerve Fibre Growth in Endometriosis

Several molecules are present in eutopic endometrium and endometriotic lesions in women with endometriosis and some of them may have effects on nerve fibre outgrowth. Insulin-like growth factor I (IGF-I) was present in eutopic endometrium and endometriotic lesions in women with endometriosis [123]. IGF-1 induced sensory nerve fibre growth and potentiated the NGF-induced neuritogenesis [124, 125]. Oestrogen also regulated the expression and synthesis of IGF-I and its receptor [126, 127].

Bcl-2 was present in eutopic endometrium and endometriotic lesions in women with endometriosis [128]. Bcl-2 is expressed in neurons and promoted axonal growth rates in sensory nerve fibres [129, 130]. Oestrogen up-regulated the expression of Bcl-2 [131], and oestrogen treatment increased the number of Bcl-2 immunoreactive nerve fibres [132]. Both oestrogen and progesterone can increase the expression of Bcl-2 [133, 134] and Bcl-2 has been shown to inhibit neuronal death [133]. Therefore oestrogen and progesterone may directly affect cell survival or prevent neuronal cell death in neurons by Bcl-2-induced inhibition of cell death and axonal growth, resulting in increased nerve fibre densities.

Hepatocyte growth factor (HGF) was up-regulated in eutopic endometrium in women with endometriosis [135]. HGF alone had no outgrowth-promoting activity, but it co-operated with NGF in enhancing axonal growth of sensory nerves and also enhanced the neurotrophic activities of NGF [136]. Oestrogen also increased the production of HGF by peritoneal macrophages in women with endometriosis [137].

Significantly increased expression of heat shock protein 27 (HSP 27) was reported in eutopic endometrium in women with endometriosis [138]. HSP27 was expressed by sensory nerve fibres [139, 140] and significantly increased survival for rat sensory and sympathetic nerve fibres after axotomy or NGF withdrawal [141]. HSP expression was stimulated by oestrogen in the endometrium [142].

Fibroblast growth factor 9 (FGF-9) was present in endometriotic lesions in women with endometriosis [143]. FGF-9 enhanced survival of cholinergic nerve fibres [144] and administration of 17β-estradiol induced FGF-9 expression in endometriotic lesions [143].

These molecules may be associated with increased nerve fibre densities, specially sensory and autonomic neurons in women with endometriosis to induce pain, and steroidal hormones may promote the synthesis of these molecules in women with endometriosis

13.12 Angiogenic Molecules

Novella-Maestre et al. [145] have demonstrated that antiangiogenic treatment with cabergoline significantly reduced the number of immature blood vessels, nerve fibres, mast cells and macrophages in endometriotic lesions in a mouse model of endometriosis. Vascular endothelial growth factor (VEGF) is a secreted vascular mitogen that is specific for endothelial cells and plays an important regulatory role in vascular growth during development [146]. VEGF is increased in DIE [147] and peritoneal fluid [148] in women with endometriosis compared with women without. It is accumulating evidence that VEGF acts as a neurotrophic and neuroprotective factor [149]. VEGF application to cultured peripheral adult ganglia caused significant neuritic outgrowth [150] and peripheral nerve regeneration in vivo has been shown to be enhanced by VEGF application [151]. There are some proangiogenic factors, such as IL-8 [152], hepatocyte growth factor (HGF) [153], erythropoietin [154], angiogenin [155], macrophage migration inhibitory factor [156], neutrophil-activating factor [157] and TNF-α [158], and these proangiogenic factors may also have neurotrophic effects and be involved in nerve fibre growth in endometriosis.

13.13 Conclusions

Increased numbers of nerve fibres in eutopic endometrium (both the functional layer and the basal layer), myometrium and endometriotic lesions may contribute in some way to the mediation of pain in women with endometriosis. It was always been assured that the pain of endometriosis is generated in the endometriotic lesions, but the findings in some studies allow the possibility that some of the pain may actually arise within the endometrium.

Endometriosis is an inflammatory condition and many chemical and inflammatory mediators such as bradykinin, prostaglandins as well as neurotrophins can be released from both eutopic endometrium and endometriotic lesions. These substances can directly activate and/or sensitise sensory nerve endings by interacting with cell-surface receptors and trigger the release of pain mediators from other cells and afferent nerve fibres. Those pain mediators sensitise nerve endings, resulting in an increased response to painful stimuli. Prostaglandins and other arachidonic acid derivatives can increase the sensitivity of nerve endings to bradykinin or other pain-producing substances, leading to a secondary sensitisation of nearby sensory nerve fibres.

There may be a correlation between pain severity and nerve fibre density; however, it seems that some nerve fibres in eutopic and ectopic endometrium are not associated with pain generation. Further research will be needed to better understand the roles of nerve fibres and molecules secreted from eutopic and ectopic endometrium from women with endometriosis.

References

1. Adrienne ED, Ardem P. Nociceptors: the sensors of the pain pathway. J Clin Invest. 2010;120:3760–72.
2. Harkins SW, Davis MD, Bush FM, Kasberger J. Suppression of first pain and slow temporal summation of second pain in relation to age. J Gerontol A Biol Sci Med Sci. 1996;51: M260–5.
3. Molliver DC, Wright DE, Leitner ML, Parsadanian AS, Doster K, Wen D, Yan Q, Snider WD. IB4-binding DRG neurons switch from NGF to GDNF dependence in early postnatal life. Neuron. 1997;19:849–61.
4. Miraucourt LS, Dallel R, Voisin DL. Glycine inhibitory dysfunction turns touch into pain through PKCgamma interneurons. PLoS One. 2007;2:e1116.
5. Maggi CA. Tachykinins and calcitonin gene-related peptide (CGRP) as co-transmitters released from peripheral endings of sensory nerves. Prog Neurobiol. 1995;45:1–98.

6. Steinhoff M, Stander S, Seeliger S, Ansel JC, Schmelz M, Luger T. Modern aspects of cutaneous neurogenic inflammation. Arch Dermatol. 2003;139:1479–88.
7. Le Greves P, Nyberg F, Terenius L, Hokfelt T. Calcitonin gene-related peptide is a potent inhibitor of substance P degradation. Eur J Pharmacol. 1985;115:309–11.
8. Wilissius T. Cerebri anatome nervorumque descriptio et usus. I Opra Omnia. Geneva; 1680. p. 1.
9. Kilian FM. Ztschr F Rat Med. 1851;10:41.
10. Frankenhauser F. Die nerven der Gebärmutter und ihre Endigungen in der glatten Muskelfascrn: Ein Beitrag zur Anatomie und Gynäkologie, Insug. Dissert, Jcna, Fr. Manke; 1867.
11. Patenko T. Zentralbl F Gynäk. 1880;19:442.
12. Kostlin R. Die Nervendigungen in den weiblichen Geschlechtsorganen. Fortschr Med. 1894;12:411–21.
13. Clivio I. Contributo alla conoscenza delle terminazioni nervose dell'utero, Pavia, tipog e legat.coop; 1894.
14. Von Gawronsky N. Arch F Gynäk. 1894;47:271.
15. Labhardt A. Arch F Gynäk. 1906;80:135.
16. Mabuchi K. Mitt. a. d. med. Fak. d. k. Univ. Tokyo; 1924. 81: 385.
17. Dahl W. Ztschr F Geburtsh U Gynäk. 1916;78:539.
18. Stöhr P. In: von Möllendorff W, editors. Handbuch der mikroscopischen Anatomie des Menschen. Berlin: Julius Springer; 1928. 4(1):393.
19. Davis AA. J Obst Gynaec Brit Emp. 1933;40:481.
20. Brown WH, Hirch EF. The intrinsic nerves of the immature human uterus. Am J Pathol. 1941;17:731–9.
21. State D, Hirsch E. The distribution of the nerves to the adult endometrium. Arch Pathol. 1941;32:939.
22. Koppen K. Results of a histologic study of uterine innervation. Arch Gynakol. 1950;177:354–91.
23. Stöhr PH Jr. Mikroskopische Anatomie des vegetativcn Nervensystems. In: Handbuch der mikroskopischen Anatomic des Menschen, Bd.IV/5, Nervensystem. Berlin-Göttingen-Haidelberg: Springer; 1957.
24. Krantz KE. Innervation of the human uterus. Ann N Y Acad Sci. 1959;75:770–84.
25. Witt HJ. Strunkturelementc und funktionelle Gesamtheit des Endometriuma. Lichtoptische Morphologie. I. Das normale menschliche Endometrium. Hrsg. V. H. Schmidt-Matthiesen. Stuttgart: Georg Thieme; 1963.
26. Lerner EJ, Jaffe M, Ree HJ, McDuff Jr HC. Proliferation of myometrial nerves in a patient with severe dysmenorrhea. R I Med J. 1985;68:265–7.
27. Quinn MJ, Kirk N. Differences in uterine innervation at hysterectomy. Am J Obstet Gynecol. 2002;187:1515–9. discussion 1519–20.
28. Samuelson UE, Dalsgaard CJ, Lundberg JM, Hokfelt T. Calcitonin gene-related peptide inhibits spontaneous contractions in human uterus and fallopian tube. Neurosci Lett. 1985;62:225–30.
29. Heinrich D, Reinecke M, Forssmann WG. Peptidergic innervation of the human and guinea pig uterus. Arch Gynecol. 1986;237:213–9.
30. Lynch EM, Wharton J, Bryant MG, Bloom SR, Polak JM, Elder MG. The differential distribution of vasoactive intestinal polypeptide in the normal human female genital tract. Histochemistry. 1980;67:169–77.
31. Helm G, Ottesen B, Fahrenkrug J, Larsen JJ, Owman C, Sjoberg NO, Stolberg B, Sundler F, et al. Vasoactive intestinal polypeptide (VIP) in the human female reproductive tract: distribution and motor effects. Biol Reprod. 1981;25:227–34.
32. Bae SE, Corcoran BM, Watson ED. Immunohistochemical study of the distribution of adrenergic and peptidergic innervation in the equine uterus and the cervix. Reproduction. 2001;122:275–82.

33. Shew RL, Papka RE, McNeill DL. Calcitonin gene-related peptide in the rat uterus: presence in nerves and effects on uterine contraction. Peptides. 1990;11:583–9.
34. Collins JJ, Wilson K, Fischer-Colbrie R, Papka RE. Distribution and origin of secretoneurin-immunoreactive nerves in the female rat uterus. Neuroscience. 2000;95:255–64.
35. Houdeau E, Prudhomme MJ, Rousseau JP. Regional difference in the distribution of vaso-active intestinal polypeptide-immunoreactive nerve fibres along the uterus and between myometrial muscle layers in the rat. Histochem J. 1998;30:525–9.
36. Rodriguez R, Pozuelo JM, Martin R, Arriazu R, Santamaria L. Stereological quantification of nerve fibers immunoreactive to PGP 9.5, NPY, and VIP in rat prostate during postnatal development. J Androl. 2005;26:197–204.
37. Renegar RH, Rexroad Jr CE. Uterine adrenergic and cholinesterase-positive nerves and myometrial catecholamine concentrations during pregnancy in sheep. Acta Anat (Basel). 1990;137:373–81.
38. Papka RE, Cotton JP, Traurig HH. Comparative distribution of neuropeptide tyrosine-, vasoactive intestinal polypeptide-, substance P-immunoreactive, acetylcholinesterase-positive and noradrenergic nerves in the reproductive tract of the female rat. Cell Tissue Res. 1985;242:475–90.
39. Otsuka M, Konishi S, Yanagisawa M, Tsunoo A, Akagi H. Role of substance P as a sensory transmitter in spinal cord and sympathetic ganglia. Ciba Found Symp. 1982;91:13–34.
40. Sato S, Hayashi RH, Garfield RE. Mechanical responses of the rat uterus, cervix, and bladder to stimulation of hypogastric and pelvic nerves in vivo. Biol Reprod. 1989;40:209–19.
41. Shew RL, Papka RE, McNeill DL, Yee JA. NADPH-diaphorase-positive nerves and the role of nitric oxide in CGRP relaxation of uterine contraction. Peptides. 1993;14:637–41.
42. Gibson SJ, Polak JM, Bloom SR, Sabate IM, Mulderry PM, Ghatei MA, McGregor GP, Morrison JF, et al. Calcitonin gene-related peptide immunoreactivity in the spinal cord of man and of eight other species. J Neurosci. 1984;4:3101–11.
43. Onuoha GN, Alpar EK. Levels of vasodilators (SP, CGRP) and vasoconstrictor (NPY) peptides in early human burns. Eur J Clin Invest. 2001;31:253–7.
44. Adham N, Schenk EA. Autonomic innervation of the rat vagina, cervix, and uterus and its cyclic cariation. Am J Obstet Gynecol. 1964;104:508–16.
45. Traurig HH, Papka RE. Autonomic efferent and visceral sensory innervation of the female reproductive system: special reference to the functional roles of nerves in reproductive organs. In: Maggi CA, editor. Nervous control of the urogenital system. Chur: Harwood Academic; 1993. p. 103–41.
46. Houdeau E, Boyer PA, Rousseau A, Rousseau JP. Coexpression of neuropeptide Y and vasoactive intestinal polypeptide in pelvic plexus neurones innervating the uterus and cervix in the rat. Cell Tissue Res. 1997;288:285–92.
47. Stjernquist M, Owman C. Interaction of noradrenaline, NPY and VIP with the neurogenic cholinergic response of the rat uterine cervix in vitro. Acta Physiol Scand. 1987;131:553–62.
48. Kirchmair R, Marksteiner J, Troger J, Mahata SK, Mahata M, Donnerer J, Amann R, Fischer-Colbrie R, Winkler H, Saria A. Human and rat primary C-fibre afferents store and release secretoneurin, a novel neuropeptide. Eur J Neurosci. 1994;6:861–8.
49. Vera PL, HaaseE B, Schramm LP. Origins of the sympathetic innervation of the cervical end of the uterus in the rat. Brain Res. 1997;747:140–3.
50. Quinn M, Armstrong G. Uterine nerve fibre proliferation in advanced endometriosis. J Obstet Gynaecol. 2004;24:932–3.
51. Atwal G, du Plessis D, Armstrong G, Slade R, Quinn M. Uterine innervation after hysterectomy for chronic pelvic pain with, and without, endometriosis. Am J Obstet Gynecol. 2005;193:1650–5.
52. Tokushige N, Markham R, Russell P, Fraser IS. High density of small nerve fibres in the functional layer of the endometrium in women with endometriosis. Hum Reprod. 2006;21:782–7.

53. Tokushige N, Markham R, Russell P, Fraser IS. Different types of small nerve fibers in eutopic endometrium and myometrium in women with endometriosis. Fertil Steril. 2007;88:795–803.
54. Tokushige N, Markham R, Russell P, Fraser IS. Effects of hormonal treatment on nerve fibers in endometrium and myometrium in women with endometriosis. Fertil Steril. 2008;90:1589–98.
55. Palter SF, Olive DL. Office microlaparoscopy under local anesthesia for chronic pelvic pain. J Am Assoc Gynecol Laparosc. 1996;3:359–64.
56. Demco L. Mapping the source and character of pain due to endometriosis by patient-assisted laparoscopy. J Am Assoc Gynecol Laparosc. 1998;5:241–5.
57. Almeida Jr OD, Val-Gallas JM. Conscious pain mapping. J Am Assoc Gynecol Laparosc. 1997;4:587–90.
58. Howard FM, El-Minawi AM, Sanchez RA. Conscious pain mapping by laparoscopy in women with chronic pelvic pain. Obstet Gynecol. 2000;96:934–9.
59. Tamburro S, Canis M, Albuisson E, Dechelotte P, Darcha C, Mage G. Expression of transforming growth factor beta1 in nerve fibers is related to dysmenorrhea and laparoscopic appearance of endometriotic implants. Fertil Steril. 2003;80:1131–6.
60. Pizzo A, Salmeri FM, Ardita FV, Sofo V, Tripepi M, Marsico S. Behaviour of cytokine levels in serum and peritoneal fluid of women with endometriosis. Gynecol Obstet Invest. 2002;54:82–7.
61. Tulandi T, Felemban A, Chen MF. Nerve fibers and histopathology of endometriosis-harboring peritoneum. J Am Assoc Gynecol Laparosc. 2001;8:95–8.
62. Quinn M, Kirk N. Uterosacral nerve fibre proliferation in parous endometriosis. J Obstet Gynaecol. 2004;24:189–90.
63. Berkley KJ, Dmitrieva N, Curtis KS, Papka RE. Innervation of ectopic endometrium in a rat model of endometriosis. Proc Natl Acad Sci U S A. 2004;101:11094–8.
64. Tokushige N, Markham R, Russell P, Fraser IS. Nerve fibres in peritoneal endometriosis. Hum Reprod. 2006;21:3001–7.
65. Tokushige N, Markham R, Russell P, Fraser IS. Effect of progestogens and combined oral contraceptives on nerve fibers in peritoneal endometriosis. Fertil Steril. 2009;92:1234–9.
66. Mechsner S, Schwarz J, Thode J, Loddenkemper C, Salomon DS, Ebert AD. Growth-associated protein 43-positive sensory nerve fibers accompanied by immature vessels are located in or near peritoneal endometriotic lesions. Fertil Steril. 2007;88:581–7.
67. Mechsner S, Kaiser A, Kopf A, Gericke C, Ebert A, Bartley J. A pilot study to evaluate the clinical relevance of endometriosis-associated nerve fibers in peritoneal endometriotic lesions. Fertil Steril. 2009;92:1856–61.
68. Alvarez P, Chen X, Hendrich J, Irwin JC, Green PG, Giudice LC, Levine JD. Ectopic uterine tissue as a chronic pain generator. Neuroscience. 2012;225:269–82.
69. Koninckx PR, Meuleman C, Demeyere S, Lesaffre E, Cornillie FJ. Suggestive evidence that pelvic endometriosis is a progressive disease, whereas deeply infiltrating endometriosis is associated with pelvic pain. Fertil Steril. 1991;55:759–65.
70. Anaf V, Chapron C, El Nakadi I, De Moor V, Simonart T, Noël JC. Pain, mast cells, and nerves in peritoneal, ovarian, and deep infiltrating endometriosis. Fertil Steril. 2006;86:1336–43.
71. Vercellini P, Somigliana E, Viganò P, Abbiati A, Daguati R, Crosignani PG. Endometriosis: current and future medical therapies. Best Pract Res Clin Obstet Gynaecol. 2008;22:275–306.
72. Wang G, Tokushige N, Markham R, Fraser IS. Rich innervation of deep infiltrating endometriosis. Hum Reprod. 2009;24:827–34.
73. Ebert AD, Bartley J, David M. Aromatase inhibitors and cyclooxygenase-2 (COX-2) inhibitors in endometriosis: new questions–old answers? Eur J Obstet Gynecol Reprod Biol. 2005;122:144–50.
74. Bergqvist A, Nejaty H, Froysa B, Bruse C, Carlberg M, Sjoblom P, Söder O. Production of interleukins 1beta, 6 and 8 and tumor necrosis factor alpha in separated and cultured

endometrial and endometriotic stromal and epithelial cells. Gynecol Obstet Invest. 2000;50:1–6.
75. Anaf V, Simon P, El Nakadi I, Fayt I, Simonart T, Buxant F, Noel JC. Hyperalgesia, nerve infiltration and nerve growth factor expression in deep adenomyotic nodules, peritoneal and ovarian endometriosis. Hum Reprod. 2002;17:1895–900.
76. Tingåker BK, Irestedt L. Changes in uterine innervation in pregnancy and during labour. Curr Opin Anaesthesiol. 2010;23:300–3.
77. Caterina MJ, Julius D. The vanilloid receptor: a molecular gateway to the pain pathway. Annu Rev Neurosci. 2001;24:487–517.
78. Barde YA. The nerve growth factor family. Prog Growth Factor Res. 1990;2:237–48.
79. Hohn A, Leibrock J, Bailey K, Barde YA. Identification and characterization of a novel member of the nerve growth factor/brain-derived neurotrophic factor family. Nature. 1990;344:339–41.
80. Hallbook F, Ibanez CF, Persson H. Evolutionary studies of the nerve growth factor family reveal a novel member abundantly expressed in *Xenopus* ovary. Neuron. 1991;6:845–58.
81. Mantyh PW, Koltzenburg M, Mendell LM, Tive L, Shelton DL. Antagonism of nerve growth factor-TrkA signaling and the relief of pain. Anesthesiology. 2011;115:189–204.
82. Meakin SO, Shooter EM. The nerve growth factor family of receptors. Trends Neurosci. 1992;15:323–31.
83. Borghese B, Vaiman D, Mondon F, Mbaye M, Anaf V, Noël JC, de Ziegler D, Chapron C. Neurotrophins and pain in endometriosis. Gynecol Obstet Fertil. 2010;38:442–6.
84. Browne AS, Yu J, Huang RP, Francisco AM, Sidell N, Taylor RN. Proteomic identification of neurotrophins in the eutopic endometrium of women with endometriosis. Fertil Steril. 2012;98:713–9.
85. Barcena de Arellano ML, Arnold J, Lang H, Vercellino GF, Chiantera V, Schneider A, Mechsner S. Evidence of neurotrophic events due to peritoneal endometriotic lesions. Cytokine. 2013;62:253–61.
86. Levi-Montalcini R, Skaper SD, Dal Toso R, Petrelli L, Leon A. Nerve growth factor: from neurotrophin to neurokine. Trends Neurosci. 1996;19:514–20.
87. Hunter DD, Myers AC, Undem BJ. Nerve growth factor-induced phenotypic switch in guinea pig airway sensory neurons. Am J Respir Crit Care Med. 2000;161:1985–90.
88. McMahon SB, Bennett DL, Priestley JV, Shelton DL. The biological effects of endogenous nerve growth factor on adult sensory neurons revealed by a trkA-IgG fusion molecule. Nat Med. 1995;1:774–80.
89. Bennett DL, Koltzenburg M, Priestley JV, Shelton DL, McMahon SB. Endogenous nerve growth factor regulates the sensitivity of nociceptors in the adult rat. Eur J Neurosci. 1998;10:1282–91.
90. Emanueli C, Salis MB, Pinna A, Graiani G, Manni L, Madeddu P. Nerve growth factor promotes angiogenesis and arteriogenesis in ischemic hindlimbs. Circulation. 2002;106:2257–62.
91. Cantarella G, Lempereur L, Presta M, Ribatti D, Lombardo G, Lazarovici P, Zappalà G, Pafumi C, et al. Nerve growth factor-endothelial cell interaction leads to angiogenesis in vitro and in vivo. FASEB J. 2002;16:1307–9.
92. Kraemer R, Nguyen H, March KL, Hempstead B. NGF activates similar intracellular signaling pathways in vascular smooth muscle cells as PDGF-BB but elicits different biological responses. Arterioscler Thromb Vasc Biol. 1999;19:1041–50.
93. Calza L, Giardino L, Giuliani A, Aloe L, Levi-Montalcini R. Nerve growth factor control of neuronal expression of angiogenic and vasoactive factors. Proc Natl Acad Sci U S A. 2001;98:4160–5.
94. Hull MA, Thomson JL, Hawkey CJ. Expression of cyclooxygenase 1 and 2 by human gastric endothelial cells. Gut. 1999;45:529–36.

95. Lambiase A, Bracci-Laudiero L, Bonini S, Starace G, D'Elios MM, De Carli M, De Carli M, Aloe L. Human CD4+ T cell clones produce and release nerve growth factor and express high-affinity nerve growth factor receptors. J Allergy Clin Immunol. 1997;100:408–14.
96. Nilsson G, Forsberg-Nilsson K, Xiang Z, Hallbook F, Nilsson K, Metcalfe DD. Human mast cells express functional TrkA and are a source of nerve growth factor. Eur J Immunol. 1997;27:2295–301.
97. Kobayashi H, Gleich GJ, Butterfield JH, Kita H. Human eosinophils produce neurotrophins and secrete nerve growth factor on immunologic stimuli. Blood. 2002;99:2214–20.
98. Barouch R, Kazimirsky G, Appel E, Brodie C. Nerve growth factor regulates TNF-alpha production in mouse macrophages via MAP kinase activation. J Leukoc Biol. 2001;69:1019–26.
99. Frossard N, Freund V, Advenier C. Nerve growth factor and its receptors in asthma and inflammation. Eur J Pharmacol. 2004;500:453–65.
100. Healy DL, Rogers PA, Hii L, Wingfield M. Angiogenesis: a new theory for endometriosis. Hum Reprod Update. 1998;4:736–40.
101. Kim SH, Choi YM, Chae HD, Kim KR, Kim CH, Kang BM. Increased expression of endoglin in the eutopic endometrium of women with endometriosis. Fertil Steril. 2001;76:918–22.
102. Singh M, Meyer EM, Simpkins JW. The effect of ovariectomy and estradiol replacement on brain-derived neurotrophic factor messenger ribonucleic acid expression in cortical and hippocampal brain regions of female Sprague–Dawley rats. Endocrinology. 1995;136:2320–4.
103. Simpkins JW, Green PS, Gridley KE, Singh M, de Fiebre NC, Rajakumar G. Role of estrogen replacement therapy in memory enhancement and the prevention of neuronal loss associated with Alzheimer's disease. Am J Med. 1997;103:19S–25S.
104. Sohrabji F, Miranda RC, Toran-Allerand CD. Identification of a putative estrogen response element in the gene encoding brain-derived neurotrophic factor. Proc Natl Acad Sci U S A. 1995;92:11110–4.
105. Gibbs RB. Treatment with estrogen and progesterone affects relative levels of brain-derived neurotrophic factor mRNA and protein in different regions of the adult rat brain. Brain Res. 1999;844:20–7.
106. Krizsan-Agbas D, Pedchenko T, Hasan W, Smith PG. Oestrogen regulates sympathetic neurite outgrowth by modulating brain derived neurotrophic factor synthesis and release by the rodent uterus. Eur J Neurosci. 2003;18:2760–8.
107. Singer CA, Figueroa-Masot XA, Batchelor RH, Dorsa DM. The mitogen-activated protein kinase pathway mediates estrogen neuroprotection after glutamate toxicity in primary cortical neurons. J Neurosci. 1999;19:2455–63.
108. Patrone C, Andersson S, Korhonen L, Lindholm D. Estrogen receptor-dependent regulation of sensory neuron survival in developing dorsal root ganglion. Proc Natl Acad Sci U S A. 1999;96:10905–10.
109. Wilson ME, Dubal DB, Wise PM. Estradiol protects against injury-induced cell death in cortical explant cultures: a role for estrogen receptors. Brain Res. 2000;873:235–42.
110. Bjorling DE, Beckman M, Clayton MK, Wang ZY. Modulation of nerve growth factor in peripheral organs by estrogen and progesterone. Neuroscience. 2002;110:155–67.
111. Li B, Sheng X, Song M, Zhang H, Weng J, Zhang M, Hu X, Zhou J, Xu M, Weng Q, Watanabe G, Taya K. Expression of nerve growth factor and its receptors TrkA and p75 in the uterus of wild female ground squirrel (Citellus dauricus Brandt). Gen Comp Endocrinol. 2012;1(176):62–9.
112. Shi Z, Arai KY, Jin W, Weng Q, Watanabe G, Suzuki AK, Taya K. Expression of nerve growth factor and its receptors NTRK1 and TNFRSF1B is regulated by estrogen and progesterone in the uteri of golden hamsters. Biol Reprod. 2006;74:850–6.
113. Pinto FM, Armesto CP, Magraner J, Trujillo M, Martin JD, Candenas ML. Tachykinin receptor and neutral endopeptidase gene expression in the rat uterus: characterization and regulation in response to ovarian steroid treatment. Endocrinology. 1999;140(6):2526–32.

114. Sumino H, Ichikawa S, Kanda T, Sakamaki T, Nakamura T, Sato K, Kobayashi I, Nagai R. Hormone replacement therapy in postmenopausal women with essential hypertension increases circulating plasma levels of bradykinin. Am J Hypertens. 1999;12(1O Pt 1):1044–7.
115. Papka RE, Storey-Workley M. Estrogen receptor-alpha and -beta coexist in a subpopulation of sensory neurons of female rat dorsal root ganglia. Neurosci Lett. 2002;319:71–4.
116. Schaible HG, Grubb BD. Afferent and spinal mechanisms of joint pain. Pain. 1993;55:5–54.
117. Toyomoto M, Ohta M, Okumura K, Yano H, Matsumoto K, Inoue S, Hayashi K, Ikeda K. Prostaglandins are powerful inducers of NGF and BDNF production in mouse astrocyte cultures. FEBS Lett. 2004;562:211–5.
118. Kanda N, Koike S, Watanabe S. Prostaglandin E2 enhances neurotrophin-4 production via EP3 receptor in human keratinocytes. J Pharmacol Exp Ther. 2005;315:796–804.
119. Ota H, Igarashi S, Sasaki M, Tanaka T. Distribution of cyclooxygenase-2 in eutopic and ectopic endometrium in endometriosis and adenomyosis. Hum Reprod. 2001;16:561–6.
120. Bartley J, Mechsner S, Beutler C, Halis G, Lange J, Ebert AD. COX-2-expression in extragenital endometriosis lesions as a novel therapeutical approach? Zentralbl Gynakol. 2003;125:252–5.
121. Fagotti A, Ferrandina G, Fanfani F, Legge F, Lauriola L, Gessi M, Castelli P, Barbieri F, et al. Analysis of cyclooxygenase-2 (COX-2) expression in different sites of endometriosis and correlation with clinico-pathological parameters. Hum Reprod. 2004;19:393–7.
122. Buchweitz O, Staebler A, Wulfing P, Hauzman E, Greb R, Kiesel L. COX-2 overexpression in peritoneal lesions is correlated with nonmenstrual chronic pelvic pain. Eur J Obstet Gynecol Reprod Biol. 2006;124:216–21.
123. Chang SY, Ho YS. Immunohistochemical analysis of insulin-like growth factor I, insulin-like growth factor I receptor and insulin-like growth factor II in endometriotic tissue and endometrium. Acta Obstet Gynecol Scand. 1997;76:112–7.
124. Kimpinski K, Mearow K. Neurite growth promotion by nerve growth factor and insulin-like growth factor-1 in cultured adult sensory neurons: role of phosphoinositide 3-kinase and mitogen activated protein kinase. J Neurosci Res. 2001;63:486–99.
125. Jones DM, Tucker BA, Rahimtula M, Mearow KM. The synergistic effects of NGF and IGF-1 on neurite growth in adult sensory neurons: convergence on the PI 3-kinase signaling pathway. J Neurochem. 2003;86:1116–28.
126. Ghahary A, Murphy LJ. Uterine insulin-like growth factor-I receptors: regulation by estrogen and variation throughout the estrous cycle. Endocrinology. 1989;125(2):597–604.
127. Wilson ME. Effects of estradiol and exogenous insulin-like growth factor I (IGF-I) on the IGF-I axis during growth hormone inhibition and antagonism. J Clin Endocrinol Metab. 1998;83:4013–21.
128. Watanabe H, Kanzaki H, Narukawa S, Inoue T, Katsuragawa H, Kaneko Y, Mori T. Bcl-2 and Fas expression in eutopic and ectopic human endometrium during the menstrual cycle in relation to endometrial cell apoptosis. Am J Obstet Gynecol. 1997;176:360–8.
129. Merry DE, Korsmeyer SJ. Bcl-2 gene family in the nervous system. Annu Rev Neurosci. 1997;20:245–67.
130. Hilton M, Middleton G, Davies AM. Bcl-2 influences axonal growth rate in embryonic sensory neurons. Curr Biol. 1997;7:798–800.
131. Fernandez AM. Gonzalez de la Vega AG, Planas B, Torres-Aleman I. Neuroprotective actions of peripherally administered insulin-like growth factor I in the injured olivo-cerebellar pathway. Eur J Neurosci. 1999;11:2019–30.
132. Cardona-Gomez GP, Mendez P, DonCarlos LL, Azcoitia I, Garcia-Segura LM. Interactions of estrogens and insulin-like growth factor-I in the brain: implications for neuroprotection. Brain Res Brain Res Rev. 2001;37:320–34.
133. Nilsen J, Brinton RD. Impact of progestins on estrogen-induced neuroprotection: synergy by progesterone and 19-norprogesterone and antagonism by medroxyprogesterone acetate. Endocrinology. 2002;143:205–12.

134. Singh M. Mechanisms of progesterone-induced neuroprotection. Ann N Y Acad Sci. 2005;1052:145–51.
135. Sugawara J, Fukaya T, Murakami T, Yoshida H, Yajima A. Increased secretion of hepatocyte growth factor by eutopic endometrial stromal cells in women with endometriosis. Fertil Steril. 1997;68:468–72.
136. Maina F, Hilton MC, Ponzetto C, Davies AM, Klein R. Met receptor signaling is required for sensory nerve development and HGF promotes axonal growth and survival of sensory neurons. Genes Dev. 1997;11:3341–50.
137. Khan KN, Masuzaki H, Fujishita A, Kitajima M, Sekine I, Matsuyama T, Ishimaru T. Estrogen and progesterone receptor expression in macrophages and regulation of hepatocyte growth factor by ovarian steroids in women with endometriosis. Hum Reprod. 2005;20:2004–13.
138. Ota H, Igarashi S, Hatazawa J, Tanaka T. Distribution of heat shock proteins in eutopic and ectopic endometrium in endometriosis and adenomyosis. Fertil Steril. 1997;68:23–8.
139. Plumier JC, Hopkins DA, Robertson HA, Currie RW. Constitutive expression of the 27-kDa heat shock protein (Hsp27) in sensory and motor neurons of the rat nervous system. J Comp Neurol. 1997;384:409–28.
140. Costigan M, Mannion RJ, Kendall G, Lewis SE, Campagna JA, Coggeshall RE, Meridith-Middleton J, Tate S, et al. Heat shock protein 27: developmental regulation and expression after peripheral nerve injury. J Neurosci. 1998;18:5891–900.
141. Lewis SE, Mannion RJ, White FA, Coggeshall RE, Beggs S, Costigan M, Martin JL, Dillmann WH, et al. A role for HSP27 in sensory neuron survival. J Neurosci. 1999;19:8945–53.
142. Tang PZ, Gannon MJ, Andrew A, Miller D. Evidence for oestrogenic regulation of heat shock protein expression in human endometrium and steroid-responsive cell lines. Eur J Endocrinol. 1995;133:598–605.
143. Wing LY, Chuang PC, Wu MH, Chen HM, Tsai SJ. Expression and mitogenic effect of fibroblast growth factor-9 in human endometriotic implant is regulated by aberrant production of estrogen. J Clin Endocrinol Metab. 2003;88:5547–54.
144. Kanda T, Iwasaki T, Nakamura S, Kurokawa T, Ikeda K, Mizusawa H. Self-secretion of fibroblast growth factor-9 supports basal forebrain cholinergic neurons in an autocrine/paracrine manner. Brain Res. 2000;876:22–30.
145. Novella-Maestre E, Herraiz S, Vila-Vives JM, Carda C, Ruiz-Sauri A, Pellicer A. Effect of antiangiogenic treatment on peritoneal endometriosis-associated nerve fibers. Fertil Steril. 2012;98:1209–17.
146. Ferrara N, Davis-Smyth T. The biology of vascular endothelial growth factor. Endocr Rev. 1997;18:4–25.
147. Machado DE, Abrao MS, Berardo PT, Takiya CM, Nasciutti LE. Vascular density and distribution of vascular endothelial growth factor (VEGF) and its receptor VEGFR-2 (Flk-1) are significantly higher in patients with deeply infiltrating endometriosis affecting the rectum. Fertil Steril. 2008;90:148–55.
148. Pupo-Nogueira A, de Oliveira RM, Petta CA, Podgaec S, Dias Jr JA, Abrao MS. Vascular endothelial growth factor concentrations in the serum and peritoneal fluid of women with endometriosis. Int J Gynaecol Obstet. 2007;99:33–7.
149. Sondell M, Sundler F, Kanje M. Vascular endothelial growth factor is a neurotrophic factor which stimulates axonal outgrowth through the flk-1 receptor. Eur J Neurosci. 2000;12:4243–54.
150. Sondell M, Lundborg G, Kanje M. Vascular endothelial growth factor has neurotrophic activity and stimulates axonal outgrowth, enhancing cell survival and Schwann cell proliferation in the peripheral nervous system. J Neurosci. 1999;19:5731–40.
151. Hobson MI, Green CJ, Terenghi G. VEGF enhances intraneural angiogenesis and improves nerve regeneration after axotomy. J Anat. 2000;197(Pt 4):591–605.

152. Barcz E, Rózewska ES, Kaminski P, Demkow U, Bobrowska K, Marianowski L. Angiogenic activity and IL-8 concentrations in peritoneal fluid and sera in endometriosis. Int J Gynaecol Obstet. 2002;79:229–35.
153. Khan KN, Masuzaki H, Fujishita A, Kitajima M, Hiraki K, Miura S, Sekine I, Ishimaru T. Peritoneal fluid and serum levels of hepatocyte growth factor may predict the activity of endometriosis. Acta Obstet Gynecol Scand. 2006;85:458–66.
154. Matsuzaki S, Murakami T, Uehara S, Yokomizo R, Noda T, Kimura Y, Okamura K. Erythropoietin concentrations are elevated in the peritoneal fluid of women with endometriosis. Hum Reprod. 2001;16:945–8.
155. Suzumori N, Zhao XX, Suzumori K. Elevated angiogenin levels in the peritoneal fluid of women with endometriosis correlate with the extent of the disorder. Fertil Steril. 2004;82:93–6.
156. Kats R, Collette T, Metz CN, Akoum A. Marked elevation of macrophage migration inhibitory factor in the peritoneal fluid of women with endometriosis. Fertil Steril. 2002;78:69–76.
157. Szamatowicz J, Laudański P, Tomaszewska I, Szamatowicz M. Chemokine growth-regulated-alpha: a possible role in the pathogenesis of endometriosis. Gynecol Endocrinol. 2002;16:137–41.
158. Maas JW, Groothuis PG, Dunselman GA, de Goeij AF, Struijker-Boudier HA, Evers JL. Development of endometriosis-like lesions after transplantation of human endometrial fragments onto the chick embryo chorioallantoic membrane. Hum Reprod. 2001;16:627–31.

Chapter 14
Endometriosis in Experimental Models

Fuminori Taniguchi and Tasuku Harada

Abstract To investigate the factors involved in the initiation and progression of endometriosis, an animal model of this disease has been employed. Animal models are often used to investigate factors affecting the initiation and progression of endometriosis. This chapter describes these models and focuses on the murine model of endometriosis as a potential tool to evaluate therapies. The traditional explanation for the existence of endometrium in ectopic locations is based on the common occurrence of retrograde menstruation. This implantation hypothesis is widely accepted as the etiology of endometriosis. Animal models are crucial for elucidating the mechanisms underlying endometriosis. Several animal models of endometriosis have been used in the past, most of which consist of transplanting endometrium into the peritoneal cavity. Because primates spontaneously develop endometriosis, primate models most closely resemble the disease in women; however, rodent models are more cost effective and readily available. Nevertheless, since rodents do not menstruate, rodent models used for the research in endometriosis have certain limitations. We addressed the question whether a murine endometriosis model is suitable for evaluating drugs employed in human endometriosis. We concluded that the murine endometriosis model may be a valuable and reliable tool for evaluating new therapeutic approaches in human endometriosis.

Keywords Cystic lesion • Experimental model • Mouse endometriosis-like lesion • Parthenolide

---

The authors have no conflicts to disclose relative to this work.

F. Taniguchi, M.D., Ph.D. (✉) • T. Harada, M.D., Ph.D.
Department of Obstetrics and Gynecology, Faculty of Medicine, Tottori University,
36-1 Nishi-cho, Yonago 683-8504, Japan
e-mail: tani4327@med.tottori-u.ac.jp

T. Harada (ed.), *Endometriosis: Pathogenesis and Treatment*,
DOI 10.1007/978-4-431-54421-0_14, © Springer Japan 2014

14.1 Introduction

Endometriosis is commonly believed to occur via retrograde menstruation, also known as the Sampson hypothesis [1], in which viable endometrial tissue flows retrograde through the fallopian tube and into the peritoneal cavity where it can attach to and invade tissues and organs within the cavity. At least 90 % of women experience retrograde menstruation, but endometriosis occurs in only 10–14 % of reproductive age women, suggesting that additional elements impact its etiology [2]. Since endometriosis impairs the quality of life of severely affected women, improved research and new treatment paradigms are needed.

Current medical therapies for endometriosis aim to decrease ovarian estrogen production and/or counteract estrogen effects with the use of GnRH agonists, progestins (including oral contraceptives), and androgens, but undesirable side effects limit their long-term use [2]. Likewise, the scope of surgical treatment is also limited by a high recurrence rate, which may eventually lead to extreme measures, such as removal of the uterus and ovaries. There is therefore a need for focused mechanistic research that can be translated into expanded therapeutic capability for this widely prevalent disease.

Animal models, which are important for elucidating the mechanisms underlying endometriosis and are used in the early stages of drug testing, usually rely on non-menstruating rodents with induced endometriosis-like lesions. One of the major limitations in endometriosis research is the paucity of robust animal disease models. Ideally, a disease model should mimic human disease and allow scientific investigation into the effects of both intrinsic (e.g., genes) and extrinsic (e.g., environment) factors on disease progression.

Several animal models of endometriosis have been established, most consisting of transplantation of endometrium into the peritoneal cavity, which is by far the most common site of disease. Besides rodents, primates, such as monkeys that spontaneously develop endometriosis or that have been transplanted intraperitoneally with endometrium, can be used to study drug candidates. Indeed, because endometriosis occurs spontaneously in monkeys, the only nonhuman animal model that has cyclic menstrual periods, such an animal model is undoubtedly the most reliable one [3–7]. However, high cost and difficulties maintaining these animals have led most researchers to concentrate their studies on smaller mammalian models, such as rats [8–12] and rabbits [13, 14]. Nevertheless, the murine model was considered as a possible candidate for this purpose, and these studies were restricted to nude [15, 16] or SCID mice [17], which were implanted with human endometrium (xenotransplantation). Since mice are much smaller than rabbits or rats, microsurgical procedures of tissue transplantation become even more complicated.

The murine model may provide advantages in terms of new therapeutic approaches. In recent decades, many knockout or transgenic mice have been generated. The availability of an endometriosis model in mice is crucial because it can be used to investigate some aspects of endometriosis.

14.2 Murine Endometriosis Model

Mice are the most common animal models capable of investigating the pathophysiology of endometriosis; however, they do not spontaneously develop endometriosis. To induce endometriosis in mice, endometrial tissue must be transplanted into the peritoneal cavity using several methods [18–21], which can be classified into two basic types, homologous and heterologous. Both models produce comparable phenotypes, which are then morphometrically evaluated.

In homologous or autologous models, normal endometrial tissue is transplanted into the peritoneal cavity of immunocompetent recipients and starts to grow in an estrogen-dependent manner. In almost all models, uterine endometrial fragments from a donor mouse are directly introduced via injection into the peritoneal cavity of an immunocompetent syngeneic recipient without suturing the implants. In heterologous models, human endometriotic lesions are transplanted into the peritoneal cavity of immunodeficient mice [22, 23]. Human endometriotic implants were sutured to the peritoneum of immunocompromised mice [24, 25]. This xenotransplantation model using the nude mouse is also used, but is limited by the lack of a normal immune system. Despite the advantage of being based on human endometrial tissues, the number of endometriotic lesions in the heterologous model that will develop varies from one animal to another. In both models, with or without suturing the endometrial implant, the drug's influence on growth of endometrial or endometriotic transplants is evaluated.

These established endometriosis models in mice are under discussion. Indeed, mice do lack a menstrual cycle and do not develop spontaneous endometriosis. It should be established whether transplanting normal endometrium into the peritoneal cavity of a non-menstruating species reflects all pathophysiological aspects of human endometriosis. Although the murine endometriosis model is not exactly the same as human endometriosis, their endometriotic lesions develop in some ways the same as human endometriotic lesions.

The murine model of endometriosis is a versatile one used to study how the immune system, hormones, and environmental factors affect endometriosis and how endometriosis affects fertility and pain. A novel study design also enables the evaluation of molecular mechanisms that are critical for disease initiation [26, 27]. In Table 14.1, the recent representatives of mouse endometriosis models are shown. Additional and ideal models of endometriosis are needed. In the next section, we demonstrate the results in a murine endometriosis model that expands the capability of conducting both mechanistic and translational research.

Table 14.1 Representatives of mouse endometriosis models

Author (year)	Donor	Host	Drug	Characteristics of models	References
Takai et al. (2013)	M	M	Parthenolide	Large cyst formation	[28]
Sokalska et al. (2013)	H	M	Simvastatin		[29]
Daftary et al. (2013)	M	M		Adhesion scoring system	[30]
Rudzitis-Auth et al. (2013)	M	M	Resveratrol		[31]
Burns et al. (2012)	M	M		Estrogen receptor KO	[27]
Novella-Maestre et al. (2012)	H	NM	Cabergoline	Assessment nerve fibers	[32]
Han et al. (2012)	M	M		SRC-1 KO	[33]
Mariani et al. (2012)	M	M	Vitamin D receptor agonist		[34]
Wieser et al. (2012)	M	M	Retinoic acid	GFP mice	[35]
Cakmak et al. (2012)	M	M	Statins		[36]
Leconte et al. (2011)	M	M	Temsirolimus	Deep infiltrating implants	[37]
Olivares et al. (2011)	M	M	Celecoxib, Rosiglitazone		[38]
Kulak Jr et al. (2011)	M	M	Bazedoxifene		[39]
Lu et al. (2010)	M	M	Trichostatin A	Autotransplant model	[40]
Styer et al. (2008)	M	M	Leptin receptor antagonist		[26]
Hirata et al. (2005)	M	M		GFP mice	[21]

M mouse, *H* human, *NM* nude mouse, *KO* knockout mouse, *GFP* green fluorescent protein

14.3 Our Animal Model of Endometriosis Using Homologous Mice

14.3.1 Care and Treatment

According to the implantation theory, we established the readily available murine model to evaluate the development of endometriosis-like lesions [27, 28]. Female mice (6 weeks of age, BALB/c) were purchased. Before initiating the experiments, animals were allowed to acclimate to the following conditions for 7 days. Mice were in a controlled temperature range (72–74 F) on a 12-h light, 12-h dark cycle. Mice were given food and water ad libitum. Recipient mice were ovariectomized through two 0.5-cm dorsolateral skin incisions and were then divided into two treatment groups, estradiol valerate (0.5 μg/mouse · week) in corn oil or only corn oil vehicle. Mice were dosed subcutaneously once per week for 2 weeks before inducing experimental endometriosis. Donor mice were primed 41 h before removing the uterus with pregnant mare serum gonadotropin (10 IU intraperitoneally). The donor uterus was removed en bloc after euthanasia, cleaned of excess tissue, and washed thrice in sterile PBS. The uterus was slit with a linear incision longitudinally and minced ($\leq$1.5 mm). Recipient mice were anesthetized using isoflurane/oxygen and given buprenorphine (0.1 mg/kg) for pain management. A 0.5-cm right dorsolateral incision was made; minced donor tissue (1:2 donor uterus to host ratio) in 500 μL PBS was injected into the peritoneal cavity of the recipient and gently massaged to disperse the tissue. An equivalent amount (~100 mg) of minced tissue was transferred into all recipients. Mice were treated for 4 additional weeks with estradiol valerate or the vehicle. After 4 weeks, mice were euthanized with CO_2, the peritoneal cavity was opened, and endometriosis-like lesions were removed. To assess the effects of drug candidates on ectopic uterine tissue, ectopic lesions were photographed to document in situ endometriosis-like lesions. Endometriosis-like lesions were visualized, dissected, measured, and weighed. Endometriosis-like lesions were removed and either fixed in 10 % formalin or snap-frozen on dry ice and stored at −80 °C until use.

14.4 Effects of Parthenolide on the Endometriosis-Like Lesions in a Murine Model

We undertook a study of feverfew as a potential therapy for endometriosis that illustrated the effectiveness of the murine model. The medical herb feverfew has long been used as a folk medicine for treating fevers, migraine, rheumatoid arthritis, and dysmenorrhea. Parthenolide is considered the primary bioactive compound in feverfew having antitumor and anti-inflammatory properties [41]. Parthenolide has produced anti-tumorigenesis effects against human acute myeloid leukemia and solid tumors, such as breast and pancreatic cancer [42–44]. We therefore used an experimental mouse model to evaluate the effect of parthenolide as therapy for endometriosis [28].

A murine model was established by injecting tissue suspension intraperitoneally. Endometriosis-like lesions had grown in the abdominal cavity of all mice. The deposits appeared as cystic lesions bulging under the serosal coat. Most of the lesions were observed around the abdominal incision, the intestinal membrane, and the renal capsule (Fig. 14.1a). The size of lesions ranged from approximately 2 to 8 mm in diameter (Fig. 14.1b). Histologic sections stained with hematoxylin and eosin were endometriotic in character. The monolayer epithelial cell lining of the cyst was revealed by HE staining (Fig. 14.1c, d) [28]. We confirmed that cytokeratin (a marker of epithelial cells) and vimentin (a marker of stromal cells) in the mouse endometriosis-like lesions were positive, whereas calretinin (that of mesothelial cells) was negative, indicating that these cystic lesions originated from the injected endometrial tissues, not the peritoneal cells.

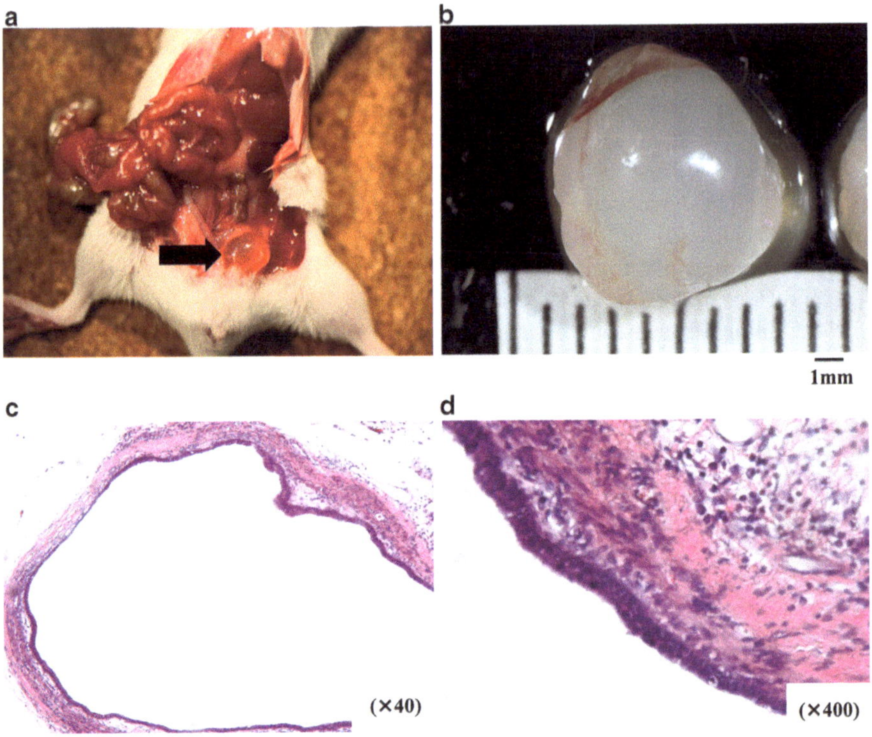

Fig. 14.1 Cystic lesion in the murine endometriosis model. (**a**) An endometriosis-like lesion developed in the murine abdominal cavity. (**b**) Representative of a large excised lesion. (**c**) and (**d**) HE staining of lesion

In view of the above considerations, we proposed a hypothesis that parthenolide may have an inhibitory effect on the development of endometriosis. After parthenolide treatment for 4 weeks, the total number of lesions (5.8 vs. 3.9/mouse) was significantly reduced, and the average weight (65.6 vs. 29.6 mg/mouse) and the surface area (50.3 vs. 25.7 mm^2/mouse) of lesions were decreased by approximately 50 % of controls. To evaluate the proliferative activity of lesions, the ratio of Ki67-stained cells was calculated. In endometrial glands epithelia, the percentage of Ki67-positive cells decreased after parthenolide treatment (17.8 vs. 8.5 %).

14.5 Discussion

Convenient and reliable endometriosis animal models are needed to accelerate emerging therapeutic alternatives. According to the Sampson "implantation theory," we established the syngeneic immunocompetent mice model. In this model, we and the other investigators provided crucial evidence of both the development of endometriosis-like lesion growth and donor tissue responsiveness. Recently, Pelch et al. described a detailed method of a mouse surgically induced endometriosis model by autotransplantation of uterine tissue [45].

The rodent endometriosis models using mice or rats are widely used in research, but may have limitations and may not mimic all aspects of human pathophysiology. For example, in homologous rodent models, "healthy" uterus is cut into fragments and transplanted into the peritoneum, whereas it has been suggested that the eutopic endometrium of women suffering from endometriosis may already be abnormal [2]. Nude mice lacking an intact immune system are employed in the heterologous model, which cannot mimic the inflammatory response normally seen in human endometriotic lesions [23]. Although heterologous rodent endometriosis models are responsive to drugs and manipulations that induce a hypoestrogenic state, such as ovariectomy, GnRH agonists, aromatase inhibitors, danazol, and selective estrogen receptor modulators, it may be difficult to analyze novel target families in which, for example, the murine ligand does not bind to the receptor of the human transplant.

Whereas cell-based in vitro experiments provide a framework for testing molecular mechanisms, eventually confirming their role in disease causality in vivo can only be accomplished by a suitable animal model. For a disease as diverse as endometriosis, a single animal model would unlikely be sufficient to represent the entire diversity in etiology, pathogenesis, and pathology. Each model has design-related strengths and limitations. For example, a recently described disease model consists of introducing endometrial tissue via direct injection into the peritoneal cavity of immunocompetent mice without suturing [21, 27, 28]. In mice, the injected tissue forms cyst-like endometriosis lesions; however, the injection method does not seem to work in rats because the tissue fails to attach to and invade the peritoneal cavity [9]. Since all endometriosis lesions in each model are attached to the peritoneum and/or mesenterium with or without suturing, evaluating attachment or invasion of lesions would be difficult. Furthermore, to quantify the injected endometrial fragments, this model may be insufficient to evaluate precisely the endometriotic lesions.

The rodent model is used extensively to study the etiology, pathology, and risk factors of endometriosis [21, 22, 27, 30, 33, 35, 46, 47] as well as to explore novel therapeutics [28, 29, 31, 32, 34, 36–40, 48–51]. In conclusion, this murine model of endometriosis provides an important tool to evaluate a therapeutic approach to the disease. This model will help to better understand disease evolution in the living animal and permit faster and more accurate characterization of a drug's effect on experimental endometriosis.

References

1. Sampson JA. Metastatic or embolic endometriosis, due to the menstrual dissemination of endometrial tissue into the venous circulation. Am J Pathol. 1927;3:93–110.43.
2. Giudice LC, Kao LC. Endometriosis. Lancet. 2004;364:1789–99.
3. MacKenzie WF, Casey HW. Animal model of human disease. Endometriosis. Animal model: endometriosis in rhesus monkeys. Am J Pathol. 1975;80:341–4.
4. Scott RB, Te Linde RW, Wharton Jr LR. Further studies on experimental endometriosis. Am J Obstet Gynecol. 1953;66:1082–103.
5. Donnez O, Soares M, Defrere S, Dehoux JP, van Langendonckt A, et al. Nerve fiber density in deep nodular endometriotic lesions induced in a baboon experimental model. Fertil Steril. 2013;100(4):1144–50.
6. Langoi D, Pavone ME, Gurates B, Chai D, Fazleabas A, et al. Aromatase inhibitor treatment limits progression of peritoneal endometriosis in baboons. Fertil Steril. 2013;99(656–662): e653.
7. Lebovic DI, Mwenda JM, Chai DC, Santi A, Xu X, et al. Peroxisome proliferator-activated receptor-(gamma) receptor ligand partially prevents the development of endometrial explants in baboons: a prospective, randomized, placebo-controlled study. Endocrinology. 2010;151:1846–52.
8. Golan A, Dargenio R, Winston RM. The effect of treatment on experimentally produced endometrial peritoneal implants. Fertil Steril. 1986;46:954–8.
9. Vernon MW, Wilson EA. Studies on the surgical induction of endometriosis in the rat. Fertil Steril. 1985;44:684–94.
10. Abbas MA, Taha MO, Disi AM, Shomaf M. Regression of endometrial implants treated with vitamin D in a rat model of endometriosis. Eur J Pharmacol. 2013;715:72–5.
11. Stilley JA, Sharpe-Timms KL. TIMP1 contributes to ovarian anomalies in both an MMP-dependent and -independent manner in a rat model. Biol Reprod. 2012;86:47.
12. Yuan P, Chen B, Huang Y, Xin X. Long-term regression of experimental endometriosis in a rat model treated with local application of levonorgestrel-loaded biodegradable microspheres. Hum Reprod. 2012;27:2089–95.
13. Rock JA, Prendergast RA, Bobbie D, Green WR, Parmley TH, et al. Intraocular endometrium in the rabbit as a model for endometriosis. Fertil Steril. 1993;59:232–5.
14. Yuan P, Huang Y, Wu H, Teng Z, Zhang J, et al. Induction of a local pseudo-pregnancy via levonorgestrel-loaded microspheres for the treatment of endometriosis in a rabbit model. Hum Reprod. 2010;25:462–9.
15. Zamah NM, Dodson MG, Stephens LC, Buttram Jr VC, Besch PK, et al. Transplantation of normal and ectopic human endometrial tissue into athymic nude mice. Am J Obstet Gynecol. 1984;149:591–7.
16. Fortin M, Lepine M, Merlen Y, Thibeault I, Rancourt C, et al. Quantitative assessment of human endometriotic tissue maintenance and regression in a noninvasive mouse model of endometriosis. Mol Ther. 2004;9:540–7.
17. Aoki D, Katsuki Y, Shimizu A, Kakinuma C, Nozawa S. Successful heterotransplantation of human endometrium in SCID mice. Obstet Gynecol. 1994;83:220–8.
18. Cummings AM, Metcalf JL. Induction of endometriosis in mice: a new model sensitive to estrogen. Reprod Toxicol. 1995;9:233–8.
19. Grummer R, Schwarzer F, Bainczyk K, Hess-Stumpp H, Regidor PA, et al. Peritoneal endometriosis: validation of an in-vivo model. Hum Reprod. 2001;16:1736–43.
20. Rossi G, Somigliana E, Moschetta M, Santorsola R, Cozzolino S, et al. Dynamic aspects of endometriosis in a mouse model through analysis of implantation and progression. Arch Gynecol Obstet. 2000;263:102–7.
21. Hirata T, Osuga Y, Yoshino O, Hirota Y, Harada M, et al. Development of an experimental model of endometriosis using mice that ubiquitously express green fluorescent protein. Hum Reprod. 2005;20:2092–6.

22. Story L, Kennedy S. Animal studies in endometriosis: a review. ILAR J. 2004;45:132–8.
23. Tirado-Gonzalez I, Barrientos G, Tariverdian N, Arck PC, Garcia MG, et al. Endometriosis research: animal models for the study of a complex disease. J Reprod Immunol. 2010;86:141–7.
24. Lee B, Du H, Taylor HS. Experimental murine endometriosis induces DNA methylation and altered gene expression in eutopic endometrium. Biol Reprod. 2009;80:79–85.
25. Bruner-Tran KL, Eisenberg E, Yeaman GR, Anderson TA, McBean J, et al. Steroid and cytokine regulation of matrix metalloproteinase expression in endometriosis and the establishment of experimental endometriosis in nude mice. J Clin Endocrinol Metab. 2002;87:4782–91.
26. Styer AK, Sullivan BT, Puder M, Arsenault D, Petrozza JC, et al. Ablation of leptin signaling disrupts the establishment, development, and maintenance of endometriosis-like lesions in a murine model. Endocrinology. 2008;149:506–14.
27. Burns KA, Rodriguez KF, Hewitt SC, Janardhan KS, Young SL, et al. Role of estrogen receptor signaling required for endometriosis-like lesion establishment in a mouse model. Endocrinology. 2012;153:3960–71.
28. Takai E, Taniguchi F, Nakamura K, Uegaki T, Iwabe T, et al. Parthenolide reduces cell proliferation and prostaglandin E synthesis in human endometriotic stromal cells and inhibits development of endometriosis in the murine model. Fertil Steril. 2013;100(4):1170–8.
29. Sokalska A, Anderson M, Villanueva J, Ortega I, Bruner-Tran KL, et al. Effects of simvastatin on retinoic acid system in primary human endometrial stromal cells and in a chimeric model of human endometriosis. J Clin Endocrinol Metab. 2013;98:E463–71.
30. Daftary GS, Zheng Y, Tabbaa ZM, Schoolmeester JK, Gada RP, et al. A novel role of the Sp/KLF transcription factor KLF11 in arresting progression of endometriosis. PLoS One. 2013;8:e60165.
31. Rudzitis-Auth J, Menger MD, Laschke MW. Resveratrol is a potent inhibitor of vascularization and cell proliferation in experimental endometriosis. Hum Reprod. 2013;28:1339–47.
32. Novella-Maestre E, Herraiz S, Vila-Vives JM, Carda C, Ruiz-Sauri A, et al. Effect of antiangiogenic treatment on peritoneal endometriosis-associated nerve fibers. Fertil Steril. 2012;98:1209–17.
33. Han SJ, Hawkins SM, Begum K, Jung SY, Kovanci E, et al. A new isoform of steroid receptor coactivator-1 is crucial for pathogenic progression of endometriosis. Nat Med. 2012;18:1102–11.
34. Mariani M, Vigano P, Gentilini D, Camisa B, Caporizzo E, et al. The selective vitamin D receptor agonist, elocalcitol, reduces endometriosis development in a mouse model by inhibiting peritoneal inflammation. Hum Reprod. 2012;27:2010–9.
35. Wieser F, Wu J, Shen Z, Taylor RN, Sidell N. Retinoic acid suppresses growth of lesions, inhibits peritoneal cytokine secretion, and promotes macrophage differentiation in an immunocompetent mouse model of endometriosis. Fertil Steril. 2012;97:1430–7.
36. Cakmak H, Basar M, Seval-Celik Y, Osteen KG, Duleba AJ, et al. Statins inhibit monocyte chemotactic protein 1 expression in endometriosis. Reprod Sci. 2012;19:572–9.
37. Leconte M, Nicco C, Ngo C, Chereau C, Chouzenoux S, et al. The mTOR/AKT inhibitor temsirolimus prevents deep infiltrating endometriosis in mice. Am J Pathol. 2011;179:880–9.
38. Olivares C, Ricci A, Bilotas M, Baranao RI, Meresman G. The inhibitory effect of celecoxib and rosiglitazone on experimental endometriosis. Fertil Steril. 2011;96:428–33.
39. Kulak Jr J, Fischer C, Komm B, Taylor HS. Treatment with bazedoxifene, a selective estrogen receptor modulator, causes regression of endometriosis in a mouse model. Endocrinology. 2011;152:3226–32.
40. Lu Y, Nie J, Liu X, Zheng Y, Guo SW. Trichostatin A, a histone deacetylase inhibitor, reduces lesion growth and hyperalgesia in experimentally induced endometriosis in mice. Hum Reprod. 2010;25:1014–25.
41. Jain NK, Kulkarni SK. Antinociceptive and anti-inflammatory effects of Tanacetum parthenium L. extract in mice and rats. J Ethnopharmacol. 1999;68:251–9.

42. Guzman ML, Rossi RM, Karnischky L, Li X, Peterson DR, et al. The sesquiterpene lactone parthenolide induces apoptosis of human acute myelogenous leukemia stem and progenitor cells. Blood. 2005;105:4163–9.
43. Liu JW, Cai MX, Xin Y, Wu QS, Ma J, et al. Parthenolide induces proliferation inhibition and apoptosis of pancreatic cancer cells in vitro. J Exp Clin Cancer Res. 2010;29:108.
44. Sweeney CJ, Mehrotra S, Sadaria MR, Kumar S, Shortle NH, et al. The sesquiterpene lactone parthenolide in combination with docetaxel reduces metastasis and improves survival in a xenograft model of breast cancer. Mol Cancer Ther. 2005;4:1004–12.
45. Pelch KE, Sharpe-Timms KL, Nagel SC. Mouse model of surgically-induced endometriosis by auto-transplantation of uterine tissue. J Vis Exp. 2012;59:e3396 doi 10.3791/3396.
46. Cummings AM, Hedge JM, Birnbaum LS. Effect of prenatal exposure to TCDD on the promotion of endometriotic lesion growth by TCDD in adult female rats and mice. Toxicol Sci. 1999;52:45–9.
47. Sharpe-Timms KL, Piva M, Ricke EA, Surewicz K, Zhang YL, et al. Endometriotic lesions synthesize and secrete a haptoglobin-like protein. Biol Reprod. 1998;58:988–94.
48. Yavuz E, Oktem M, Esinler I, Toru SA, Zeyneloglu HB. Genistein causes regression of endometriotic implants in the rat model. Fertil Steril. 2007;88:1129–34.
49. Dmitrieva N, Nagabukuro H, Resuehr D, Zhang G, McAllister SL, et al. Endocannabinoid involvement in endometriosis. Pain. 2010;151:703–10.
50. Efstathiou JA, Sampson DA, Levine Z, Rohan RM, Zurakowski D, et al. Nonsteroidal antiinflammatory drugs differentially suppress endometriosis in a murine model. Fertil Steril. 2005;83:171–81.
51. Becker CM, Sampson DA, Short SM, Javaherian K, Folkman J, et al. Short synthetic endostatin peptides inhibit endothelial migration in vitro and endometriosis in a mouse model. Fertil Steril. 2006;85:71–7.

Chapter 15
Malignant Transformation of Endometriosis: Underlying Mechanisms

Masaki Mandai, Ken Yamaguchi, Noriomi Matsumura, and Ikuo Konishi

Abstract Although it is well known that ovarian cancer, especially clear cell and endometrioid carcinoma, sometimes develops from endometriotic cyst, the precise mechanism of carcinogenesis is not clarified yet. Recently, several molecules, including HNF-1β, AKT/PI3K/Met, and ARID1A, have been shown to be involved in this carcinogenic process. Some of them are included in the "OCCC signature genes" which we identified as a gene group specifically expressed in clear cell carcinoma among ovarian cancers. "OCCC signature genes" contain many stress-related genes and were induced by treatment with the fluid of endometriotic cysts. The fluid of endometriotic cysts contained significantly high concentration of free iron and oxidative stress-related products. These findings suggest that microenvironment within the endometriotic cyst may play an important role in the malignant transformation of endometriosis and development of clear cell carcinoma, a rare histotype among ovarian cancers.

Keywords Carcinogenesis • Clear cell carcinoma • Iron • Microenvironment • Ovarian cancer

---

M. Mandai (✉)
Department of Obstetrics and Gynecology, Faculty of Medicine, Kinki University, 377-2 Ono-Higashi, Osaka-Sayama, Osaka 589-5811, Japan
e-mail: mandai@med.kindai.ac.jp

K. Yamaguchi • N. Matsumura • I. Konishi
Department of Gynecology and Obstetrics, Graduate School of Medicine, Kyoto University, Kyoto, Japan

T. Harada (ed.), *Endometriosis: Pathogenesis and Treatment*,
DOI 10.1007/978-4-431-54421-0_15, © Springer Japan 2014

15.1 Introduction

Endometriosis affects approximately 5–10 % of women of reproductive age and is estimated to be increasing due to late marriage and low birth rates in some countries including Japan. Although the causes of endometriosis have been extensively investigated, as shown in detail in this book, we do not have definite answers yet. Endometriosis is clinically associated with three major disorders, namely, endometriosis-associated pain, endometriosis-associated infertility, and endometriosis-associated ovarian cancer (EAOC). The former two are disorders that occur during reproductive age, but EAOC frequently occurs after menopause when endometriosis itself regresses. This fact indicates two issues: Clinically, it is very important to follow the patient with endometriosis even after menopause, and if there is a sign of malignant transformation, prompt surgery should be considered. From the basic science perspective, it is possible that the menopausal status may somehow contribute to the occurrence of EAOC.

EAOC primarily consists of endometrioid and clear cell subtypes, both of which are relatively rare histotypes among ovarian cancers (Fig. 15.1). However, there is no clear explanation why these particular histologies are associated with endometriosis. As described in detail in another section of this book, the frequency of malignant transformation of endometriotic cysts is apparently higher than that of other benign epithelial ovarian cysts, including serous and mucinous cystadenoma. However, again, the reason is unclear. In this chapter, by reviewing possible mechanisms responsible for the malignant transformation of endometriosis, we will discuss the characteristic carcinogenesis of endometriosis.

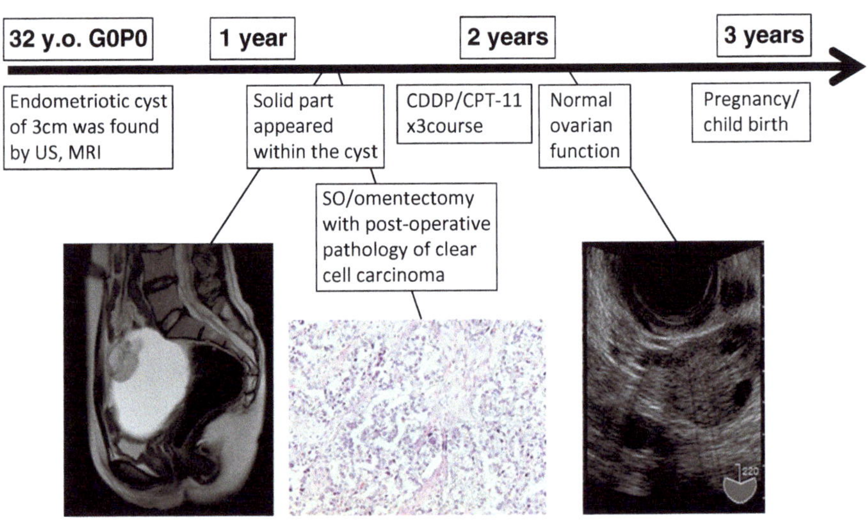

Fig. 15.1 Typical case of malignant transformation of endometriotic cyst

15.2 Endometriosis as a Precursor of Ovarian Cancer

15.2.1 Molecular Evidence

Endometriosis is currently classified as a tumorlike lesion according to the WHO classification, although it is not fully described. However, a variety of genetic analyses have demonstrated that endometriosis, especially the endometriotic cyst of the ovary, is a monoclonal lesion. In the late 1990s, X chromosome-linked polymorphism analysis revealed that an endometriotic cyst consisted of monoclonal epithelium [1–3]. Later, fluorescence in situ hybridization (FISH) analysis demonstrated the possibility that specific chromosomal loss or gain plays a role in the development and/or progression of endometriosis [4]. Similarly, another FISH study indicated that perturbations of chromosome 17 and the *p53* locus occur frequently in severe, late-stage endometriosis [5]. In an analysis of DNA from 40 cases of endometriosis, 11 cases (28 %) demonstrated LOH at one or more loci, although no mutations were detected in the *p53* or K-*ras* genes [6]. Most other similar analyses [1–3, 7, 8] revealed the monoclonal nature of endometriotic epithelium, except for one paper [9] in which the interpretation of the data may be inadequate. These findings clearly demonstrated that a majority of the endometriotic cysts are monoclonal and neoplastic. Moreover, genetic events may accumulate in endometriotic epithelia in parallel with the development of endometriosis.

15.2.2 Pathological View

Given the fact that endometriosis is a neoplastic disorder, it may have precancerous potential. Most endometrioses show a benign character, but malignant transformation may accompany some morphologic and genetic alterations. In pathology, we sometimes encounter the so-called atypical endometriosis, a putative intermediate between benign endometriosis and endometriosis-associated ovarian cancer (EAOC). Sampson first described ovarian cancer in endometriosis and defined a criterion for EAOC [10]. In a review of 194 cases of ovarian endometriosis, Czernobilsky and Morris found severe cytological atypia in 3.6 % of the cases [11]. Moreover, in their study, 2.0 % of the cases showed adenomatous, hyperplasia-like lesions. LaGrenade and Silverberg presented four cases of ovarian carcinomas contiguous with atypical glandular epithelial changes in endometriosis [12]. Subsequently, Fukunaga et al. reported that as many as 61 % of the cases of endometriosis coexisting with ovarian cancer had atypical endometriosis foci, while only 1.7 % of the cases of endometriosis without ovarian cancer exhibited atypical lesions [13]. Ogawa et al. reported that atypical endometriosis was found in 78 % of the cases with EAOC [14]. In their investigations, the transition from typical to atypical endometriosis was detected in 22 of 37 cases, and the transition from atypical endometriosis to carcinoma was found in 23 cases. These pathological observations suggest that benign endometriosis develops into ovarian cancer in some cases via atypical endometriosis, a premalignant stage.

15.2.3 Links Between the Pathology and Molecular Findings

Several studies have demonstrated that atypical endometriosis, which is a putative pathological transition between benign endometriosis and EAOC, has actually shown an intermediate nature by molecular analyses. Sáinz de la Cuesta et al. evaluated the immunohistochemical expression of p53 in normal endometrium, endometriosis, atypical endometriosis, and ovarian cancer associated with endometriosis. They found that 82.4 % of cancers associated with endometriosis and all the atypical endometriosis samples showed P53 overexpression, whereas only 11.8 % of the endometriosis samples, and none of the endometrium samples, showed P53 overexpression [15]. In the report by Obata et al., frequent LOH was observed on chromosome 6q (60.0 %) and chromosome 10q (40.0 %) in ovarian atypical endometriosis [16]. However, not all the endometriosis cases that are coincident with ovarian cancer have atypical endometriosis lesions, and the biological significance of atypical endometriosis is still unclear.

15.3 Molecular Events Associated with Malignant Transformation of Endometriosis

15.3.1 Loss of Heterozygosity (LOH)

There are several ways of analyzing LOH. LOH is usually used to estimate the locus of a tumor suppressor gene associated with a corresponding event, the development and malignant transformation of endometriosis in this case. Using DNA from 40 cases of endometriosis, Jiang et al. analyzed candidate ovarian tumor suppressor loci on chromosome arms 6q, 9p, 11q, 17p, 17q, and 22q [17]. LOH was detected on chromosomes 9p (18 %), 11q (18 %), and 22q (15 %), and, in total, 11 of 40 (28 %) cases demonstrated LOH at one or more of these loci. The same investigators subsequently examined 14 cases of endometriosis synchronous with ovarian cancer for LOH on 12 chromosome arms and for X chromosome inactivation. In all four of the cases in which the carcinoma had arisen within the endometriosis and in five of the seven cases in which the carcinoma was adjacent to the endometriosis, common genetic lesions were detected to be consistent with a common lineage [17]. Prowse et al. analyzed LOH in 10 EAOCs with coexisting endometriosis using 82 microsatellite markers and found that, of 63 LOH events detected in the carcinoma samples, 22 were also detected in the corresponding endometriosis samples [18]. Goumenou et al. reported that LOH in *p16*, *GALT*, and *p53*, as well as *APOA2*, a region frequently lost in ovarian cancer, occurred in endometriosis, even in stage II of the disease [19]. Sato et al. examined 20 ovarian endometrioid carcinomas, 24 clear cell carcinomas, and 34 solitary endometrial cysts of the ovary for LOH at 10q23.3 [20]. In five endometrioid carcinomas synchronous with endometriosis, three cases displayed LOH events common to both the carcinoma and the endometriosis. In seven clear cell carcinomas that are synchronous with endometriosis, three displayed LOH events common to both the carcinoma and the endometriosis. No LOH events were found in solitary endometriosis. These findings indicate that attenuation of tumor suppressor genes is associated with the malignant transformation of endometriosis.

15.3.2 Mutation and Altered Expression of Oncogenes and Tumor Suppressor Genes

Mutations and altered expression of several genes have been implicated in the malignant transformation of endometriosis.

15.3.2.1 Augmented Expression of HNF-1β

Hepatocyte nuclear factor-1β is a transcription factor that is expressed specifically in clear cell carcinoma. Kato et al. examined expression of HNF-1β in 30 clear cell tumors (26 malignant, three borderline, and one benign) and in 40 endometriotic cysts [21]. All of the 30 clear cell tumors expressed HNF-1β. In 9 of 12 cases with the endometriotic epithelium, expression of HNF-1β was detected in the endometriotic epithelium as well as in the clear cell tumor. Furthermore, 16 of 40 (40 %) endometriotic cysts without neoplasms also expressed HNF-1β. They concluded that early differentiation into the clear cell lineage takes place in ovarian endometriosis, not only in atypical endometriosis but also in endometriosis with degenerative and regenerative changes.

15.3.2.2 The AKT/PI3K/Met Pathway

An array-based comparative genomic hybridization (CGH) analysis by Yamashita et al. revealed Met gene amplification in 4/13 ovarian clear cell carcinomas and 2/8 cell lines [22]. Amplification of the AKT2 gene was also observed in 5/21 samples. In 73 ovarian clear cell cases, 37.0 % demonstrated Met gene amplification (>4 copies), and 8.2 % had AKT2 amplification, suggesting that the Met signaling pathway plays an important role in clear cell carcinogenesis.

According to Yamamoto et al., exons 9 and 20 of the PIK3CA gene were analyzed in 23 clear cell carcinomas with synchronous putative precursor lesions [23]. Somatic mutations of the PIK3CA gene were detected in 10/23 (43 %) carcinomas and in the coexisting endometriotic epithelium adjacent to the carcinoma in 9/10 (90 %) cases. Moreover, in six of the nine lesions, the mutation was identified even in the endometrioses lacking cytological atypia. The authors suggested that mutations of the PIK3CA gene are early events in tumorigenesis, most likely initiating the malignant transformation of endometriosis.

15.3.2.3 ARID1A Mutations

ARID1A encodes BAF250a, one of the components of the SW1/SNF chromatin remodeling complex. In 2010, two groups identified mutations of the ARID1A gene in EAOC and in ovarian clear cell carcinoma. Genome-wide mutational analysis exhibited ARID1A mutations in almost one half of the clear cell carcinomas, one third of the endometrioid carcinomas, and none of the serous carcinomas of the ovary [24]. BAF250a protein expression was also lost in these cases. In some cases, loss of BAF1a expression was also found in atypical endometriosis adjacent to the cancer lesions. In another study, ARID1A mutations were detected in 57 % of the cases as well as PI3CA mutations in 40 % of the cases [25]. Although ARID1A is thought to play a role as a tumor suppressor gene [26], the precise effects of mutations in this gene are not fully understood.

Clinically, loss of ARID1A expression was significantly correlated with advanced FIGO stage, high CA125 levels, and with shorter progression-free survival of patients with clear cell carcinomas treated with platinum-based chemotherapy [27]. Although loss of ARID1A protein expression is thought to be an early event in the development of ovarian clear cell adenocarcinoma [28], its biological effect on the malignant transformation of endometriosis should be further clarified.

15.4 Environmental Factors That Affect Malignant Transformation of Endometriosis

15.4.1 Microenvironments in Endometriotic Cysts

15.4.1.1 Oxidative Stress and Carcinogenesis

In our bodies, live cells are continuously exposed to oxidative stresses, which are produced internally or externally. Internal stress consists of mitochondrial respiratory stress, cytochrome P450 metabolism, and inflammatory responses. External stresses are generated by various agents, including chemicals, xenobiotics, irradiation, and metal ions, including Fe ions. One of the well-known mechanisms

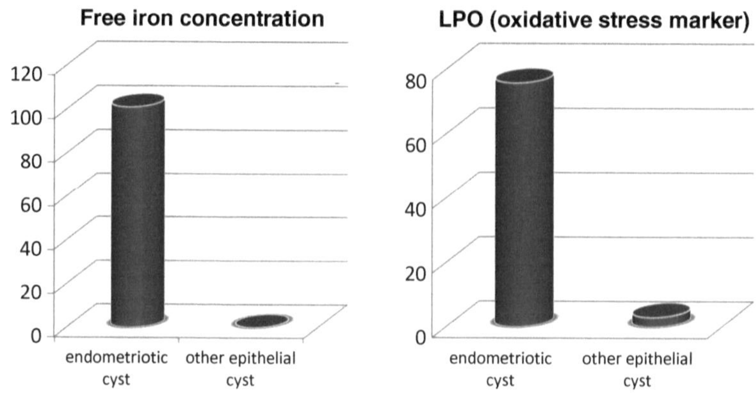

Fig. 15.2 Differences in Fe concentration/oxidative stress between endometriotic cysts and other benign epithelial cysts

by which metal ions produce intracellular ROS is called the Fenton reaction [29]. During this reaction, highly toxic dOH and anoxidized metal ions are generated from H_2O_2. Metal-induced ROS causes DNA damage, including single- or double-strand breaks, base modifications, deoxyribose modifications, and DNA cross-linking, which ultimately contributes to carcinogenesis.

In normal conditions, ROS overproduction is avoided by endogenous antioxidants, including superoxide dismutase (SOD), catalase (CAT), and glutathione peroxidase (GPx). If the balance between the cellular antioxidant defense and ROS generation is impaired, excessive ROS can cause oxidative stress. Prolonged and excessive oxidative stress mediates a variety of chronic and degenerative diseases, including cancers, inflammation, aging, and neuronal disorders [29].

15.4.1.2 Oxidative Stress in Endometriotic Cysts

The content of endometriotic cysts consists of old blood containing a high concentration of iron derived from hemoglobin. We compared the concentrations of free iron in endometriotic cysts with those in other ovarian cysts, including serous and mucinous cystadenoma, and found that the concentrations were significantly higher in endometriotic cysts [30] (Fig. 15.2). Likewise, lactose dehydrogenase (LDH) (a marker of tissue damage), potential antioxidant (PAI) (an antioxidant marker), lipid peroxidase (LPO) (Fig. 15.2) (a marker of oxidative stress), and 8-hydroxy-2-deoxyguanosine (a marker of DNA damage) were all significantly elevated in endometriotic cysts compared with other ovarian cysts. These data strongly suggest that the epithelial cells of the endometriotic cyst are constantly exposed to excessive oxidative stress and are subjected to cellular and DNA damage (Fig. 15.3).

To elucidate the mutagenic property of the fluid in chocolate cysts, we conducted an experiment in vitro, which demonstrated that the fluid in chocolate

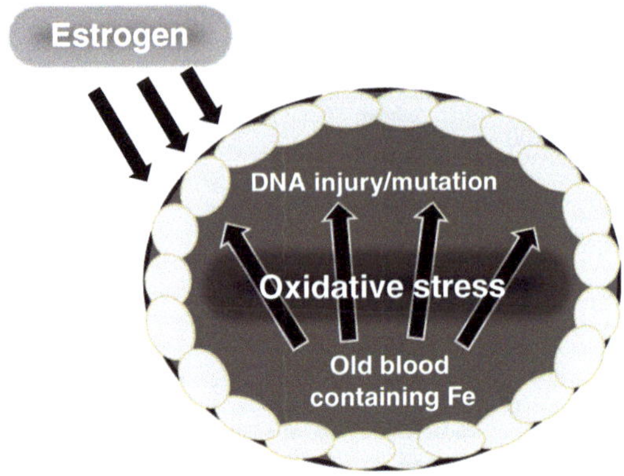

Fig. 15.3 Intrinsic and extrinsic factors affecting malignant transformation of endometriotic cyst

cysts is more mutagenic than that in other cysts [30]. There are several reports suggesting a link between a stressful microenvironment and cancer development. (1) Chromosomal aberrations are more frequent in ovarian endometriotic cysts than in extra-gonadal endometriosis [31]. (2) Malignant transformation of endometriotic cysts increases with the duration of endometriosis [32].

15.4.2 Clear Cell Carcinoma and the Stress Response

If the microenvironment in endometriotic cysts affects cancer development, is it also associated with the phenotype of the ovarian cancer that arises as a result of malignant transformation? To assess this possibility, we began by identifying the gene signature that distinguishes clear cell carcinoma from other types of ovarian cancer using microarray datasets [33]. The signature composed of 437 genes was designated as the ovarian clear cell carcinoma (OCCC) signature. By using a categorical analysis, we demonstrated that the OCCC signature contains genes in three major categories, that is, stress response, sugar metabolism, and coagulation. Stress-related genes were estimated to play a central role, suggesting that the stress response is the fundamental feature of clear cell carcinoma. Actually, the OCCC signature was shown to involve a signal network consisting of many stress-related genes, including HIF1-α, IL-6, and SOD2. Moreover, when ovarian surface epithelial cells were treated with the contents of endometriotic cysts, the OCCC signature was increased in a time-dependent manner. The constitutive expression of the OCCC signature in clear cell carcinoma may reflect gene induction in response to the microenvironment in endometriotic cysts.

These data raise a novel and important concept that the specific microenvironment induces unique gene expression and leads to a cancer of a special phenotype. The local microenvironment, including ROS or inflammation, is likely not only to be implicated in cancer development [34], but it is also likely to be related to the occurrence of a specific cancer phenotype.

15.5 The Carcinogenic Scheme of Endometriotic Cysts and Future Applications

15.5.1 The Natural History of Endometriosis and Malignant Transformation

As mentioned earlier, endometriosis itself is largely a monoclonal, neoplastic disorder and has a potential for malignant transformation. Because endometriotic epithelium is a mullerian-type epithelium, it may be subject to mullerian organ carcinogenesis, leading to the development of various types of cancers, including serous carcinoma, mucinous carcinoma, and borderline tumors such as mucinous mullerian borderline tumors [35]. However, these types of cancer are relatively rare. A major type of cancer that develops from endometriosis is endometrioid carcinoma. The carcinogenic process of development of endometrioid carcinoma from endometriosis may resemble that in the endometrium under the influence of (unopposed) estrogen. In this case, progestin may play a prophylactic role, although no definite data are available yet.

The third mechanism, which is associated with the occurrence of clear cell carcinomas, is strongly influenced by the unique microenvironment within the chocolate cyst [35]. Continuous exposure to oxidative stress, partly caused by iron, results in the expression of stress-responsive genes, the OCCC signature. Constitutive expression of the OCCC signature genes is closely associated with the stress-resistant and slow-growing phenotype of malignancy, that is, clear cell carcinoma [36] (Fig. 15.4). Regarded as the prevention of clear cell carcinoma, surgical treatment to improve the microenvironment may be the best option.

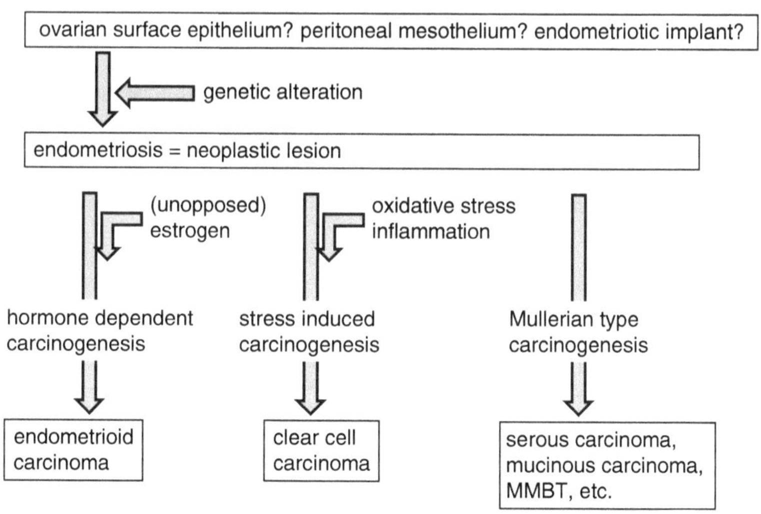

Fig. 15.4 Hypothetical mechanism of malignant transformation of endometriotic cyst

Thus, clarification of the precise natural course of malignant transformation of endometriotic cysts should lead to the proper management of endometriosis in terms of malignant transformation.

15.5.2 Future Treatment Strategy of EAOC, Especially Ovarian Clear Cell Carcinoma

Recent advances in understanding the molecular and biological features of clear cell carcinoma enable us to consider several new treatment strategies. Frequent activation of the AKT/PI3K/Met pathway in EAOC suggests that mTOR inhibitors may be effective in the treatment of these cancers. Mabuchi et al. showed that the mTOR inhibitor RAD001 is effective in the treatment of clear cell carcinoma of the ovary [37]. We have shown that sorafenib, a multikinase inhibitor, showed therapeutic effects in the RMG-2 clear cell cancer cell line, which is resistant to cisplatin [38]. In the future, the exploration of more precise mechanisms of malignant transformation of endometriosis may lead not only to various molecular targeted therapies but also to therapies targeting neovascularization or cancer metabolism [36].

References

1. Jimbo H, Hitomi Y, Yoshikawa H, Yano T, Momoeda M, Sakamoto A, Tsutsumi O, Taketani Y, Esumi H. Evidence for monoclonal expansion of epithelial cells in ovarian endometrial cysts. Am J Pathol. 1997;150(4):1173–8.
2. Nilbert M, Pejovic T, Mandahl N, Iosif S, Willén H, Mitelman F. Monoclonal origin of endometriotic cysts. Int J Gynecol Cancer. 1995;5(1):61–3.
3. Tamura M, Fukaya T, Murakami T, Uehara S, Yajima A. Analysis of clonality in human endometriotic cysts based on evaluation of X chromosome inactivation in archival formalin-fixed, paraffin-embedded tissue. Lab Invest. 1998;78(2):213–8.
4. Shin JC, Ross HL, Elias S, Nguyen DD, Mitchell-Leef D, Simpson JL, Bischoff FZ. Detection of chromosomal aneuploidy in endometriosis by multi-color fluorescence in situ hybridization (FISH). Hum Genet. 1997;100(3–4):401–6.
5. Bischoff FZ, Heard M, Simpson JL. Somatic DNA alterations in endometriosis: high frequency of chromosome 17 and p53 loss in late-stage endometriosis. J Reprod Immunol. 2002;55(1–2):49–64.
6. Jiang X, Hitchcock A, Bryan EJ, Watson RH, Englefield P, Thomas EJ, Campbell IG. Microsatellite analysis of endometriosis reveals loss of heterozygosity at candidate ovarian tumor suppressor gene loci. Cancer Res. 1996;56(15):3534–9.
7. Nabeshima H, Murakami T, Yoshinaga K, Sato K, Terada Y, Okamura K. Analysis of the clonality of ectopic glands in peritoneal endometriosis using laser microdissection. Fertil Steril. 2003;80(5):1144–50.
8. Wu Y, Basir Z, Kajdacsy-Balla A, Strawn E, Macias V, Montgomery K, Guo SW. Resolution of clonal origins for endometriotic lesions using laser capture microdissection and the human androgen receptor (HUMARA) assay. Fertil Steril. 2003;79 Suppl 1:710–7.

9. Mayr D, Amann G, Siefert C, Diebold J, Anderegg B. Does endometriosis really have premalignant potential? A clonal analysis of laser-microdissected tissue. FASEB J. 2003;17(6):693–5.
10. Sampson J. Endometrial carcinoma of the ovary, arising in endometrial tissue in that organ. Arch Surg. 1925;10:1–72.
11. Czernobilsky B, Morris WJ. A histologic study of ovarian endometriosis with emphasis on hyperplastic and atypical changes. Obstet Gynecol. 1979;53(3):318–23.
12. LaGrenade A, Silverberg SG. Ovarian tumors associated with atypical endometriosis. Hum Pathol. 1988;19(9):1080–4.
13. Fukunaga M, Nomura K, Ishikawa E, Ushigome S. Ovarian atypical endometriosis: its close association with malignant epithelial tumours. Histopathology. 1997;30(3):249–55.
14. Ogawa S, Kaku T, Amada S, Kobayashi H, Hirakawa T, Ariyoshi K, Kamura T, Nakano H. Ovarian endometriosis associated with ovarian carcinoma: a clinicopathological and immunohistochemical study. Gynecol Oncol. 2000;77(2):298–304.
15. Sáinz de la Cuesta R, Izquierdo M, Cañamero M, Granizo JJ, Manzarbeitia F. Increased prevalence of p53 overexpression from typical endometriosis to atypical endometriosis and ovarian cancer associated with endometriosis. Eur J Obstet Gynecol Reprod Biol. 2004;113(1):87–93.
16. Obata K, Hoshiai H. Common genetic changes between endometriosis and ovarian cancer. Gynecol Obstet Invest. 2000;50 Suppl 1:39–43.
17. Jiang X, Morland SJ, Hitchcock A, Thomas EJ, Campbell IG. Allelotyping of endometriosis with adjacent ovarian carcinoma reveals evidence of a common lineage. Cancer Res. 1998;58(8):1707–12.
18. Prowse AH, Manek S, Varma R, Liu J, Godwin AK, Maher ER, Tomlinson IP, Kennedy SH. Molecular genetic evidence that endometriosis is a precursor of ovarian cancer. Int J Cancer. 2006;119(3):556–62.
19. Goumenou AG, Arvanitis DA, Matalliotakis IM, Koumantakis EE, Spandidos DA. Microsatellite DNA assays reveal an allelic imbalance in p16(Ink4), GALT, p53, and APOA2 loci in patients with endometriosis. Fertil Steril. 2001;75(1):160–5.
20. Sato N, Tsunoda H, Nishida M, Morishita Y, Takimoto Y, Kubo T, Noguchi M. Loss of heterozygosity on 10q23.3 and mutation of the tumor suppressor gene PTEN in benign endometrial cyst of the ovary: possible sequence progression from benign endometrial cyst to endometrioid carcinoma and clear cell carcinoma of the ovary. Cancer Res. 2000;60(24):7052–6.
21. Kato N, Sasou S, Motoyama T. Expression of hepatocyte nuclear factor-1beta (HNF-1beta) in clear cell tumors and endometriosis of the ovary. Mod Pathol. 2006;19(1):83–9.
22. Yamashita Y, Akatsuka S, Shinjo K, Yatabe Y, Kobayashi H, Seko H, Kajiyama H, Kikkawa F, Takahashi T, Toyokuni S. Met is the most frequently amplified gene in endometriosis-associated ovarian clear cell adenocarcinoma and correlates with worsened prognosis. PLoS One. 2013;8(3):e57724.
23. Yamamoto S, Tsuda H, Takano M, Iwaya K, Tamai S, Matsubara O. PIK3CA mutation is an early event in the development of endometriosis-associated ovarian clear cell adenocarcinoma. J Pathol. 2011;225(2):189–94.
24. Jones S, Wang TL, Shih IM, Mao TL, Nakayama K, Roden R, Glas R, Slamon D, Diaz Jr LA, Vogelstein B, Kinzler KW, Velculescu VE, Papadopoulos N. Frequent mutations of chromatin remodeling gene ARID1A in ovarian clear cell carcinoma. Science. 2010;330(6001):228–31.
25. Wiegand KC, Shah SP, Al-Agha OM, Zhao Y, Tse K, Zeng T, Senz J, McConechy MK, Anglesio MS, Kalloger SE, Yang W, Heravi-Moussavi A, Giuliany R, Chow C, Fee J, Zayed A, Prentice L, Melnyk N, Turashvili G, Delaney AD, Madore J, Yip S, McPherson AW, Ha G, Bell L, Fereday S, Tam A, Galletta L, Tonin PN, Provencher D, Miller D, Jones SJ, Moore RA, Morin GB, Oloumi A, Boyd N, Aparicio SA, Shih IM, Mes-Masson AM, Bowtell DD, Hirst M, Gilks B, Marra MA, Huntsman DG. ARID1A mutations in endometriosis-associated ovarian carcinomas. N Engl J Med. 2010;363(16):1532–43.

26. Guan B, Wang TL, Shih IM. ARID1A, a factor that promotes formation of SWI/SNF-mediated chromatin remodeling, is a tumor suppressor in gynecologic cancers. Cancer Res. 2011;71 (21):6718–27.
27. Katagiri A, Nakayama K, Rahman MT, Rahman M, Katagiri H, Nakayama N, Ishikawa M, Ishibashi T, Iida K, Kobayashi H, Otsuki Y, Nakayama S, Miyazaki K. Loss of ARID1A expression is related to shorter progression-free survival and chemoresistance in ovarian clear cell carcinoma. Mod Pathol. 2012;25(2):282–8.
28. Yamamoto S, Tsuda H, Takano M, Tamai S, Matsubara O. PIK3CA mutations and loss of ARID1A protein expression are early events in the development of cystic ovarian clear cell adenocarcinoma. Virchows Arch. 2012;460(1):77–87.
29. Lee JC, Son YO, Pratheeshkumar P, Shi X. Oxidative stress and metal carcinogenesis. Free Radic Biol Med. 2012;53(4):742–57.
30. Yamaguchi K, Mandai M, Toyokuni S, Hamanishi J, Higuchi T, Takakura K, Fujii S. Contents of endometriotic cysts, especially the high concentration of free iron, are a possible cause of carcinogenesis in the cysts through the iron-induced persistent oxidative stress. Clin Cancer Res. 2008;14(1):32–40.
31. Körner M, Burckhardt E, Mazzucchelli L. Higher frequency of chromosomal aberrations in ovarian endometriosis compared to extragonadal endometriosis: a possible link to endometrioid adenocarcinoma. Mod Pathol. 2006;19(12):1615–23.
32. Melin A, Sparén P, Persson I, Bergqvist A. Endometriosis and the risk of cancer with special emphasis on ovarian cancer. Hum Reprod. 2006;21(5):1237–42.
33. Yamaguchi K, Mandai M, Oura T, Matsumura N, Hamanishi J, Baba T, Matsui S, Murphy SK, Konishi I. Identification of an ovarian clear cell carcinoma gene signature that reflects inherent disease biology and the carcinogenic processes. Oncogene. 2010;29(12):1741–52.
34. Gonda TA, Tu S, Wang TC. Chronic inflammation, the tumor microenvironment and carcinogenesis. Cell Cycle. 2009;8(13):2005–13.
35. Mandai M, Yamaguchi K, Matsumura N, Baba T, Konishi I. Ovarian cancer in endometriosis: molecular biology, pathology, and clinical management. Int J Clin Oncol. 2009;14(5):383–91.
36. Mandai M, Matsumura N, Baba T, Yamaguchi K, Hamanishi J, Konishi I. Ovarian clear cell carcinoma as a stress-responsive cancer: influence of the microenvironment on the carcinogenesis and cancer phenotype. Cancer Lett. 2011;310(2):129–33.
37. Mabuchi S, Kawase C, Altomare DA, Morishige K, Sawada K, Hayashi M, Tsujimoto M, Yamoto M, Klein-Szanto AJ, Schilder RJ, Ohmichi M, Testa JR, Kimura T. mTOR is a promising therapeutic target both in cisplatin-sensitive and cisplatin-resistant clear cell carcinoma of the ovary. Clin Cancer Res. 2009;15(17):5404–13.
38. Matsumura N, Mandai M, Okamoto T, Yamaguchi K, Yamamura S, Oura T, Baba T, Hamanishi J, Kang HS, Matsui S, Mori S, Murphy SK, Konishi I. Sorafenib efficacy in ovarian clear cell carcinoma revealed by transcriptome profiling. Cancer Sci. 2010;101(12):2658–63.

Chapter 16
Potential New Drugs for Endometriosis: Experimental Evidence

Kaei Nasu, Yukie Kawano, Masakazu Nishida, Akitoshi Tsuno, Akitoshi Yuge, Wakana Abe, Kentaro Kai, Mamiko Okamoto, and Hisasshi Narahara

Abstract Endometriosis, a disease affecting 3–10 % of women of reproductive age, is characterized by the ectopic growth of endometrial tissue. Recent basic studies have revealed that the dysregulation of apoptosis, fibrosis, and epigenetic factors plays important roles in the pathogenesis of this enigmatic disease.

Contraceptive steroids, progestogens, agonists of gonadotropin-releasing hormone, androgens, and nonsteroidal anti-inflammatory agents have been used to treat endometriosis. Endometriosis treatments designed to lower circulating estradiol concentrations can be used only for a limited time due to unacceptable side effects. The development of medical treatments based on novel strategies to prevent or treat endometriosis has thus become a research priority.

Regarding the development of novel medical treatments for endometriosis, many researchers have been evaluating new drugs including molecular-targeting agents and herbal medicine as well as the newly developed hormonal agents. This chapter is a review of the findings from recent basic research on the pathogenesis of endometriosis and the evaluations of novel medical treatments for this disease, especially focusing on the inhibitors of nuclear factor-κB, the mevalonate-Rho/ROCK pathway, and histone deacetylase. These agents are now considered promising agents for the treatment and prevention of endometriosis.

Keywords Endometriosis • Histone deacetylase inhibitor • Mevalonate-Rho/ROCK pathway • Nuclear factor-κB

K. Nasu, M.D., Ph.D. (✉) • Y. Kawano • M. Nishida • A. Tsuno • A. Yuge • W. Abe
K. Kai • M. Okamoto • H. Narahara
Department of Obstetrics and Gynecology, Faculty of Medicine, Oita University,
Idaigaoka 1-1, Hasama-machi, Yufu-shi, Oita 879-5593, Japan
e-mail: nasu@oita-u.ac.jp

T. Harada (ed.), *Endometriosis: Pathogenesis and Treatment*,
DOI 10.1007/978-4-431-54421-0_16, © Springer Japan 2014

16.1 Introduction

Endometriosis—the benign, estrogen-dependent, tumorlike disease characterized by chronic pelvic pain, dysmenorrhea, dyspareunia, and/or subfertility—is due to the uncontrolled ectopic growth of proliferative endometrial tissue. Women of reproductive age are most commonly affected by endometriosis, which usually occurs in the peritoneum, ovaries, and rectovaginal septum [1]. The symptoms of endometriosis may markedly reduce a woman's quality of life.

Several surgical and medical strategies have been used to treat endometriosis. Contraceptive steroids, progestogens, and agonists of gonadotropin-releasing hormone, androgens, and nonsteroidal anti-inflammatory agents have been attempted [2]. Endometriosis treatments designed to lower circulating estradiol concentrations can be used only for a limited time due to unacceptable side effects. The current medical treatments inhibit the growth of endometriotic implants by suppressing ovarian steroids and inducing a hypoestrogenic state; they have been demonstrated to be effective in relieving endometriosis-associated pain [2]. However, high recurrence rates, up to 45 %, after the completion of medical treatments remain a significant problem [3]. An international consensus group proposed the development of nonhormonal medical treatments to prevent or treat endometriosis as a research priority [4]. In addition, many research groups have been evaluating new drugs for endometriosis such as molecular-targeting agents and herbal medicine, as well as the newly developed hormonal agents.

In this chapter, we review the recent basic studies on the development of novel medical treatments for endometriosis based on distinct strategies. We focus on the recent publications about the nuclear factor (NF)-κB inhibitors, mevalonate-Ras homology (Rho)/Rho-associated coiled-coil-forming protein kinase (ROCK) inhibitors, and histone deacetylase (HDAC) inhibitors (HDACIs) as potential candidates for the next era in endometriosis treatment and prevention.

16.2 Potential New Drugs

16.2.1 NF-κB Inhibitors

Apoptosis plays a critical role in maintaining tissue homeostasis, and its function is to eliminate excess cells and dysfunctional cells. Apoptosis can be initiated by extracellular or intracellular "death signals," and it results from a series of related morphologic and biochemical processes. Morphologically, apoptotic cells present with condensed chromatin, multiple membrane-bound organelles (apoptotic bodies), and shrunken appearance. Biochemically, apoptosis is characterized by monomeric or multimeric 180-base pair nucleosomal fragments resulting from the cleavage of double-stranded nuclear DNA [5]. Apoptosis is controlled by the expression of a number of regulatory genes, including c-myc, p53, Fas, NF-κB, and members of the B-cell lymphoma/leukemia (Bcl)-2 family [6–11].

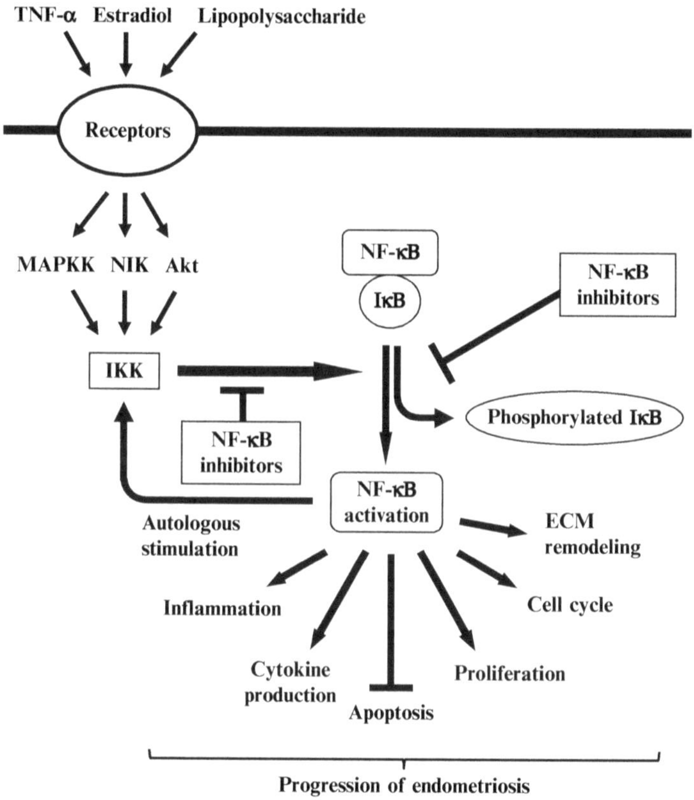

Fig. 16.1 Involvement of the NF-κB-mediated pathway in the pathogenesis of endometriosis. *ECM* extracellular matrix, *IκB* inhibitor κB, *IKK* IκB kinase, *NIK* NF-κB-inducing kinase, *MAPKK* MAPK kinase, *TNF* tumor necrosis factor

Histologically, endometriotic tissues and normal proliferative endometrium are similar. However, endometriosis is increasingly being recognized as a condition in which endometriotic cells at the ectopic sites exhibit abnormal proliferative and apoptotic regulation in response to appropriate stimuli [12–22]. It has been demonstrated that the degree of apoptosis in endometriotic lesions is less than that in the endometrium of the same patients and that of healthy women [13–15, 23–25]. The resistance of endometriotic cells to apoptosis is suspected to be either intrinsic or brought about by environmental factors. Aberrantly expressed proliferation-related and apoptosis-related molecules in endometriosis include the decreased expressions of homeobox (HOX) A10 [26] and caspase-1 [27] and the enhanced expressions of c-myc [28], cellular inhibitor of apoptosis protein (cIAP) 1 [29], X chromosome-linked IAP [29], B-cell lymphoma/leukemia (Bcl)-2 [19], Bcl-X_L [19], and NF-κB [30, 31] in endometriotic cells.

The pleiotropic transcription factor NF-κB has been identified as a critical component of several signal transduction pathways [29]. Figure 16.1 shows the proposed functions of NF-κB in the pathogenesis of endometriosis. One important function of NF-κB is its ability to protect cells from apoptosis by activating antiapoptotic genes [9, 10]. Wieser et al. [32] demonstrated the constitutive activation of NF-κB in endometriotic cells. It is suggested that NF-κB has a significant role in the proliferation of endometriotic lesions [30, 31]. The activation of NF-κB by lipopolysaccharide (LPS) induces the proliferation of endometriotic stromal cells [33].

A number of substances have been presented in the endometriosis literature as NF-κB inhibitors. The reported selective inhibitors of NF-κB include an IκB protease inhibitor, *N*-tosyl-L-phenylalanine chloromethyl ketone (TPCK) [33], thalidomide [34], BAY 11–7085 [35], pyrrolidine dithiocarbamate (PDTC) [36–38], costunolide [39], and parthenolide [40]. The urinary preparation human chorionic gonadotropin A (hCG-A) [41], gonadotropin-releasing hormone (GnRH) agonists [30], progesterone [42], and danazol [42] have been demonstrated to inhibit NF-κB activity in endometriosis. NF-κB inhibitors have been shown to significantly block the proliferation of endometriotic stromal cells [33, 35, 40] and they induce apoptosis and the G0/G1 phase cell-cycle arrest of endometriotic stromal cells [35, 38, 39]. Additionally, after endometriotic stromal cells were treated with NF-κB inhibitors, the downregulation of the expression of antiapoptotic factors (Bcl-2 and Bcl-X_L), inflammatory cytokines (interleukin-6 [IL-6], IL-8, monocyte chemoattractant protein-1 [MCP-1], and granulocyte-macrophage colony-stimulating factor [GM-CSF]), inflammatory mediators (COX-2 and PGE2), extracellular matrix remodeling mediators (MMP-2, MMP-3, MMP-7, MMP-9), CD44, and vascular endothelial growth factor [VEGF] with simultaneous activation of caspase-3, caspase-8, and caspase-9 was observed [30, 34–41].

The suppression of NF-κB activity by proteasome inhibitors also suppresses the proliferation of endometriotic cells in vitro [31]. The NF-κB inhibitors BAY 11–7085 and SN-50 significantly reduced the development of endometriotic lesions in a nude mice model [43]. Takai et al. [40] also demonstrated that parthenolide reduced the growth of endometriotic lesions in a murine model. The antioxidant PDTC reduced the growth and vascularity of experimental peritoneal endometriotic lesions in a rat model [44].

16.2.2 Mevalonate-Rho/ROCK Inhibitors

During the development and progression of endometriotic lesions, excess fibrosis may lead to scarring, chronic pain, and the alterations of tissue function that are characteristic of this disease [45–48]. It has been suggested that type I collagen is a major contributor to endometriosis-associated fibrosis [46, 49], whereas α-smooth muscle actin (SMA)-positive fibroblastic cells were frequently detected in the fibrotic areas associated with endometriosis of the peritoneum, ovary, rectovaginal septum, and uterosacral ligaments [45, 48, 50]. An immunohistochemical analysis led Anaf et al. [50] to suggest that endometriotic stromal cells can differentiate to α-SMA-positive myofibroblasts.

To establish a model of fibrosis formation in endometriosis, we used a 3D collagen culture system with human endometriotic stromal cells [51, 52]. We cultured the cells in floating collagen lattices to reorganize the collagen fibers and make them compact, resulting in contraction of the collagen gels. This culture system provided a model for mechanically relaxed tissue with low tensile strength, comparable to the early stages of an endometriotic lesion. We found that endometriotic stromal cells cultured in floating 3D gels have an enhanced contractile profile compared to normal endometrial stromal cells [51]. This suggested that endometriotic stromal cells may acquire fibrogenetic ability or fail to avoid fibrogenesis during the pathogenesis of endometriosis.

Members of the Rho family of small guanosine triphosphatase (GTPase) are known to regulate cell shape, motility, cell-substratum adhesion, and cell contraction through the reorganization of actin cytoskeletons [53–65]. The active form of Rho is GTP-bound [54, 62], and many polypeptides have been reported as targets of activated Rho, including ROCK-I/p160ROCK and Rho-kinase/ROCK-II [66]. ROCKs phosphorylate the myosin light chain (MLC) [67] and the myosin-binding subunit of myosin phosphatase [68], and they inhibit myosin II regulatory light chain phosphatase activity [68] in cultured fibroblasts. Rho and ROCKs have been implicated in myosin II-dependent force generation [69]. Thus, the activation of ROCKs by Rho can promote the assembly of focal adhesions, actin stress fiber formation, and contraction of non-muscle cells [62, 68], in which RhoA regulates α-SMA expression [70].

Based on these observations in fibroblasts, we have investigated the signaling pathway underlying endometriotic stromal cell-mediated contractility by using 3D cultures. Our data indicated that human endometriotic stromal cells undergo myofibroblastic differentiation and show increased expression of RhoA, ROCK-I, and ROCK-II proteins, resulting in enhanced contractility [51]. Thus, we evaluated several inhibitors of mevalonate-Rho/ROCK pathways as candidate drugs for the treatment and prevention of endometriosis-associated fibrosis [51, 52, 71–73].

16.2.3 Statins

Statins are potent inhibitors of cholesterol biosynthesis that are widely used to reduce serum cholesterol levels in hyperlipidemic patients [74, 75]. Statins are divided into three categories: natural statins (i.e., lovastatin and pravastatin), semisynthetic statins (i.e., simvastatin), and synthetic statins (i.e., atorvastatin, fluvastatin, and cerivastatin) [75, 76]. These three subtypes of statin exhibit markedly different hydrophobicities, with simvastatin as the most hydrophobic and pravastatin as the most hydrophilic.

Statins competitively inhibit 3-hydroxy-3-methylglutarylcoenzyme A (HMG-CoA) reductase to block the conversion of HMG-CoA to L-mevalonate, a rate-limiting step in cholesterol synthesis [77]. By inhibiting the initial step of the cholesterol synthesis pathway, statins reduce the synthesis of several important lipid intermediate compounds including isoprenoids such as farnesyl pyrophosphate (FPP), a precursor of cholesterol, and geranylgeranyl pyrophosphate (GGPP), which is synthesized from FPP [78]. Both FPP and GGPP are important isoprenoid intermediates and serve as lipid attachments for a variety of intercellular proteins to the plasma membrane, including Rho proteins, resulting in their activation [59, 79]. By inhibiting the activation of Rho proteins, statins also regulate both the Rho/ROCK pathways and the mevalonate pathway [80, 81].

Simvastatin has been demonstrated to inhibit the proliferation of endometriotic stromal cells as well as the collagen gel contraction mediated by these cells [71]. Attenuation of the endometriotic stromal cell attachment to collagen fibers is involved in this mechanism. Lovastatin also inhibited cell proliferation and angiogenesis in endometriosis [82], whereas simvastatin and mevastatin inhibited the MCP-1 production by endometriotic cells [83]. Atorvastatin also exhibited antiproliferative and anti-inflammatory effects in endometriotic cells [84]. Oktem et al. [85] demonstrated that atorvastatin induced the regression of endometriotic implants in a rat model. Similarly, Bruner-Tran et al. [86] demonstrated that simvastatin induced the regression of endometriotic implants in a nude mouse model.

16.2.4 ROCK Inhibitors

Several selective ROCK inhibitors including Y-27632 and fasudil hydrochloride are now available for basic and clinical studies [58, 63, 87, 88]. We demonstrated that Y-27632, a pyridine derivative that acts as a specific inhibitor of ROCK-I and ROCK-II [58, 63], inhibits endometriotic stromal cell-mediated contractility [51]. Interestingly, Y-27632 was found to exert a greater effect on the contractility of endometriotic stromal cells than on the contractility of normal eutopic endometrial stromal cells, whereas fasudil hydrochloride also inhibited endometriotic stromal cell-mediated contractility, myofibroblastic differentiation, and cell proliferation [72].

16.2.5 Heparin

Heparin is an analog of heparan sulfate, a unique class of macromolecules that is widely expressed on the cell surface and in the extracellular matrix [89]. It is a commonly used anticoagulant drug [90]. Heparin was shown to inhibit the gel contraction mediated by dermal fibroblasts [91, 92]. We demonstrated that heparin attenuates the contractility of endometriotic stromal cells by suppressing the cells' attachment to collagen fibers, the inhibition of myofibroblastic differentiation, and the suppression of the Rho/ROCK-mediated pathway [73]. However, the precise target molecule of heparin's action on endometriotic stromal cells has not yet been elucidated.

16.2.6 HDACIs

Epigenetics refers to the stable inheritance of phenotypes of cells and organisms without changes in DNA sequence or DNA content [93]. The epigenetic phenotypes are conferred via nuclear processes such as DNA methylation and chromatin modifications (e.g., acetylation, biotinylation, isomerization, methylation, phosphorylation, ribosylation, sumoylation, and ubiquitination of histones) and underlie the regulation of all genome functions, including gene expression, DNA replication, and genome stability [94–96]. Epigenetic phenotypes are also conferred via microRNA and double-stranded noncoding RNA, which are interconnected and may work together to establish and/or maintain specific gene activity states in normal cells [93, 96, 97]. Epigenetic processes are known to be involved in development, health, disease, and aging and are responsible for phenomena such as X-chromosome inactivation and genomic imprinting [98, 99]. Of these epigenetic regulatory mechanisms, histone acetylation is the most studied.

The acetylation levels of histone are controlled by a balance between histone acetyltransferases and histone deacetylases (HDACs). Histone acetyltransferases transfer acetyl groups from acetyl-CoA to lysine residues on the aminoterminal region of histones and activate genetic transcription. Conversely, HDACs restore the positive charge on lysine residues (by removing the acetyl groups) and prevent transcription. HDACs are large multiprotein complexes that target promoter sites through their interaction with sequence-specific transcription. They play an important role in the regulation of gene transcription through the remodeling of chromatin structure and dynamic changes in the nucleosomal packaging of DNA [100].

The hyperacetylation of histones H3 and H4 is often associated with activated transcription, and the hypoacetylation of histones H3 and H4 correlates with transcriptional silencing or repression [101], whereas Choi et al. [102] suggested that the substrates of HDACs are not restricted to histones but include transcriptional regulators, such as p53, E2F-1, Mad-1, BCL-6, and ETO. In this regard, global gene expression analyses have shown that HDACIs affect the expression levels of 2–20 % of genes in the genome, of which about half are upregulated and half downregulated [103].

Accumulating evidence indicates that several epigenetic aberrations are involved in the pathogenesis of endometriosis [104–110]. We observed that the levels of acetylated histones H3 and H4 were significantly lower in unstimulated endometriotic stromal cells compared to normal endometrial stromal cells, suggesting that aberrant histone modifications are present in endometriosis [108]. This initial finding encouraged us to evaluate the efficacy of HDACIs for the treatment of endometriosis. Our subsequent experiments demonstrated that

HDACIs significantly inhibited the proliferation of endometriotic stromal cells, and they also induced significant levels of cell-cycle arrest at the G0/G1 or G2/M phases and significant apoptosis of these cells [108].

Interestingly, HDACIs showed marginal to weak effects on normal endometrial stromal cells compared to endometriotic stromal cells. Moreover, HDACI treatment significantly inhibited HDAC activity and resulted in the accumulation of acetylated histones H3 and H4 in total cellular chromatin and in the promoter regions of the $p16^{INK4a}$, $p21^{Waf1/Cip1}$, $p27^{Kip1}$, and cell-cycle checkpoint kinase 2 (chk2) genes in these cells. A Western blot analysis revealed the increased protein levels of $p16^{INK4a}$, $p21^{Waf1/Cip1}$, $p27^{Kip1}$, and chk2, the suppression of Bcl-2 and Bcl-X_L protein levels, and the activation of caspase-3 and caspase-9 in endometriotic stromal cells after treatment with HDACIs [108]. Recently, we found that the expression of CCAAT/enhancer-binding protein (C/EBP)-α, a tumor suppressor gene, and death receptor 6, a TNF receptor superfamily gene, was epigenetically suppressed by histone deacetylation (our unpublished data).

Histone deacetylation appears to be a potent regulator of gene expression in endometriosis, which raises the prospect of using HDACIs as therapeutic tools in endometriosis [108]. Several classes of HDACIs have been identified, including (a) organic hydroxamic acids [e.g., trichostatin A and suberoylanilide bishydroxamine (SAHA)], (b) short-chain fatty acids [e.g., butyrates and valproic acid (VPA)], (c) benzamides (e.g., MS-275), (d) cyclic tetrapeptides (e.g., trapoxin), and (e) sulfonamide anilides [108]. The molecular events that mediate the biological effects of HDACIs are incompletely understood. Inhibition of HDAC by HDACIs increases histone acetylation and maintains chromatin structure in a more open conformation, resulting in the reactivation of transcriptionally silenced pathways or the suppression of aberrantly expressed genes through the recruitment of repressors [111, 112]. HDACIs can reactivate genes silenced by promoter hypermethylation as well as the demethylation agents [113]. HDACIs also cause mitotic defects through non-transcriptional mechanisms [114].

We demonstrated that HDACIs, including VPA, SAHA, and apicidin, can inhibit the proliferation, induce cell differentiation and cell-cycle arrest, and stimulate the apoptosis of endometriotic cells [108]. Guo and his colleagues have demonstrated that HDACIs, such as VPA and trichostatin A, can suppress the proliferation, induce cell-cycle arrest, inhibit IL-1β-induced cyclooxygenase-2 expression and NF-κB activation, upregulate peroxisome proliferator-activated receptor γ, $p21^{Waf1/Cip1}$ and PR-B expression, attenuate invasiveness, and reactivate the silenced E-cadherin gene expression of endometriotic cells [115–120]. Romidepsin, an HDACI, was shown to specifically reduce HDAC enzymatic activity, resulting in inhibited cell proliferation, cell-cycle arrest, increased apoptosis, and reduced expression of VEGF mRNA and protein in endometriotic cells [121, 122]. Treatment with trichostatin A and VPA has been shown to significantly reduce the growth of endometriotic lesions in a murine model [123, 124]. Histone deacetylation appears to be a potent regulator of gene expression in endometriosis, which raises the prospect of using HDACIs as therapeutic tools in endometriosis [108, 117].

VPA was used in a pilot study of three patients with endometriosis and adenomyosis who had moderate to severe dysmenorrhea [125]. A VPA dose of 1,000 mg/day was used for 3 months. Complete relief of pain in all cases and an average reduction of one-third in uterine size were reported. The disappearance or reduction of palpable tender nodules in the cul-de-sac was also reported.

16.3 Conclusions

Basic research on endometriosis offers new opportunities to understand the pathogenesis of this enigmatic disease and to provide novel medical treatments other than hormonal therapy. As shown in this chapter, NF-κB inhibitors and mevalonate-Rho/ROCK inhibitors as well as HDACIs seem to be promising therapeutic strategies for the treatment of endometriosis.

Acknowledgments This work was supported in part by a Grant-in-Aid for Scientific Research from the Japan Society for the Promotion of Science (no. 13237327 to K. Nasu, no. 25861500 to Y. Kawano, and no. 23592407 to H. Narahara).

References

1. Giudice LC, Kao LC. Endometriosis. Lancet. 2004;364:1789–99.
2. Practice Committee of the American Society for Reproductive Medicine. Endometriosis and infertility. Fertil Steril. 2004;81:1441–6.
3. Bergqvist A. A comparative study of the acceptability and effect of goserelin and nafarelin on endometriosis. Gynecol Endocrinol. 2000;14:425–32.
4. Rogers PA, D'Hooghe TM, Fazleabas A, Gargett CE, Giudice LC, Montgomery GW, Rombauts L, Salamonsen LA, Zondervan KT. Priorities for endometriosis research: recommendations from an international consensus workshop. Reprod Sci. 2009;16:335–46.
5. Oberhammer F, Wilson JW, Dive C, et al. Apoptotic death in epithelial cells: cleavage of DNA to 300 and/or 50 kb fragments prior to or in the absence of internucleosomal fragmentation. EMBO J. 1993;12:3679–84.
6. White E. Death-defying acts: a meeting review on apoptosis. Genes Dev. 1993;7:2277–84.
7. Osborne BA, Schwartz LM. Essential genes that regulate apoptosis. Trends Cell Biol. 1994;4:394–8.
8. Nagata S, Golstein P. The Fas death factor. Science. 1995;267:1449–56.
9. Beg AA, Baltimore D. An essential role for NF-κB in preventing TNF-α-induced cell death. Science. 1996;274:782–4.
10. Van Antwerp DJ, Martin SJ, Kafri T, Green DR, Verma IM. Suppression of TNF-α-induced apoptosis by NF-κB. Science. 1996;274:787–9.
11. Sattler M, Liang H, Nettesheim D, et al. Structure of Bcl-xL-BaK peptide complex: recognition between regulators of apoptosis. Science. 1997;225:983–6.
12. Harada M, Suganuma N, Furuhashi M, Nagasaka T, Nakashima N, Kikkawa F, Tomoda Y, Furui K. Detection of apoptosis in human endometriotic tissues. Mol Hum Reprod. 1996;2:307–15.

13. Dmowski WP, Gebel H, Braun DP. Decreased apoptosis and sensitivity to macrophage mediated cytolysis of endometrial cells in endometriosis. Hum Reprod Update. 1998;4:696–701.
14. Gebel HM, Braun DP, Tambur A, Frame D, Rana N, Dmowski WP. Spontaneous apoptosis of endometrial tissue is impaired with endometriosis. Fertil Steril. 1998;69:1042–7.
15. Imai A, Takagi A, Tamaya T. Gonadotropin-releasing hormone analog repairs reduced endometrial cell apoptosis in endometriosis in vitro. Am J Obstet Gynecol. 2000;182:1142–6.
16. Selam B, Arici A. Implantation defect in endometriosis: endometrium or peritoneal fluid. J Reprod Fertil Suppl. 2000;55:121–8.
17. Peiro G, Diebold J, Buretton GB, Kimmig R, Lohrs U. Cellular apoptosis susceptibility gene expression in endometrial carcinoma: correlation with Bcl-2, Bax, and Caspase-3 expression and outcome. Int J Gynecol Pathol. 2001;20:359–67.
18. Harada T, Kaponis A, Iwabe T, Taniguchi F, Makrydimas G, Sofikitis N, et al. Apoptosis in human endometrium and endometriosis. Hum Reprod Update. 2004;10:29–38.
19. Nishida M, Nasu K, Ueda T, Fukuda J, Takai N, Miyakawa I. Endometriotic cells are resistant to interferon-γ-induced cell growth inhibition and apoptosis: a possible mechanism involved in the pathogenesis of endometriosis. Mol Hum Reprod. 2005;11:29–34.
20. Dufournet C, Uzan C, Fauvet R, Cortez A, Siffroi J-P, Daria E. Expression of apoptosis-related proteins in peritoneal, ovarian and colorectal endometriosis. J Reprod Immunol. 2006;70:151–62.
21. Izawa M, Harada T, Deura I, Taniguchi F, Iwabe T, Terakawa N. Drug-induced apoptosis was markedly attenuated in endometriotic stromal cells. Hum Reprod. 2006;21:600–4.
22. Klemmt PAB, Carver JG, Kennedy SH, Koninckx PR, Mardon HJ. Stromal cells from endometriotic lesions and endometrium from women with endometriosis have reduced decidualization capacity. Fertil Steril. 2006;85:564–72.
23. Suganuma N, Harada M, Furuhashi M, Nawa A, Kikkawa F. Apoptosis in human and endometriotic tissues. Horm Res. 1997;48:42–7.
24. Jones RK, Searle RF, Bulmer JN. Apoptosis and bcl-2 expression in normal human endometrium, endometriosis and adenomyosis. Hum Reprod. 1998;13:3496–502.
25. Beliard A, Noel A, Foidart J-M. Reduction of apoptosis and proliferation in endometriosis. Fertil Steril. 2004;82:80–5.
26. Taylor HS, Bagot C, Kardana A, Olive D, Arici A. HOX gene expression is altered in the endometrium of women with endometriosis. Hum Reprod. 1999;14:1328–31.
27. Braun DP, Ding J, Shaheen F, Willey JC, Rana N, Dmowski WP. Quantitative expression of apoptosis-regulating genes in endometrium from women with and without endometriosis. Fertil Steril. 2007;87:263–8.
28. Pellegrini C, Gori I, Achtari C, Hornung D, Chardonnens E, Wunder D, Fiche M, Canny GO. The expression of estrogen receptors as well as GREB1, c-MYC, and Cyclin D1, estrogen-regulated genes implicated in proliferation, is increased in peritoneal endometriosis. Fertil Steril. 2012;98:1200–8.
29. Watanabe A, Taniguchi F, Izawa M, Suou K, Uegaki T, Takai E, et al. The role of survivin in the resistance of endometriotic stromal cells to drug-induced apoptosis. Hum Reprod. 2009;24:3172–9.
30. Sakamoto Y, Harada T, Horie S, Iba Y, Taniguchi F, Yoshida S, et al. Tumor necrosis factor-a-induced interleukin-8 (IL-8) expression in endometriotic stromal cells, probably through nuclear factor-κB activation: gonadotropin releasing hormone agonist treatment reduced IL-8 expression. J Clin Endocrinol Metab. 2003;88:730–5.
31. Guo S-W. Nuclear factor-κB (NF-κB): an unsuspected major culprit in the pathogenesis of endometriosis that is still at large? Gynecol Obstet Invest. 2007;63:71–97.
32. Wieser F, Vigne J-L, Ryan I, Hornung D, Djalali S, Taylor RN. Sulindac suppresses nuclear factor-κB activation and RANTES gene and protein expression in endometrial stromal cells from women with endometriosis. J Clin Endocrinol Metab. 2005;90:6441–7.

33. Iba Y, Harada T, Horie S, Deura I, Iwabe T, Terakawa N. Lipopolysaccharide-promoted proliferation of endometriotic stromal cells via induction of tumor necrosis factor a and interleukin-8 expression. Fertil Steril. 2004;82 Suppl 3:1036–42.
34. Yagyu T, Kobayashi H, Matsuzaki H, Wakahara K, Kondo T, Kurita N, et al. Thalidomide inhibits tumor necrosis factor-a-induced interleukin-8 expression in endometriotic stromal cells, possibly through suppression of nuclear factor-κB activation. J Clin Endocrinol Metab. 2005;90:3017–21.
35. Nasu K, Nishida M, Ueda T, Yuge A, Takai N, Narahara H. Application of the selective nuclear factor-κB inhibitor, BAY 11–7085, for the treatment of endometriosis: an in vitro study. Am J Physiol Endocrinol Metab. 2007;293:E16–23.
36. Zhang JJ, Xu ZM, Dai HY, Ji XQ, Duan YY, Zhang CM, et al. Application of the nuclear factor-κB inhibitor pyrrolidine dithiocarbamate for the treatment of endometriosis: an in vitro study. Fertil Steril. 2010;94:2942–4.
37. Zhang HI, Li M, Wang F, Liu S, Li J, Wen Z, et al. Endometriotic epithelial cells induce MMPs expression in endometrial stromal cells via an NFκB-dependent pathway. Gynecol Endocrinol. 2010;26:456–67.
38. Zhang JJ, Xu ZM, Zhang CM, Dai HY, Ji XQ, Wang XF, et al. Pyrrolidine dithiocarbamate inhibits nuclear factor-κB pathway activation and regulates adhesion, migration, invasion and apoptosis of endometriotic stromal cells. Mol Hum Reprod. 2011;17:175–81.
39. Kim JH, Yang YI, Lee KT, Park HJ, Choi JH. Costunolide induces apoptosis in human endometriotic cells through inhibition of the prosurvival Akt and nuclear factor kappa B signaling pathway. Biol Pharm Bull. 2011;34:580–5.
40. Takai E, Taniguchi F, Uegaki T, Iwabe T, Terakawa N, Harada T. Parthenolide reduces cell proliferation and PGE2 synthesis in human endometriotic stromal cells and inhibits development of endometriosis in murine mode. J Endometriosis. 2012;4:165.
41. Huber AV, Saleh L, Prast J, Haslinger P, Knöfler M. Human chorionic gonadotropin attenuates NF-κB activation and cytokine expression of endometriotic stromal cells. Mol Hum Reprod. 2007;13:595–604.
42. Horie S, Harada T, Mitsunari M, Taniguchi F, Iwabe T, Terakawa N. Progesterone and progestational compounds attenuate tumor necrosis factor alpha-induced interleukin-8 production via nuclear factor kappaB inactivation in endometriotic stromal cells. Fertil Steril. 2005;83:1530–5.
43. Gonzalez-Ramos R, Van Langendonckt A, Defrere S, Lousse JC, Mettlen M, Guillet A, Donnez J. Agents blocking the nuclear factor-κB pathway are effective inhibitors of endometriosis in an in vivo experimental model. Gynecol Obstet Invest. 2008;65:174–86.
44. Celik O, Hascalik S, Elter K, Tagluk ME, Gurates B, Aydin NE. Combating endometriosis by blocking proteasome and nuclear factor-κB pathways. Hum Reprod. 2008;23:2458–65.
45. Nisolle M, Donnez J. Peritoneal endometriosis, ovarian endometriosis, and adenomyotic nodules of the rectovaginal septum are three different entities. Fertil Steril. 1997;68:585–96.
46. Matsuzaki S, Canis M, Darcha C, Dechelotte P, Pouly J-L, Bruhat MA. Fibrogenesis in peritoneal endometriosis. Gynecol Obstet Invest. 1998;47:197–9.
47. Bonte H, Chapron C, Vieira M, Fauconnier A, Barakat H, Fritel X, Vacher-Lavenu M-C, Dubuisson J-B. Histologic appearance of endometriosis infiltrating uterosacral ligaments in women with painful symptoms. J Am Assoc Gynecol Laparosc. 2002;9:519–24.
48. Itoga T, Matsumoto T, Takeuchi H, Yamasaki S, Sasahara N, Hoshi T, Kinoshita K. Fibrosis and smooth muscle metaplasia in rectovaginal endometriosis. Pathol Int. 2003;53:371–5.
49. Stovall DW, Anners JA, Halme J. Immunohistochemical detection of type I, III, and IV collagen in endometriotic implants. Fertil Steril. 1992;57:984–9.
50. Anaf V, Simon P, Fayt I, Noel J-C. Smooth muscles are frequent components of endometriotic lesions. Hum Reprod. 2000;15:767–71.
51. Yuge A, Nasu K, Matsumoto H, Nishida M, Narahara H. Collagen gel contractility is enhanced in human endometriotic stromal cells: a possible mechanism underlying the pathogenesis of endometriosis-associated fibrosis. Hum Reprod. 2007;22:938–44.

52. Nasu K, Yuge A, Tsuno A, Narahara H. Mevalonate-Ras homology (Rho)/Rho-associated coiled-coil-forming protein kinase (ROCK)-mediated signaling pathway as a therapeutic target for the treatment of endometriosis-associated fibrosis. Curr Signal Transduct Ther. 2010;5:141–8.
53. Ridley AJ, Hall A. The small GTP-binding protein rho regulates the assembly of focal adhesions and actin stress fibers in response to growth factors. Cell. 1992;70:389–99.
54. Lee T-L, Lin Y-C, Mochitate K, Grinnell F. Stress-relaxation of fibroblasts in collagen matrices triggers ectocytosis of plasma membrane vesicles containing actin, annexins II and VI, and β_1 integrin receptors. J Cell Sci. 1993;105:167–77.
55. Amano M, Mukai H, Ono Y, Chihara K, Matsui T, Hamajima Y, Okawa K, Iwamatsu A, Kaibuchi K. Identification of a putative target for Rho as the serine-threonine kinase protein kinase N. Science. 1996;271:648–50.
56. Kimura K, Ito M, Amano M, Chihara K, Fukata Y, Nakafuku M, Yamamori B, Feng J, Nakano T, Okawa K, Iwamatsu A, Kaibuchi K. Regulation of myosin phosphatase by Rho and Rho-associated kinase (Rho-kinase). Science. 1996;273:245–8.
57. Nakagawa O, Fujisawa K, Ishizaki T, Saito Y, Nakao K, Narumiya S. ROCK-I and ROCK-II, two isoforms of Rho-associated coiled-coil forming protein serine/threonine kinase in mice. FEBS Lett. 1996;39:189–93.
58. Uehata M, Ishizaki T, Satoh H, Ono T, Kawahara T, Morishita T, Tamakawa H, Yamagami K, Inui J, Maekawa M, Narumiya S. Calcium sensitization of smooth muscle mediated by a Rho-associated protein kinase in hypertension. Nature. 1997;389:990–4.
59. Van Aelst L, D'Souza-Schorey C. Rho GTPases and signaling networks. Genes Dev. 1997;11:2295–322.
60. Hall A. Rho GTPases and the actin cytoskeleton. Science. 1998;279:509–14.
61. Park HJ, Galper JB. 3-Hydroxy-3-methylglutaryl CoA reductase inhibitors up-regulate transforming growth factor-beta signaling in cultured heart cells via inhibition of geranylgeranylation of RhoA GTPase. Proc Natl Acad Sci U S A. 1999;96:11525–30.
62. Ravanti L, Heino J, Lopez-Otin C, Kahari VM. Induction of collagenase-3 (MMP-13) expression in human skin fibroblasts by three-dimensional collagen is mediated by p38 mitogen-activated protein kinase. J Biol Chem. 1999;274:2446–55.
63. Ishizaki T, Uehata M, Tamechika I, Keel J, Nonomura K, Maekawa M, Narumiya S. Pharmacological properties of Y-27632, a specific inhibitor of rho-associated kinases. Mol Pharmacol. 2000;57:976–83.
64. Mack CP, Somlyo AV, Hautmann M, Somlyo AP, Owens GK. Smooth muscle differentiation marker gene expression is regulated by RhoA-mediated actin polymerization. J Biol Chem. 2001;276:341–7.
65. Etienne-Manneville S, Hall A. Rho GTPases in cell biology. Nature. 2002;420:629–35.
66. Rosenfeldt H, Grinnell F. Fibroblast quiescence and the disruption of ERK signaling in mechanically unloaded collagen matrices. J Biol Chem. 2000;275:3088–92.
67. Grundstrom G, Mosher DF, Sakai T, Rubin K. Integrin αvβ3 mediates platelet-derived growth factor-BB-stimulated collagen gel contraction in cells expressing signaling deficient integrin α2β1. Exp Cell Res. 2003;291:463–73.
68. Fringer J, Grinnell F. Fibroblast quiescence in floating or released collagen matrices. J Biol Chem. 2001;276:31047–52.
69. Carnevali S, Mio T, Adachi Y, Spurzem JR, Striz I, Romberger DJ, Illig M, Rennard SI. Gamma radiation inhibits fibroblast-mediated collagen gel retraction. Tissue Cell. 2003;35:459–69.
70. Galois L, Hutasse S, Cortial D, Rousseau CF, Grossin L, Ronziere MC, Herbage D, Freyria AM. Bovine chondrocytes behaviour in three-dimensional type I collagen gel in terms of gel contraction, proliferation and gene expression. Biomaterials. 2006;27:79–90.
71. Nasu K, Yuge A, Tsuno A, Narahara H. Simvastatin inhibits the proliferation and the contractility of human endometriotic stromal cells: a promising agent for the treatment of endometriosis. Fertil Steril. 2009;92:2097–9.

72. Tsuno A, Nasu K, Kawano Y, Yuge A, Li H, Abe W, Narahara H. Fasudil inhibits the proliferation and contractility and induces cell cycle arrest and apoptosis of human endometriotic stromal cells: a promising agent for the treatment of endometriosis. J Clin Endocrinol Metab. 2011;96:E1944–52.
73. Nasu K, Tsuno A, Hirao M, Kobayashi H, Yuge A, Narahara H. Heparin is a promising agent for the treatment of endometriosis-associated fibrosis. Fertil Steril. 2010;94:46–51.
74. Molgaard J, Von Schenck H, Olsson AG. Effects of simvastatin on plasma lipid, lipoprotein and apolipoprotein concentrations in hypercholesterolaemia. Eur Heart J. 1988;9:541–51.
75. Hamelin BA, Turgeon J. Hydrophilicity/lipophilicity: relevance for the pharmacology and clinical effects of HMG-CoA reductase inhibitors. Trends Pharmacol. 1998;19:26–37.
76. Davidson M, McKenney J, Stein E, Schrott H, Bakker-Arkema R, Fayyad R, Black D. Comparison of one-year efficacy and safety of atorvastatin versus lovastatin in primary hypercholesterolemia. Atorvastatin Study Group I. Am J Cardiol. 1997;79:1475–81.
77. Goldstein JL, Brown MS. Regulation of the mevalonate pathway. Nature. 1990;343:425–30.
78. Graaf MR, Richel DJ, Van Noorden CJ, Guchelaar HJ. Effects of statins and farnesyltransferase inhibitors on the development and progression of cancer. Cancer Treat Rev. 2004;30:609–41.
79. Casey PJ, Seabra MC. Protein prenyltransferases. J Biol Chem. 1996;271:5289–92.
80. Auer J, Berent R, Weber T, Eber B. Clinical significance of pleiotropic effects of statins: lipid reduction and beyond. Curr Med Chem. 2002;9:1831–50.
81. Menge T, Hartung HP, Stuve O. Statins – a cure-all for the brain? Nat Rev Neurosci. 2005;6:325–31.
82. Esfandiari N, Khazaei M, Ai J, Bielecki R, Gotlieb L, Casper RF. Effect of a statin on an in vitro model of endometriosis. Fertil Steril. 2007;87:257–62.
83. Cakmak H, Basar M, Seval-Celik Y, Osteen KG, Duleba AJ, Taylor HS, Lockwood CJ, Arici A. Statins inhibit monocyte chemotactic protein 1 expression in endometriosis. Reprod Sci. 2012;19:572–9.
84. Sharma I, Dhawan V, Mahajan N, Saha SC, Dhaliwal LK. In vitro effects of atorvastatin on lipopolysaccharide-induced gene expression in endometriotic stromal cells. Fertil Steril. 2010;94:1639–46.
85. Oktem M, Esinler I, Eroglu D, Haberal N, Bayraktar N, Zeyneloglu HB. High-dose atorvastatin causes regression of endometriotic implants: a rat model. Hum Reprod. 2007;22:1474–80.
86. Bruner-Tran KL, Osteen KG, Duleba AJ. Simvastatin protects against the development of endometriosis in a nude mouse model. J Clin Endocrinol Metab. 2009;94:2489–94.
87. Mraiche F, Cena J, Das D, Vollrath B. Effects of statins on vascular function of endothelin-1. Br J Pharmacol. 2005;144:715–26.
88. Ruperez M, Rodrigues-Diez R, Blanco-Colio LM, Sanchez-Lopez E, et al. HMG-CoA reductase inhibitors decrease angiotensin II-induced vascular fibrosis. Role of RhoA/ROCK and MAPK pathways. Hypertension. 2007;50:377–83.
89. Hirsh J, Raschke R, Warrkentin TE, Dalen JE, Deykin D, Poller L. Heparin: mechanism of action, pharmacokinetics, dosing considerations, monitoring, efficacy, and safety. Chest. 1995;108:258–75.
90. Becker RC. Optimizing heparin compounds: a working construct for future antithrombotic drug development. J Thromb Thrombolysis. 2004;18:55–8.
91. Guidry C, Grinnell F. Heparin modulates the organization of hydrated collagen gels and inhibits gel contraction by fibroblasts. J Cell Biol. 1987;104:1097–103.
92. Schaefer T, Roux M, Stuhlsatz HW, Herken R, Coulomb B, Krieg T, Smola H. Glycosaminoglycans modulate cell-matrix interactions of human fibroblasts and endothelial cells in vitro. J Cell Sci. 1996;109:479–88.
93. Goldberg AD, Allis CD, Bernstein E. Epigenetics: a landscape takes shape. Cell. 2007;128:635–8.
94. Turner BM. Cellular memory and the histone code. Cell. 2002;111:285–91.

95. Jaenisch R, Bird A. Epigenetic regulation of gene expression: how the genome integrates intrinsic and environmental signals. Nat Genet. 2003;33(Suppl):245–54.
96. Kouzarides T. Chromatin modifications and their function. Cell. 2007;128:693–705.
97. Bartel DP. MicroRNAs: genomics, biogenesis, mechanism, and function. Cell. 2004;116:281–97.
98. Robertson KD, Wolffe AP. DNA methylation in health and disease. Nat Rev Genet. 2000;1:11–9.
99. Rodenhiser D, Mann M. Epigenetics and human disease: translating basic biology into clinical applications. CMAJ. 2006;174:341–8.
100. Marks PA, Rifkind RA, Richon VM, Breslow R. Inhibitors of histone deacetylase are potentially effective anticancer agents. Clin Cancer Res. 2001;7:759–60.
101. Norton VG, Imai BS, Yau P, Bradbury EM. Histone acetylation reduces nucleosome core particle linking number change. Cell. 1989;57:449–57.
102. Choi CH, Burton ZF, Usheva A. Auto-acetylation of transcription factors as a control mechanism in gene expression. Cell Cycle. 2004;3:114–5.
103. Joseph J, Mudduluru G, Antony S, Vashistha S, Ajitkumar P, Somasundaram K. Expression profiling of sodium butyrate (NaB)-treated cells: identification of regulation of genes related to cytokine signaling and cancer metastasis by NaB. Oncogene. 2004;23:6304–15.
104. Wu Y, Strawn E, Basir Z, Halverson G, Guo SW. Promoter hypermethylation of progesterone receptor isoform B (PR-B) in endometriosis. Epigenetics. 2006;1:106–11.
105. Wu Y, Strawn E, Basir Z, Halverson G, Guo SW. Aberrant expression of deoxyribonucleic acid methyltransferases DNMT1, DNMT3A, and DNMT3B in women with endometriosis. Fertil Steril. 2007;87:24–32.
106. Xue Q, Lin Z, Yin P, Milad MP, Cheng Y-H, Confino E, Reierstad S, Bulun SE. Transcriptional activation of steroidogenic factor-1 by hypomethylation of the 5′ CpG island in endometriosis. J Clin Endocrinol Metab. 2007;92:3261–7.
107. Xue Q, Lin Z, Cheng YH, Huang CC, Marsh E, Yin P, Milad MP, Confino E, Reierstad S, Innes J, Bulun SE. Promoter methylation regulates estrogen receptor 2 in human endometrium and endometriosis. Biol Reprod. 2007;77:681–7.
108. Kawano Y, Nasu K, Li H, Tsuno A, Abe W, Takai N, Narahara H. Application of the histone deacetylase inhibitors for the treatment of endometriosis: histone modifications as pathogenesis and novel therapeutic target. Hum Reprod. 2011;26:2486–98.
109. Nasu K, Kawano Y, Tsukamoto Y, Takano M, Takai N, Li H, Furukawa Y, Abe W, Moriyama M, Narahara H. Aberrant DNA methylation status of endometriosis: epigenetics as the pathogenesis, biomarker and therapeutic target. J Obstet Gynaecol Res. 2011;37:683–95.
110. Abe W, Nasu K, Nakada C, Kawano Y, Moriyama M, Narahara H. miR-196b targets c-myc and Bcl-2 expression, inhibits proliferation and induces apoptosis in endometriotic stromal cells. Hum Reprod. 2013;28:750–61.
111. Richon VM, O'Brien JP. Histone deacetylase inhibitors: a new class of potential therapeutic agents for cancer treatment. Clin Cancer Res. 2002;8:662–4.
112. Verdin E, Dequiedt F, Kasler HG. Class II histone deacetylases: versatile regulators. Trends Genet. 2003;19:286–93.
113. Cameron EE, Bachman KE, Myohanen S, Herman JG, Baylin SB. Synergy of demethylation and histone deacetylase inhibition in the re-expression of genes silenced in cancer. Nat Genet. 1999;21:103–7.
114. Warrener R, Beamish H, Burgess A, Waterhouse NJ, Giles N, Fairlie D, Gabrielli B. Tumor cell-selective cytotoxicity by targeting cell cycle checkpoints. FASEB J. 2003;17:1550–2.
115. Wu Y, Guo SW. Suppression of IL-1β-induced COX-2 expression by trichostatin A (TSA) in human endometrial stromal cells. Eur J Obstet Gynecol Reprod Biol. 2007;135:88–93.
116. Wu Y, Starzinski-Powitz A, Guo SW. Trichostatin A, a histone deacetylase inhibitor, attenuates invasiveness and reactivates E-cadherin expression in immortalized endometriotic cells. Reprod Sci. 2007;14:374–82.

117. Wu Y, Guo SW. Histone deacetylase inhibitors trichostatin A and valproic acid induce cell cycle arrest and p21 expression in immortalized human endometrial stromal cells. Eur J Obstet Gynecol Reprod Biol. 2008;137:198–203.
118. Wu Y, Starzinski-Powitz A, Guo S-W. Prolonged stimulation with tumor necrosis factor-α induced partial methylation at PR-B promoter in immortalized epithelial-like endometriotic cells. Fertil Steril. 2008;90:234–7.
119. Wu Y, Guo SW. Peroxisome proliferator-activated receptor-gamma and retinoid X receptor agonists synergistically suppress proliferation of immortalized endometrial stromal cells. Fertil Steril. 2009;91(Suppl):2142–7.
120. Wu Y, Starzinski-Powitz A, Guo S-W. Constitutive and tumor necrosis factor-alpha-stimulated activation of nuclear factor-kappab in immortalized endometriotic cells and their suppression by trichostatin A. Gynecol Obstet Invest. 2010;70:23–33.
121. Imesch P, Fink D, Fedier A. Romidepsin reduces histone deacetylase activity, induces acetylation of histones, inhibits proliferation, and activates apoptosis in immortalized epithelial endometriotic cells. Fertil Steril. 2010;94:2838–42.
122. Imesch P, Samartzis EP, Schneider M, Fink D, Fedier A. Inhibition of transcription, expression, and secretion of the vascular epithelial growth factor in human epithelial endometriotic cells by romidepsin. Fertil Steril. 2011;95:1579–83.
123. Lu Y, Nie J, Liu X, Zheng Y, Guo SW. Trichostatin A, a histone deacetylase inhibitor, reduces lesion growth and hyperalgesia in experimentally induced endometriosis in mice. Hum Reprod. 2010;25:1014–25.
124. Liu M, Liu X, Zhang Y, Guo SW. Valproic acid and progestin inhibit lesion growth and reduce hyperalgesia in experimentally induced endometriosis in rats. Reprod Sci. 2012;19:360–73.
125. Liu X, Guo SW. A pilot study on the off-label use of valproic acid to treat adenomyosis. Fertil Steril. 2008;89:246–50.

Chapter 17
Altered Biological Characteristics of Eutopic and Ectopic Endometrium

Cássia G.T. Silveira, Admir Agic, Geraldine O. Canny, and Daniela Hornung

Abstract As it has been presented thus far, the pathogenesis of endometriosis is complex and multifactorial. The intrinsic endometrial abnormalities thought to be associated with endometriosis include abnormal gene expression, altered endometrial responses to hormones such as progesterone, impaired immunological response, increased nerve density, and oxidative stress. Also interesting is the fact that such biological alterations have also been observed in the eutopic endometrium of patients with endometriosis, which strongly indicates their critical role in the pathophysiology of the disease. Indeed, it has been suggested that the evaluation of eutopic endometrium is an important line of investigation which may help to achieve a fuller understanding of endometriosis pathogenesis. Hence, we present herein a literature review and a comprehensive evaluation of the involvement of the eutopic endometrium in endometriosis. The biological characteristics of both eutopic and ectopic endometrial tissues as well as their clinical correlations with the disease are highlighted, with the primary objective of understanding the role of the eutopic endometrium in this enigmatic gynecological disorder.

Keywords Apoptosis • Endometrium • Estrogen Signaling • Inflammation • Invasion • L1CAM • YB-1

C.G.T. Silveira
Department of Gynecology and Obstetrics, University of Lübeck, Lübeck, Germany

A. Agic
Department of Gynecology and Obstetrics, Diakonissenkrankenhaus Karlsruhe Rüppurr, Diakonissenstr. 28, 76199 Karlsruhe, Germany

G.O. Canny
Geneva Foundation for Medical Education and Research, Versoix, Switzerland

D. Hornung (✉)
Department of Gynecology and Obstetrics, University of Lübeck, Lübeck, Germany

Department of Gynecology and Obstetrics, Diakonissenkrankenhaus Karlsruhe Rüppurr, Diakonissenstr. 28, 76199 Karlsruhe, Germany
e-mail: D.Hornung@gmx.de

T. Harada (ed.), *Endometriosis: Pathogenesis and Treatment*,
DOI 10.1007/978-4-431-54421-0_17, © Springer Japan 2014

17.1 Introduction

17.1.1 The Biology of Eutopic and Ectopic Endometria

The endometrium is a highly specialized tissue composed of a surface epithelium and associated glands surrounded by a cell-rich connective tissue stroma containing a rich supply of blood vessels. Within the endometrium, two distinct layers can be clearly distinguished: the first layer is the transient superficial functionalis, which comprises the upper-two-thirds of the endometrium and which includes loose stroma and differentiating glands; it is constantly regulated by sequential changes in circulating sex steroid hormones through the menstrual cycle and is shed during menstruation; the second layer is the basalis (germinal layer), which comprises undifferentiated glands embedded in stroma and which is responsible for producing a new functionalis in the subsequent cycle; it is relatively insensitive to hormonal changes persisting from cycle to cycle [1–4].

Remarkably, the human endometrium is a dynamic tissue that undergoes cycles of regeneration (proliferative phase), differentiation (secretory phase), and shedding (menstrual phase) over the reproductive life of women. These successive events of cellular proliferation and differentiation are finely orchestrated by sequential changes in circulating sex steroid hormones across the menstrual cycle, which is also accompanied by significant variations in histological and gene expression profiles [5] and by immune mediators [6].

Prior to ovulation, increasing levels of ovarian estrogens produced in response to follicle-stimulating hormone promotes the reepithelialization of the luminal edge and growth of stromal and glandular components, preparing the tissue for the subsequent secretory transformation of the glands triggered by the post-ovulation production of progesterone. In addition to glandular cell differentiation, progesterone also mediates growth and coiling of spiral arteries, influx of distinct immune cells, and pre-decidualization of stromal compartments. Subsequently, in the absence of implantation and upon steroid hormone withdrawal, the stromal compartment signals the activation of matrix-degrading enzymes to mediate tissue desquamation and endometrial bleeding [7].

The actions of estrogen and progesterone are mediated by specific intracellular and membrane bound receptor proteins in stromal and epithelial endometrial cells [8]. In particular, estrogen-related effects on endometrial cell proliferation and survival are predominantly mediated via estrogen receptor α (ER1) [9], while its isoform β (ER2), expressed at low levels in the endometrium, promotes epithelial differentiation through negative regulation of ER1-mediated responses [10]. In the secretory phase, the antiproliferative effect of progesterone on the endometrial epithelium is mediated via progesterone receptor A (PR-A) [11].

During the menstrual cycle, locally produced growth factors also participate in endometrial regeneration exerting mitogenic effects of estrogen and differentiating effects of progesterone through autocrine and/or paracrine interactions between epithelial and stromal cells. For instance, the synthesis and secretion of transforming growth factor β (TGFβ), epidermal growth factor (EGF) and EGF receptors, as well as insulin-like growth factor-1 (IGF-1) in response to estrogen were shown and associated with endometrial cell proliferation and decidualization. Interestingly, these growth factors are also believed to modulate the effects of estrogen or progesterone or each other by altering growth factor receptor or binding protein expression [12–14].

Indeed, the architecture and function of the endometrium are maintained by the dynamic relationship between epithelial and stromal cells and the complex microenvironment that includes the extracellular matrix (ECM), diffusible growth factors, cytokines, and other paracrine messengers, as well as a variety of other cell types such as endothelial cells, lymphocytes, and macrophages [15, 16]. Thus, it has become evident that the abnormal interactions between these cellular components and their microenvironments may disrupt tissue homeostasis and precede the development of several endometrial pathologies, including endometriosis. So far, numerous studies have pointed out that the onset and progression of endometriosis are potentially supported by the interruption of this well-balanced cellular equilibrium [15, 17–21] potentially resulting from genetic [22] and epigenetic changes [23].

Similar to intrauterine endometrium, ectopic endometrial tissue consists of endometrial-like epithelial and stromal cells although cases of only stromal endometriosis have also been reported [24]. In ectopic loci, such as the peritoneum and ovary, both endometriotic epithelial and stromal cells are functional and respond actively to steroid hormones during the menstrual cycle. On the other hand, endometriotic tissue displays a distinct production of cytokines and prostaglandins, diverse estrogen biosynthesis and metabolic pathways, as well as an altered response to progesterone, e.g., progesterone resistance [25], that seem to favor ectopic endometrial growth and maintenance.

In addition to altered steroid content and metabolism, ectopic endometrium also retains other peculiar characteristics that contribute to disease development. Although peritoneal, ovarian, and rectovaginal endometriotic lesions are considered distinct entities with a different pathogenesis [26–28], a general consensus exists regarding the critical role of the cross talk between endometriotic cells, host peritoneum and infiltrating leukocytes, endothelial cells, and fibroblasts. This all appears to support the development of the disease [16].

17.1.2 Eutopic Endometrium in Endometriosis: Villain or Victim?

Although a number of studies have been focused on elucidating the etiology of endometriosis, a unifying theory regarding its origin has remained elusive. Instead, several theories have emerged to account for the disparate observations regarding the pathogenesis, and these can generally be categorized as those suggesting that implants originate from uterine endometrium and those proposing that implants arise from tissues or cells other than the uterus. Intrinsic to these theories are inciting factors (i.e., immune, endocrine, and environmental factors) and genetic susceptibilities whose roles are beginning to be delineated, although they are still insufficient to fully explain the cause and development of disease. For instance, acquired genomic alterations and several physiological changes were shown to represent a potential source for a conferred proliferation and survival advantage to endometriotic implants [29].

In this context, the potential involvement of eutopic endometrium seems to be particularly critical in the pathogenesis of endometriosis, evinced by Sampson's retrograde menstruation theory in 1921 [30], the most widely accepted hypothesis, which nonetheless does not fully explain the etiology. In accordance with this theory, it is presumed that the establishment of endometrial cells from refluxed menses in ectopic sites is supported by the following characteristics: (a) the endometrial debris, including both epithelial and stromal cells, must exist in the reflux menses; (b) these two cellular components must be viable and able to evade immune attack within the pelvic cavity; (c) both epithelial and stromal cells must have the potential ability to attach and implant into the pelvic mesothelium; and (d) ultimately, once implanted at an ectopic location, endometriotic cells must be able to survive and develop a neovascular system [31]. Indeed, the link between altered eutopic endometrium and the risk for developing endometriosis may possibly justify the morbidity of the disease in only 10–15 % of the women with menstrual reflux [32, 33] and at least partially explain the high rate of recurrence after medical and/or surgical treatment [34].

In fact, important functional and biochemical differences between eutopic endometrium of women with and without endometriosis have been reported in the literature [35, 36]. In particular, a large number of differentially expressed gene transcripts, miRNAs, and proteins have been detected and they appear to mostly encode molecular signals mediating cross talk between epithelial and stromal cells, cell proliferation, differentiation and survival, as well as endometrial receptivity [37–43]. For instance, aberrant production of cytokines, growth and angiogenic factors, different steroid receptor expression and signaling, and abnormal expression of specific cancer-related genes presented in eutopic endometrial cells are thought to predispose to growth and survival of endometrial foci outside the uterus and to produce disease-related symptoms such as reduced fertility and implantation failures.

The role of the eutopic endometrium as a major and active contributor for the development of endometriotic lesions has also been supported by the accumulating evidence implying the involvement of stem cells. Stem cells are rare undifferentiated cells characterized by high proliferative, self-renewal, and differentiation potential that are present in virtually all adult tissues and organs [44]. The presence of aberrant stem cells has been associated with the pathogenesis of several tumors and proliferative disorders in female reproductive organs [45]. As thoroughly addressed in Chap. 4, endometrium-derived stem/progenitor cells residing in the basalis and/or functionalis have been suggested to reach the peritoneal cavity via menstrual reflux or lymphovascular dissemination and establish endometriotic implants [46, 47].

Bearing in mind that the eutopic endometrium of women with endometriosis shows a wide variety of anomalies both in the tissue architecture and biochemistry and this tissue being a potential source of endometrial stem cells, it is plausible that the primary defect in endometriosis may be the eutopic endometrium [48–50]. Nevertheless, it is becoming increasingly apparent that interplay between eutopic endometrium and endometriotic lesions is more complex than abnormal eutopic endometrium resulting in establishment of endometriotic lesions [51]. In addition to critical interactions between shed endometrial fragments and peritoneum (i.e., peritoneal mesothelium and environment) during lesion establishment [16, 52], it is likely that the biology of eutopic endometrium is altered in response to the presence of endometriotic lesions as it has currently been demonstrated in in vivo models of endometriosis [51].

So far, the abnormalities described in endometriotic endometrium and suggested to predispose to endometriosis were in fact identified when the disease was already present, thus making it difficult to define whether these endometrial changes are a cause or an effect of endometriosis. Alternatively, by using mouse and non-primate models with no previous history of disease, it was possible to evaluate the endometrium before and after induction of endometriosis and to obtain strong evidence that the presence of endometriotic lesions directly influences the endometrial environment.

In particular, data obtained from baboon models of experimentally induced endometriosis indicate that a complex series of changes in endometrial gene and protein expression occurs at different time points during disease progression [53, 54], potentially as a result of epigenetic modifications triggered in the presence of ectopic lesions [55]. Similar to anomalies in eutopic endometrium of women with endometriosis, collective findings in this model show a local increase in proliferation and angiogenesis and a significant alteration in steroid hormone receptor distribution and signaling with an evident progesterone resistance [53, 54, 56–60]. Moreover, it has recently been demonstrated in a mouse model of endometriosis that cells from endometriotic lesions can migrate to and preferentially populate the endometrial basal layer, thus further supporting the bidirectional interaction between eutopic and ectopic endometrial tissue [61].

In women with endometriosis, the effects of ectopic lesions on eutopic endometrium remain uncertain, and due to a range of reasons (mainly ethics-related issues), this relationship is extremely difficult to study. However, the interaction between lesions and eutopic endometrium is likely to occur and contribute to both endometriosis establishment and progression. From animal model data, it is speculated that the interconnecting roles of the vascular, lymphatic, and nervous systems in both the uterine and peritoneal environments with concurrent participation of eutopic endometrium, ovarian steroids, and inflammatory mediators may favor the development of endometriosis and its associated symptoms. A hypothesized pathway has been suggested [51].

17.2 Eutopic and Ectopic Endometria: Similarities and Dissimilarities

As addressed above, eutopic endometrium of endometriosis patients retains several abnormalities that in fact resemble the biological characteristics found in ectopic endometrial tissues such as augmented proliferation, aromatase activity, unusual cytokine expression, decreased apoptosis, as well as altered local hormone metabolism [62, 63].

Although the morphological appearance of endometriotic implants may reflect that of eutopic endometrium, these similarities are often only limited. Indeed, a variety of investigations have also revealed important differences between eutopic and ectopic endometria involving cell structure, gene expression, and responsiveness of various proteins [16, 63–68].

Morphologically, both endometriotic glandular and stromal cells retain ultrastructural features that are recognizably different from those of eutopic endometrium of patients with endometriosis. In contrast to eutopic tissue, endometriotic tissue was shown to encompass a wide range of morphological development from poorly to highly differentiated glands [69]. Interestingly, such variations were detected not only from gland to gland but also within the same gland. Moreover, while complete proliferative development has been detected in some endometriosis patients, full secretory transformation seems to frequently be absent in ectopic implants [69]. Additionally, the comparative observations of Yu et al. [70] of eutopic and ectopic endometrial cells cultured in vitro described an enlarged nucleus and manifold chromatin in endometriotic glandular cells, whereas endometriotic stromal cells appeared to be smaller and characterized by many tiny villi and protuberances on the plasma membrane.

Apart from morphological features, the dissimilarities between endometriotic lesions and eutopic endometrium are even more evident at the molecular level. With the advent of microarray-based technologies, several investigators were able to explore the distinct pattern of gene expression in eutopic and ectopic endometrium. Large-scale transcriptional profiling analyses using microarrays are widely employed for analyzing the expression of thousands of genes simultaneously in a single experiment supported by the availability of the complete nucleotide sequence of the human genome. Microarray studies provide extremely important information enabling a better understanding of the etiology and pathophysiology of a variety of diseases and the development of new diagnostic and therapeutic strategies [71, 72].

To date, a considerable number of studies comparing the global expression profiles of paired eutopic endometrium and endometriosis specimens have been published although the data available in the public domain is still restricted and occasionally divergent. In fact, it is important to note that some discrepancies may be a result of the potential impact of one or more factors such as demographic characteristics, site of endometriosis, fertility history, severity of stages, and phases of the menstrual cycle that were not fully considered in most studies despite their well-known influences on gene expression in eutopic and ectopic tissues [73–75].

In spite of these limitations, significant and interesting findings have been provided by microarray-based analyses of eutopic and ectopic endometrium which have been confirmed by subsequent investigations using other conventional and sophisticated methodologies. Collectively, these published data highlight differences in the expression of gene-encoding proteins involved in multiple biological process and hypothesized to be responsible for the establishment of ectopic endometrial implants, including cell adhesion, extracellular matrix remodeling, migration, proliferation, apoptosis, immune system regulation, inflammatory pathways, sex hormone-related signaling and neuroangiogenesis [16, 64–68, 75] that will be thoroughly addressed in the following sections.

Also noteworthy are the observations on the differential expression pattern of microRNAs (miRNAs) in ectopic versus eutopic endometrium [76, 77]. miRNAs are small noncoding RNA molecules that have a critical role in posttranscriptional regulation of gene expression by repression of target mRNA translation. A relatively recent microarray-based investigation in paired eutopic and ectopic endometria has identified more than 80 differentially expressed miRNAs. Interestingly, most of them are predicted to regulate a large fraction of protein-coding genes associated with genetic (i.e., cancer) and immunological disorders and involved in cellular growth and proliferation, apoptosis, cellular movement, cell-mediated immune response, cell-to-cell signaling and interaction, as well as gene expression regulation [78].

Evidence for molecular abnormalities in eutopic and ectopic endometria has also been revealed through proteomic approaches. In particular, large-scale proteomic studies including mass spectrometry and protein microarray-based technologies have enabled the simultaneous evaluation of several hundred proteins in eutopic and ectopic endometrium as well as biological fluids and provided valuable information regarding their expression pattern, functions, localization, posttranslational modifications, and interactions [79]. Investigations focusing on the comparative proteomic analysis of paired eutopic and ectopic endometrial tissues are still limited although they are currently gaining more attention. For instance, a recent study combining two-dimensional electrophoresis and mass spectrometry demonstrated a remarkable difference in the protein repertoire of endometriotic lesions compared with its uterine counterpart [80]. Interestingly, significant differences comprised proteins primarily involved in cellular spreading and attachment, cell homeostasis and survival, mRNA processing and transport, immune response, and protein trafficking [80].

In addition to differences between eutopic and ectopic endometrium, increasing evidence in the literature has also suggested that the biological characteristics of endometriotic cells might differ between different forms of endometriosis [28, 81]. These findings may possibly account for the high heterogeneity observed in endometriosis pathogenesis and disease-related symptoms and imply that a single universal treatment is perhaps not effective for all forms of endometriosis.

17.3 Endometrial Cell Proliferation, Survival, and Invasion

Endometriosis could result from increased cellular proliferation or decreased apoptosis in response to appropriate stimuli. Eutopic endometrium from women with endometriosis has several differences compared with normal endometrium of women without endometriosis. These differences may contribute to the survival of retrograded endometrial cells into the peritoneal cavity and thus to the development of endometriosis.

Nearly all women of reproductive age exhibit some degree of endometrial debris reflux [82]. Menstrual effluent retrogradely shed into the peritoneal cavity was observed to contain viable endometrial cells [83–87]. Summarizing previous knowledge of the disease, Vinatier et al. [88] presented two theories to explain why only some patients develop the disease. The first theory is based on disorders of the ectopic endometrial tissue whereby it resists normal peritoneal "cleaning." The second suggests that the disease is secondary to abnormalities of cellular and humoral immunity, which induces excessive receptivity of the peritoneal mesothelium, hyperactivated macrophages, and NK cell abnormalities. Mediators in the peritoneal environment may alter a genetically predisposed endometrium which then exhibits increased invasion. It is also possible that an excess of refluxed endometrium or altered endometrium has the potential to contribute to the development of a proinflammatory environment favorable to disease establishment [88].

17.3.1 Apoptosis in Endometriosis

Accumulating evidence suggests that endometrial cells from women with and without endometriosis exhibit fundamental differences in their apoptotic capacity. Endometrial cells from women with endometriosis have enhanced proliferation and an increased ability to implant and survive in ectopic locations. Impaired sensitivity of endometrial tissue to spontaneous apoptosis contributes to the abnormal implantation and growth of endometrium at ectopic sites.

The inability of endometrial cells to transmit a "death" signal or their ability to avoid cell death is associated with increased expression of anti-apoptotic factors (Bcl-2) and decreased expression of pre-apoptotic factors (BAX) [89]. However, it remains unclear whether abnormal apoptosis in the eutopic endometrium from patients with endometriosis is a primary or a secondary process after establishment of the pelvic endometriosis process. This could be attributed to the fact that at the time of clinical presentation and diagnosis, most women already have established disease and, therefore, it is difficult to investigate the early developmental stages of endometriosis.

Reflux of endometrial fragments during menstruation into the peritoneal cavity is a common phenomenon. Under normal conditions, cells which do not adhere to their extracellular matrix enter apoptosis as they receive different signals from their adhesion receptors [90]. However, in women with endometriosis, these cells have the ability to adhere to mesothelial cells of the peritoneum, proliferate, and induce neoangiogenesis resulting in the development of active endometriotic implants. The effect of MMPs on apoptotic factors and their regulation by steroid hormones may provide a link between endometrial turnover and the invasive process necessary for the development of disease.

Recent studies from González-Ramos et al. [91, 92] showed constitutive NF-κB activation in peritoneal endometriosis. They reported that the NF-κB pathway is implicated in the development of endometriotic lesions in vivo and that NF-κB inhibition reduces intracellular adhesion molecule-1 expression and cell proliferation, but increases apoptosis of endometriotic lesions, diminishing the initial development of endometriosis in an animal model. This and other observations support the notion that endometriosis is characterized by persistent inflammation and proliferation.

Murk et al. [93] described extracellular signal-regulated kinase (ERK1/2) activity in human endometrium. ERK1/2 plays key intracellular roles in activating cellular survival and differentiation processes. The authors found that ERK1/2-mediated steroid inhibition in endometrial stromal cells reduced proliferation and increased apoptosis. They suggested that abnormally high levels of ERK1/2 activity may be involved in endometriosis, possibly by stimulating endometrial cell survival.

Some studies have suggested that genetic factors are likely to influence individual susceptibility to endometriosis. Genetic alterations in somatic chromosomes [94] and DNA deletions that inactivate some tumor suppressor genes (e.g. PTEN) are likely to be involved in the initiation, persistence, and progression of endometriosis [95, 96].

cDNA microarray analysis provided an interesting insight into altered gene expression profiles in endometriosis patients. Using this method, Arimoto et al. [37] found 97 upregulated and 337 downregulated genes in women with endometriosis. Genes related to apoptosis (GADD34, GADD45A, GADD45B, PIG11) and the tumor suppressor TP53 gene were downregulated in endometriotic tissues. On the other hand, Eyster et al. [66] found that only a few genes in apoptosis resistance pathways were differentially expressed in endometriosis cells compared to normal endometrial cells. They suggested that the presence of ligands to activate the apoptotic pathway or the apoptosis resistance pathways may be more important than whether specific members of the pathway are over- or underexpressed.

Braun et al. [97] demonstrated that the transcript abundance ratio of anti-apoptotic to pro-apoptotic isoforms of the Bcl-X gene favors survival in eutopic and ectopic endometrial cells from women with endometriosis, but not control endometrial cells. This was found throughout the menstrual cycle for ectopic endometrial cells. Eutopic but not ectopic endometrial cells also expressed increased transcript abundance of the anti-apoptotic DAD-1 gene in endometriosis. Eutopic and ectopic endometrial cells from women with endometriosis expressed decreased transcript abundance of p53 and caspase-1 compared to endometrial cells from women without endometriosis. Dysregulation of pro- and anti-apoptotic regulatory gene expression characterized eutopic and ectopic endometrial cells from women with endometriosis, consistent with apoptotic resistance and enhanced survival of endometrial cells in endometriosis. This data should provide useful information for finding candidate genes whose products might regulate the apoptotic machinery in endometriosis and, additionally, could serve as molecular targets for diagnosis or treatment of endometriosis.

Othman et al. [98] reported that mutants of estrogen receptor genes delivered to endometriotic cells via an adenovirus vector (Ad-DNER) decreased cell proliferation, induced apoptosis, and decreased cytokine production. The authors suggested that adenovirus-mediated gene therapy may represent a potential therapeutic option for endometriosis in the future.

17.3.2 Invasion in Endometriosis

Endometriosis is a benign and frequently progressive disease with a high prevalence in the female population of reproductive age. Nevertheless, endometriosis shows behavior similar to malignant tumors. Deep invasion in different tissues such as the peritoneum, ovary, and intestines is presumably occurs as a result of migrating epithelial and stromal cells of modified endometrium adhering to distant tissues [99]. Endometriotic cells are capable of attaching to the peritoneal mesothelium, breaking the peritoneal lining, and destroying ECM, thereby invading surrounding tissue.

Endometriosis is associated with an increased risk for several types of malignant diseases [100, 101]. Especially the endometrioid subtype of ovarian cancer has a high probability for developing on the basis of existing endometriosis [102–105]. Like malignancy, endometriosis displays features of atypia, adherence, invasion, and metastases. The risk of direct malignant transformation of ovarian endometriosis has been estimated as 0.7–1.6 % over an average of 8 years.

Among several investigated potential invasion markers, two proteins, YB-1 and L1CAM, seem to have very important roles in the progression of endometriosis.

17.3.2.1 Cold Shock Domain Family Member YB-1 Expression in Endometrium and Endometriosis

The Y-box binding protein YB-1, an evolutionarily conserved 48 kDa protein, belongs to the superfamily of cold shock domain proteins with pleiotropic biological functions. Eukaryotic YB proteins are involved in the regulation of DNA transcription and repair, in translational control of protein synthesis, as well as in cellular responses to a wide variety of stressors [106–108].

The YB-1 protein is highly expressed in a number of malignant diseases, and it seems to promote tumor growth and multidrug resistance [109] through the induction of specific growth factors [110–113].

Based on multiple biological functions of YB-1 and its close association with tumorigenesis, YB-1 expression in human endometrium, ovarian endometriosis, and peritoneal macrophages was investigated [114]. YB-1 gene and protein expression was significantly higher in ovarian lesions, eutopic endometrium, and peritoneal macrophages of patients with endometriosis in comparison to the control group. Interestingly, the strongest YB-1 expression was observed in the epithelial compartment of endometrial tissues. In the 12Z endometriotic epithelial cell line, YB-1 knockdown resulted in significant cell growth inhibitory effects including reduced cell proliferation and increased spontaneous and TNFα-induced apoptosis rate. Significantly higher RANTES (regulated upon activation, normal T cell expressed and secreted chemokine) expression and decreased cell invasion in vitro were also associated with YB-1 inactivation. Elevated YB-1 expression seems to have an impact on the development and progression of endometriosis [114].

17.3.2.2 L1 Cell Adhesion Molecule (L1CAM) as a Pathogenic Factor in Endometriosis

L1 cell adhesion molecule (L1CAM, CD171) is a type I transmembrane glycoprotein (200–220 kDa) which belongs to the immunoglobulin superfamily [115]. Initial studies showed that L1CAM plays an important role in the development of the nervous system [115–117] and have implicated L1CAM also in the ontogeny of human tumors including melanomas, neural tumors, renal carcinomas, colon carcinoma, and endometrial and ovarian carcinomas [118–121]. The expression of L1CAM in carcinomas augments dissemination of tumor cells by enabling cell migration and invasion [122–124].

Given the role of L1 in endometrial and ovarian carcinomas, L1CAM was also investigated as a pathogenetic factor in endometriosis [125].

L1CAM was found present in endometriotic tissue of women with endometriosis and increased at gene and protein levels using short-term cultures of endometriosis lesions. A significantly higher expression of L1CAM Significantly higher L1CAM expression in the epithelial cell fraction in rAFS stages III and IV (AFS 1997) of endometriosis was found. The nerve growth-promoting activity of the conditioned medium of endometrial epithelial cell cultures from women with endometriosis was studied using a chicken ganglion assay. The conditioned medium of endometrial epithelial cell cultures from patients with endometriosis stimulated strong neurite growth which was blocked by co-incubation with anti-L1-mAb in a dose-dependent fashion [125].

17.4 Estrogen-Related Signaling and Progesterone Resistance in Endometrium and Endometriotic Lesions

It is well known that endometriosis is a hormone-responsive disease and that disease progression is inhibited by an antiestrogenic environment. In postmenopausal women undergoing in vitro fertilization with donor eggs, the exogenous administration of only estradiol (E2) and progesterone is sufficient to prepare the endometrium for implantation in the absence of ovarian function. This observation underscores the essential roles of these steroids in uterine physiology. Indeed, both E2 and progesterone are master regulators of endometrial tissue [25]. Each hormone is estimated to regulate expression of hundreds of genes during various phases of the menstrual cycle [126]. Endometriotic and eutopic endometrial tissues respond to E2 and progesterone with apparently similar histological changes, and both tissues contain immunoreactive ERs and PRs. The eutopic endometrium predictably becomes atrophic in response to prolonged progestin therapy or oral contraceptives that contain progestins. Treatment with these agents, however, does not predictably suppress endometriotic tissue growth. Endometriotic tissue in ectopic locations, such as the peritoneum or ovary, is fundamentally different from eutopic endometrium within the uterus in terms of production of cytokine and prostaglandin production, estrogen biosynthesis and metabolism, and clinical response to progestins [127–129].

17.4.1 Estrogen Action in the Endometrium and Endometriosis

Both circumstantial and laboratory evidence strongly supports the notion that estrogen is an extremely strong mitogen for endometriotic tissue. The biologically active estrogen 17 beta estradiol (E2), which is secreted by the ovary or locally produced by in endometriotic tissue, acts as a classical steroid hormone to regulate growth of endometrial or endometriotic tissue. E2 enters cells and binds to the ER in estrogen-responsive cells. ER subtypes α and β are proteins with high affinity for E2 and are encoded by separate genes. The classical human ERα was cloned in 1986, and a second estrogen receptor, ERβ, was cloned from rat prostate and human testis in 1996 [130–132]. Although both ERα and ERβ are present in the endometrium, ERα seems to be the primary mediator of estrogenic action in this tissue [133]. Studies using ERα-deficient mice have revealed the central role of this receptor in reproductive function, at all levels of the hypothalamic–pituitary–gonadal axis [134]. Despite its sensitivity to estrogen, endometriosis appears to have an altered steroid hormone receptor profile compared with that of its normal tissue counterpart, the eutopic endometrium. For example, several investigators reported markedly higher levels of ERβ and lower levels of ERα in human endometriotic tissues and primary stromal cells compared with eutopic endometrial tissues and cells [56, 135, 136]. Moreover, the levels of both isoforms of PR, particularly PR-B, are significantly lower in endometriosis compared with eutopic endometrium [137, 138].

The E2-receptor complex acts as a transcription factor that becomes associated with the promoters of E2-responsive genes via direct DNA binding or binding to other docking transcription factors at basal promoter regions [139]. This interaction brings about ER-specific initiation of gene transcription, which promotes the synthesis of specific mRNAs and proteins [139]. PR is one of many E2-responsive genes, and E2 acts in eutopic endometrial tissues and stromal cells to promote endometrial responsiveness to progesterone [140]. In contrast, PR mRNA and protein levels are not elevated in biopsied endometriotic tissues exposed to high E2 levels during late proliferative phase or in endometriotic cells treated with E2, indicating that E2 induction of PR expression in endometriosis is markedly blunted [138].

17.4.2 Progesterone Resistance in Eutopic Endometrium and Endometriotic Lesions

E2 is the best-defined mitogen for growth and inflammation processes in ectopic endometriotic tissue that commonly resides on pelvic organs. Progesterone and progestins may relieve pain by limiting growth and inflammation in endometriosis, but some patients with pelvic pain do not respond to treatment with progestins. Moreover, progesterone-induced molecular changes in eutopic endometrial tissue of women with endometriosis are either blunted or undetectable. These in vivo observations are indicative of resistance to progesterone action in endometriosis. The molecular basis of progesterone resistance in endometriosis may be related to an overall reduction in levels of progesterone receptors (PRs) and the lack of the PR isoform progesterone receptor B (PR-B). In normal endometrium, progesterone acts on stromal cells to induce secretion of paracrine factor(s). These unknown factor(s) act on neighboring epithelial cells to induce the expression of the enzyme 17β-hydroxysteroid dehydrogenase type 2 (17β-HSD-2), which metabolizes E2 to the less active estrone (E1). In endometriotic tissue, progesterone does not induce epithelial 17β-HSD-2 expression due to a stromal cell defect. The inability of endometriotic stromal cells to produce progesterone-induced paracrine factors that stimulate 17β-HSD-2 may be due to the lack of PR-B and very low levels of progesterone receptor A (PR-A) observed in vivo in endometriotic tissue. The end result is deficient E2 metabolism in endometriosis giving rise to high local concentrations of this mitogen [137].

Other mechanisms proposed to explain progesterone resistance are altered expression or function of chaperone proteins like FKBP52 [141] and co-regulators such as HIC-5/ARA55 [142].

PR is a target gene of ERα in several cell types including breast cancer epithelial cells. ERα mediates E2-induced PR expression. It has been reported that two distinct E2-regulated promoters generate transcripts encoding two functionally different human PR isoforms, PR-A and PR-B [143]. Previous studies have demonstrated that maximal PR mRNA and protein levels are reached after human breast cancer cells have been exposed to E2 for 3 days [144–146]. Two major transcriptional start sites have been identified. The upstream transcription start site gives rise to a full-length mRNA species that encodes the PR-B protein. Another mRNA species with a further downstream transcription initiation site gives rise to the truncated PR-A form. Despite the fact that both proposed PR promoter sequences are E2 responsive, neither contains a classical palindromic ERE sequence [147]. Several nonclassic regulatory elements (e.g., AP1, Sp1) in the human PR promoter have been reported. These sites have been shown to bind ERα and on one occasion ERβ [140, 147–155]. Bulun et al. speculate that a critical level of ERα may be necessary for E2-dependent induction of PR in endometrial stromal cells. The occupancy of the PR promoter regions with varying ratios of ERα to ERβ may be critical in determining the effect of E2 on PR expression. A strikingly lower ERα-to-ERβ ratio in endometriotic stromal cells may be responsible for a shift from E2 stimulation to E2 inhibition of PR expression in endometriotic stromal cells [25].

17.5 The Inflammatory Response in Eutopic and Ectopic Endometria

The immune status has been suggested to play an important role in both initiation and progression of endometriosis. T and B lymphocytes and natural killer cells seem to play essential roles in determining if endometrial and endometriotic cells accept or reject survival, implantation, and proliferation [156, 157]. Several studies have shown a reduced activity of cytotoxic T cells and NK cells, cytokine secretion by helper T cells, and autoantibody production by B lymphocytes in women with endometriosis [156–158]. As alluded to in a previous section, NF-κB transcriptional activity modulates inflammatory key cell processes contributing to the initiation and progression of endometriosis [159]. It has further been shown that immune–endocrine interactions are likely to be involved in the pathogenesis of endometriosis.

Endometriosis is associated with an increased inflammatory activity, as seen by elevated serum levels of inflammatory markers such as CA-125 [160] and C-reactive protein [161]. Changes in peritoneal fluid inflammatory markers of peritoneal fluid have also been observed in women with endometriosis [162]. The generalized inflammatory activity may lead to more generalized clinical effects where some women with endometriosis suffer from fever and a general feeling of sickness, especially AT times when they experience more pain.

17.6 Neurogenesis in Endometrial and Endometriotic Tissue

Recent evidence indicates that ectopic endometriotic implants recruit their own unique neural and vascular supplies through neuroangiogenesis. It is believed that these nascent nerve fibers in endometriotic implants influence dorsal root neurons within the central nervous system, increasing pain perception in patients [163].

Several studies have suggested that endometrial biopsies with the detection of nerve fibers provide a reliability of diagnosing endometriosis [164, 165]. Newer studies however were not able to demonstrate any differences in the amount of nerve fibers or neuronal markers in endometrium of women with endometriosis compared to women without endometriosis. The neuronal markers, PGP9.5, NGFp75, and VR1, are expressed in the endometrium at levels that do not differ between women with and without endometriosis [166].

Endometrial functional layer nerve fibers were identified in 22 % of biopsies overall including 19 % of cases with histologically confirmed peritoneal endometriosis and 29 % of cases without endometriosis. There was no correlation between the presence of functional layer nerve fibers and the presenting symptoms, endometrial histology, or current hormonal therapy. Endometrial functional layer nerve fibers assessment performed using standard immunohistochemical techniques on routine biopsy specimens proved neither sensitive nor specific for the diagnosis of endometriosis [167]. In conclusion, much rigorous research to better understanding this complex pathology and to find specific and sensitive biomarkers remains to be done.

References

1. Ferenczy A, Bertrand G, Gelfand MM. Proliferation kinetics of human endometrium during the normal menstrual cycle. Am J Obstet Gynecol. 1979;133(8):859–67.
2. Padykula HA. Regeneration in the primate uterus: the role of stem cells. Ann N Y Acad Sci. 1991;622:47–56.
3. Brenner RM, Slayden OD, Rodgers WH, et al. Immunocytochemical assessment of mitotic activity with an antibody to phosphorylated histone H3 in the macaque and human endometrium. Hum Reprod. 2003;18(6):1185–93.
4. Slayden OD, Brenner RM. Hormonal regulation and localization of estrogen, progestin and androgen receptors in the endometrium of nonhuman primates: effects of progesterone receptor antagonists. Arch Histol Cytol. 2004;67:393–409.
5. Ponnampalam AP, Weston GC, Trajstman AC, et al. Molecular classification of human endometrial cycle stages by transcriptional profiling. Mol Hum Reprod. 2004;10(12):879–93.
6. Thiruchelvam U, Dransfield I, Saunders PT, et al. The importance of the macrophage within the human endometrium. J Leukoc Biol. 2013;93(2):217–25.
7. Giudice LC, Irwin JC. Roles of the insulin-like growth factor family in nonpregnant human endometrium and at the decidual: trophoblast interface. Semin Reprod Endocrinol. 1999;17 (1):13–21.

8. Healy DL, Hodgen GD. The endocrinology of human endometrium. Obstet Gynecol Surv. 1983;38(8):509–30.
9. Couse JF, Korach KS. Estrogen receptor null mice: what have we learned and where will they lead us? Endocr Rev. 1999;20(3):358–417.
10. Wada-Hiraike O, Imamov O, Hiraike H, et al. Role of estrogen receptor beta in colonic epithelium. Proc Natl Acad Sci U S A. 2006;103(8):2959–64.
11. Conneely OM, Mulac-Jericevic B, Lydon JP, et al. Reproductive functions of the progesterone receptor isoforms: lessons from knock-out mice. Mol Cell Endocrinol. 2001;179:97–103.
12. Giudice LC. Growth factors and growth modulators in human uterine endometrium: their potential relevance to reproductive medicine. Fertil Steril. 1994;61(1):1–17.
13. Smith CL. Cross-talk between peptide growth factor and estrogen receptor signaling pathways. Biol Reprod. 1998;58:627–32.
14. Gargett CE, Chan RW, Schwab KE. Hormone and growth factor signaling in endometrial renewal: role of stem/progenitor cells. Mol Cell Endocrinol. 2008;288(1–2):22–9.
15. Arnold JT, Kaufman DG, Seppälä M, et al. Endometrial stromal cells regulate epithelial cell growth in vitro: a new co-culture model. Hum Reprod. 2001;16(5):836–45.
16. Hull ML, Escareno CR, Godsland JM, et al. Endometrial-peritoneal interactions during endometriotic lesion establishment. Am J Pathol. 2008;173(3):700–15.
17. Donjacour AA, Cunha GR. Stromal regulation of epithelial function. Cancer Treat Res. 1991;53:335–64.
18. Cooke PS, Buchanan DL, Young P, et al. Stromal estrogen receptors mediate mitogenic effects of estradiol on uterine epithelium. Proc Natl Acad Sci U S A. 1997;94(12):6535–40.
19. Witz CA. Pathogenesis of endometriosis. Gynecol Obstet Invest. 2002;53:52–62.
20. Griffith JS, Rodgers AK, Schenken RS. Reviews: in vitro models to study the pathogenesis of endometriosis. Reprod Sci. 2010;17(1):5–12.
21. Zhang H, Li M, Zheng X, et al. Endometriotic stromal cells lose the ability to regulate cell-survival signaling in endometrial epithelial cells in vitro. Mol Hum Reprod. 2009;15 (10):653–63.
22. Silveira CG, Abrão MS, Dias Jr JA, et al. Common chromosomal imbalances and stemness-related protein expression markers in endometriotic lesions from different anatomical sites: the potential role of stem cells. Hum Reprod. 2012;27(11):3187–97.
23. Guo SW. Epigenetics of endometriosis. Mol Hum Reprod. 2009;15(10):587–607.
24. Clement PB, Young RH, Scully RE. Stromal endometriosis of the uterine cervix. A variant of endometriosis that may simulate a sarcoma. Am J Surg Pathol. 1990;14(5):449–55.
25. Bulun SE, Cheng YH, Pavone ME, et al. Estrogen receptor-beta, estrogen receptor-alpha, and progesterone resistance in endometriosis. Semin Reprod Med. 2010;28(1):36–43.
26. Donnez J, Nisolle M, Smoes P, et al. Peritoneal endometriosis and "endometriotic" nodules of the rectovaginal septum are two different entities. Fertil Steril. 1996;66(3):362–8.
27. Nisolle M, Donnez J. Progesterone receptors (PR) in ectopic endometrium? Fertil Steril. 1997;68(5):943–4.
28. Matsuzaki S, Maleysson E, Darcha C. Analysis of matrix metalloproteinase-7 expression in eutopic and ectopic endometrium samples from patients with different forms of endometriosis. Hum Reprod. 2010;25(3):742–50.
29. Burney RO, Giudice LC. Pathogenesis and pathophysiology of endometriosis. Fertil Steril. 2012;98(3):511–9.
30. Sampson JA. Metastatic or embolic endometriosis, due to the menstrual dissemination of endometrial tissue into the venous circulation. Am J Pathol. 1927;3(2):93–110.
31. Ulukus M, Cakmak H, Arici A. The role of endometrium in endometriosis. J Soc Gynecol Investig. 2006;13(7):467–76.
32. Eskenazi B, Warner ML. Epidemiology of endometriosis. Obstet Gynecol Clin North Am. 1997;24(2):235–58.
33. Cramer DW, Missmer SA. The epidemiology of endometriosis. Ann N Y Acad Sci. 2002;955:11–22.

34. Guo SW. Recurrence of endometriosis and its control. Hum Reprod Update. 2009;15 (4):441–61.
35. Bromer JG, Aldad TS, Taylor HS. Defining the proliferative phase endometrial defect. Fertil Steril. 2009;91(3):698–704.
36. Jones CJ, Inuwa IM, Nardo LG, et al. Eutopic endometrium from women with endometriosis shows altered ultrastructure and glycosylation compared to that from healthy controls - a pilot observational study. Reprod Sci. 2009;16(6):559–72.
37. Arimoto T, Katagiri T, Oda K, et al. Genome-wide cDNA microarray analysis of gene-expression profiles involved in ovarian endometriosis. Int J Oncol. 2003;22(3):551–60.
38. Kao LC, Germeyer A, Tulac S, et al. Expression profiling of endometrium from women with endometriosis reveals candidate genes for disease-based implantation failure and infertility. Endocrinology. 2003;144(7):2870–81.
39. Matsuzaki S, Canis M, Vaurs-Barrière C, et al. DNA microarray analysis of gene expression in eutopic endometrium from patients with deep endometriosis using laser capture microdissection. Fertil Steril. 2005;84:1180–90.
40. Matsuzaki S, Canis M, Pouly JL, et al. Analysis of aromatase and 17beta-hydroxysteroid dehydrogenase type 2 messenger ribonucleic acid expression in deep endometriosis and eutopic endometrium using laser capture microdissection. Fertil Steril. 2006;85(2):308–13.
41. Burney RO, Talbi S, Hamilton AE, et al. Gene expression analysis of endometrium reveals progesterone resistance and candidate susceptibility genes in women with endometriosis. Endocrinology. 2007;148(8):3814–26.
42. Sherwin JR, Sharkey AM, Mihalyi A, et al. Global gene analysis of late secretory phase, eutopic endometrium does not provide the basis for a minimally invasive test of endometriosis. Hum Reprod. 2008;23(5):1063–8.
43. Laudanski P, Szamatowicz J, Kowalczuk O, et al. Expression of selected tumor suppressor and oncogenes in endometrium of women with endometriosis. Hum Reprod. 2009;24 (8):1880–90.
44. Roobrouck VD, Ulloa-Montoya F, Verfaillie CM. Self-renewal and differentiation capacity of young and aged stem cells. Exp Cell Res. 2008;314(9):1937–44.
45. Sasson IE, Taylor HS. Stem cells and the pathogenesis of endometriosis. Ann N Y Acad Sci. 2008;1127:106–15.
46. Maruyama T, Masuda H, Ono M, et al. Human uterine stem/progenitor cells: their possible role in uterine physiology and pathology. Reproduction. 2010;140(1):11–22.
47. Figueira PG, Abrão MS, Krikun G, et al. Stem cells in endometrium and their role in the pathogenesis of endometriosis. Ann N Y Acad Sci. 2011;1221:10–7.
48. Vinatier D, Cosson M, Dufour P. Is endometriosis an endometrial disease? Eur J Obstet Gynecol Reprod Biol. 2000;91(2):113–25.
49. Sharpe-Timms KL. Endometrial anomalies in women with endometriosis. Ann N Y Acad Sci. 2001;943:131–47.
50. Wu Y, Strawn E, Basir Z, et al. Genomic alterations in ectopic and eutopic endometria of women with endometriosis. Gynecol Obstet Invest. 2006;62(3):148–59.
51. Hey-Cunningham AJ, Peters KM, Zevallos HB, et al. Angiogenesis, lymphangiogenesis and neurogenesis in endometriosis. Front Biosci (Elite Ed). 2013;5:1033–56.
52. Kyama CM, Mihalyi A, Simsa P, et al. Role of cytokines in the endometrial-peritoneal cross-talk and development of endometriosis. Front Biosci (Elite Ed). 2009;1:444–54.
53. Hapangama DK, Turner MA, Drury J, et al. Aberrant expression of regulators of cell-fate found in eutopic endometrium is found in matched ectopic endometrium among women and in a baboon model of endometriosis. Hum Reprod. 2010;25(11):2840–50.
54. Afshar Y, Hastings J, Roqueiro D, et al. Changes in eutopic endometrial gene expression during the progression of experimental endometriosis in the baboon, Papio anubis. Biol Reprod. 2013;88(2):44.
55. Lee B, Du H, Taylor HS. Experimental murine endometriosis induces DNA methylation and altered gene expression in eutopic endometrium. Biol Reprod. 2009;80(1):79–85.

56. Pellegrini C, Gori I, Achtari C, et al. The expression of estrogen receptors as well as GREB1, c-MYC, and cyclin D1, estrogen-regulated genes implicated in proliferation, is increased in peritoneal endometriosis. Fertil Steril. 2012;98(5):1200–8.
57. Gashaw I, Hastings JM, Jackson KS, et al. Induced endometriosis in the baboon (Papio anubis) increases the expression of the proangiogenic factor CYR61 (CCN1) in eutopic and ectopic endometria. Biol Reprod. 2006;74(6):1060–6.
58. Hastings JM, Jackson KS, Mavrogianis PA, et al. The estrogen early response gene FOS is altered in a baboon model of endometriosis. Biol Reprod. 2006;75(2):176–82.
59. Hastings JM, Fazleabas AT. A baboon model for endometriosis: implications for fertility. Reprod Biol Endocrinol. 2006;4:S7.
60. Jackson KS, Brudney A, Hastings JM, et al. The altered distribution of the steroid hormone receptors and the chaperone immunophilin FKBP52 in a baboon model of endometriosis is associated with progesterone resistance during the window of uterine receptivity. Reprod Sci. 2007;14(2):137–50.
61. Santamaria X, Massasa EE, Taylor HS. Migration of cells from experimental endometriosis to the uterine endometrium. Endocrinology. 2012;153(11):5566–74.
62. Garai J, Molnar V, Varga T, et al. Endometriosis: harmful survival of an ectopic tissue. Front Biosci. 2006;11:595–619.
63. Huhtinen K, Desai R, Ståhle M, et al. Endometrial and endometriotic concentrations of estrone and estradiol are determined by local metabolism rather than circulating levels. J Clin Endocrinol Metab. 2012;97(11):4228–35.
64. Hu WP, Tay SK, Zhao Y. Endometriosis-specific genes identified by real-time reverse transcription-polymerase chain reaction expression profiling of endometriosis versus autologous uterine endometrium. J Clin Endocrinol Metab. 2006;91(1):228–38.
65. Wu Y, Kajdacsy-Balla A, Strawn E, et al. Transcriptional characterizations of differences between eutopic and ectopic endometrium. Endocrinology. 2006;47(1):232–46.
66. Eyster KM, Klinkova O, Kennedy V, et al. Whole genome deoxyribonucleic acid microarray analysis of gene expression in ectopic versus eutopic endometrium. Fertil Steril. 2007;88 (6):1505–33.
67. Honda H, Barrueto FF, Gogusev J, et al. Serial analysis of gene expression reveals differential expression between endometriosis and normal endometrium. Possible roles for AXL and SHC1 in the pathogenesis of endometriosis. Reprod Biol Endocrinol. 2008;6:59.
68. Meola J, Rosa e Silva JC, Dentillo DB, et al. Differentially expressed genes in eutopic and ectopic endometrium of women with endometriosis. Fertil Steril. 2010;93(6):1750–73.
69. Schweppe KW, Wynn RM, Beller FK. Ultrastructural comparison of endometriotic implants and eutopic endometrium. Am J Obstet Gynecol. 1984;148(7):1024–39.
70. Yu CQ, Shi SF, Liu YH, et al. Primary culture and morphologic observation of eutopic and ectopic endometrial cells from patients with endometriosis. Zhong Xi Yi Jie He Xue Bao. 2006;4(2):189–93.
71. Chen HW, Tzeng CR. Applications of microarray in reproductive medicine. Chang Gung Med J. 2006;29(1):15–24.
72. Matsuzaki S. DNA microarray analysis in endometriosis for development of more effective targeted therapies. Front Biosci (Elite Ed). 2011;3:1139–53.
73. Bulun SE, Adashi EY. The physiology and pathology of the female reproductive axis. In: Larsen PR, Kronenberg HM, Melmed S, et al., editors. Williams textbook of endocrinology. 10th ed. Philadelphia: WB Saunders; 2003. p. 587–664.
74. Rogers PAW, D'Hooghe TM, Fazleabas A, et al. Priorities for endometriosis research: recommendations from an International consensus workshop. Reprod Sci. 2009;16:335–46.
75. Khan MA, Sengupta J, Mittal S, et al. Genome-wide expressions in autologous eutopic and ectopic endometrium of fertile women with endometriosis. Reprod Biol Endocrinol. 2012;10:84.

76. Pan Q, Luo X, Toloubeydokhti T, et al. The expression profile of micro-RNA in endometrium and endometriosis and the influence of ovarian steroids on their expression. Mol Hum Reprod. 2007;13(11):797–806.
77. Teague EM, Print CG, Hull ML. The role of microRNAs in endometriosis and associated reproductive conditions. Hum Reprod Update. 2010;16(2):142–65.
78. Filigheddu N, Gregnanin I, Porporato PE, et al. Differential expression of microRNAs between eutopic and ectopic endometrium in ovarian endometriosis. J Biomed Biotechnol. 2010;2010(369549).
79. Bharadwaj Siva A, Srivastava P, Shivaji S. Understanding the pathogenesis of endometriosis through proteomics: recent advances and future prospects. Proteomics Clin Appl. 2014;8(1–2):86–98
80. Chehna-Patel N, Sachdeva G, Gajbhiye R, et al. "Spot"-ting differences between the ectopic and eutopic endometrium of endometriosis patients. Fertil Steril. 2010;94(6):1964–71.
81. Klemmt PA, Carver JG, Koninckx P, et al. Endometrial cells from women with endometriosis have increased adhesion and proliferative capacity in response to extracellular matrix components: towards a mechanistic model for endometriosis progression. Hum Reprod. 2007;22 (12):3139–47.
82. Halme J, Hammond MG, Hulka JF, Raj S, Talbert LM. Increased activation of pelvic macrophages in infertile women with endometriosis. Obstet Gynecol. 1984;64:151–4.
83. Keettel WC, Stein RJ. The viability of the cast-off menstrual endometrium. Am J Obstet Gynecol. 1951;61:440.
84. Nisolle M, Berliere M, Paindaveine B, Casanas-Roux F, Bourdon A, Donnez J. Histologic study of peritoneal endometriosis in infertile women. Fertil Steril. 1990;53:984–8.
85. Kruitwagen RFPM, Poels LG, Willemsen WNP, de Ronde IJ, Jap PH, Rolland R. Endometrial epithelial cells in peritoneal fluid during the early follicular phase. Fertil Steril. 1991;55:297–303.
86. Arumugam K, Lim JM. Menstrual characteristics associated with endometriosis. Br J Obstet Gynecol. 1997;104:948–50.
87. Vercellini P, De Giorgo O, Aimi G, Panazza S, Uglietti A, Crosignani PG. Menstrual characteristics in women with and without endometriosis. Obstet Gynecol. 1997;90:264–8.
88. Vinatier D, Orazi G, Cosson M, Dufour P. Theories of endometriosis. Eur J Obstet Gynecol Reprod Biol. 2001;96:21–34.
89. Meresman GF, Vighi S, Buquet RA, Contreras-Ortiz O, Tesone M, Rumi LS. Apoptosis and expression of Bcl-2 and Bax in eutopic endometrium from women with endometriosis. Fertil Steril. 2000;74:760–6.
90. Aplin AE, Howe A, Alahari SK, Juliano RL. Signal transduction and signal modulation by cell adhesion receptors: the role of integrins, cadherins, immunoglobulin-cell adhesion molecules, and selectins. Pharmacol Rev. 1998;50:197–263.
91. González-Ramos DJ, Defrère S, et al. Nuclear factor-kappa B is constitutively activated in peritoneal endometriosis. Mol Hum Reprod. 2007;13:503–9.
92. González-Ramos R, Van Langendonckt A, Defrère S, et al. Agents blocking the nuclear factor-kappaB pathway are effective inhibitors of endometriosis in an in vivo experimental model. Gynecol Obstet Invest. 2008;65(3):174–86.
93. Murk W, Atabekoglu CS, Cakmak H, et al. Extracellularly signal-regulated kinase activity in the human endometrium: possible roles in the pathogenesis of endometriosis. J Clin Endocrinol Metab. 2008;93(9):3532–40.
94. Kosugi Y, Elias S, Malinak LR, et al. Increased heterogeneity of chromosome 17 aneuploidy in endometriosis. Am J Obstet Gynecol. 1999;180:792–7.
95. Jiang X, Morland SJ, Hitchcock A, Thomas EJ, Campbell IG. Allelotyping of endometriosis with adjacent ovarian carcinoma reveals evidence of a common lineage. Cancer Res. 1998;58:1707–12.
96. Obata K, Morland SJ, Watson RH, et al. Frequent PTEN/MMAC mutations in endometrioid, but not serous or mucinous epithelial ovarian tumors. Cancer Res. 1998;58:2095–7.

97. Braun DP, Ding J, Shaheen F, Willey JC, Rana N, Dmowski WP. Quantitative expression of apoptosis-regulating genes in endometrium from women with and without endometriosis. Fertil Steril. 2007;87(2):263–8.
98. Othman EE, Salama S, Ismail N, Al-Hendy A. Toward gene therapy of endometriosis: adenovirus-mediated delivery of dominant negative estrogen receptor genes inhibits cell proliferation, reduces cytokine production, and induces apoptosis of endometriotic cells. Fertil Steril. 2007;88(2):462–71.
99. Witz CA, Allsup KT, Montoya-Rodriguez IA, Vaughan SL, Centonze VE, Schenken RS. Pathogenesis of endometriosis–current research. Hum Fertil (Camb). 2003;6:34–40.
100. Sherman ME, Bitterman P, Rosenshein NB, Delgado G, Kurman RJ. Uterine serous carcinoma. A morphologically diverse neoplasm with unifying clinicopathologic features. Am J Surg Pathol. 1992;16:600–10.
101. Blumenfeld Z. Hormonal suppressive therapy for endometriosis may not improve patient health. Fertil Steril. 2004;81:487–92.
102. Ridley JH. Primary adenocarcinoma in implant of endometriosis. Obstet Gynecol. 1966;27:261–7.
103. Czernobilsky B, Silverman BB, Mikuta JJ. Endometrioid carcinoma of the ovary. A clinicopathologic study of 75 cases. Cancer. 1970;26:1141–52.
104. Czernobilsky B, Silverman BB, Enterline HT. Clear-cell carcinoma of the ovary. A clinicopathologic analysis of pure and mixed forms and comparison with endometrioid carcinoma. Cancer. 1970;25:762–72.
105. Czernobilsky B, Morris WJ. A histologic study of ovarian endometriosis with emphasis on hyperplastic and atypical changes. Obstet Gynecol. 1979;53:318–23.
106. Matsumoto K, Wolffe AP. Gene regulation by Y-box proteins: coupling control of transcription and translation. Trends Cell Biol. 1998;8:318–23.
107. Kohno K, Izumi H, Uchiumi T, Ashizuka M, Kuwano M. The pleiotropic functions of the Y-box binding protein, YB-1. Bioessays. 2003;25:691–8.
108. Lage H, Surowiak P, Holm PS. YB-1 as a potential target in cancer therapy. Pathologe. 2008;29:187–90.
109. Chatterjee M, Rancso C, Stuhmer T, et al. The Y-box binding protein YB-1 is associated with progressive disease and mediates survival and drug resistance in multiple myeloma. Blood. 2008;111:3714–22.
110. Bargou RC, Jurchott K, Wagener C, et al. Nuclear localization and increased levels of transcription factor YB-1 in primary human breast cancers are associated with intrinsic MDR1 gene expression. Nat Med. 1997;3:447–50.
111. Wu J, Lee C, Yokom D, et al. Disruption of the Y-box binding protein-1 results in suppression of the epidermal growth factor receptor and HER-2. Cancer Res. 2006;66:4872–9.
112. Fujii T, Yokoyama G, Takahashi H, et al. Preclinical and clinical studies of novel breast cancer drugs targeting molecules involved in protein kinase C signaling, the putative metastasis-suppressor gene Cap43 and the Y-box binding protein-1. Curr Med Chem. 2008;15:528–37.
113. Habibi G, Leung S, Law JH, et al. Redefining prognostic factors for breast cancer: YB-1 is a stronger predictor of relapse and disease-specific survival than estrogen receptor or HER-2 across all tumor subtypes. Breast Cancer Res. 2008;10:R86.
114. Silveira CG, Krampe J, Ruhland B, Diedrich K, Hornung D, Agic A. Cold Shock Domain Family Member YB-1 Expression in Endometrium and Endometriosis. Hum Reprod. 2012;27(1):173–82.
115. Schachner M. Neural recognition molecules and synaptic plasticity. Curr Opin Cell Biol. 1997;9:627–34.
116. Montgomery AM, Becker JC, Siu CH, et al. Human neural cell adhesion molecule L1 and rat homologue NILE are ligands for integrin alpha v beta 3. J Cell Biol. 1996;132:475–85.
117. Hortsch M. Structural and functional evolution of the L1 family: are four adhesion molecules better than one? Mol Cell Neurosci. 2000;15:1–10.

118. Meier F, Busch S, Gast D, et al. The adhesion molecule L1 (CD171) promotes melanoma progression. Int J Cancer. 2006;119:549–55.
119. Huszar M, Moldenhauer G, Gschwend V, et al. Expression profile analysis in multiple human tumors identifies L1 (CD171) as a molecular marker for differential diagnosis and targeted therapy. Hum Pathol. 2006;37:1000–8.
120. Kaifi JT, Strelow A, Schurr PG, et al. L1 (CD171) is highly expressed in gastrointestinal stromal tumors. Mod Pathol. 2006;19:399–406.
121. Fogel M, Gutwein P, Mechtersheimer S, et al. L1CAM expression as a predictor of progression and survival in patients with uterine and ovarian carcinomas. Lancet. 2003;362:869–75.
122. Ohnishi T, Matsumura H, Izumoto S, et al. A novel model of glioma cell invasion using organotypic brain slice culture. Cancer Res. 1998;58:2935–40.
123. Mechtersheimer S, Gutwein P, Agmon-Levin N, et al. Ectodomain shedding of L1 adhesion molecule promotes cell migration by autocrine binding to integrins. J Cell Biol. 2001;155:661–73.
124. Felding-Habermann B, Silletti S, Mei F, et al. A single immunoglobulin-like domain of the human neural cell adhesion molecule L1 supports adhesion by multiple vascular and platelet integrins. J Cell Biol. 1997;139:1567–81.
125. Finas D, Huszar M, Agic A, et al. L1 cell adhesion molecule (L1CAM) as a pathogenetic factor in endometriosis. Hum Reprod. 2008;23(5):1053–62.
126. Kao LC, Tulac S, Lobo S, et al. Global gene profiling in human endometrium during the window of implantation. Endocrinology. 2002;143(6):2119–38.
127. Vercellini P, Cortesi I, Crosignani PG. Progestins for symptomatic endometriosis: a critical analysis of the evidence. Fertil Steril. 1997;68(3):393–401.
128. Hornung D, Ryan IP, Chao VA, Vigne JL, Schriock ED, Taylor RN. Immunolocalization and regulation of the chemokine RANTES in human endometrial and endometriosis tissues and cells. J Clin Endocrinol Metab. 1997;82(5):1621–8.
129. Zeitoun KM, Bulun SE. Aromatase: a key molecule in the pathophysiology of endometriosis and a therapeutic target. Fertil Steril. 1999;72(6):961–9.
130. Kuiper GG, Enmark E, Pelto-Huikko M, Nilsson S, Gustafsson JA. Cloning of a novel receptor expressed in rat prostate and ovary. Proc Natl Acad Sci U S A. 1996;93 (12):5925–30.
131. Mosselman S, Polman J, Dijkema R. ER beta: identification and characterization of a novel human estrogen receptor. FEBS Lett. 1996;392(1):49–53.
132. Green S, Walter P, Kumar V, et al. Human oestrogen receptor cDNA: sequence, expression and homology to verb-A. Nature. 1996;320(6058):134–9.
133. Hewitt SC, Harrell JC, Korach KS. Lessons in estrogen biology from knockout and transgenic animals. Annu Rev Physiol. 2005;67:285–308.
134. Korach KS, Emmen JM, Walker VR, et al. Update on animal models developed for analyses of estrogen receptor biological activity. J Steroid Biochem Mol Biol. 2003;86(3–5):387–91.
135. Brandenberger AW, Lebovic DI, Tee MK, et al. Oestrogen receptor (ER)-alpha and ER-beta isoforms in normal endometrial and endometriosis-derived stromal cells. Mol Hum Reprod. 1999;5(7):651–5.
136. Fujimoto J, Hirose R, Sakaguchi H, Tamaya T. Expression of oestrogen receptor-alpha and -beta in ovarian endometriomata. Mol Hum Reprod. 1999;8:742–7.
137. Bulun SE, Cheng YH, Yin P, et al. Progesterone resistance in endometriosis: link to failure to metabolize estradiol. Mol Cell Endocrinol. 2006;248(1–2):94–103.
138. Attia GR, Zeitoun K, Edwards D, Johns A, Carr BR, Bulun SE. Progesterone receptor isoform A but not B is expressed in endometriosis. J Clin Endocrinol Metab. 2000;85(8):2897–902.
139. Lin Z, Reierstad S, Huang CC, Bulun SE. Novel estrogen receptor-alpha binding sites and estradiol target genes identified by chromatin immunoprecipitation cloning in breast cancer. Cancer Res. 2007;67(10):5017–24.

140. Schultz JR, Petz LN, Nardulli AM. Cell- and ligand-specific regulation of promoters containing activator protein-1 and Sp1 sites by estrogen receptors alpha and beta. J Biol Chem. 2005;280(1):347–54.
141. Tranguch S, Wang H, Daikoku T, Xie H, Smith DF, Dey SK. FKBP52 deficiency-conferred uterine progesterone resistance is genetic background and pregnancy stage specific. J Clin Invest. 2007;117:1824–34.
142. Aghajanova L, Velarde MC, Giudice LC. The progesterone receptor coactivator Hic-5 is involved in the pathophysiology of endometriosis. Endocrinology. 2009;150:3863–70.
143. Kastner P, Krust A, Turcotte B, et al. Two distinct estrogen-regulated promoters generate transcripts encoding the two functionally different human progesterone receptor forms A and B. EMBO J. 1990;9(5):1603–14.
144. Nardulli AM, Greene GL, O'Malley BW, Katzenellenbogen BS. Regulation of progesterone receptor messenger ribonucleic acid and protein levels in MCF-7 cells by estradiol: analysis of estrogen's effect on progesterone receptor synthesis and degradation. Endocrinology. 1988;122(3):935–44.
145. Wei LL, Krett NL, Francis MD, et al. Multiple human progesterone receptor messenger ribonucleic acids and their autoregulation by progestin agonists and antagonists in breast cancer cells. Mol Endocrinol. 1988;2(1):62–72.
146. Read LD, Snider CE, Miller JS, Greene GL, Katzenellenbogen BS. Ligand-modulated regulation of progesterone receptor messenger ribonucleic acid and protein in human breast cancer cell lines. Mol Endocrinol. 1988;2(3):263–71.
147. Petz LN, Ziegler YS, Schultz JR, Nardulli AM. Fos and Jun inhibit estrogen-induced transcription of the human progesterone receptor gene through an activator protein-1 site. Mol Endocrinol. 2004;18(3):521–32.
148. Matthews J, Wihlén B, Tujague M, Wan J, Ström A, Gustafsson JA. Estrogen receptor (ER) beta modulates ERalpha-mediated transcriptional activation by altering the recruitment of c-Fos and c-Jun to estrogen-responsive promoters. Mol Endocrinol. 2006;20(3):534–43.
149. Petz LN, Ziegler YS, Schultz JR, Kim H, Kemper JK, Nardulli AM. Differential regulation of the human progesterone receptor gene through an estrogen response element half site and Sp1 sites. J Steroid Biochem Mol Biol. 2004;88(2):113–22.
150. Petz LN, Nardulli AM. Sp1 binding sites and an estrogen response element half-site are involved in regulation of the human progesterone receptor A promoter. Mol Endocrinol. 2000;14(7):972–85.
151. Petz LN, Ziegler YS, Loven MA, Nardulli AM. Estrogen receptor alpha and activating protein-1 mediate estrogen responsiveness of the progesterone receptor gene in MCF-7 breast cancer cells. Endocrinology. 2002;143(12):4583–91.
152. Schultz JR, Petz LN, Nardulli AM. Estrogen receptor alpha and Sp1 regulate progesterone receptor gene expression. Mol Cell Endocrinol. 2003;201(1–2):165–75.
153. Savouret JF, Bailly A, Misrahi M, et al. Characterization of the hormone responsive element involved in the regulation of the progesterone receptor gene. EMBO J. 1991;10(7):1875–83.
154. Montano MM, Kraus WL, Katzenellenbogen BS. Identification of a novel transferable cis element in the promoter of an estrogen-responsive gene that modulates sensitivity to hormone and antihormone. Mol Endocrinol. 1997;11(3):330–41.
155. Scott RE, Wu-Peng XS, Yen PM, Chin WW, Pfaff DW. Interactions of estrogen- and thyroid hormone receptors on a progesterone receptor estrogen response element (ERE) sequence: a comparison with the vitellogenin A2 consensus ERE. Mol Endocrinol. 1997;11(11):1581–92.
156. Osuga Y, Koga K, Hirota Y, Hirata T, Yoshino O, Taketani Y. Lymphocytes in endometriosis. Am J Reprod Immunol. 2011;65:1–10.
157. Berbic M, Fraser IS. Regulatory T cells and other leukocytes in the pathogenesis of endometriosis. J Reprod Immunol. 2011;88:149–55.
158. Sikora J, Mielczarek-Palacz A, Kondera-Anasz Z. Role of natural killer cell activity in the pathogenesis of endometriosis. Curr Med Chem. 2011;18:200–8.

159. Gonzalez-Ramos R, Van Langendonckt A, Defrere S, et al. Involvement of the nuclear factorκB pathway in the pathogenesis of endometriosis. Fertil Steril. 2010;94:1985–94.
160. Barbieri RL, Niloff JM, Bast Jr RC, Scaetzl E, Kistner RW, Knapp RC. Elevated serum concentrations of CA-125 in patients with advanced endometriosis. Fertil Steril. 1986;45:630–4.
161. Abrao MS, Podgaec S, Filho BM, Ramos LO, Pinotti JA, de Oliveira RM. The use of biochemical markers in the diagnosis of pelvic endometriosis. Hum Reprod. 1997;12:2523–7.
162. Koninckx PR, Kennedy SH, Barlow DH. Endometriotic disease: the role of peritoneal fluid. Hum Reprod Update. 1998;4:741–51.
163. Asante A, Taylor RN. Endometriosis: the role of neuroangiogenesis. Annu Rev Physiol. 2011;73:163–82.
164. Al-Jefout M, Dezarnaulds G, Cooper M, et al. Diagnosis of endometriosis by detection of nerve fibres in an endometrial biopsy: a double blind study. Hum Reprod. 2009;24 (12):3019–24.
165. Bokor A, Kyama CM, Vercruysse L, et al. Density of small diameter sensory nerve fibres in endometrium: a semi-invasive diagnostic test for minimal to mild endometriosis. Hum Reprod. 2009;24(12):3025–32.
166. Newman TA, Bailey JL, Stocker LJ, Woo YL, Macklon NS, Cheong YC. Expression of neuronal markers in the endometrium of women with and those without endometriosis. Hum Reprod. 2013;28(9):2502–10.
167. Leslie C, Ma T, McElhinney B, Leake R, Stewart CJ. Is the detection of endometrial nerve fibers useful in the diagnosis of endometriosis? Int J Gynecol Pathol. 2013;32(2):149–55.

Part III
Clinical Science

Chapter 18
Prevention of Endometriosis

Ebru H. Biberoglu and Kutay O. Biberoglu

Abstract There is an association between the presence of endometriosis and common autoimmune and atopic diseases and some of the cancers. There are also concerns about the risk for birth defects in the children of women with endometriosis. Prevention of endometriosis may also reduce the risk for these other health problems and their sequelae. To be able to prevent or delay the development of endometriosis and hopefully other associated comorbidities, risk factors for endometriosis should be defined. Exposure to environmental chemicals recently has been proposed to contribute to several gynecologic pathologies including endometriosis, especially when exposures occur during critical periods of development. Although potential role in the pathogenesis of endometriosis has not been established, exposure to certain endocrine-disrupting chemicals is shown to be higher in women affected by endometriosis compared to women without the disease. Although there is extensive scientific and clinical data applicable to endometriosis when it is regarded as a systemic inflammatory, endocrine, and immunological disease, the prevention of endometriosis per se, have not been addressed fully in the medical literature.

Keywords Chemicals • Endometriosis • Environment • Life style • Nutrition • Prevention

E.H. Biberoglu (✉)
Dr. Zekai Tahir Burak Women Health Care, Education and Research Hospital Ankara, Turkey
e-mail: ebru2513@gmail.com

K.O. Biberoglu
Gazi University Medical School, Professor of Obstetrics and Gynecology, Gynecological Endocrinology and Infertility Unit Besevler, Ankara, Turkey
e-mail: kobiber@gmail.com

T. Harada (ed.), *Endometriosis: Pathogenesis and Treatment*,
DOI 10.1007/978-4-431-54421-0_18, © Springer Japan 2014

18.1 Risk Factors

Although science has not yet addressed directly, there are extensive scientific and clinical resources applicable to the prevention of endometriosis, especially when regarded as the systemic inflammatory, autoimmune and endocrine disease. Further, dioxin and endocrine-disrupting environmental toxicants that modify the inflammatory process have been strongly associated with endometriosis [1].

Endometriosis shares pathophysiological characteristics such as immune response alterations, increased inflammation, elevated levels of tissue-remodeling components, altered apoptosis, increased local and/or systemic levels of cytokines.

Growth factors including fibroblast growth factor (FGF), vascular endothelial growth factor (VEGF), platelet-derived growth factor (PDGF), epidermal growth factor (EGF), transforming growth factor-h (IGF-h) and granulocyte/macrophage-colony-stimulating factor (GM-CSF) and inflammatory mediators like IL-1, TNF-a, IL-2, IL-6, IL-8, IL-10, IL-11, MCP-1, and interferon-g (IFN-g) produced by peritoneal leukocytes are all elevated in the peritoneal fluid of women with endometriosis.

There is an association between the presence of endometriosis and common autoimmune and atopic diseases, such as systemic lupus erythematosus, Sjögren's syndrome, rheumatoid arthritis, Crohn's disease, psoriasis. chronic fatigue immune dysfunction syndrome, multiple sclerosis, hypothyroidism and fibromyalgia. Research has suggested that endometriosis may increase the risk of ovarian and breast cancer, non Hodgkin's lymphoma, melanoma, thyroid, kidney and brain tumors. There are also concerns about the risk for birth defects in the children of women with endometriosis. Therefore, prevention of the disease processes involving endometriosis may also reduce the risk for these other health problems and their sequelae [1–3].

To be able to prevent or delay the development of endometriosis and hopefully other associated comorbidities, known risk factors for endometriosis should be defined at the first place. The plethora of risk factors for endometriosis may reflect varying methodologies such as study populations, definitions utilized for risk factors, and diagnostic accuracy. Infertility by itself is a significant risk factor for endometriosis. An infertility history increases the odds of an endometriosis diagnosis in both the operative (OR, 2.43; 95 % CI, 1.57–3.76) and population (OR, 7.91; 95 % CI, 1.69–37.2) cohorts [4]. Increasing age, alcohol use, early menarche, family history of endometriosis, infertility, intercourse during menses, low body weight, prolonged menstrual flow, and short cycle interval are known risk factors [5–8]. Endometriosis has been negatively associated with exercise and smoking [9]. Recently, red hair [10], blue or green eyes, and freckles have been reported to increase the odds of diagnosis [11]. It is possible that there may not be a classic set of risk factors generic to all women with endometriosis. Rather, risk factors may need tailoring to the subgroups of women by their behavioral and clinical characteristics.

18.1.1 Family History

First degree relatives of a woman with endometriosis carry 4–10 times higher risk of also having endometriosis when compared to the general population. Candidate genes such as ESR1, COMT, IL6, IL10, CYP17A1, CYP19A1, CYP1A1, MMP1, and MMP9 studied in genomic DNA showed no association with endometriosis [12].

In more than 1,000 families with two or more members with surgically documented endometriosis from Australia and the UK, significant linkage to 10q26 and 20p13 was demonstrated. However, no causative gene was identified [13]. It is likely that endometriosis is a common polygenic/multifactorial disease caused by an interaction between genes as well as the environment [14, 15].

18.1.2 Menstrual Cycle Characteristics

Early age at menarche ($\leq$11 years old) might increase a woman's exposure to menstruation during her reproductive lifetime and consequently increase the risk of endometriosis. The data, however, do not present strong evidence for the clinical utility of a history of early menarche in the evaluation of endometriosis [16]. The lowest risk was seen in those whose age at menarche was 15 years [17].

Increased exposure to menstruation in terms of short cycle length, long duration of flow, and low parity have frequently been identified as possible risk factors. The use of tampons does not seem to confer a risk for endometriosis.

Dysmenorrhea is likely to be a precursor to disease development, and shorter cycles may possibly suggest increased risk [18, 19].

In contrast to past studies, data of a recent study found no relationship between endometriosis and menstrual cycle history, including age at menarche, average cycle length, and number of menstrual cycles in the past 12 months. However, >80 % of the women in all groups in this study had a history of oral contraceptive use. This contraceptive use may have altered both recent menstrual cycle patterns or possibly the presence or absence of endometriosis [4].

Therefore, the potential role of menstrual cycle characteristics in the actual development of endometriosis remains an open question. At best they may be used to guide diagnostic and therapeutic strategies if other symptoms point to endometriosis as a possible diagnosis.

18.1.3 Lean Body Mass

Several studies have found that a lower body mass index (BMI) during adolescence and early adulthood is a risk factor for endometriosis. Taller women tend to have higher follicular-phase estradiol levels and thus may have an increased risk of endometriosis. This evidence was supported by a retrospective study that found that women with endometriosis have lower BMI and are less frequently obese than control subjects [20]. Indeed, for every unit increase in BMI, 12–14 % decrease in the likelihood of having endometriosis was claimed [21]. In a recent study, BMI (OR, 0.95; 95 % CI, 0.93–0.98) was found to decrease the odds of diagnosis of endometriosis [4]. The 20 years follow-up within the Nurses' Health Study II prospective cohort revealed that BMI at age 18 and current BMI were each significantly inversely associated with endometriosis ($P < 0.0001$). Both associations were stronger among infertile women. Obese infertile women with current BMIs of 35–39.9 kg/m^2 and ≥40 kg/m^2 had a 55 % (95 % CI 0.30–0.67) and a 62 % (95 % CI 0.23–0.62) lower risk of endometriosis, respectively, compared with the low-normal BMI referent (18.5–22.4 kg/m^2). Rates of endometriosis were nearly threefold higher in women with waist-to-hip ratios,0.60 (RR = 2.78, 95 % CI 1.38–5.60) compared with those with waist-to-hip ratios between 0.70 and 0.79 [22].

18.1.4 DES Exposure

The incidence rates of diagnosis of laparoscopically confirmed endometriosis was found to be 80 % greater among women exposed to diethylstilbestrol (DES) (RR = 1.8, CI = 1.2–2.8) [23]. Exposure to DES in utero has been associated with cervical stenosis, uterine smooth muscle abnormalities, and altered estrogen receptor expression in both mice and women [24]. In addition, it was reported that exposed women with vaginal epithelial changes had 50 % more autoimmune disease than exposed women without vaginal epithelial changes [25]. Therefore the relation between DES exposure and endometriosis may result from a combined effect of increased retrograde menstruation, immune dysfunction, and exogenous estrogen exposure.

18.1.5 Environmental Exposures

Endocrine-disrupting chemicals (EDC) directly through induction of gene expression or indirectly impair female reproduction by interfering with the production, release, transportation, metabolism, action, or elimination of natural hormones. Also the neuroendocrine (monitoring the environment and sending signals to the endocrine system) and the epigenetic (altering transcriptional capabilities without changing DNA sequence) routes could have been involved in the pathogenesis. In epigenetic disruption, the chemicals modify histones altering the DNA–nuclear protein interactions or promote DNA methylation. Most importantly, the resultant chromatin modifications can be passed on to future generations and increase the likelihood of a disease state later in life across several generations [26, 27].

Although potential role in the pathogenesis of endometriosis has not been established, exposure to certain EDCs is shown to be higher in women affected by endometriosis compared to women without the disease [28–31].

A recent study demonstrated that infertile patients affected by endometriosis had higher percentage of serum sample with bisphenol A (BPA), perfluorooctane sulfonate (PFOS), perfluorooctanoic acid (PFOA), di-(2-ethylhexyl) phthalate (DEHP) and mono-ethylhexyl phthalate (MEHP) levels compared with infertile patients without endometriosis. The study group of infertile patients had also a significantly higher expression of several nuclear receptors that represent potential EDC targets, namely, estrogen receptor alpha (ERa) and beta (Erb), androgen receptor (AR), pregnane X receptor (PXR), aryl hydrocarbon receptor (AhR), and peroxisome proliferator-activated receptor gamma (PPARg) [32].

While some evidence from laboratory animal studies suggests that endometriosis can be promoted by many organochlorines, a class of xenobiotic chemicals including the dioxin TCDD, the pesticides methoxychlor and dichlorodiphenyltrichloroethane (DDT), and many polychlorinated biphenyls (PCBs) with dioxin-like effects, some others fail to find any significant relationship between the two. The hypothesis that EDC exposure during embryogenesis increases susceptibility for endometriosis, but subsequent adult hormone, immune, and/or EDC irregularities are required for disease onset was supported by the finding of larger implanted endometriotic lesions when exposure of the fetus to the dioxin 2,3,7,8-tetrachlorodibenzo-*p*-dioxin (TCDD) on gestational day 8 was combined with the adult exposure in the mouse model [33, 34].

It is possible that fetal exposure to TCDD promotes adult endometriosis through altered P action, because PR expression is reduced in the uterus of adult mice that were exposed to TCDD in utero [35]. It is also possible that TCDD which is an immunosuppressant promotes endometriosis through altered immune function enabling establishment and growth of peritoneal endometriosis under the influence of E2, proangiogenic, proliferative, and antiapoptotic factors [36]. Alternatively, TCDD could activate specific signaling pathways causing overexpression of K-ras thereby promoting peritoneal endometriosis [37].

Endometriotic lesions have increased expression of aromatase and 17β-HSD type 1 and decreased expression of 17β-HSD types 2 and 4, resulting in an increase in production of E2 [38]. If this expression pattern is established during fetal development via epigenetic mechanisms, then endometriosis could manifest during adulthood after estrogenic exposures [39].

Studies have found increased risk of endometriosis-associated infertility among workers exposed to formaldehyde, video display terminals, chemical dusts, or organic solvents, and among workers in agricultural industries and occupations, in particular farmworkers. Having ever worked as a flight attendant, service station attendant, or health worker, particularly as a nurse or health aide, is associated with increased risk of endometriosis (flight attendant: OR 9.80, 95 % CI 1.08–89.02; service station attendant: OR 5.77, 95 % CI 1.03–32.43; health worker: OR 1.49, 95 % CI 1.03–2.15) [40].

18.1.6 Cigarette Smoking, Alcohol, and Caffeine

Active cigarette smoking in adulthood or adolescence, with the known antiestrogenic effect of inhaled tobacco smoke, has generally been associated with decreased endometriosis risk in previous research [9]. Whereas, a deleterious effect on endometriosis risk through exposure to polycyclic aromatic hydrocarbons [41] or dioxins [42] in tobacco smoke may dominate. A negative effect of passive smoking during childhood on endometriosis risk has also been suggested but further research is needed to confirm this relationship [43]. In a recent study where smoking habits in endometriosis patients are studied, no correlation between smoking habits and the risk of any form of endometriosis (superficial peritoneal endometriosis, ovarian endometriomas, and deep infiltrating endometriosis) and with the revised American Fertility Society stages or scores have been demonstrated [44]. Alcohol and caffeine consumption have also been shown to increase the risk of endometriosis. It is known that alcohol increases estrogen levels in the body and may disrupt the immune response during the menstrual cycle. The effect of caffeine is likely related to its influence on the immune system as well [45].

18.1.7 History of Allergic, Inflammatory, and Autoimmune Diseases

Alterations in inflammatory response and in both cellular/humoral immunity ends up with overproduction of prostaglandins, metalloproteinases, cytokines, and chemokines, thus favoring an optimal environment for the survival and proliferation of endometriotic implants [46]. This might explain why women with endometriosis report symptoms of not only pain but also of nervousness, tension, anxiety, headaches, depression, fatigue, insomnia, indigestion, bloating, recurrent vaginitis, recurrent cystitis, autoimmune diseases, asthma, and allergies [47, 48].

Women with endometriosis have a higher prevalence of allergies on medications, allergic rhinitis, asthma, and family history of allergic diseases compared to control subjects. In epidemiological studies, 48 % of women with endometriosis were reported to be allergic to at least one medication. Of these, 85 % had complaints of sinus and 14 % had suffered from asthma. Additionally, 80 % had a parent with allergic disease [49]. In another study, 61 % of the women with endometriosis reported allergies (compared with 18 % of the general female population), and 12 % had asthma (compared with 5 % of the general female population) [50]. In a recent study, a 4.6-fold increased frequency of allergic women with endometriosis compared with the control group was reported and the most prevalent allergen was found to be penicillin in this group [51].

Evidence available to date indicates that immune and inflammatory factors, whether they are released by immune or peritoneal, endometrial, and endometriotic cells, may play a critical role in the ectopic survival, implantation, and growth of endometrial tissue. Higher incidence of autoimmune diseases, abnormalities in T- and B-cell function, increased polyclonal B cell activity, high B-cell and T-cell counts, reduced natural killer (NK) cell activity, and the familial inheritance pattern and its recurring nature support an autoimmune aspect of endometriosis [47]. A recent genome-wide study suggests that endometriosis exhibits a gene expression signature in terms of increased presence and activation of plasma cells and macrophages and upregulation of complement system [52]. A macrophage product B lymphocyte stimulator (BLyS) which is a member of TNF superfamily is found to be elevated in the serum of women with in rheumatoid arthritis, systemic lupus erythematosus, and Sjögren's syndrome [52] and with endometriosis in association with BLyS-817C/T polymorphism [53].

Recent studies support the contributing role of inflammation in endometriosis-related pain. The proinflammatory peptides facilitate endometriotic cell survival by stimulating cell proliferation and inhibiting apoptosis of endometriotic cells. The main cell processes that NF-κB regulates, contributing to endometriosis development, are inflammation, cell proliferation, and inhibition of apoptosis. Iron overload in the pelvic cavity of endometriosis patients is very probably an important facilitator or inductor of chronic NF-κB activation, enhancing the NF-κB-mediated inflammatory reaction and endometriotic cell survival and growth [54].

From the clinical perspective, patients with endometriosis have been shown to have a higher prevalence of several generalized autoimmune diseases, including systemic lupus, erythematosus, rheumatoid arthritis, and Sjogren's syndrome, and also of irritable bowel syndrome, painful bladder syndrome, migraine head ache, and fibromyalgia [55–57].

18.1.8 Fibromyalgia, Chronic Fatigue Syndrome, Irritable Bowel Syndrome, Painful Bladder Syndrome, and Migraine

In recent years, epidemiologic studies have identified an association between endometriosis and some other pain syndromes (such as fibromyalgia, chronic fatigue syndrome, interstitial cystitis, and irritable bowel syndrome) as well as various autoimmune and atopic conditions as already been discussed [50]. A recent study described a high prevalence of comorbid chronic pain syndromes (56 %) and mood disorders (48 %) in adolescents and young women with endometriosis [58]. Nevertheless, irritable bowel syndrome, painful bladder syndrome, and chronic headache were detected in 25 % versus 65 % [59]; in 16 % versus 65 % [60] and 19 % versus 38 % [61] in adolescent/young women compared to adult endometriosis patients, respectively. Fibromyalgia and chronic fatigue syndrome prevalences were found in 7 % and 4 % of young girls versus 6 % and 5 % of adult endometriosis women, respectively [50]. Women with endometriosis have a 30 % increased risk of migraines. There is also an increased prevalence of endometriosis in women with migraine. The subgroup of migraineurs with endometriosis is more likely to have other comorbid conditions affecting mood and pain [56]. Angiogenic cytokines are hypothesized to play a critical role in the pathogenesis of endometriosis and migraine, possibly by stimulating matrix metalloproteinases (MMPs) [62]. There may also be a neuro-immuno-endocrine link between endometriosis and migraine, fibromyalgia, irritable bowel syndrome, chronic fatigue syndrome, interstitial cystitis (painful bladder), and mood disorder through increased mast cell activation [63]. Mast cell activation without allergic degranulation has been documented to occur in response to stress and lead to painful sterile inflammatory states [64]. An increased prevalence of hypothyroidism, fibromyalgia and chronic fatigue syndrome, and autoimmune inflammatory diseases in women with endometriosis compared with the general female population was previously reported. The coexistence of all these conditions suggests an underlying role for the immune system in fibromyalgia and chronic fatigue syndrome [50].

18.1.9 Anatomical Obstruction of the Uterus and Surgical Scar Endometriosis

Sampson's theory of retrograde menstruation and implantation is supported by evidence that obstructive Mullerian anomalies that enhance retrograde menstruation such as a narrowed or completely blocked cervix, a malformed or absent cervix, absence of the vagina, or a completely blocking hymen have been associated with endometriosis in adolescent women, and repair of these anomalies has been associated with resolution of endometriosis [65–68].

Endometriosis has been reported at or near the site of surgical scars at the perineum, abdominal wall, even at the laparoscopic trocar port site, likely due to the mechanical transplantation of endometrial tissue during previous episiotomy, cesarean section, hysterectomy, hysteroscopy, tubal ligation, vulvar surgery, and accidental trauma [69–73].

Timing of abdominal surgery was suggested to play role in the development of the disease. In women with endometriosis, the recurrence rate was higher in those who had surgery near the end of the menstrual cycle (days 22–28) than in those who had surgery earlier in their cycle [74].

18.1.10 Contraception

If nonsteroidal anti-inflammatory drugs fail in alleviating dysmenorrhea, oral contraceptive pills (OCP) are commonly offered to young women. The symptoms of dysmenorrhea usually disappear with the suppression of ovulation but recur once pill taking is discontinued [75]; therefore long-term use is recommended [76].

The risk of endometriosis appears to rise with greater lifetime number of ovulatory cycles. Besides suppressing ovulation, OCPs increase the low apoptotic activity of the endometrium of women with endometriosis [77]; progestins in OCPs prevent implantation of regurgitated endometrium, inhibit angiogenesis and also expression of matrix metalloproteinases, and reduce the inflammation of the endometriotic implants and the consequent immune response [78].

The findings of the reports studying the link between OCP and endometriosis are contradictory. Decreased [17, 79, 80] or increased [81, 82] risk of endometriosis among OCP users have been published. On the other hand, some of the studies failed to find any association between the two [83, 84].

A cross-sectional study on a large series of patients revealed that past use of OCP if particularly given for treating severe dysmenorrhea was associated with all stages of endometriosis, especially deep infiltrative endometriosis (DIE) whereas no association was shown with endometriosis and current OCP use [85]. Meta-analysis are in agreement with decreased endometriosis prevalence in current but increased prevalence in past OCP users. Data from cohort studies (excluding case–control studies) demonstrate a protective effect of current OC use (relative reduction, 43 %; 95 % CI, 20–60 %), whereas previous use seems to increase the risk by 60 % (95 % CI from 40 to 82 %) [86]. The pill may reduce the risk of endometriosis by suppressing ovulation.

On the other hand, it was experimentally demonstrated that the regurgitated endometrial tissue into the peritoneum of castrated female monkeys survived only if estradiol was supplemented [87]. Therefore, it is quite possible that the estrogen in the pill may act as a rescue factor for regurgitated endometrial glands that would otherwise be resorped during hypo-estrogenic menstrual milieu.

The observed link might not be a causal one. It is well known that hormonal therapies are effective on pain symptoms [88], and women who receive OCP especially following failed NSAIDs for dysmenorrhea may already have developed endometriosis, but is still undiagnosed [89]. Since OCP use reduces pelvic pain symptoms, current users tend not to be investigated for endometriosis. On the other hand, women with endometriosis-induced dysmenorrhea might have been selectively excluded from the "never OC users" category, with a consequent increased risk for past users as a group.

In the end, it appears unlikely that OCs influence the risk of endometriosis to any great extent, because a consistent dose–response effect for lifetime duration of use has not been observed. Furthermore, also the pattern of risk with time since last use does not support a causal relationship [86].

If retrograde menstruation is involved in the etiology of endometriosis, exposure to nonhormonal intrauterine devices (IUD), by increasing the menstrual flow, may be a risk factor for endometriosis. The results of the studies are contradictory. Several studies have suggested that IUD use does not influence the development of endometriosis [81, 90–92]. Others have reported an increased prevalence of endometriosis among former IUD users [9, 93, 94]. Even a weak protection has been observed in a subgroup for subjects who stopped using IUD more than 10 years ago [90].

There is no question that levonorgestrel-containing intrauterine systems (LNG IUS) which induce endometrial atrophy and decidual transformation of the stroma downregulate endometrial cell proliferation, increase apoptotic activity, which also has anti-inflammatory and immunomodulatory effects, and play a definite role in the treatment of endometriosis-associated symptoms [95, 96]. The LNG IUS also reduce the risk of recurrence of dysmenorrhea after conservative surgery for endometriosis [97].

Tubal ligation has been linked to development of endometriosis. Overall, no relationship between tubal ligation and prevalence of endometriosis was found in a group of women. On the other hand, tubal ligation was significantly associated with severity of disease [$P = 0.036$, crude OR (95 % CI) = 0.17 (0.02–0.85), adjusted OR (95 % CI) = 0.21 (0.04–1.08)]. In subgroups, moderate–severe endometriosis was found in 8.7 % and 36.4 % among patients with and without sterilization, respectively [98]. In another group of 3384 multiparous women who underwent tubal sterilization, endometriosis was detected in 126 patients (3.7 %), which was not different from the control group [92].

18.2 Boosting the Immune System and Reducing the Inflammation Stress

Activation of the hypothalamo–pituitary–adrenal (HPA) and sympathetic–adrenal–medullary axes in the presence of stress lead to abnormal corticotropin-releasing factor (CRF) secretion pattern, overexpression of glucocorticoid receptors, and chronic overreaction of the body's stress system [99]. The release of cortisol also affects the immune system, in addition to its effects on the brain. Acute stressors are associated with an upregulation of the immune system, while prolonged increase in cortisol levels has been shown to depress immunologic function [100].

In women with chronic diseases such as gastrointestinal (GI) disorders causing chronic pelvic pain, chronic fatigue syndrome, dysmenorrhea, and mood disorders (e.g., anxiety, depression, posttraumatic stress syndrome), besides elevated levels of inflammatory cytokines, findings reflecting abnormal HPA responses and decreased cortisol levels have been reported. Chronic stress and hypocortisolism have been hypothesized to cause a deregulation in the neuroendocrine–immune axis leading to diseases including endometriosis. In fact, women with endometriosis have lower salivary and follicular fluid cortisol levels [101], but higher serum cortisol levels are detected in infertile women with advanced endometriosis [102]. It might be that other neuroendocrine factors, like CRF levels, could be more accurate and informative markers of HPA axis deregulation than systemic cortisol levels.

It is hypothesized that stressful life events can impact the immunological health of an individual. It is also known that endometriosis is associated with increased secretion of cytokines and impaired cell-mediated immunity, modulating the growth of ectopic endometrial implants [103]. The fibrosis and inflammation, particularly the mast cells in the infiltrate surrounding ectopic endometrial tissue, suggest that a hypersensitivity reaction, specifically, is strongly related to endometriosis [104, 105]. Increased activated and degranulating mast cells and its histological relationship with nerves in deeply infiltrating endometriosis lesions may be contributing to intense and typical deep pelvic pain [106, 107]

The increased frequency of having shorter cycle length which is a known risk factor for endometriosis in women with stressful jobs compared with those who did not consider their jobs stressful and twofold elevated dysmenorrhea prevalence in women reporting high levels of stress in the preceding menstrual cycle are indirect evidences supporting the link between stress and endometriosis [108, 109]. Although it is unknown whether stress is a causal or exacerbating factor in the development of endometriosis, establishment of psychological, behavioral, and stress-reduction interventions as part of multidisciplinary preventive management should be taken into consideration.

18.2.1 Vaccines

The use of bacillus Calmette–Guérin (BCG) and granulocyte–macrophage colony-stimulating factor (GM-CSF), among others, as boosters for the immune system in oncology cases, stimulated researchers to study their possible role in the prevention of endometriosis. In animal studies, systemic prophylaxis with BCG caused an inhibitory effect on endometrial transplantation [110].

The effects of mycobacteria in altering the ability of peripheral blood mononuclear cells (PBMCs) and natural killer (NK) cells to kill endometrial stromal cells have been assessed in in vitro model and endometrial stromal cell susceptibility to killer cells has been demonstrated [111].

Research on possible immunomodulatory role of pentoxifylline did not show any impact on future fertility in infertile women with asymptomatic minimal and mild endometriosis [112].

After vaccination with RESAN which is a complex of molecules extracted from xenogeneic tissues containing glycoproteins, peptides, and carbohydrate fragments of more than 40 different common tumor antigens, a reduction in endometriosis induction from 69.6 to 4.3 % was obtained in the rat model [113].

18.2.2 Retinoic Acid

Cytokines, chemokines, proteases, and angiogenic factors in the peritoneal cavity which are derived mainly from activated peritoneal macrophages promote the development and progression of endometriosis [114]. Defects in macrophage activation may lead to chronic immune activation with accompanying reduction in immune response contributing to the growth of endometriotic lesions [115]. Retinoic acid (RA) has been shown to modulate inflammation in autoimmune disease by enhancing regulatory T-cell (Treg) suppression of proinflammatory cells [116, 117]. In model systems involving activated monocytes/macrophages, RA decreases proinflammatory cytokines while increasing anti-inflammatory proteins such as interleukin-10 [118] also decrease the peritoneal fluid levels of interleukin-6 (IL-6) and macrophage chemotactic factor-1(MCP-1), which have been implicated in its pathogenesis of endometriosis [119]. These in vivo findings emphasize the potential use of retinoids to prevent and to treat women with endometriosis [120].

18.2.3 Melatonin as an Antioxidant

Proper regulation of matrix metalloproteinases (MMPs) is essential for physiological functioning of the endometrium, for invasion characteristics, and for remodeling of the extracellular matrix. Derangement of MMP regulation is critical in the development of endometriosis. Both MMP-2 and MMP-9 are activated by reactive oxygen species (ROS), and their expressions seem to be regulated by oxidant stress [121]. In the animal model, antioxidant enzymes like superoxide dismutase and catalase prevent intraperitoneal adhesions of endometriotic tissues in the peritoneal cavity [122].

Melatonin and its metabolites as antioxidants protect cellular components, stimulate secretion of progesterone, and have oncostatic, antiproliferative, and antiestrogenic effects [123, 124].

The role of melatonin in prevention and regression of endometriotic lesions is through upregulation of proMMP-9 and antiestrogenic activities. Also a new diagnostic marker, MMP-9/TIMP-1 (tissue inhibitors of matrix metalloproteinases) expression ratio in judging disease progression and severity have been demonstrated in animal model [125].

18.2.4 Anti-inflammatory Modulators

Endometriotic cells respond to TNF-α with increased secretion of MCP-1, which is a factor found to be elevated in peritoneal fluid of patients with endometriosis [126]. Experimental data emerging from treatments with anti-inflammatory modulators such as cyclooxygenase 2 inhibitors [127], peroxisome proliferator-activated receptor-γ agonist [128], and TNF-α inhibitors like TNFα-binding protein (TBP)-1, TNF-soluble high-affinity receptor complex, infliximab, and etanercept [129, 130] are promising and suggest potential for targeting the immune system to treat patients with endometriosis.

Macrophage migration inhibitory factor (MIF), an important regulator of the host immune system that promotes the proinflammatory functions of immune cells, plays a role in angiogenesis, tumorigenesis, as well as in many inflammatory and autoimmune diseases. Circulating and local peritoneal levels and expression of MIF which is a product of activated peritoneal macrophages are found to be elevated in the presence of early, vascularized, and most active endometriotic lesions. In in vivo model of endometriosis, ISO-1 [(S,R) 3-(4-hydroxyphenyl)-4,5-dihydro-5-isoxazoleacetic methyl ester)], a highly specific inhibitor of MIF, has been shown to lead to regression of ectopic endometrial implants; downregulation of angiogenic, tissue remodeling, and survival factors such as integrins αv and β3, VEGF, IL8 and COX2; and the expressions of MMP2 and MMP9 and Bcl2 [131].

Several previous studies showed the benefit of targeting MIF and also of managing inflammatory diseases such as asthma, sepsis, and viral infection [132, 133].

18.2.5 25-Hydroxyvitamin D and Selective Vitamin D Receptor Agonist (VDR) as Immunoregulatory and Anti-inflammatory Agents

Endometriosis risk may be influenced by dietary vitamin D intake and plasma 25-hydroxyvitamin D concentration through immunomodulatory effects [134]. In a large prospective study, a significantly lower rate of laparoscopically confirmed endometriosis among women with greater predicted plasma 25(OH)D levels and among women with a higher intake of dairy foods has been demonstrated. Calcium, vitamin D, and magnesium intakes from foods were also inversely related to endometriosis [135]. Several other studies reported contradictory results [136–138]. Moreover, data in humans suggest that high magnesium intake may be associated with lower levels of inflammatory markers, including interleukin-6 and tumor necrosis factor alpha receptor 2 [139]. Magnesium has also been shown to relax smooth muscles [140] and as a result may influence endometriosis through its effect on retrograde menstruation.

Several immunomodulatory effects could be mediated by the capacity of VDR agonists to inhibit the NF-κB [141, 142]. In addition, the inhibition of leucocyte infiltration into inflammatory sites by treatment with VDR agonists is associated with their capacity to inhibit chemokine production by cells in the target organ via the inhibition of NF-κB activation which results in interference with the growth of experimentally induced endometriosic lesions [142, 143].

It has been shown that the VDR agonist, elocalcitol, inhibits lesion development in a mouse model of endometriosis [144].

By administering elocalcitol during the perimenstrual and menstrual phase of the cycle, inhibition of inflammation, endometrial cell adhesion, and lesion organization could be exerted with the maximal efficacy; thereby prevention of the development of endometriotic implants could be feasible in subjects at high risk of disease recurrence.

18.2.6 Simvastatin

Statins reduce the rate of endometrial stromal growth and angiogenesis, interfere with the development and attachment of endometriotic implants, and also protect the subject from the development of endometriosis by virtue of their anti-inflammatory and antioxidant properties [145]. Considering its safety and minimal side effects, use of statins in treatment of endometriosis holds promise [146].

18.2.7 Pentoxifylline

A methylxanthine acting as a phosphodiesterase inhibitor, an anti-inflammatory agent, and also an immunomodulator which has been used for many years to modify blood viscosity and improve tissue oxygen delivery in the management of defective microcirculation reduces the production and action of cytokines such as TNF-α and interleukin-1 and thereby inhibits the inflammatory activation of polymorphonuclear neutrophils and also inhibits phagocytosis and the generation of toxic oxygen species and proteolytic enzymes by macrophages and granulocytes. Experimentally it has been shown that pentoxifylline can modulate rat endometriotic implant growth and production of implant-specific proteins [147]. Therefore, immunomodulation of peritoneal inflammatory cell hyperactivation with pentoxifylline may represent a new modality to specifically manage the pathophysiology of endometriosis. On the other hand, up until now, there still appears to be little evidence to support using pentoxifylline in the management of endometriosis [112, 148].

18.2.8 Sorafenib: An Antiangiogenic and Tyrosine Kinase Inhibitor

Various epigenetic aberrations have been described in endometriosis [149]. Mesenchymal stem cells (MSC), located in the microenvironment of the ectopic endometriotic lesion, may be modulated epigenetically and lead to the survival of the MSC cells with enhanced migratory, proliferative, and angiogenic properties. Since endometrial MSC do not express ER [150], the current use of antiestrogenic medications is likely to spare MSC and target only ER-positive cells which explains why symptom relief is just temporary and eradication of the disease is not possible.

Researchers just recently observed that sorafenib treatment inhibited the increased phosphorylation of ezrin which plays a major role in the regulation of cell morphology, migration, and attachment in ectopic MSC, and consequently limited the increased migration of ectopic MSC. Targeting the stem cell population may be relevant in achieving the complete eradication of endometriotic implants [151].

18.2.9 Curcumin as an Antioxidant, Anti-inflammatory, and Antiproliferative Agent

Curcumin is a naturally occurring polyphenolic yellow-/turmeric-colored compound derived from the rhizome of Curcuma longa which is widely used as a spice and coloring agent in several foods such as curry, mustard, and potato chips and also in cosmetics and drugs. The anti-inflammatory effects are mediated through interference with multiple key signaling molecules, including nuclear factor-kappaB (NF-κB). The increased MMP-9 activity and expression of tumor necrosis factor-alpha (TNF-α) in endometriotic tissues can be reversed by administration of curcumin in experimental models. Moreover, lipid peroxidation and protein oxidation in endometriotic tissues are prevented by curcumin [152]. Another study documents the Curcumin's effect on regulation of matrix metalloproteinase (MMP-2) activity by tissue inhibitor of MMP (TIMP-2) during the early phase of endometriosis development [153]. It has also been demonstrated that curcumin can effectively suppress ICAM-1 and VCAM-1 gene and protein expression, as well as secretion of IL-6, IL-8, and MCP-1, by inhibiting the activation of NF-κB induced by TNF-α in human ectopic endometriotic stromal cells [154]. All these findings provide a novel rationale for the potential of curcumin in the prevention and treatment of endometriotic disease in humans.

18.2.10 Green Tea as a Potent Antiangiogenesis Agent

Endometriosis is an angiogenesis-dependent disorder. Since endometriotic lesions require new vessel formation to deliver the nutrient supply, dense vascularization is a typical pathological feature of endometriosis. Antiangiogenesis is one of the most well-characterized biological properties of green tea. The polyphenols, especially epigallocatechin-3-gallate (EGCG) in the leaves of the tea plant Camellia sinensis, have potent antioxidative, antimitotic, and antiangiogenic properties [155, 156].

In mice experimental endometriosis model, pro-EGCG, inhibits the development, growth, and angiogenesis of the implants [157, 158]. EGCG selectively suppresses vascular endothelial growth factor C (VEGFC) and tyrosine kinase receptor VEGF receptor 2 (VEGFR2) expressions in experimental endometriosis in vivo and endothelial cells in vitro [158].

Antiangiogenesis for the management of endometriosis has the potential advantage of lower recurrence rates and less endocrine side effects compared to conventional surgical and hormonal therapies.

18.2.11 Resveratrol: A Phytochemical Compound

Resveratrol (*trans*-3,5,4′-trihydroxystilbene) is a phytochemical compound of grapes, red wine, nuts, and different berries, affecting multiple cellular processes, including proliferation, apoptosis, and oxygen radical formation [159], and also suppressing the development of new blood vessels. Moreover, resveratrol dose-dependently suppresses the development of new blood vessels [160]. The most significant concentrations of resveratrol are found in the skin of grapes and therefore in red wines but not white wines. Resveratrol has been suggested as a promising therapeutic agent for the treatment of cancer [161] as well as several inflammatory, metabolic [162], and cardiovascular diseases [163]. A group of researchers just recently have shown in mice that resveratrol inhibits the establishment of endometriotic lesions by decreasing proliferative activity and by upregulating apoptotic cell death inside the lesions [164]. Another group have also demonstrated that resveratrol treatment suppresses the development of new microvessels and inhibits the proliferation of both stromal and glandular endometrial cells in peritoneal and mesenteric lesions [165]. Better understanding of the basic mechanisms of action of EGCG and resveratrol, as well as their bioavailability, is needed to determine the potential usefulness of these natural compounds as endometriosis-preventive agents [166].

18.2.12 Chinese Herbal Medicine: Puerarin as a Phytoestrogen

Puerarin, the main isoflavone glycoside derived from the Chinese medicinal herb Radix puerariae, exhibits antiestrogenic activity by suppressing P450arom and interferes with the invasion of endometrial stromal cells (ESC) and angiogenesis of ectopic tissues, in a model of endometriosis. This might be a good option for avoiding the relapse of endometriosis after the initial surgical and/or medical therapy, since it can be used for long periods without severe side effects, unlike the classical antiestrogenic medical treatment modalities [167].

According to several clinical studies in the medical literature, treatment with Chinese herbal medicine (CHM) involving formulae of between 10 and 20 separate herbal ingredients selected from a materia medica of several hundred commonly herbs that are administered as pills, enemas, and intramuscular injections prevents the recurrence of endometriosis after a conservative operation with fewer adverse reactions when compared with conventional "western medicine." Better quality randomized controlled trials are needed to investigate a possible role for CHM in the prevention and management of endometriosis [168, 169].

18.3 Life Style

18.3.1 Pregnancy and Vaginal Parturition

It has been established that there is a higher prevalence of endometriosis in infertile women (48 %) than in fertile women (5 %) [170], and infertile women are 6–8 times more likely to have endometriosis than fertile women [171]. Gravidity (OR, 0.49; 95 % CI, 0.32–0.75) and parity (OR, 0.42; 95 % CI, 0.28–0.64) decrease the odds of diagnosis of endometriosis [4]. It is possible that pregnancy may indeed suppress the growth and inflammation of endometriotic lesions due to elevated progesterone levels.

Among parous women, parity and lifetime duration of lactation are associated with decreased risk. Among parous women, there is a linear decrease in risk with the number of liveborn children (rate ratio of 0.5 comparing >3 with 2 children; 95 % CI 0.4–0.7) and lifetime duration of lactation if time since last birth is less than 5 years (rate ratio of 0.2 comparing >23 months with never; 95 % CI 0.1–0.4) [17]. The recurrence rate of endometriosis has been found to be significantly lower in women who had vaginal parturition than in nulliparous women and those who delivered by cesarean section. Enlargement of the internal cervical ostium has been inversely related to the recurrence of endometriosis, confirming the role of retrograde bleeding in the occurrence and recurrence of the disease. Regardless of the presence of endometriosis, a relief in dysmenorrhea has been observed only in women who deliver vaginally [172].

18.3.2 Diet

Over the past decade, many studies have provided evidence that higher intakes of fruit and vegetables, rich in antioxidants, among other micronutrients, improve the function of the immune system and fight free radical damage [173]. Manipulation of dietary polyunsaturated fatty acid (PUFA) composition demonstrably affects the proinflammatory activities of many cell types involved in the immune response, inflammatory reactions, and cytokine network and on the synthesis and biological activity of prostaglandins and cytokines such as IL-1, IL-2, IL-6, TNF, and interferon [174, 175]. In the presence of high n-6:n-3 PUFA ratios of dietary intake, biosynthesis of their metabolites steadies a prominent production of 2-series prostaglandins (PGE2, PGF2a), thromboxane A2, and 4-series leukotrienes, in contrast to high n-3:n-6 PUFA ratios. Moreover, a diet based on vitamin B, vegetables, fibers, and antioxidants decreases estrogenic state-related body fat excess implicated in the estrogen-dependent growth of endometriotic tissue [174]. Dietary supplementation induces enzymes of estradiol metabolism, and the subsequent defective formation and metabolism of steroid hormones are responsible for the promotion and development of endometriosis [176]. Although not well characterized, some observational studies have shown that plant-based and high in fiber diets decrease concentrations of bioavailable estrogen by increasing its excretion and thus lower endometriosis risk [177, 178]. Additionally, high-fat diets have been associated with increased estradiol levels in premenopausal women [177, 179], suggesting that diets low in fat and high in fiber may modify endometriosis risk by altering steroid hormone metabolism. The published reports on this issue are somewhat contradictory [34, 173]. A recent large cohort study using 12 years of prospectively collected data have failed to show any association between total dietary fat intake and endometriosis risk, but a decreased risk with increased long-chain n-3 fatty acid consumption and an increased risk with trans-fat intake have been demonstrated [180]. A recently published population-based case–control study [181] suggests a possible inverse risk of disease with dietary fat and dairy consumption and an increased risk of endometriosis with β-carotene and higher servings of fruit, but these findings have not been confirmed elsewhere and require further evaluation in a prospective investigation. Unfortunately, there are only few well-designed, randomized, controlled trials to evaluate the efficacy and safety of complementary dietary therapy to manage endometriosis. From the accumulated data, one can conclude that the effect of dietary fat on the risk and incidence of endometriosis, if any, is marginal and is not clinically relevant. There is no adequate scientific support to the suggestion that fish oil consumption is beneficial for the prevention of endometriosis. Keeping in mind that the diagnosis of endometriosis can be made by laparoscopy especially in women with pain and that women with a high fatty acid intake are less likely to undergo a laparoscopy since a high fatty acid intake can reduce menstrual pain, the association between the risk of undergoing a laparoscopy and fatty acid intake will therefore probably be as significant as the association between endometriosis and fatty acid intake. The impact of diet on endometriosis risk is urgently needed to be further studied before development of population-based strategies to prevent endometriosis can be suggested.

18.3.3 Physical Activity

Physical activity has been hypothesized to be protective since endometriosis is an estrogen-dependent disease, and physical activity may increase levels of sex hormone-binding globulin (SHBG), which would reduce estrogens. Regular exercise has been associated with a 40–80 % reduction in risk for endometriosis in several case–control studies. Four case–control studies have found inverse associations between physical activity and the risk of endometriosis, with relative risks ranging from 0.2 to 0.6 [9, 34, 182]. 70 % decreased risk of developing an endometrioma with recent, frequent, and regular high intensity physical activity, as characterized by $\geq$3 times/week, $\geq$30 min/episode, $\geq$10 month/year for 2 years. Another study found a 40 % lower risk for women who reported "regular exercise" for 3–7 h/week and an 80 % risk reduction for those who exercised more than 7 h/week when compared with nonexercisers [183]. On the contrary to the others, in the Nurses' Health Study II, activity reported 6 years prior to diagnosis and inactivity have not been found to be associated with endometriosis [184].

Although adult physical activity has been mostly associated with lower endometriosis risk [9, 34, 182, 183, 185], little is known about the influence of childhood or adolescent physical activity on endometriosis.

One of the studies reported a 27 % increased risk of endometrioma for any physical activity at 12–21 years of age [182], and the other one, the Nurses' Health Study II, also found a positive linear relationship between strenuous physical activity at 12–13 years of age and endometriosis risk [186], suggesting that the early adolescent period is a critical window of exposure for the implantation of endometriosis lesions, which physical activity might promote at that age.

18.4 The Timing of Exposure to Environmental Factors

Exposure to environmental chemicals recently has been proposed to contribute to several gynecologic pathologies including endometriosis, especially when exposures occur during critical periods of development. There are limited data on the prevalence of conditions that affect women's reproductive health. Hormone-related diseases such as endometriosis and uterine fibroids, pubertal developmental abnormalities, and polycystic ovary syndrome are more common, although few data on population-based trends are available. The toxic chemicals altering reproductive health in females have been demonstrated by the consequences of diethylstilbestrol (DES) use by pregnant women. Other synthetic chemicals which are called endocrine-disrupting compounds (EDCs) used in commerce are known to mimic hormones and have been shown to contribute to disease onset [187].

The impact of the environment on reproductive physiology can be a direct inducer of gene expression, acting directly as hormones or disrupting the metabolism or synthesis of endogenous hormones, or through a neuroendocrine route, whereby the nervous system monitors the environment sending signals to the endocrine system, and an epigenetic route could have been chosen, whereby altering transcriptional capabilities without changing DNA sequence [188].

The data collected from the Nurses' Health Study have revealed that DES daughters have an 80 % increased risk (relative risk [RR] 1.8, [CI] 1.2–2.8) of the development of endometriosis [23]. At the same time, in mice model, exposure to the dioxin 2,3,7,8-tetrachlorodibenzo-*p*-dioxin (TCDD) on gestational day 8 increases the size of implanted endometriotic lesions when combined with an adult exposure [33]. Based on these evidences, one can hypothesize that during embryogenesis, EDC exposure has an organizational effect that increases susceptibility for endometriosis, but subsequent adult hormone, immune, and/or EDC irregularities are required for disease onset.

Although estrogen is necessary for the progression of endometriosis, other factors also influence this progression. The most toxic dioxin, TCDD, induces endometriosis, not in ovariectomized mice but with an intact ovary [34]. Also, in women with peritoneal endometriosis, immune dysfunction by TCDD has been blamed since the immune system fails to prevent implantation of endometrial debris, despite high levels of activated macrophages and inflammatory cytokines in the peritoneal environment [189], suggesting that the progression of endometriosis is dependent on both hormonal and immune environments.

Increasing experimental evidence suggests an influence of environmental organochlorines, a class of xenobiotic chemicals on endometriosis development, including dioxin or dioxin-like compounds [190, 191] which are known to disrupt endocrine and immune functions [192].

Human endometrium is a known site for estrogen, and many environmental chemicals have been detected there [193] or may induce inflammation and the chronic stimulation of proinflammatory cytokines. At the same time, they have been associated with immunologic changes, downregulating natural killer cells or interleukin-1β and interleukin-12 [194].

Recently, organochlorine pesticides have also been shown to increase endometriosis risk in a laparoscopic cohort of US women [195] and other studies have reported increased risks with higher concentration of phthalates [196, 197], polychlorinated dibenzodioxins and polychlorinated dibenzofurans, and polychlorinated biphenyls [198, 199].

Experiments on rodents suggest that both adult and in utero exposure to dioxin can promote endometriosis during adulthood. Increased endometriotic lesion size was observed in mice exposed to TCDD during both perinatal and adult life stages [33].

Since in utero and lactational exposure to TCDD reduces circulating estradiol in vivo [200] and decreases ovarian estradiol production in cultures [201], and also causes degradation of ER-α [202], it is possible that fetal exposure to TCDD promotes adult endometriosis through altered P action, because PR expression is reduced in the uterus of adult mice that were exposed to TCDD in utero [35] and P insensitivity is characteristic of women with endometriosis [189, 203]. TCDD which is an immunosuppressant [36] might promote endometriosis by altering the immune function, thereby enabling establishment and growth of peritoneal endometriosis under the influence of E2, proangiogenic, proliferative, and antiapoptotic factors. Alternatively, TCDD could activate the expression of K-ras in the ovarian surface resulting in peritoneal endometriosis [37]. Endometriotic lesions have increased expression of aromatase and 17β-HSD type 1 and decreased expression of 17β-HSD types 2 and 4, resulting in an increase in production of estradiol [39]. If this expression pattern is established during fetal development via epigenetic mechanisms, then endometriosis could manifest during adulthood after estrogenic exposures. In ectopic endometrial tissue, ER-β is upregulated and acts as the mediator of endometrial proliferation [204, 205]. Therefore, adult exposures to high doses of ER-β agonists are hypothesized to promote ectopic endometrium growth after retrograde menstruation.

18.4.1 The "Developmental Origins of Adult Disease" Hypothesis

According to Barker hypothesis, adverse influences early in development, particularly during intrauterine life, can result in permanent changes in physiology and metabolism resulting in increased disease risk in adulthood, which is speculated to occur largely through epigenetic mechanisms [206]. As a typical example, low birth weight (LBW) is associated with a list of chronic diseases ranging from coronary artery disease (CAD), type II diabetes mellitus (T2DM), cancer, and osteoporosis to various psychiatric illnesses [207]. As stated by Dr. Ian Donald, "The first 38 weeks of human life spent in the allegedly protected environment of the amniotic sac are medically more eventful and more fraught with danger than the next 38 years in the lifespan of most human individuals" [208].

Regarding endometriosis, development of permanent increased estrogen sensitivity due to imprinting the regulatory gene HOXA10, in offspring exposed to bisphenol A (BPA) during pregnancy, has been reported [209].

Unfortunately, placenta instead of being a protective barrier for the fetus allows many toxic chemicals to pass to the fetus. BPA, for example, in animal model, passes to the fetus reaching to higher than maternal blood levels in less than 30 min after exposure [210, 211]. The embryo or fetus also cannot or partially detoxify the chemicals since the key enzyme, cytochrome P450 activity, is lacking or not fully developed in the fetus, even in young children [212].

Breastfed infants exposed to EDCs have much higher blood levels than formula-fed infants [213]. It has also been emphasized that breastfed infants receives about 50 times the daily PCB intake of adults and up to 18 % higher than those of formula-fed infants [214].

It is unknown whether breastfeeding can counteract or not, the detrimental effects of prenatal toxicant exposure. Given that toxic chemicals are being removed from the mother's stores during lactation and that the longer the lactation, the more toxins removed, it might be expected that breastfeeding reduces breast cancer and endometriosis risk. In fact, among the benefits of breastfeeding to the mother are reduced risk of breast cancer and reduced risk of recurrence of endometriosis in women who have had children, not longer than 5 years ago [215, 216].

In addition to the recommendations to choose breastfeeding or not, mother to be should be as healthy as possible even before conception, lose weight if necessary, eat organically, be supplemented with antioxidants and other detoxifiers, and avoid all toxic exposures possible while breastfeeding [217, 218]. By losing weight in the postpartum period, whether there will be any remobilization or not of adipose tissue resulting in increased circulating levels of previously stored EDCs, thereby increasing the levels in breast milk, is unknown [219].

Parents should be advised to avoid plastic bottles and not to store foods including breast milk or formula for baby in plastics to avoid bisphenol A. There are also toxins including dioxin, xylene, ethylbenzene, and styrene in disposable diapers made of bleached paper and plastic [220]. Infants whose skin are exposed to lotion, powder, and shampoo reveal increased urinary concentrations of phthalates [221].

Since food is the primary exposure to EDCs, eating organic instead of genetically modified foods is very critical [222]. Another way to reduce exposure is to eat more vegetables, grains, fruits, and less animal products [223]. One might skip meat completely and go vegetarian. On the other hand, soy, corn, potatoes, squash, canola oil, cottonseed oil, papaya, and tomatoes are among the most commonly genetically engineered foods. Consuming lignin-containing vegetables like cabbage, cauliflower, broccoli, and Brussels sprouts, which helps in the removal of excess estrogen, is another way to reduce exposure [224]. In brief, contaminated fish, meats, dairy, eggs, processed oils and fast foods, fried foods, and refined processed foods should better be reduced or even avoided.

Avoiding pesticides and herbicides from other, non-food, sources is also important. Pesticides have been linked to some immune abnormalities seen in endometriosis, infections, asthma, and allergies. PVC, a source of phthalates, is prevalent worldwide in building materials, plumbing, shoes, rain gear, shower curtains, flooring, and toys. Dental sealants, used to protect teeth from decay-causing bacteria, typically contain bisphenol A [225]. Children who have been exposed to pesticides are 3–7 times more likely to develop non-Hodgkin's lymphoma than children who have not been exposed to pesticides and this risk was similar for pesticide exposure to the mother during pregnancy and direct exposure after birth [226]. Since women with endometriosis have 40 % higher risk for developing hematopoietic malignancies, mainly non-Hodgkin lymphoma, this may be a problem which requires extra caution [227].

Menarche is correlated to percent body fat with about 17 % body fat required for menarche and 22 % body fat reported to be required to maintain or restore menstruation [228]. Since fat cells produce estrogen, heavier girls usually begin sexual development and periods earlier [229]. Fat cells also make cytokines, therefore keeping down fat should also avoid inflammation [230]. The fat consumed as a child may be even more an important risk than the fat consumed as an adult. Exercise is another way to keep body fat low and achieve the goal of delaying puberty and menarche [231].

The Nurses' Health Study II (NHS II), in a well-characterized cohort, has reported that low birth weight, multiple gestation, and DES are associated with a diagnosis of endometriosis [23]. Another study demonstrated lower odds of the diagnosis with in utero exposure to cigarette smoking [232]. Women eventually diagnosed with endometriosis were leaner from childhood through diagnosis relative to women without endometriosis [21]. This finding was subsequently corroborated in the large Nurses Health III Cohort Study [233]. Despite some indirect evidence suggestive of an early origin for endometriosis, some recent studies failed to demonstrate an association between in utero exposures and increased odds of an endometriosis diagnosis [234, 235].

18.5 Conclusion

In conclusion, medical literature have not yet addressed the prevention of endometriosis. However, there is extensive scientific and clinical data applicable to prevention of endometriosis when it is regarded as a systemic inflammatory, endocrine, and immunological disease. We hope this review will stimulate further basic and clinical research on this very critical health problem of women.

References

1. Ballweg ML. Prevention of endometriosis: it might be possible. In: Matalliotakis I, Arici A, editors. New Developments in Endometriosis. CreateSpace; 2011. p. 1–44.
2. Ballweg ML. Impact of endometriosis on women's health: comparative historical data show that the earlier the onset, the more severe the disease. Best Pract Res Clin Obstet Gynaecol. 2004;18(2):201–18.
3. Biberoglu K. Prevention of endometriosis: Is it possible? J Endometriosis. 2012;4(3):129–30.
4. Peterson CM, Johnstone EB, Hammoud AO, Stanford JB, Varner MW, Kennedy A, et al. ENDO Study Working Group. Risk factors associated with endometriosis: importance of study population for characterizing disease in the ENDO study. Am J Obstet Gynecol. 2013;208:451. e1–11.
5. Matalliotakis IM, Cakmak H, Fragouli YG, Goumenou AG, Mahutte NG, Arici A. Epidemiological characteristics in women with and without endometriosis in the Yale series. Arch Gynecol Obstet. 2008;277:389–93.
6. Vercellini P, De Giorgi O, Aimi G, Panazza S, Uglietti A, Crosignani PG. Menstrual characteristics in women with and without endometriosis. Obstet Gynecol. 1997;90:264–8.
7. Nouri K, Ott J, Krupitz B, Huber JC, Wenzl R. Family incidence of endometriosis in first-, second-, and third-degree relatives: case–control study. Reprod Biol Endocrinol. 2010;8:85.
8. Filer RB, Wu CH. Coitus during menses: its effect on endometriosis and pelvic inflammatory disease. J Reprod Med. 1989;34:887–90.
9. Cramer DW, Wilson E, Stillman RJ, Berger MJ, Belisle S, Schiff I, et al. The relation of endometriosis to menstrual characteristics, smoking, and exercise. JAMA. 1986;255:1904–8.
10. Woodworth SH, Singh M, Yussman MA, Sanfilippo JS, Cook CL, Lincoln SR. A prospective study on the association between red hair color and endometriosis in infertile patients. Fertil Steril. 1995;64:651–2.
11. Somigliana E, Vigano P, Abbiati A, Gentilini D, Parazzini F, Benaglia L, et al. 'Here comes the sun': pigmentary traits and sun habits in women with endometriosis. Hum Reprod. 2010;25:728–33.
12. Ewens KG, Stewart DR, Ankener W, Urbanek M, McAllister JM, Chen C, et al. Family-based analysis of candidate genes for polycystic ovary syndrome. J Clin Endocrinol Metab. 2010;95:2306–15.

13. Treloar SA, Wicks J, Nyholt DR, Montgomery GW, Bahlo M, Smith V, et al. Genomewide linkage study in 1176 affected sister pair families identifies a significant susceptibility locus for endometriosis on chromosome 10q26. Am J Hum Genet. 2005;77:365–76.
14. Matalliotakis IM, Arici A, Cakmak H, Goumenou AG, Koumantakis G, Mahutte NG. Familial aggregation of endometriosis in the Yale Series. Arch Gynecol Obstet. 2008;278(6):507–11.
15. Layman LC. The genetic basis of female reproductive disorders: etiology and clinical testing. Mol Cell Endocrinol. 2013;370(1–2):138–48.
16. Nnoaham KE, Webster P, Kumbang J, Kennedy SH, Zondervan KT. Is early age at menarche a risk factor for endometriosis? A systematic review and meta-analysisof case–control studies. Fertil Steril. 2012;98(3):702–12.
17. Missmer SA, Hankinson SE, Spiegelman D, Barbieri RL, Malspeis S, Willet WC, et al. Reproductive history and endometriosis among premenopausal women. Obstet Gynec. 2004;5(1):965–74.
18. Treloar SA, Bell TA, Nagle CM, Purdie DM, Green AC. Early menstrual characteristics associated with subsequent diagnosis of endometriosis. Am J Obstet Gynecol. 2010;202:534. e1–6.
19. Eskenazi B, Warner ML. Epidemiology of endometriosis. Obstet Gynecol Clin North Am. 1997;24:235–58.
20. Ferrero S, Anserini P, Remorgida V, Ragni N. Body mass index in endometriosis. Eur J Obstet Gynecol Reprod Biol. 2005;121:94–8.
21. Hediger ML, Hartnett J, Buck Louis GM. Association of endometriosis with body size and figure. Fertil Steril. 2005;84(5):1366–74.
22. Shah DK, Correia KF, Vitonis AF, Missmer SA. Body size and endometriosis: results from 20 years of follow-up within the Nurses' Health Study II prospective cohort. Hum Reprod. 2013;28:1783 [Epub ahead of print].
23. Missmer SA, Hankinson SE, Spiegelman D, Barbieri RL, Michels KB, Hunter DJ. In utero exposures and the incidence of endometriosis. Fertil Steril. 2004;82(6):1501–8.
24. Newbold R. Cellular and molecular effects of developmental exposure to diethylstilbestrol: implications for other environmental estrogens. Environ Health Perspect. 1995;103:83–7.
25. Noller KL, Blair PB, O'Brien PC, Melton 3rd LJ, Offord JR, Kaufman RH, et al. Increased occurrence of autoimmune disease among women exposed in utero to diethylstilbestrol. Fertil Steril. 1988;49:1080–2.
26. Jirtle RL, Skinner MK. Environmental epigenomics and disease susceptibility. Nat Rev Genet. 2007;8:253–62.
27. Edwards TM, Myers JP. Environmental exposures and gene regulation in disease etiology. Environ Health Perspect. 2007;115:1264–70.
28. Anway MD, Skinner MK. Epigenetic transgenerational actions of endocrine disruptors. Endocrinology. 2006;147:S43–9.
29. Simsa P, Mihalyi A, Schoeters G, Koppen G, Kyama CM, Den Hond EM, et al. Increased exposure to dioxin-like compounds is associated with endometriosis in a case–control study in women. Reprod Biomed Online. 2010;20:681–8.
30. Cobellis L, Colacurci N, Trabucco E, Carpentiero C, Grumetto L. Measurement of bisphenol A and bisphenol B levels in human blood sera from healthy and endoemtriotic women. Biomed Chromatogr. 2009;23:1186–90.
31. Weuve J, Hauser R, Calafat AM, Missmer SA, Wise LA. Association of exposure to phthalates with endometriosis and uterine leiomyomata: findings from NHANES, 1999–2004. Environ Health Perspect. 2010;118:825–8.
32. Caserta D, Bordi G, Ciardo F, Marci R, La Rocca C, Tait S, et al. The influence of endocrine disruptors in a selected population of infertile women. Gynecol Endocrinol. 2013;29 (5):444–7.
33. Cummings AM, Hedge JM, Birnbaum LS. Effect of prenatal exposure to TCDD on the promotion of endometriotic lesion growth by TCDD in adult female rats and mice. Toxicol Sci. 1999;52:45–9.

34. Cummings AM, Metcalf JL, Birnbaum L. Promotion of endometriosis by 2,3,7,8-tetrachlorodibenzo-*p*-dioxin in rats and mice: time-dose dependence and species comparison. Toxicol Appl Pharmacol. 1996;138:131–9.
35. Nayyar T, Bruner-Tran KL, Piestrzeniewicz-Ulanska D, Osteen KG. Developmental exposure of mice to TCDD elicits a similar uterine phenotype in adult animals as observed in women with endometriosis. Reprod Toxicol. 2007;23:326–36.
36. Mueller MD, Vigne JL, Streich M, Tee MK, Raio L, Dreher E, et al. 2,3,7,8-Tetrachlorodibenzo-*p*-dioxin increases glycodelin gene and protein expression in human endometrium. J Clin Endocrinol Metab. 2005;90:4809–15.
37. Dinulescu DM, Ince TA, Quade BJ, Shafer SA, Crowley D, Jacks T. Role of K-ras and Pten in the development of mouse models of endometriosis and endometrioid ovarian cancer. Nat Med. 2005;11:63–70.
38. Maia Jr H, Haddad C, Coelho G, Casoy J. Role of inflammation and aromatase expression in the eutopic endometrium and its relationship with the development of endometriosis. Womens Health (Lond Engl). 2012;8(6):647–58.
39. Dassen H, Punyadeera C, Kamps R, Delvoux B, Van Langendonckt A, Donnez J, et al. Estrogen metabolizing enzymes in endometrium and endometriosis. Hum Reprod. 2007;22:3148–58.
40. Marino JL, Holt VL, Chen C, Davis S. Lifetime occupational history and risk of endometriosis. Scand J Work Environ Health. 2009;35(3):233–40.
41. Zhong Y, Carmella SG, Upadhyaya P, Hochalter JB, Rauch D, Oliver A, et al. Immediate consequences of cigarette smoking: rapid formation of polycyclic aromatic hydrocarbon diol epoxides. Chem Res Toxicol. 2011;24:246–52.
42. Sadeu JC, Hughes CL, Agarwal S, Foster WG. Alcohol, drugs, caffeine, tobacco, and environmental contaminant exposure: reproductive health consequences and clinical implications. Crit Rev Toxicol. 2010;40:633–52.
43. Kvaskoff M, Bijon A, Clavel-Chapelon F, Mesrine S, Boutron-Ruault MC. Childhood and adolescent exposures and the risk of endometriosis. Epidemiology. 2013;24(2):261–9.
44. Chapron C, Souza C, de Ziegler D, Lafay-Pillet MC, Ngô C, Bijaoui G, et al. Smoking habits of 411 women with histologically proven endometriosis and 567 unaffected women. Fertil Steril. 2010;94(6):2353–5.
45. McLeod BS, Retzloff MG. Epidemiology of endometriosis: an assessment of risk factors. Clin Obstet Gynecol. 2010;53(2):389–96.
46. Olovsson M. Immunological aspects of endometriosis: an update. Am J Reprod Immunol. 2011;66:101–4.
47. Matarese G, De Placido G, Nikas Y, Alviggi C. Pathogenesis of endometriosis: natural immunity dysfunction or autoimmune disease? Trends Mol Med. 2003;9:223–8.
48. Kyama CM, Debrock S, Mwenda JM, D' Hooghe TM. Potential involvement of the immune system in the development of endometriosis. Reprod Biol Endocrinol. 2003;1(123):1–9.
49. Mabray CR, Burditt ML, Martin TL, Jaynes CR, Hayes JR. Treatment of common gynecologic-endocrinologic symptoms by allergy management procedures. Obstet Gynecol. 1982;59:560–4.
50. Sinaii N, Cleary SD, Ballweg ML, Nieman LK, Stratton P. High rates of autoimmune and endocrine disorders, fibromyalgia, chronic fatigue syndrome and atopic diseases among women with endometriosis: a survey analysis. Hum Reprod. 2002;17:2715–24.
51. Matalliotakis I, Cakmak H, Matalliotakis M, Kappou D, Arıcı A. High rate of allergies among women with endometriosis. J Obstet Gynaecol. 2012;32(3):291–3.
52. Hever A, Roth RB, Hevezi P, Marin ME, Acosta JA, Acosta H, et al. Human endometriosis is associated with plasma cells and overexpression of B lymphocyte stimulator. Proc Natl Acad Sci U S A. 2007;104:12451–6.
53. Christofolini DM, Cavalheiro CM, Teles JS, Lerner TG, Brandes A, Bianco B, et al. Promoter -817C>T variant of B lymphocyte stimulator gene (BLyS) and susceptibility to

endometriosis-related infertility and idiopathic infertility in Brazilian population. Scand J Immunol. 2011;74(6):628–31.
54. González-Ramos R, Defrère S, Devoto L. Nuclear factor-kappaB: a main regulator of inflammation and cell survival in endometriosis pathophysiology. Fertil Steril. 2012;98 (3):520–8.
55. Keller JJ, Liu SP, Lin HC. A case–control study on the association between rheumatoid arthritis and bladder pain syndrome/interstitial cystitis. Neurourol Urodyn. 2013;32 (7):980–5.
56. Tietjen GE, Bushnell CD, Herial NA, Utley C, White L, Hafeez F. Endometriosis is associated with prevalence of comorbid conditions in migraine. Headache. 2007;47 (7):1069–78.
57. Seaman SE, Ballard KD, Wright JT, de Vries CS. Endometriosis and its coexistence with irritable bowel syndrome and pelvic inflammatory disease: findings from a national case–control study- part 2. BJOG. 2008;115:1392–6.
58. Smorgick N, Marsh CA, As-Sanie S, Smith YR, Quint EH. Prevalence of pain syndromes, mood conditions, and asthma in adolescents and young women with endometriosis. J Pediatr Adolesc Gynecol. 2013;26(3):171–5.
59. Issa B, Onon TS, Agrawal A, Shekhar C, Morris J, Hamdy S, et al. Visceral hypersensitivity in endometriosis:a new target for treatment? Gut. 2012;61:367–72.
60. Butrick CW. Patients with chronic pelvic pain: endometriosis or interstitial cystitis/painful bladder syndrome? JSLS. 2007;11:182–9.
61. Ferrero S, Pretta S, Bertoldi S, Anserini P, Remorgida V, Del Sette M, et al. Increased frequency of migraine among women with endometriosis. Hum Reprod. 2004;19:2927–32.
62. Tamburro S, Canis M, Albuisson E, Dechelotte P, Darcha C, Mage G. Expression of transforming growth factor β1 in nerve fibers is related to dysmenorrhea and laparoscopic appearance of endometriotic implants. Fertil Steril. 2003;80:1131–6.
63. Kempuraj D, Papadopoulou N, Stanford EJ, Christodoulou S, Madhappan B, Sant GR, et al. Increased numbers of activated mast cells in endometriosis lesions positive for corticotropin releasing hormone and urocortin. Am J Reprod Immunol. 2004;52:267–75.
64. Theoharides TC. Mast cells and stress—a psychoneuroimmunological perspective. J Clin Psychopharmacol. 2002;22:103–8.
65. Laufer MR, Sanfilippo J, Rose G. Adolescent endometriosis: diagnosis and treatment approaches. J Pediatr Adolesc Gynecol. 2003;16:S3.
66. Bricou A, Batt RE, Chapron C. Peritoneal fluid flow influences anatomical distribution of endometriotic lesions: Why Sampson seems to be right. Eur J Obstet Gynecol Reprod Biol. 2008;138:127.
67. Mok-Lin EY, Wolfberg A, Hollinquist H, Laufer MR. Endometriosis in a patient with Mayer–Rokitansky–Küster–Hauser syndrome and complete uterine agenesis: evidence to support the theory of coelomic metaplasia. J Pediatr Adolesc Gynecol. 2010;23(1):e35–7.
68. Uğur M, Turan C, Mungan T, Kuşçu E, Senöz S, Ağiş HT, et al. Endometriosis in association with müllerian anomalies. Gynecol Obstet Invest. 1995;40(4):261–4.
69. Nasu K, Okamoto M, Nishida M, Narahara H. Endometriosis of the perineum. J Obstet Gynaecol Res. 2013;39(5):1095–7.
70. Emre A, Akbulut S, Yilmaz M, Bozdag Z. Laparoscopic trocar port site endometriosis: a case report and brief literature review. Int Surg. 2012;97(2):135–9.
71. Horton JD, Dezee KJ, Ahnfeldt EP, Wagner M. Abdominal wall endometriosis: a surgeon's perspective and review of 445 cases. Am J Surg. 2008;196(2):207–12.
72. Odobasic A, Pasic A, Iljazovic-Latifagic E, Arnautalic L, Odobasic A, Idrizovic E, et al. Perineal endometriosis: a case report and review of the literature. Tech Coloproctol. 2010;14 Suppl 1:S25–7.
73. Nominato NS, Prates LF, Lauar I, Morais J, Maia L, Geber S. Caesarean section greatly increases risk of scar endometriosis. Eur J Obstet Gynecol Reprod Biol. 2010;152(1):83–5.

74. Schweppe KW, Ring D. Peritoneal defects and the development of endometriosis in relation to the timing of endoscopic surgery during the menstrual cycle. Fertil Steril. 2002;78(4):763–6.
75. Harada T, Momoeda M, Taketani Y, Hoshiai H, Terakawa N. Low-dose oral contraceptive pill for dysmenorrhea associated with endometriosis: a placebo-controlled, double-blind, randomized trial. Fertil Steril. 2008;90:1583–8.
76. ACOG Committee Opinion. Number 310, April 2005. Endometriosis in adolescents. Obstet Gynecol. 2005;105:921–7.
77. Meresman GF, Auge L, Baranao RI, Lombardi E, Tesone M, Sueldo C. Oral contraceptive suppress cell proliferation and enhance apoptosis of eutopic endometrial tissue from patients with endometriosis. Fertil Steril. 2002;77:1141–7.
78. Vercellini P, Fedele L, Pietropaolo G, Frontino G, Somigliana E, Crosignani PG. Progestogens for endometriosis: forward to the past. Hum Reprod Update. 2003;9:387–96.
79. Vessey MP, Villard-Mackintosh L, Painter R. Epidemiology of endometriosis in women attending family planning clinics. BMJ. 1993;306:182–4.
80. Fraser IS, Kovacs GT. The efficacy of non-contraceptive uses for hormonal contraceptives. Med J Aust. 2003;178:621–3.
81. Parazzini F, Ferraroni M, Bocciolone L, Tozzi L, Rubessa S, La Vecchia C. Contraceptive methods and risk of pelvic endometriosis. Contraception. 1994;49:47–55.
82. Italian Endometriosis Study Group. Oral contraceptive use and risk of endometriosis. BJOG. 1999;106:695–9.
83. Darrow SL, Vena JE, Batt RE, Zielezny MA, Michalek AM, Selman S. Menstrual cycle characteristics and the risk of endometriosis. Epidemiology. 1993;4:135–42.
84. Heilier JF, Donnez J, Nackers F, Rousseau R, Verougstraete V, Rosenkranz K, et al. Environmental and host-associated risk factors in endometriosis and deep endometriotic nodules: a matched case–control study. Environ Res. 2007;103:121–9.
85. Chapron C, Souza C, Borghese B, Lafay-Pillet MC, Santulli P, Bijaoui G, et al. Oral contraceptives and endometriosis: the past use of oral contraceptives for treating severe primary dysmenorrhea is associated with endometriosis, especially deep infiltrating endometriosis. Hum Reprod. 2011;26(8):2028–35.
86. Vercellini P, Eskenazi B, Consonni D, Somigliana E, Parazzini F, Abbiati A, et al. Oral contraceptives and risk of endometriosis: a systematic review and meta-analysis. Hum Reprod Update. 2011;17:159–70.
87. Di Zerega GB, Barber DL, Hodgen GD. Endometriosis: role of ovarian steroids in initiation, maintenance and suppression. Fertil Steril. 1980;33:649–53.
88. Seracchioli R, Mabrouk M, Frasca C, Manuzzi L, Savelli L, Venturoli S. Long-term oral contraceptive pills and postoperative pain management after laparoscopic excision of ovarian endometrioma: a randomized controlled trial. Fertil Steril. 2010;94:464–71.
89. Somigliana E, Vercellini P, Vigano P, Abbiati A, Benaglia L, Fedele L. Endometriosis and estroprogestins: the chicken or the egg causality dilemma. Fertil Steril. 2011;95:431–3.
90. Hemmings R, Rivard M, Olive DL, Poliquin-Fleury J, Gagné D, Hugo P, et al. Evaluation of risk factors associated with endometriosis. Fertil Steril. 2004;81(6):1513–21.
91. Moen MH. Endometriosis in women at interval sterilization. Acta Obstet Gynecol Scand. 1987;66:451–4.
92. Sangi-Haghpeykar H, Poindexter AN. Epidemiology of endometriosis among parous women. Obstet Gynecol. 1995;85(6):983–92.
93. Mahmood TA, Templeton A. Prevalence and genesis of endometriosis. Hum Reprod. 1991;6:544–9.
94. Kirshon B, Poindexter AN. Contraception: a risk factor for endometriosis. Obstet Gynecol. 1988;71:829–31.
95. Lan S, Ling L, Jianhong Z, Xijing J, Lihui W. Analysis of the levonorgestrel-releasing intrauterine system in women with endometriosis. J Int Med Res. 2013;41(3):548–58.

96. ESHRE Capri Workshop Group. Intrauterine devices and intrauterine systems. Hum Reprod Update. 2008;14(3):197–208.
97. Vercellini P, Frontino G, De Giorgi O, Aimi G, Zaina B, Crosignani PG. Comparison of a levonorgestrel-releasing intrauterine device versus expectant management after conservative surgery for symptomatic endometriosis: a pilot study. Fertil Steril. 2003;80:305–9.
98. Cheewadhanaraks S. Effect of tubal ligation on pelvic endometriosis externa in multiparous women with chronic pelvic pain. J Med Assoc Thai. 2004;87(7):735–9.
99. Kudielka BM, Kirschbaum C. Sex differences in HPA axis responses to stress: a review. Biol Psychol. 2005;69(1):113–32.
100. De Longis A, Folkman S, Lazarus RS. The impact of daily stress on health and mood: psychological and social resources as mediators. J Pers Soc Psychol. 1988;54(3):486–95.
101. Petrelluzzi KF, Garcia MC, Petta CA, Grassi-Kassisse DM, Spadari-Bratfisch RC. Salivary cortisol concentrations, stress and quality of life in women with endometriosis and chronic pelvic pain. Stress. 2008;11(5):390–7.
102. Lima AP, Moura MD, Rosa e Silva AAM. Prolactin and cortisol levels in women with endometriosis. Braz J Med Biol Res. 2006;39(8):1121–7.
103. Christodoulakos G, Augoulea A, Lambrinoudaki I, Sioulas V, Creatsas G. Pathogenesis of endometriosis: the role of defective ‘immunosurveillance’. Eur J Contracept Reprod Health Care. 2007;12(3):194–202.
104. Tariverdian N, Theoharides TC, Siedentopf F, Gutiérrez G, Jeschke U, Rabinovich GA, et al. Neuroendocrine-immune disequilibrium and endometriosis: an interdisciplinary approach. Semin Immunopathol. 2007;29(2):193–210.
105. Cuevas M, Flores I, Thompson KJ, Ramos-Ortolaza DL, Torres-Reveron A, Appleyard CB. Stress exacerbates endometriosis manifestations and inflammatory parameters in an animal model. Reprod Sci. 2012;19(8):851–62.
106. Sugamata M, Ihara T, Uchiide I. Increase of activated mast cells in human endometriosis. Am J Reprod Immunol. 2005;53(3):120–5.
107. Anaf V, Chapron C, Nakadi IE, De Moor V, Simonart T, Noel JC. Pain, mast cells, and nerves in peritoneal, ovarian and deep infiltrating endometriosis. Fertil Steril. 2006;86(5):1336–43.
108. Fenster L, Waller K, Chen J, Hubbard AE, Windham GC, Elkin E, et al. Psychological stress in the workplace and menstrual function. Am J Epidemiol. 1999;149(2):127–34.
109. Wang L, Wang X, Wang W, Chen C, Ronnennberg AG, Guang W, et al. Stress and dysmenorrhoea: a population based prospective study. Occup Environ Med. 2004;61 (12):1021–6.
110. Gul A, Yaspar T, Ugras S. BCG vaccination to prevent implantation of endometriosis: an experimental study in rats. Eur J Obstet Gynecol Reprod Biol. 2001;98:209–12.
111. Clayton RD, Duffy SR, Wilkinson N, Garry R, Jackson AM. Increase in peripheral blood mononuclear cell (PBMC)- and CD56+ cell-mediated killing of endometrial stromal cells by mycobacteria; a possible role in endometriosis immunotherapy? Hum Reprod. 2004;19 (8):1886–93.
112. Balasch J, Creus M, Fabregas F, Carmona F, Martínez-Román S, Manau D, et al. Pentoxifylline versus placebo in the treatment of infertility associated with minimal or mild endometriosis: a pilot randomized clinical trial. Hum Reprod. 1997;12:2046–50.
113. Szymanowski K, Chmaj-Wierzchowska K, Yantczenko A, Niepsuj-Biniaś J, Florek E, Opala T, et al. Endometriosis prophylaxis and treatment with the newly developed xenogenic immunomodulator RESAN in an animal model. Eur J Obstet Gynecol Reprod Biol. 2009;142 (2):145–8.
114. Chuang PC, Wu MH, Shoji Y, Tsai SJ. Downregulation of CD36 results in reduced phagocytic ability of peritoneal macrophages of women with endometriosis. J Pathol. 2009;219:232–41.
115. Sidell N, Han SW, Parthasarathy S. Regulation and modulation of abnormal immune responses in endometriosis. Ann N Y Acad Sci. 2002;955:159–73. 99–200, 396–406.

116. Jadidi-Niaragh F, Mirshafiey A. Th17 cell, the new player of neuroinflammatory process in multiple sclerosis. Scand J Immunol. 2011;74:1–13.
117. Elias KM, Laurence A, Davidson TS, Stephens G, Kano Y, Shevach EM, et al. Retinoic acid inhibits Th17 polarization and enhances FoxP3 expression through a Stat-3/Stat-5 independent signaling pathway. Blood. 2008;111:1013–20.
118. Wang X, Allen C, Ballow M. Retinoic acid enhances the production of IL-10 while reducing the synthesis of IL-12 and TNF-alpha from LPS-stimulated monocytes/macrophages. J Clin Immunol. 2007;27:193–200.
119. Kalu E, Sumar N, Giannopoulos T, Patel P, Croucher C, Sherriff E, et al. Cytokine profiles in serum and peritoneal fluid from infertile women with and without endometriosis. J Obstet Gynaecol Res. 2007;33:490–5.
120. Wieser F, Wu J, Shen Z, Taylor RN, Sidell N. Retinoic acid suppresses growth of lesions, inhibits peritoneal cytokine secretion, and promotes macrophage differentiation in an immunocompetent Mouse model of endometriosis. Fertil Steril. 2012;97(6):1430–7.
121. Alpay Z, Saed GM, Diamond MP. Female infertility and free radicals: potential role in adhesions and endometriosis. J Soc Gynecol Invest. 2006;13:390–8.
122. Portz DM, Elkins TE, White R, Warren J, Adadevoh S, Randolph J. Oxygen free radicals and pelvic adhesion formation: I. Blocking oxygen free radical toxicity to prevent adhesion formation in an endometriosis model. Int J Fertil. 1991;36:39–42.
123. Del Río B, García Pedrero JM, Martínez-Campa C, Zuazua P, Lazo PS, Ramos S. Melatonin, an endogenous-specific inhibitor of estrogen receptor alpha via calmodulin. J Biol Chem. 2004;279:38294–302.
124. Rato AG, Pedrero JG, Martinez MA, del Rio B, Lazo PS, Ramos S. Melatonin blocks the activation of estrogen receptor for DNA binding. FASEB J. 1999;13:857–68.
125. Paul S, Sharma AV, Mahapatra PD, Bhattacharya P, Reiter RJ, Swarnakar S. Role of melatonin in regulating matrix metalloproteinase-9 via tissue inhibitors of metalloproteinase-1 during protection against endometriosis. J Pineal Res. 2008;44 (4):439–49.
126. Akoum A, Lemay A, McColl S, Turcot-Lemay L, Maheux R. Elevated concentration and biologic activity of monocyte chemotactic protein-1 in the peritoneal fluid of patients with endometriosis. Fertil Steril. 1996;66:17–23.
127. Matsuzaki S, Canis M, Darcha C, Dallel R, Okamura K, Mage G. Cyclooxygenase-2 selective inhibitor prevents implantation of eutopic endometrium to ectopic sites in rats. Fertil Steril. 2004;82:1609–15.
128. Lebovic DI, Mwenda JM, Chai DC, Mueller MD, Santi A, Fisseha S, et al. PPAR-gamma receptor ligand induces regression of endometrial explants in baboons: a prospective, randomized, placebo- and drug-controlled study. Fertil Steril. 2007;88:1108–19.
129. Barrier BF, Bates GW, Leland MM, Leach DA, Robinson RD, Propst AM. Efficacy of anti-tumor necrosis factor therapy in the treatment of spontaneous endometriosis in baboons. Fertil Steril. 2004;81 Suppl 1:775–9.
130. Altan ZM, Denis D, Kagan D, Grund EM, Palmer SS, Nataraja SG. A long-acting tumor necrosis factor alpha-binding protein demonstrates activity in both in vitro and in vivo models of endometriosis. J Pharmacol Exp Ther. 2010;334(2):460–6.
131. Khoufache K, Bazin S, Girard K, Guillemette J, Roy MC, Verreault JP, et al. Macrophage migration inhibitory factor antagonist blocks the development of endometriosis in vivo. PLoS One. 2012;7(5):e37264.
132. Chen PF, Luo YL, Wang W, Wang JX, Lai WY, Hu SM, et al. ISO-1, a macrophage migration inhibitory factor antagonist, inhibits airway remodeling in a murine model of chronic asthma. Mol Med. 2010;16:400–8.
133. Hou XQ, Gao YW, Yang ST, Wang CY, Ma ZY, Xia XZ. Role of macrophage migration inhibitory factor in influenza H5N1 virus pneumonia. Acta Virol. 2009;53:225–31.
134. Arnson Y, Amital H, Shoenfeld Y. Vitamin D and autoimmunity: new aetiological and therapeutic considerations. Ann Rheum Dis. 2007;66(9):1137–42.

135. Harris HR, Chavarro JE, Malspeis S, Willett WC, Missmer SA. Dairy-food, calcium, magnesium, and vitamin D intake and endometriosis: a prospective cohort study. Am J Epidemiol. 2013;177(5):420–30.
136. Hartwell D, Rodbro P, Jensen SB, Thomsen K, Christiansen C. Vitamin D metabolites—relation to age, menopause and endometriosis. Scand J Clin Lab Invest. 1990;50(2):115–21.
137. Somigliana E, Panina-Bordignon P, Murone S, Di Lucia P, Vercellini P, Vigano P. Vitamin D reserve is higher in women with endometriosis. Hum Reprod. 2007;22(8):2273–8.
138. Agic A, Xu H, Altgassen C, Noack F, Wolfler MM, Diedrich K, et al. Relative expression of 1,25-dihydroxyvitamin D3 receptor, vitamin D 1α-hydroxylase, vitamin D 24-hydroxylase, and vitamin D 25-hydroxylase in endometriosis and gynecologic cancers. Reprod Sci. 2007;14(5):486–97.
139. Chacko SA, Song Y, Nathan L, Tinker L, de Boer IH, Tylavsky F, et al. Relations of dietary magnesium intake to biomarkers of inflammation and endothelial dysfunction in an ethnically diverse cohort of postmenopausal women. Diabetes Care. 2010;33(2):304–10.
140. D'Angelo EK, Singer HA, Rembold CM. Magnesium relaxes arterial smooth muscle by decreasing intracellular Ca^{2+} without changing intracellular Mg^{2+}. J Clin Invest. 1992;89 (6):1988–94.
141. Shand AW, Nassar N, Von Dadelszen P, Innis SM, Green TJ. Maternal vitamin D status in pregnancy and adverse pregnancy outcomes in a group at high risk for pre-eclampsia. BJOG. 2010;13:1593–8.
142. Gonzalez-Ramos R, Van Langendonckt A, Defrere S, Lousse JC, Mettlen M, Guillet A, et al. Agents blocking the nuclear factor-kappa B pathway are effective inhibitors of endometriosis in an in vivo experimental model. Gynecol Obstet Invest. 2008;3:174–86.
143. Griffin MD, Xing N, Kumar R. Vitamin D and its analogs as regulators of immune activation and antigen presentation. Annu Rev Nutr. 2003;23:117–45.
144. Mariani M, Viganò P, Gentilini D, Camisa B, Caporizzo E, Di Lucia P, et al. The selective vitamin D receptor agonist, elocalcitol, reduces endometriosis development in a mouse model by inhibiting peritoneal inflammation. Hum Reprod. 2012;27(7):2010–9.
145. Bruner-Tran KL, Osteen KG, Duleba AJ. Simvastatin protects against the development of endometriosis in a nude mouse model. J Clin Endocrinol Metab. 2009;94(7):2489–94.
146. Sokalska A, Cress A, Bruner-Tran KL, Osteen KG, Taylor HS, Ortega I, et al. Simvastatin decreases invasiveness of human endometrial stromal cells. Biol Reprod. 2012;87(1):2. 1–6.
147. Nothnick WB, Curry TE, Vernon MW. Immunomodulation of rat endometriotic implant growth and protein production. Am J Reprod Immun. 1994;31:151–62.
148. Lu D, Song H, Li Y, Clarke J, Shi G. Pentoxifylline for endometriosis. CochrDatabase Syst Rev. 2012; (1): CD007677.
149. Guo SW. Epigenetics of endometriosis. Mol Hum Reprod. 2009;15:587–607.
150. Olive DL. Medical therapy of endometriosis. Semin Reprod Med. 2003;21:209–22.
151. Moggio A, Pittatore G, Cassoni P, Marchino GL, Revelli A, Bussolati B. Sorafenib inhibits growth, migration, and angiogenic potential of ectopic endometrial mesenchymal stem cells derived from patients with endometriosis. Fertil Steril. 2012;98(6):1521–30. e2.
152. Swarnakar S, Paul S. Curcumin arrests endometriosis by downregulation of matrix metalloproteinase-9 activity. Indian J Biochem Biophys. 2009;46(1):59–65.
153. Jana S, Rudra DS, Paul S, Snehasikta S. Curcumin delays endometriosis development by inhibiting MMP-2 activity. Indian J Biochem Biophys. 2012;49(5):342–8.
154. Kim KH, Lee EN, Park JK, Lee JR, Kim JH, Choi HJ, et al. Curcumin attenuates TNF-α-induced expression of intercellular adhesion molecule-1, vascular cell adhesion molecule-1 and proinflammatory cytokines in human endometriotic stromal cells. Phytother Res. 2012;26(7):1037–47.
155. Xu H, Lui WT, Chu CY, Ng PS, Wang CC, Rogers MS. Anti-angiogenic effects of green tea catechin on an experimental endometriosis mouse model. Hum Reprod. 2009;24:608–18.
156. Hull ML, Charnock-Jones DS, Chan CL, Bruner-Tran KL, Osteen KG, Tom BD, et al. Antiangiogenic agents are effective inhibitors of endometriosis. J Clin Endocrinol Metab. 2003;88:2889–99.

157. Wang CC, Xu H, Man GC, Zhang T, Chu KO, Chu CY, et al. Prodrug of green tea epigallocatechin-3-gallate (Pro-EGCG) as a potent anti-angiogenesis agent for endometriosis in mice. Angiogenesis. 2013;16(1):59–69.
158. Xu H, Becker CM, Lui WT, Chu CY, Davis TN, Kung AL, et al. Green tea epigallocatechin-3-gallate inhibits angiogenesis and suppresses vascular endothelial growth factor C/vascular endothelial growth factor receptor 2 expression and signaling in experimental endometriosis in vivo. Fertil Steril. 2011;96:1021–8.
159. Athar M, Back JH, Kopelovich L, Bickers DR, Kim AL. Multiple molecular targets of resveratrol: anti-carcinogenic mechanisms. Arch Biochem Biophys. 2009;486:95–102.
160. Chen Y, Tseng SH. Review. Pro- and anti-angiogenesis effects of resveratrol. In Vivo. 2007;21:365–70.
161. Aluyen JK, Ton QN, Tran T, Yang AE, Gottlieb HB, Bellanger RA. Resveratrol: potential as anticancer agent. J Diet Suppl. 2012;9:45–56.
162. Beaudeux JL, Nivet-Antoine V, Giral P. Resveratrol: a relevant pharmacological approach for the treatment of metabolic syndrome? Curr Opin Clin Nutr Metab Care. 2010;13:729–36.
163. Petrovski G, Gurusamy N, Das DK. Resveratrol in cardiovascular health and disease. Ann N Y Acad Sci. 2011;1215:22–33.
164. Bruner-Tran KL, Osteen KG, Taylor HS, Sokalska A, Haines K, Duleba AJ. Resveratrol inhibits development of experimental endometriosis *in vivo* and reduces endometrial stromal cell invasiveness in vitro. Biol Reprod. 2011;84:106–12.
165. Rudzitis-Auth J, Menger MDM, Laschke MW. Resveratrol is a potent inhibitor of vascularization and cell proliferation in experimental endometriosis. Hum Reprod. 2013;28 (5):1339–47.
166. Ricci AG, Olivares CN, Bilotas MA, Bastón JI, Singla JJ, Meresman GF, et al. Natural therapies assessment for the treatment of endometriosis. Hum Reprod. 2013;28(1):178–88.
167. Wang D, Liu Y, Han J, Zai D, Ji M, Cheng W, et al. Puerarin suppresses invasion and vascularization of endometriosis tissue stimulated by 17β-estradiol. PLoS One. 2011;6(9): e25011.
168. Flower A, Liu JP, Lewith G, Little P, Li Q. Chinese herbal medicine for endometriosis. Cochrane Database of Systematic Reviews. 2012;(5):CD006568.
169. Zhao RH, Hao ZP, Zhang Y, Lian FM, Sun WW, Liu Y, Wang R, Long L, Cheng L, Ding YF, Song DR, Meng QW, Wang AM. Controlling the recurrence of pelvic endometriosis after a conservative operation: comparison between Chinese herbal medicine and western medicine. Chin J Integr Med. 2013;19(11):820–5.
170. Strathy JH, Molgaard CA, Coulam CB, Melton 3rd LJ. Endometriosis and infertility: a laparoscopic study of endometriosis among fertile and infertile women. Fertil Steril. 1982;38:667–72.
171. Verkauf BS. The incidence, symptoms, and signs of endometriosis in fertile and infertile women. J Fla Med Assoc. 1987;74:671–5.
172. Bulletti C, Montini A, Setti PL, Palagiano A, Ubaldi F, Borini A. Vaginal parturition decreases recurrence of endometriosis. Fertil Steril. 2010;94(3):850–5.
173. Parazzini F, Chiaffarino F, Surace M, Chatenoud L, Cipriani S, Chiantera V, et al. Selected food intake and risk of endometriosis. Hum Reprod. 2004;19:1755–9.
174. Kidd PM. Omega-3 DHA and EPA for cognition, behavior, and mood: clinical findings and structural-functional synergies with cell membrane phospholipids. Altern Med Rev. 2007;12:207–27.
175. Halliwell B, Gutteridge JM. Role of free radicals and catalytic metal ions in human disease: an overview. Methods Enzymol. 1990;186:1–85.
176. Harel Z, Biro FM, Kottenhahn RK, Rosenthal SL. Supplementation with omega-3 polyunsaturated fatty acids in the management of dysmenorrhea in adolescents. Am J Obstet Gynecol. 1996;174:1335–8.
177. Kaneda N, Nagata C, Kabuto M, Shimizu H. Fat and fiber intakes in relation to serum estrogen concentration in premenopausal Japanese women. Nutr Cancer. 1997;27:279–83.

178. Armstrong BK, Brown JB, Clarke HT, Crooke DK, Hähnel R, Masarei JR, et al. Diet and reproductive hormones: a study of vegetarian and nonvegetarian postmenopausal women. J Natl Cancer Inst. 1981;67:761–7.
179. Longcope C, Gorbach S, Goldin B, et al. The effect of a low fat diet on estrogen metabolism. J Clin Endocrinol Metab. 1987;64:1246–50.
180. Missmer SA, Chavarro JE, Malspeis S, Bertone-Johnson ER, Hornstein MD, Spiegelman D, et al. A prospective study of dietary fat consumption and endometriosis risk. Hum Reprod. 2010;25:1528–35.
181. Trabert B, Peters U, De Roos AJ, Scholes D, Holt VL. Diet and risk of endometriosis in a population-based case–control study. Br J Nutr. 2011;105(3):459–67.
182. Dhillon PK, Holt VL. Recreational physical activity and endometrioma risk. Am J Epidemiol. 2003;158:156–64.
183. Missmer SA, Cramer DW. The epidemiology of endometriosis. Obstet Gynecol Clin North Am. 2003;30:1–19.
184. Vitonis AF, Hankinson SE, Hornstein MD, Missmer SA. Adult physical activity and endometriosis risk. Epidemiology. 2010;21(1):16–23.
185. Signorello LB, Harlow BL, Cramer DW, Spiegelman D, Hill JA. Epidemiologic determinants of endometriosis: a hospital-based case–control study. Ann Epidemiol. 1997;7:267–741.
186. Vitonis AF, Maruti SS, Se H, Hornstein MD, Missmer SA. Adolescent physical activity and endometriosis risk. J Endometriosis. 2009;1:157–63.
187. Crain DA, Janssen SJ, Edwards TM, Heindel J, Ho SM, Hunt P, et al. Female reproductive disorders: the roles of endocrine- disrupting compounds and developmental timing. Fertil Steril. 2008;90(4):911–40.
188. Gilbert SF. Mechanisms for the environmental regulation of gene expression: ecological aspects of animal development. J Biosci. 2005;30:65–74.
189. Bumey RO, Giudice LC. The pathogenesis of endometriosis. In: Nezhat's operative gynecologic laparoscopy and hysteroscopy. 3rd ed. New York: Cambridge University Press; 2008. p. 251–7.
190. Dl A, Foster WG. The link between environmental toxicant exposure and endometriosis. Front Biosci. 2008;13:1578–93.
191. Kl B-T, Yeaman GR, Crispens MA, Igarashi TM, Osteen KG. Dioxin may promote inflammation-related development of endometriosis. Fertil Steril. 2008;89(5 suppl):1287–98.
192. Herington JL, Bruner-Tran KL, Lucas JA, Osteen KG. Immune interactions in endometriosis. Expert Rev Clin Immunol. 2011;7:611–26.
193. Schaefer WR, Hermann T, Meinhold-Heerlein I, Deppert WR, Zahradnik HP. Exposure of human endometrium to environmental estrogens, antiandrogens, and organochlorine compounds. Fertil Steril. 2000;74:558–63.
194. Quaranta MG, Porpora MG, Mattioli B, Giordani L, Libri I, Ingelido AM, et al. Impaired NK-cell-mediated cytotoxic activity and cytokine production in patients with endometriosis: a possible role for PCBs and DDE. Life Sci. 2006;79:491–8.
195. Cooney MA, Buck Louis GM, Hediger ML, Vexler A, Kostyniak PJ. Organochlorine pesticides and endometriosis. Reprod Toxicol. 2010;30:365–9.
196. Cobellis L, Latini G, De Felice C, Razzi S, Paris I, Ruggieri F, et al. High plasma concentrations of di-(2-ethylhexyl)-phthalate in women with endometriosis. Hum Reprod. 2003;18:1512–5.
197. Reddy BS, Rozati R, Reddy S, Kodampur S, Reddy P, Reddy R. High plasma concentrations of polychlorinated biphenyls and phthalate esters in women with endometriosis: a prospective case control study. Fertil Steril. 2006;85:775–9.
198. Buck Louis GM, Weiner JM, Whitcomb BW, Sperrazza R, Schisterman EF, Lobdell DT, et al. Environmental PCB exposure and risk of endometriosis. Hum Reprod. 2005;20:279–85.
199. Buck Louis GM, Chen Z, Peterson CM, Hediger ML, Croughan MS, Sundaram R, et al. Persistent lipophilic environmental chemicals and endometriosis : the ENDO Study. Environ Health Perspect. 2012;120(6):811–6.

200. Myllymaki SA, Haavisto TE, Brokken LJ, Viluksela M, Toppari J, Paranko J. In utero and lactational exposure to TCDD; steroidogenic outcomes differ in male and female rat pups. Toxicol Sci. 2005;88:534–44.
201. Pesonen SA, Haavisto TE, Viluksela M, Toppari J, Paranko J. Effects of in utero and lactational exposure to 2,3,7,8-tetrachlorodibenzo-*p*-dioxin (TCDD) on rat follicular steroidogenesis. Reprod Toxicol. 2006;22:521–8.
202. Wormke M, Stoner M, Saville B, Safe S. Crosstalk between estrogen receptor alpha and the aryl hydrocarbon receptor in breast cancer cells involves unidirectional activation of proteasomes. FEBS Lett. 2000;478:109–12.
203. Osteen KG, Bruner-Tran KL, Eisenberg E. Reduced progesterone action during endometrial maturation: a potential risk factor for the development of endometriosis. Fertil Steril. 2005;83:529–37.
204. Fazleabas AT, Brudney A, Chai D, Langoi D, Bulun SE. Steroid receptor and aromatase expression in baboon endometriotic lesions. Fertil Steril. 2003;80 Suppl 2:820–7.
205. Hudelist G, Keckstein J, Czerwenka K, Lass H, Walter I, Auer M, et al. Estrogen receptor beta and matrix metalloproteinase 1 are coexpressed in uterine endometrium and endometriotic lesions of patients with endometriosis. Fertil Steril. 2005;84 Suppl 2:1249–56.
206. Daxinger L, Whitelaw E. Understanding transgenerational epigenetic inheritance via the gametes in mammals. Nat Rev Genet. 2012;13:153–62.
207. Calkins K, Devaskar SU. Fetal origins of adult disease. Curr Probl Pediatr Adolesc Health Care. 2011;41(6):158–76.
208. Genuis SJ. The chemical erosion of human health: adverse environmental exposure and in-utero pollution- determinants of congenital disorders and chronic disease. J Perinat Med. 2006;34:185–95.
209. Taylor HS M.D. Endocrine disruptors affect developmental programming of HOX gene expression. Fertil Steril. 2008;89(1):e57–8.
210. Takahashi O, Oishi S. Disposition of orally administered 2,2-Bis (4-hydroxyphenyl) propane (Bisphenol A) in pregnant rats and the placental transfer to fetuses. Environ Health Perspect. 2000;108:931–5.
211. Zalko D, Soto AM, Dolo L, Dorio C, Rathahao E, Debrauwer L, et al. Biotransformations of bisphenol A in a mammalian model: answers and new questions raised by low-dose metabolic fate studies in pregnant CDI mice. Environ Health Perspect. 2003;111:309–19.
212. Oesterheld J. A review of developmental aspects of cytochrome P450. J Child Adolesc Psychopharm. 1998;8:161–74.
213. Kreuzer PE, Csanady GA, Baur C, Kessler W, Papke O, Greim H, et al. 2,3,7,8,-tetrachlorodibenzo-*p*-dioxin (TCDD) and congeners in infants. A toxicokinetic model of human lifetime body burden by TCDD with special emphasis on its uptake by nutrition. Arch Toxicol. 1997;71:383–400.
214. Jorissen J. Literature review: outcomes associated with postnatal exposure to polychlorinated biphenyls (PCBs) via breast milk. Adv Neonatal Care. 2007;7(5):230–7.
215. Boersema ER, Lanting CI. Environmental exposure to polychlorinated biphenyls (PCBs) and dioxins. Consequences for longterm neurological and cognitive development of the child lactation. Adv Exp Med Biol. 2000;478:271–87.
216. Lee SY, Kim MT, Kim SW, Song MS, Yoon SJ. Effect of lifetime lactation on breast cancer risk: a Korean women's cohort study. Int J Canc. 2003;105:390–3.
217. Daniels JL, Jen-Pan I, Jones R, Anderson S, Patterson DG, Needham LL, et al. Individual characteristics associated with PBDE levels in U.S. human milk samples. Environ Health Perspect. 2010;118(1):155–60.
218. Miyata H, Takenaka T, Nakao T, Aozasa O, Ohta S, Fujimine Y, et al. Investigation of the main source of halogenated environmental pollutants in human breast milk (The Third Report)- Influence by fasting. Organohalogen Comp. 2006;68:145–8.
219. LaKind JS. Recent global trends and physiologic origins of dioxins and furans in human milk. J Expo Sci Environ Epidemiol. 2007;17(6):510–24.

220. Anderson RC, Anderson JH. Acute respiratory effects if diaper emissions. Arch Environ Health. 1999;54(5):353.
221. Sathyanarayana S, Karr CJ, Lozano P, Brown E, Calafat AM, Liu F, et al. Baby care products: possible sources of infant phthalate exposure. Pediatrics. 2008;121(2):e260–8.
222. Curl C, Fenske RA, Elgethun K. Organophosphorus pesticide exposure of urban and suburban preschool children with organic and conventional diets. Environ Health Perspect. 2003;111(3):377–82.
223. Kimbrell A. Fatal harvest: the tragedy of industrial agriculture. Washington: Foundation for Deep Ecology and Island Press; 2002. p. 211.
224. Zeligs MA. Diet and estrogen status: the cruciferous connection. J Med Food. 1998;1(2):67–82.
225. Estrogenic agents leach from dental sealant. Science News April 11, 1996;49:214.
226. Buckley JD, Meadows AT, Kadin ME, Le Beau MM, Siegel S. Pesticide exposures in children with non Hodgkin's Lymphoma. Cancer. 2000;89(11):2315–21.
227. Kokcu A. Relationship between endometriosis and cancer from current perspective. Arch Gynecol Obstet. 2011;284(6):1473–9.
228. Frisch RE. Body fat, menarche and fertility. Hum Reprod. 1987;2(6):521–33.
229. Stark O, Peckham CS, Moynihan C. Weight and age at menarche. Arch Dis Child. 1989;64:383–7.
230. Diamond F. The function of adipose tissue. Growth Genet Horm. 2002;18(2):17–22.
231. Chavarro JE, Peterson KE, Sobol AM, Wiecha JL, Gortmaker SL. Effect of a school-based obesity-prevention on menarche. Cancer Causes Control. 2005;16:1245–52.
232. Buck Louis GM, Hediger ML, Peña JB. Intrauterine exposures and risk of endometriosis. Hum Reprod. 2007;22:3232–6.
233. Vitonis AF, Baer HJ, Hankinson SE, Laufer MR, Missmer SA. A prospective study of body size during childhood and early adulthood and the incidence of endometriosis. Hum Reprod. 2010;25:1325–34.
234. Somigliana E, Vigano P, Abbiati A, Paffoni A, Benaglia L, Vercellini P, et al. Perinatal environment and endometriosis. Gynecol Obstet Invest. 2011;72:135–40.
235. Wolff EF, Sun L, Hediger ML, Sundaram R, Peterson CM, Chen Z, et al. In utero exposures and endometriosis: the Endometriosis, Natural History, Disease, Outcome(ENDO) Study. Fertil Steril. 2013;99(3):790–5.

Chapter 19
MR Imaging of Endometriosis

Shinya Fujii

Abstract MR imaging has played a significant role as a noninvasive method, although laparoscopy is the gold standard for diagnosis. We describe MR imaging findings about endometriotic cyst, endometriotic implant, adhesion, deep endometriosis, decidualized endometriotic cyst, and malignant neoplasms arising from endometriosis.

Keywords Endometriosis • MRI • Ovary

19.1 Endometriotic Cyst

The signal intensity of endometriotic cysts is hyperintense on T1-weighted imaging similar to that of fat. T2-weighted imaging finding of endometriotic cyst is hypointense (shading) in most cases (Fig. 19.1), but can be hyperintense. Besides, multiplicity of the cysts is another important finding. MR imaging for the diagnosis of endometriotic cysts has a sensitivity of 90–92 %, a specificity of 91–98 %, and an accuracy of 91–96 % [1–4]. Therefore, MR imaging is very important and useful for the diagnosis of endometriotic cysts. This characteristic signal intensity is considered to reflect aged blood and its viscosity [1]. The signal intensity of endometriotic cysts on T2-weighted imaging has a significant relationship with the iron concentration, although there is no significant relationship with the signal intensity on T1-weighted imaging [5]. Fat-suppressed T1-weighted imaging should always be performed for not only the differentiation from mature cystic teratoma showing hyperintensity on T1-weighted imaging but also the detection of small lesions such as endometriotic implants. Another characteristic finding is thick wall with hypointensity on both T1- and T2-weighted imaging. This finding reflects the fibrous nature of the cyst wall with

S. Fujii (✉)
Division of Radiology, Department of Pathophysiological and Therapeutic Science,
Faculty of Medicine, Tottori University, Yonago, Japan
e-mail: sfujii@med.tottori-u.ac.jp

T. Harada (ed.), *Endometriosis: Pathogenesis and Treatment*,
DOI 10.1007/978-4-431-54421-0_19, © Springer Japan 2014

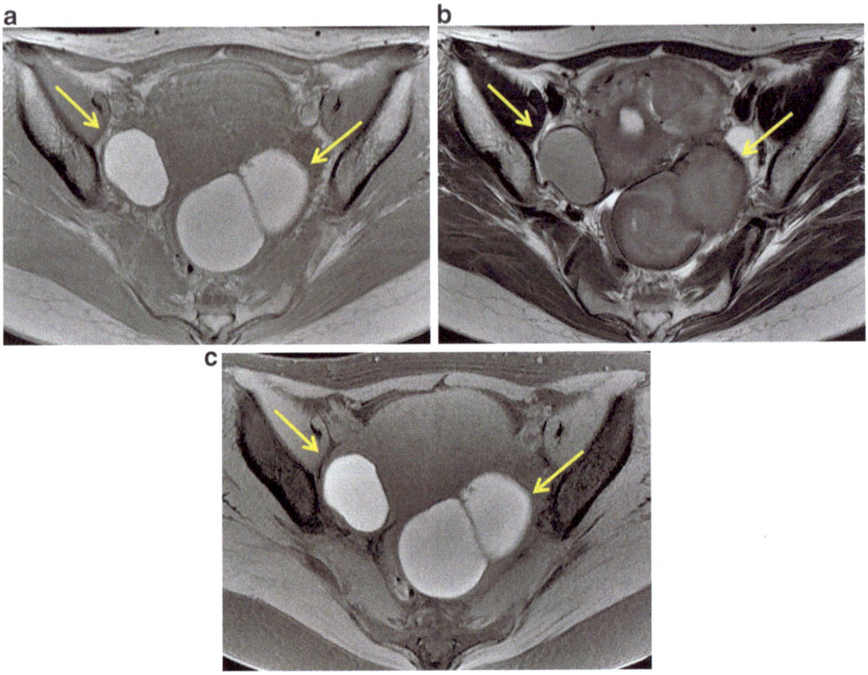

Fig. 19.1 A 39-year-old woman with bilateral ovarian endometriotic cysts. Axial T1-weighted MR image (**a**) shows bilateral hyperintense ovarian masses (*arrows*). T2-weighted image shows shading with hyperintensity in both lesions (*arrows*) (**b**). On fat-suppressed T1-weighted image, these masses remain hyperintense (**c**)

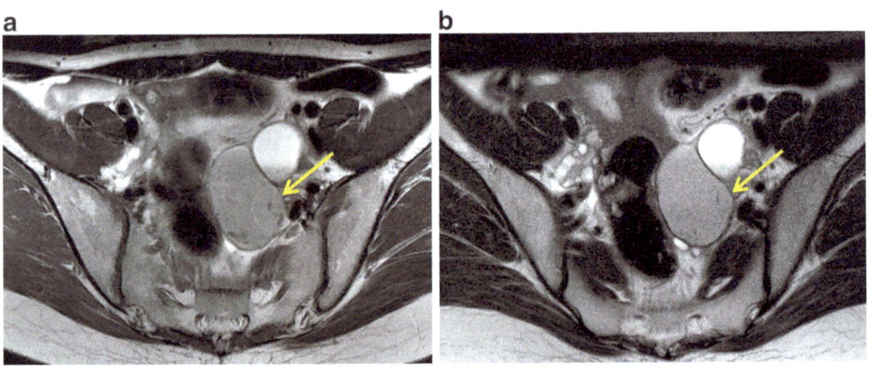

Fig. 19.2 A 32-year-old woman with left ovarian endometriotic cyst. Axial T2-weighted images demonstrate left ovarian hypointense cystic mass (*arrow*). The shading sign is more prominent at 3 T (**a**) than at 1.5 T (**b**)

hemosiderin-laden macrophages [6]. Susceptibility weighted imaging can detect this hemosiderin deposit [7]. Meanwhile, 3.0 T MR imaging is more useful for the diagnosis of endometriotic cysts than that of 1.5 T, because 3.0 T MR imaging can demonstrate shading sign on T2-weighted images [8] (Fig. 19.2).

19.2 Endometriotic Implants

Fat-suppressed T1-weighted imaging is mandatory sequence for the detection of endometriotic implants [2, 3, 9–11]. The sensitivity in detecting peritoneal implants is significantly higher with fat-suppressed T1-weighted imaging (61 %) than with conventional T1-weighted imaging (27 %) due to better visualization of hemorrhagic implants with signal suppression of surrounding fat tissue [9]. Additionally, fat-suppressed T1-weighted imaging can detect endometriotic implants that are not detected during surgery because of overlying adhesions [12, 13]. However, the sensitivity is not so high because even fat-suppressed T1-weighted images cannot detect tiny peritoneal lesions and the lesions which do not contain enough methemoglobin [12]; some small endometriotic implants can show hypointensity on T1-weighted images and hyperintensity on T2-weighted images [6].

19.3 Adhesion, Posterior Cul-de-sac Obliteration

Adhesion is diagnosed when there is obliteration of fat planes with a lack of a clear interface between adjacent organs, spiculated hypointensity stranding between the organs, and angulation and distortion of adjacent bowel loops [14]. These findings are usually subtle, and we should detect the findings carefully.

The following findings are related to posterior cul-de-sac obliteration: retroflexed uterus, elevated posterior vaginal fornix, intestinal tethering and/or a tethered appearance of the rectum in the direction of the uterus, faint strands between the uterus and intestine, and fibrotic plaque and/or nodule covering the serosal surface of the uterus [14] (Fig. 19.3). Particularly, the following findings are proposed as the major criteria for diagnosing cul-de-sac obliteration because of their good specificity: intestinal tethering and/or a tethered appearance of the rectum in the direction of the uterus, strands between the uterus and intestine, and a fibrotic plaque covering the serosal surface of the uterus. Additionally, the most accurate combination of two findings is intestinal tethering in the direction of the uterus and fibrotic plaque in the uterine serosal surface, and the next highest combination is retroflexed uterus and intestinal tethering in the direction of the uterus [14].

19.4 Deep Pelvic Endometriosis

Deep infiltrating endometriosis is defined as the presence of endometriotic implants, fibrosis, and muscular hyperplasia penetrating >5 mm into the peritoneum. Associated symptoms include dysmenorrhea, dyspareunia, noncyclical pelvic

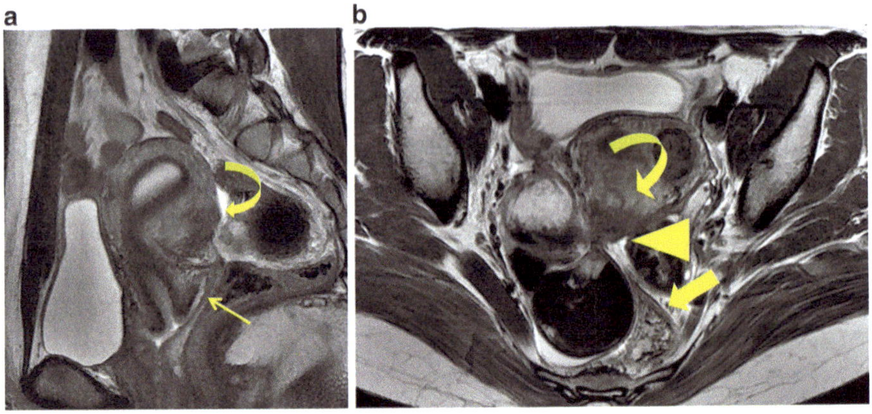

Fig. 19.3 A 34-year-old woman with bilateral ovarian endometriotic cysts and posterior cul-de-sac obliteration. The uterus is retroflexed on sagittal T2-weighted image (**a**). An irregular hypointense area at posterior serosal surface of uterus is found (*curved arrows*). The posterior vaginal fornix (*arrow*) is elevated toward this area. Axial T2-weighted image (**b**) shows faint strands between uterus and rectum (*arrowhead*), tethered appearance of the rectum in the direction of the uterus (*bold arrow*)

pain, dysuria, and lower gastrointestinal symptoms. The lesion can involve the posterior cul-de-sac, uterosacral ligaments, rectovaginal septum, ureters, bowel, and bladder. Endometriotic implants usually elicit an intense desmoplastic response in the surrounding tissues, leading to the formation of adhesions, fibrotic bands, and plaques. The histologic finding of deep pelvic endometriosis is mainly characterized by fibromuscular hyperplasia surrounding foci of endometriosis. Previous report has demonstrated the high accuracy in the prediction of deep pelvic endometriosis with a sensitivity of 90.3 %, specificity of 91 %, and accuracy of 90.8 % [15]. Additionally, 3.0 T MR imaging has high accuracy in the diagnosis and staging of deep endometriosis [16].

Deep endometriosis shows typically hypointensity with punctate hyperintensity on T1-weighted imaging, hypointensity on T2-weighted imaging, and contrast enhancement, which findings correspond to fibrous tissue. Punctate foci of hyperintensity reflect hemorrhage surrounded by solid fibrous tissue. Additionally, tiny hyperintensities within the lesion, which represent endometrial glands, can be shown on T2-weighted imaging.

Irregular fibrotic thickening and nodularity with regular or stellate margins along the course of the uterosacral ligament suggests deep pelvic endometriosis (Fig. 19.4) [15]. MR imaging for the diagnosis of uterosacral ligament endometriosis has a sensitivity of 69.2–90 % and a specificity of 76–94.3 % [17]. Thin-section oblique axial T2-weighted imaging can improve the depiction of uterosacral ligament endometriosis [18]. However, 3D T2-weighted imaging in combination with a multi-planar reconstruction technique has no significant different accuracy from that of conventional 2D axial T2-weighted imaging [17].

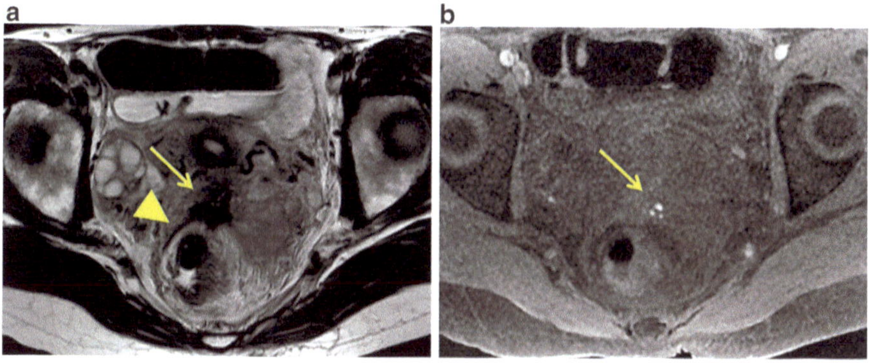

Fig. 19.4 A 29-year-old woman with deep pelvic endometriosis of bilateral uterosacral ligaments. Axial T2-weighted image (**a**) demonstrates hypointense fibrotic plaque (*arrow*) with punctate hyperintense foci on fat-suppressed T1-weighted image (*arrow*) (**b**) and irregular thickening of the right uterosacral ligament (*arrowheads*)

Endometriosis of rectovaginal septum is mainly classified to massive lesion of the deepest portion of the pouch of Douglas and retroperitoneal deep endometriotic lesion originating from the metaplasia of müllerian remnants located in the rectovaginal septum. Laparoscopic diagnosis is difficult because of complete obliteration of the cul-de-sac. The lesion demonstrates ill-defined hypointense mass between posterior vaginal fornix and rectum and can cause rectal stenosis and hydronephrosis.

The rectum and distal sigmoid colon account for most of the bowel endometriosis. The endometriotic implants are usually serosal, but can eventually erode through the subserosal layers and cause marked thickening and fibrosis of the muscularis propria. Inflammatory response to cyclic hemorrhage can lead to adhesions, bowel stricture, and gastrointestinal obstruction. Bowel endometriosis shows mushroom or fan-shaped configuration, demonstrating isointensity compared to muscle and slightly hyperintense at the luminal side of the bowel wall on T2-weighted imaging [19, 20] (Fig. 19.5). The lesions sometimes demonstrate hemorrhagic foci that are hyperintense on fat-suppressed T1-weighted imaging. MR imaging has a sensitivity of 100 % and specificity of 75 % for predicting muscular infiltration [20]. Diffusion-weighted imaging depicts the lesion as hypointensity and is useful for the differentiation from colorectal cancer [21]. Additionally, contrast-enhanced imaging can allow easier recognition of colorectal endometriosis [22].

Involvement of bladder is seen in less than 1 % of patients with endometriosis. Bladder endometriosis is mostly found on the posterior wall or in the dome of the bladder. Bladder endometriosis can be demonstrated as localized or diffuse bladder wall thickening showing hypointensity on T1- and T2-weighted imaging.

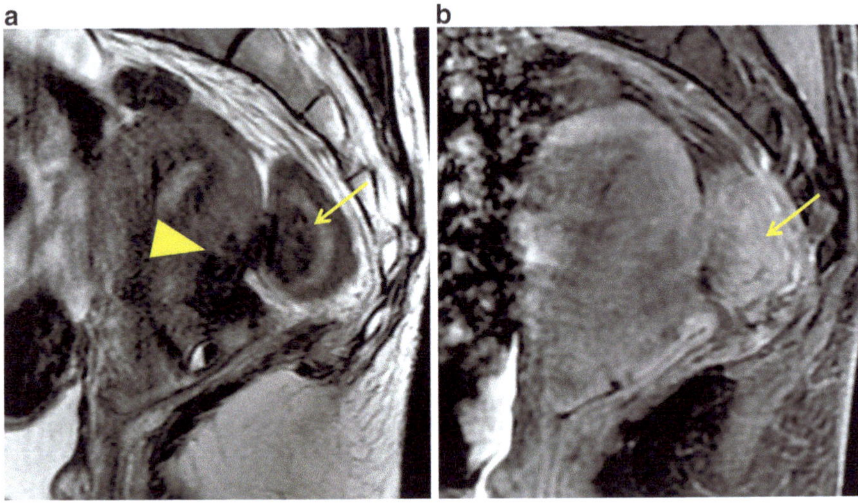

Fig. 19.5 A 30-year-old woman with deep pelvic endometriosis infiltrating the rectosigmoid. Rectosigmoid involvement shows hypointense fan-shaped configuration on sagittal T2-weighted image (**a**) and contrast enhancement on enhanced T1-weighted image (*arrow*). An irregular hypointensity area at posterior serosal surface of uterus is also found (*arrowhead*)

Hyperintense foci on fat-suppressed T1-weighted and T2-weighted imaging indicative of hemorrhage and endometrial glands may be seen within the lesion [23, 24].

Parametrial involvement can also occur, representing a severe form of endometriosis, and is important for surgical planning for deep infiltrating endometriosis because a parametrectomy can be required for the complete removal of deep infiltrating endometriosis. Recent report demonstrates the MR findings indicating parametrial involvement as follows: the presence of a hypointense area in the paracervical or paravaginal region on T2-weighted imaging or pelvic wall involvement and ureteral dilatation [25].

19.5 Prediction of Hormone Therapy Response

MR imaging can predict the hormone therapy response of endometriotic cyst. Response of the therapy is not good for endometriotic cysts with shading on T2-weighted imaging, while endometriotic cysts without shading and multiplicity indicate a good response to hormone therapy [26] (Fig. 19.6). The signal intensity of responding endometriotic cysts decreases after the therapy on T2-weighted imaging.

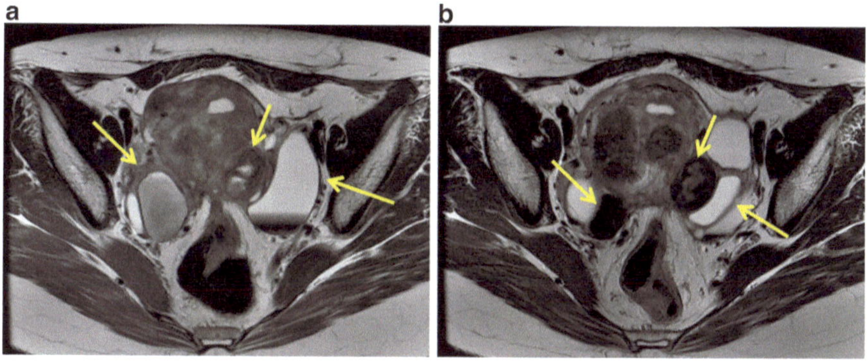

Fig. 19.6 A 34-year-old woman with bilateral ovarian endometriotic cysts. Bilateral endometriotic cysts (*arrows*) show hyperintensity with subtle shading on axial T2-weighted images obtained before hormone therapy (**a**). The size and signal intensity of the cysts (*arrows*) decreased after hormone therapy (**b**)

19.6 Decidualized Endometrioma

Decidual changes of the ectopic endometrial stroma during pregnancy are well known. Decidual changes of endometrial tissue in endometriomas during pregnancy may manifest as mural nodules and mimic malignant transformation. The mural nodules indicating decidualization are demonstrated as linear, small nodular, broad-based nodular, or polypoid structures, which show isointensity with the nomotopic decidualized endometrium on T1- and T2-weighted images, balanced fast field echo images, and diffusion-weighted images [27–29]. Additionally, the apparent diffusion coefficient of decidualized mural nodules is significantly higher than that of ovarian cancers [29]. These MR imaging characteristics can help to differentiate decidualized endometriotic cyst from malignant transformation.

19.7 Malignant Tumor Arising in Endometriotic Cyst

Malignant transformation is a rare complication of endometriosis and is estimated to occur in 0.6–0.8 % of women with ovarian endometriosis. Approximately 75 % of malignancies arising in endometriosis are found in ovarian endometriosis, and 25 % are found in extraovarian endometriosis [30]. Malignancies arising in ovarian endometriosis are composed of endometrioid carcinomas in about 70 %, clear cell carcinoma in 13.5 %, and sarcoma in 11.6 %, while malignancies arising in extraovarian endometriosis are composed of endometrioid carcinomas in 65 %, sarcoma in 25 %, and clear cell carcinoma in 4.5 % [28].

The following findings suggesting endometriotic cysts with malignant transformation are endometrioma with increasing size, larger size than those of

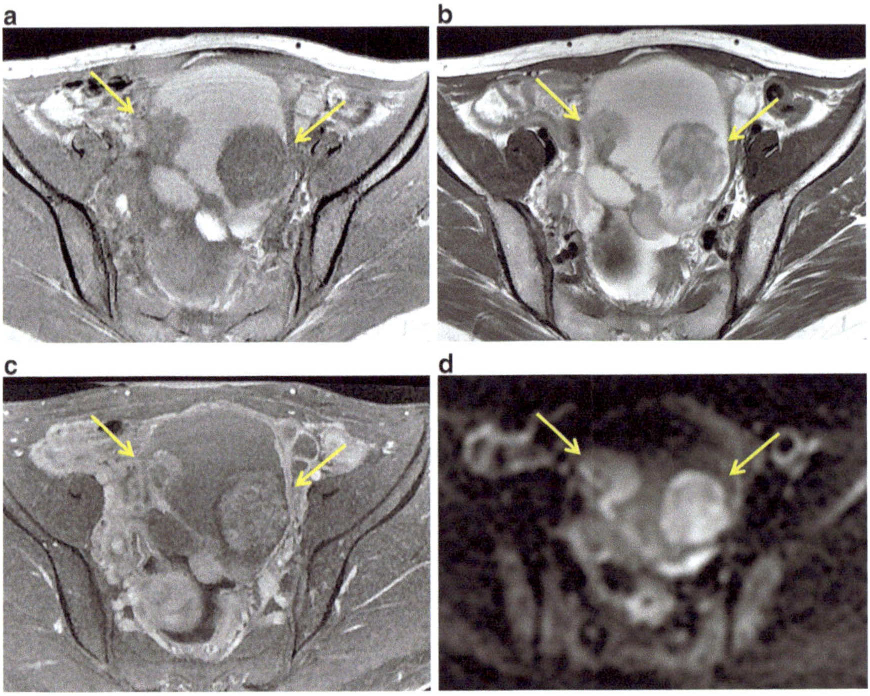

Fig. 19.7 A 45-year-old woman with endometrioid adenocarcinoma associated with endometriotic cyst. Left endometriotic cyst shows hyperintensity on axial T1-weighted image (**a**) and absence of shading on T2-weighted image (**b**). The solid component (*arrows*) demonstrates contrast enhancement on contrast-enhanced T1-weighted image (**c**) and hyperintensity on diffusion-weighted image (**d**)

contralateral endometriotic cysts, loss of shading on T2-weighted images, and enhancing mural nodules on contrast-enhanced images [31] (Fig. 19.7). The enhancement of mural nodules is sometimes difficult to evaluate on conventional contrast-enhanced T1-weighted images. Dynamic subtraction imaging can improve the detection of enhancing mural nodule against intrinsically hyperintense background signal of endometriotic cyst [31] and is useful for the differentiation of the tumors from intracystic blood clots. Meanwhile diffusion-weighted images can provide a little information about its differentiation because some clots can show hyperintensity [32]. Additionally, we should recognize that the small enhancing nodules have the possibility of benign conditions such as granulomatous tissue and benign endometriotic tissue [33].

Müllerian mucinous borderline tumor (MMBT) should be recognized as malignant tumor arising from endometriosis because of coexistence with ovarian or pelvic endometriosis in about 30 %. MMBTs are unilocular or paucilocular in 80 % of cases, bilateral in 7.7–40 %, and show prominent hyperintensity on T2-weighted images reflecting intraluminal mucinous material and stromal edema [34].

Malignant tumors arising in extraovarian endometriosis occur in various anatomic locations, such as rectovaginal sites, colorectal sites, and bladder, which seem to reflect the distribution of extraovarian endometriotic implants. Malignant tumors arising from extraovarian endometriosis typically manifest as solid lesions showing intermediate signal intensity on T1- and T2-weighted images, enhanced by contrast material, and hyperintensity on diffusion-weighted images [35].

References

1. Togashi K, Nishimura K, Kimura I, et al. Endometrial cysts: diagnosis with MR imaging. Radiology. 1991;180:73–8.
2. Sugimura K, Okizuka H, Imaoka I, et al. Pelvic endometriosis: detection and diagnosis with chemical shift MR imaging. Radiology. 1993;188:435–8.
3. Outwater EK, Dunton CJ. Imaging of the ovary and adnexa: clinical issues and applications of MR imaging. Radiology. 1995;194:1–18.
4. Scoutt LM, McCarthy SM, Lange R, et al. MR evaluation of clinically suspected adnexal masses. J Comput Assist Tomogr. 1994;18:609–18.
5. Takahashi K, Okada S, Okada M, et al. Magnetic resonance relaxation time in evaluating the cyst fluid characteristics of endometrioma. Hum Reprod. 1996;11:857–60.
6. Woodward PJ, Sohaey R, Mezzetti Jr TP. Endometriosis: radiologic-pathologic correlation. Radiographics. 2001;21:193–216.
7. Takeuchi M, Matsuzaki K, Nishitani H. Susceptibility-weighted MRI of endometrioma: preliminary results. AJR Am J Roentgenol. 2008;191:1366–70.
8. Takeuchi M, Matsuzaki K, Kubo H, Nishitani H. Magnetic resonance manifestations of endometrial cysts at 3 T compared with 1.5T. J Comput Assist Tomogr. 2008;32:369–71.
9. Ha HK, Lim YT, Kim HS, et al. Diagnosis of pelvic endometriosis: fat suppressed T1 weighted vs conventional MR images. AJR Am J Roentgenol. 1994;163:127–31.
10. Bis KG, Vrachliotis TG, Agrawal R, et al. Pelvic endometriosis: MR imaging spectrum with laparoscopic correlation and diagnostic pitfalls. Radiographics. 1997;17:639–55.
11. Ascher SM, Agrawal R, Bis KG, et al. Endometriosis: appearance and detection with conventional and contrast-enhanced fat-suppressed spin-echo techniques. J Magn Reson Imaging. 1995;5:251–7.
12. Tanaka YO, Itai Y, Anno I, et al. MR staging of pelvic endometriosis: role of fat-suppression T1-weighted images. Radiat Med. 1996;14:111–6.
13. Zanardi R, Del Frate C, Zuiani C, et al. Staging of pelvic endometriosis based on MRI findings versus laparoscopic classification according to the American Fertility Society. Abdom Imaging. 2003;28:733–42.
14. Kataoka ML, Togashi K, Yamaoka T, et al. Posterior cul-de-sac obliteration associated with endometriosis: MR imaging evaluation. Radiology. 2005;234:815–23.
15. Bazot M, Darai E, Hourani R, et al. Deep pelvic endometriosis: MR imaging for diagnosis and prediction of extension of disease. Radiology. 2004;232:379–89.
16. Hottat N, Larrousse C, Anaf V, et al. Endometriosis: contribution of 3.0-T pelvic MR imaging in preoperative assessment—initial results. Radiology. 2009;253:126–34.
17. Bazot M, Stivalet A, Daraï E, et al. Comparison of 3D and 2D FSE T2-weighted MRI in the diagnosis of deep pelvic endometriosis: preliminary results. Clin Radiol. 2013;68:47–54.
18. Bazot M, Gasner A, Ballester M, et al. Value of thin-section oblique axial T2-weighted magnetic resonance images to assess uterosacral ligament endometriosis. Hum Reprod. 2011;26:346–53.

19. Yoon JH, Choi D, Jang KT, et al. Deep rectosigmoid endometriosis: "mushroom cap" sign on T2-weighted MR imaging. Abdom Imaging. 2010;35:726–31.
20. Busard MP, van der Houwen LE, Bleeker MC, et al. Deep infiltrating endometriosis of the bowel: MR imaging as a method to predict muscular invasion. Abdom Imaging. 2012;37:549–57.
21. Busard MP, Pieters-van den Bos IC, Mijatovic V, et al. Evaluation of MR diffusion-weighted imaging in differentiating endometriosis infiltrating the bowel from colorectal carcinoma. Eur J Radiol. 2012;81:1376–80.
22. Scardapane A, Bettocchi S, Lorusso F, et al. Diagnosis of colorectal endometriosis: contribution of contrast enhanced MR-colonography. Eur Radiol. 2011;21:1553–63.
23. Del Frate C, Girometti R, Pittino M, et al. Deep retroperitoneal pelvic endometriosis: MR imaging appearance with laparoscopic correlation. Radiographics. 2006;26:1705–18.
24. Busard MP, Mijatovic V, Lüchinger AB, et al. MR imaging of bladder endometriosis and its relationship with the anterior uterine wall: experience in a tertiary referral centre. Eur J Radiol. 2012;81:2106–11.
25. Bazot M, Jarboui L, Ballester M, et al. The value of MRI in assessing parametrial involvement in endometriosis. Hum Reprod. 2012;27:2352–8.
26. Sugimura K, Okizuka H, Kaji Y, et al. MRI in predicting the response of ovarian endometriomas to hormone therapy. J Comput Assist Tomogr. 1996;20:145–50.
27. Miyakoshi K, Tanaka M, Gabionza D, et al. Decidualized ovarian endometriosis mimicking malignancy. AJR Am J Roentgenol. 1998;171:1625–6.
28. Tanaka YO, Shigemitsu S, Nagata M, et al. A decidualized endometrial cyst in a pregnant woman: a case observed with a steady-state free precession imaging sequence. Magn Reson Imaging. 2002;20:301–4.
29. Takeuchi M, Matsuzaki K, Nishitani H. Magnetic resonance manifestations of decidualized endometriomas during pregnancy. J Comput Assist Tomogr. 2008;32:353–5.
30. Heaps JM, Nieberg RK, Berek JS. Malignant neoplasms arising in endometriosis. Obstet Gynecol. 1990;75:1023–8.
31. Tanaka YO, Yoshizako T, Nishida M, et al. Ovarian carcinoma in patients with endometriosis: MR imaging findings. AJR Am J Roentgenol. 2000;175:1423–30.
32. Fujii S, Kakite S, Nishihara K, et al. Diagnostic accuracy of diffusion-weighted imaging in differentiating benign from malignant ovarian lesions. J Magn Reson Imaging. 2008;28:1149–56.
33. Tanaka YO, Okada S, Yagi T, et al. MRI of endometriotic cysts in association with ovarian carcinoma. AJR Am J Roentgenol. 2010;194:355–61.
34. Kataoka M, Togashi K, Koyama T, et al. MR imaging of mullerian mucinous borderline tumors arising from endometriotic cysts. J Comput Assist Tomogr. 2002;26:532–7.
35. McDermott S, Oei TN, Iyer VR, et al. MR imaging of malignancies arising in endometriomas and extraovarian endometriosis. Radiographics. 2012;32:845–63.

Chapter 20
Biomarkers of Endometriosis

Amelie Fassbender*, Dorien O*, Bart De Moor, Etienne Waelkens, Christel Meuleman, Carla Tomassetti, Karen Peeraer, and Thomas D'Hooghe

Abstract Endometriosis is a benign gynecological disease defined by the ectopic presence of endometrium and associated with pelvic pain and infertility. The etiology and pathogenesis remain unclear. The gold standard of diagnosing endometriosis is laparoscopy followed by histological confirmation, associated with an 8-year delay in the diagnosis of endometriosis. A clinically reliable test for endometriosis can be expected to allow early diagnosis and treatment, with profound impact on the reduction of health care and individual costs. A noninvasive diagnostic test could be developed for serum or plasma, urine, and endometrial or menstrual fluid.

---

*Amelie Fassbender and Dorien O are joint first authors

A. Fassbender • D. O (✉)
Department of Development and Regeneration, Organ systems,
KU Leuven, Leuven, Belgium

Department of Obstetrics and Gynaecology, Leuven University Fertility Centre,
University Hospital Leuven, UZ Gasthuisberg, Leuven, Belgium

B. De Moor
Department of Electrical Engineering (ESAT-SCD), KU Leuven,
Leuven, Belgium

E. Waelkens
Department of Molecular Cell Biology, Campus Gasthuisberg, Leuven, Belgium

C. Meuleman • C. Tomassetti • K. Peeraer
Department of Obstetrics and Gynaecology, Leuven University Fertility Centre,
University Hospital Leuven, UZ Gasthuisberg, Leuven, Belgium

T. D'Hooghe (✉)
Department of Development and Regeneration, Organ systems,
KU Leuven, Leuven, Belgium

Department of Obstetrics and Gynaecology, Leuven University Fertility Centre,
University Hospital Leuven, UZ Gasthuisberg, Leuven, Belgium

Division of Reproductive Biology, Institute of Primate Research, Karen, Nairobi, Kenya
e-mail: thomas.dhooghe@uzleuven.be

T. Harada (ed.), *Endometriosis: Pathogenesis and Treatment*,
DOI 10.1007/978-4-431-54421-0_20, © Springer Japan 2014

A semi-invasive test could be developed for peritoneal fluid and eutopic endometrium. The development of such a test from initial biomarker discovery to be a clinically approved biomarker assay is a long, difficult, and uncertain process and includes four different phases. A review of the existing literature is provided in this chapter. Overall, most endometriosis biomarker studies remain at the level of phase I, with only a few currently in phase II of biomarker development. There is a need for a well-designed multinational study including academic and industrial partners for phase II and phase III trials.

Keywords Diagnostic test • Endometriosis • Ultrasound negative

20.1 Introduction

Endometriosis is one of the most common gynecological disorders, affecting approximately 10 % of women in the reproductive age group and up to 50 % of all infertile women [1, 2]. This estrogen-dependent disease is characterized by the presence of endometrial-like tissue at ectopic sites like the pelvic peritoneum, the ovaries, the rectovaginal septum, and in some cases even the pericardium, the pleura, and the brain [1]. Infertility is frequently associated with endometriosis as it is estimated that up to 50 % of endometriosis patients are subfertile (any form of reduced fertility with prolonged time of unwanted non-conception) [3]. Another important symptom that accompanies endometriosis is pain. Endometriosis-associated pain typically occurs as chronic pelvic pain in 90 % of women suffering from painful menstruations (dysmenorrhea), in 42 % of women suffering from pain during intercourse (dyspareunia), and in 39 % of women suffering from non-menstrual pain [4, 5]. The degree of pain and the severity of endometriosis are poorly related and the exact mechanism of endometriosis-associated pain has yet to be determined [6]. Pain might be caused by pressure of large nodules on visceral organs, pelvic adhesions, tissue damage by infiltration of lesions, or an inflammatory response in the peritoneal cavity triggered by cyclical bleeding of lesions [4, 7]. Recent evidence suggests that endometriosis-associated nerve fibers might be a pain-causing feature. Indeed, in endometriotic lesions, ingrowth of blood vessels along with nerve fibers has been observed [8, 9].

The diagnosis of endometriosis is currently made by means of laparoscopy to identify endometrial-like tissue at ectopic places [1]. The severity of the disease is determined according to the revised American Fertility Society classification system. The classification of the disease stage (stages I to IV or minimal to severe) is based on acquired information during laparoscopic surgery on the morphology and depth of the implants, the presence, place, and type of lesion, and the presence, place, and type of adhesion [10]. Although laparoscopy is considered the golden standard, it can fail to detect very small lesions and lesions might not be noticed because of their location [11]. Furthermore, an average delay of 8 years precedes an accurate diagnosis. Five to six of these years can be attributed to a delay in the search of medical help and the remainder to obtaining the correct diagnosis [12].

The etiology and pathogenesis of endometriosis is still controversial and is almost certainly multifactorial [13]. Despite several established theories such as retrograde menstruation, abnormal immune system, coelomic metaplasia, genetic and epigenetic factors, and the stem cell theory, researchers still have not found the possible mechanism and cause of endometriosis.

Treatment options are directed against endometriosis itself, against endometriosis-associated pain, or against endometriosis-related infertility. Surgery aims to remove all visible endometriotic lesions [14]. However, as it does not manage the underlying mechanisms of the disease, recurrences of endometriotic lesions are common. Currently, different medical treatments are used in the clinic as well [15]. These treatments focus on altering the hormonal environment, hereby creating a suboptimal milieu for the growth and maintenance of the lesions. Still, these medications have many side effects and their efficiency is not ideal [14]. It has been indicated that, in order to improve diagnostic tools and treatment strategies, the underlying mechanism of endometriosis needs to be clarified [16]. In recent years, new more targeted therapies are being developed, e.g., aromatase inhibitors, angiogenesis inhibitors, and immunomodulating agents [17].

A noninvasive diagnostic test could be developed for serum or plasma, urine, and endometrial or menstrual fluid that can be recovered from the posterior vaginal fornix and from the cervix during speculum examination. A semi-invasive test could be developed in peritoneal fluid, obtained after transvaginal ultrasound-guided aspiration, or in endometrial, obtained after transcervical endometrial biopsy. Whatever method is used, the most important goal of the test is that no women with endometriosis or other significant pelvic pathology are missed who might benefit from surgery [18]. To achieve this, a test with a high sensitivity is needed, which is the probability of a test of being positive when endometriosis is present. At present, such a test does not exist [19, 20].

Researchers and clinicians need to realize that a diagnostic test may do more harm than good, e.g., by subjecting patients to unnecessary or even potentially harmful procedures [21] since the benefits of treating women with asymptomatic endometriosis are unclear [19]. Therefore, we do not recommend the development or use of a blood test for screening purpose in asymptomatic women. However, up to 45 % of subfertile women with a regular cycle whose partner has normal sperm quality, with or without pelvic pain, and with normal clinical examination and a normal pelvic ultrasound may have endometriosis [20, 22].

Most gynecologists are not sure if endometriosis is present if a woman has, for example, subfertility, a regular cycle, and a partner with a normal sperm examination and if they have been unsuccessful in trying to conceive for more than 1 year without moderate severe cyclic pelvic pain. In addition, if a woman has chronic pelvic pain (requiring at least cyclic or chronic use of pain killers), combined with a normal clinical examination and a normal pelvic ultrasound, many gynecologists are in doubt about the value of a diagnostic laparoscopy. From a clinical perspective, it is unlikely that these women will have moderate–severe endometriosis, but they may have extensive peritoneal endometriosis with or without adhesions associated with subfertility and possibly mild pain [18]. For this population, a noninvasive or semi-invasive diagnostic test would be useful to discriminate between women without endometriosis who need to avoid having unnecessary surgery and those with endometriosis, most likely minimal–mild disease, who are known to benefit from surgical therapy for both subfertility and pain and from controlled ovarian stimulation in combination with intrauterine insemination for subfertility [15, 18, 20, 23]. In summary, a noninvasive test for endometriosis would be useful for women with pelvic pain and/or subfertility with normal ultrasound. This would include nearly all cases of minimal–mild endometriosis, some cases of moderate–severe endometriosis without clearly visible ovarian endometrioma, and cases with pelvic adhesions and/or other pelvic pathology, who might benefit from surgery to improve pelvic pain and/or subfertility [18, 20].

20.2 Noninvasive Test

The last few years, tremendous work has been published regarding biomarkers. In 2009 and 2013, researchers proposed that the development of reliable noninvasive test of endometriosis is one of the top research priorities in endometriosis [16, 24]. A clinically reliable test for endometriosis can be expected to have a profound impact on the reduction of health care and individual costs by:

1. Reducing time to diagnosis and the time wasted to see numerous health-care professionals
2. Subsequently reducing the time before individualized specialist care is invoked
3. Subsequently reducing expensive hit-and-miss treatments
4. Subsequently reducing expensive fertility treatments if the disease is under control before fertility is impaired [25]

Highly relevant markers known to be involved in the pathogenesis of endometriosis have been studied such as glycoproteins, inflammatory and noninflammatory cytokines, adhesions, and angiogenic and growth factors [20]. At present, neither a single biomarker nor a panel of biomarkers measurable in peripheral blood has been validated as a noninvasive test for endometriosis [19]. The measurement of serum CA-125 levels has no value as a diagnostic tool compared to laparoscopy [15]. Although previous studies have shown that various tumor markers, cytokines, and angiogenic and growth factors show altered levels in peripheral blood (plasma or serum) of women with endometriosis when compared to controls [19, 26], so far none of them, alone or in combination, have been validated as a noninvasive test for endometriosis [19]. Furthermore, at present there is no consensus on the value of inflammatory factors as biomarkers for endometriosis [20]. Comparable serum IL-6 [27, 28], IL-8 [27, 29], TNF-alpha, and IL-1 [27, 28, 30] levels were previously reported in women with and without endometriosis. However, other investigators reported elevated peripheral levels of IL-6 [30, 31], IL-8 [32, 33], TNF-alpha [31, 34], and IFN-gamma [30] in endometriosis patients compared with controls [20].

So far, studies evaluating panels of biomarkers [35–38] have been limited with respect to the number of biomarkers analyzed, the statistics used, and the lack of validation in an independent test set of patients [20]. One study proposed two panels of four biomarkers (annexin V, VEGF, CA-125, and glycodelin or sICAM-1) measured in plasma samples obtained during menstruation allowed the detection of ultrasound-negative endometriosis with high sensitivity (82 %) and acceptable specificity (63–75 %) in an independent test data set [39]. In the same study, three biomarkers (VEGF, annexin V, and CA-125) present in plasma obtained during menstruation allowed the diagnosis of endometriosis (minimal–severe endometriosis, both with and without ultrasound evidence) with 85–94 % sensitivity and 62–75 % specificity in an independent test data set [39]. These results are promising but need to be validated in a prospective study. Surprisingly, inflammatory molecules did not emerge as biomarkers in this study [39].

Recently, a diagnostic model including patient-reported clinical data derived from a validated questionnaire predicted any-stage endometriosis poorly, but stages III and IV accurately, with menstrual dyschezia and a history of benign ovarian cysts as the strongest predictive factors [40]. More research is needed to add clinical factors to diagnostic models based on plasma or endometrial analysis.

The development of a noninvasive diagnostic test, from initial biomarker discovery to a clinically approved biomarker assay, is a long, difficult, and uncertain process [41] and occurs in four different phases as described below:

Phase I—Preclinical discovery phase. This phase consists of exploratory preclinical studies aiming to identify potential biomarkers. In endometriosis research, the state of the art in this field has recently been reviewed by May et al. [19].

Phase II—Preclinical assay development and validation of a clinically useful noninvasive diagnostic test in the preclinical setting, as has been done in the context of endometriosis in our most recent paper [39].

Phase III—Prospective clinical validation and determination of clinical utility. This phase establishes the diagnostic accuracy and predictive value in the target population, but this phase has not yet been reached in endometriosis biomarker research so far.

Phase IV—Commercialization: product development by industry, which has not yet been done successfully for noninvasive endometriosis biomarkers.

Overall, most endometriosis biomarker studies remain at the level of phase I [19] and only a few have made it to phase II studies. There is a need for well-designed phase II and phase III trials to make progress in this field.

20.2.1 Nerve Fibers

The most promising efforts in developing a semi-invasive diagnostic test reported an increased nerve fiber density in the functional layer of eutopic endometrium of women with endometriosis, uniting the concept of an alternation of eutopic endometrium with the presence of nerve fibers provoking pelvic pain [42].

The first study to investigate the presence of nerve fibers in eutopic endometrium as a potential endometriosis biomarker reported a higher density of small nerve fibers in the functional layer of women with endometriosis compared with women without endometriosis [43]. Uterine curettage (endometriosis $n = 25$ and control $n = 47$) and hysterectomy samples (endometriosis $n = 10$ and control $n = 35$) were immunostained with antibodies against protein gene product 9.5 (PGP 9.5) as pan-neural marker for both unmyelinated and myelinated nerve fibers and neurofilament (NF) for myelinated nerve fibers. The most outspoken difference could be found in the functional layer of the endometrium where PGP 9.5-positive nerve fibers were observed in all endometriosis cases (on average for all cycle phases 11 ± 5 mm^{-2} for hysterectomy specimens and 10 ± 5 mm^{-2} for curettage specimens), but never in control patients ($P < 0.001$). The difference was the most obvious in the secretory phase of the cycle, but was also significant in the menstrual and proliferative phases [43].

To determine the type of small nerve fibers in the endometrium, the same research group published an additional study [44] in which uterine blocks were obtained after hysterectomy from women with endometriosis ($n = 10$) and controls ($n = 35$). Positive staining of the nerve fibers in the functional layer for SP (1.0 ± 0.2 mm^{-2}), CGRP (1.7 ± 0.4 mm^{-2}), VIP (8.5 ± 2.3 mm^{-2}), and NPY (9.6 ± 2.8 mm^{-2}) and the absence of staining with TH or VAChT antibodies indicated the presence of different types of sensory C nerve fibers in women with endometriosis. This finding might be relevant to the mechanism of pain generation in women with endometriosis.

While the previous studies [43, 44] focused on full endometrial curettage and full uterine blocks after hysterectomy, clinical relevance of an endometrial biomarker is only valid if an endometrial biopsy can generate the same sensitivity and specificity [45]. Endometrial curettage requires general anesthesia and the need for hospitalization, while endometrial biopsy sampling can be done in an outpatient setting [46]. A pilot study including 20 endometriosis patients and 17 controls compared the diagnostic value of an endometrial biopsy and a full curettage [45]. Much care was given to the correct sampling of the endometrial biopsy, using a cannula to take a tissue column representing full thickness of the endometrium. Despite the wide range in nerve fiber densities observed in the functional layer of the endometrium, previous findings of increased nerve fiber density in endometrium obtained in hysterectomy specimens were confirmed in endometrium obtained by endometrial sampling (26.7 ± 55.9 mm^{-2}) or by curettage (20.4 ± 33.1 mm^{-2}), suggesting equal diagnostic capacity of the two collection methods. Sensitivity, specificity, positive predictive value (PPV), and negative predictive value (NPV) were all 100 %.

To further prove the diagnostic relevance of the detection of nerve fibers in an endometrial biopsy, a double-blind study [47] was conducted using endometrial biopsies from 99 consecutive patients who received a laparoscopy for pelvic pain and/or infertility, including 64 cases with endometriosis and 35 controls without endometriosis. Immunohistochemical staining with PGP 9.5 showed a mean nerve fiber density of 2.7 ± 3.4 nerve fibers per mm^2 in the functional layer of endometrium from nearly all endometriosis patients and an absence of nerve fibers in most control patients (except in six cases), resulting in a statistically significant difference between the two groups ($P < 0.001$). The specificity and sensitivity of the test were 83 and 98 %. PPV and NPV were 91 and 96 %, respectively.

The accuracy of making an endometrial-based diagnosis of endometriosis was also investigated by two other independent research groups [48, 49]. In a paper from Bokor et al. [49], endometrial samples from only the secretory phase were included, because the initial Tokushige pilot study had reported a higher nerve fiber density in this phase [43]. Only patients with minimal ($n = 10$) or mild ($n = 10$) endometriosis were recruited, as they have the greatest need of a semi-invasive diagnostic test [49]. Another 20 patients with a normal pelvis were included as controls. Prevalence of pain symptoms was comparable in both groups. PGP 9.5, NF, SP, VIP, NPY, and CGRP expression was detected by immunohistochemistry and showed a 14-fold higher density of small nerve fibers in the functional layer of women with endometriosis (1.96 ± 2.73 mm^{-2}) compared with the control group (0.14 ± 0.46 mm^{-2}) ($P < 0.0001$). Multivariate analysis showed that the combined assessment of VIP, PGP 9.5, and SP had the greatest diagnostic accuracy to predict endometriosis with a sensitivity of 95 %, a specificity of 100 %, a PPV of 100 %, and an NPV of 95 %. In contrast to the Bokor study (84), results were not controlled for cycle phase or disease severity in another study [48]. In spite of this limitation, nerve fibers positive for PGP 9.5 or NF were present in all 12 endometriosis cases (mean 13.1 ± 3.3 mm^{-2}) and only in 3 of 15 patients without endometriosis (mean 2.2 ± 4.7 mm^{-2}) resulting in a significant difference between the two groups, although no exact p-value was mentioned [48]. Sensitivity and specificity were not mentioned, but can be calculated based on the published data to be 100 and 80 %, respectively. No significant differences in the pain characteristics of both groups were reported.

An alternative study showed the added value of detection of endometrial PGP 9.5-stained nerve fibers to IL-6 measurement in serum for diagnosis of minimal/mild endometriosis [50] in endometriosis patients ($n = 35$) compared with controls ($n = 40$). Specificity and sensitivity of the test for predicting minimal/mild endometriosis regarding the presence of nerve fibers were 92 and 80 %, respectively (PPV and NPV were 81 and 91 %). These values raised to 100 and 92.5 % (PPV and NPV 92.7 and 100 %) when IL-6 was added. The exact nerve fiber densities in endometriosis patients were not mentioned.

A meta-analysis of several studies [43, 47–49] included 131 women with endometriosis and 152 controls [51]. Mean nerve fiber density per mm^2 was significantly higher in endometriosis patients (5.67 ± 12.08) versus controls (0.78 ± 3.39, $P < 0.005$) [51]. This meta-analysis demonstrated that PGP 9.5 staining of eutopic endometrium can be used as a semi-invasive test and could reduce in the delay of diagnosis; however, further research is necessary [51].

Despite the promising data shown in the previously discussed papers, nerve fiber density in eutopic endometrium is not yet ready to be used in clinical practice.

The abovementioned data were not confirmed by Newman and coworkers, comparing 20 patients with endometriosis (minimal–mild $n = 20$, moderate $n = 4$, and severe $n = 4$) to 25 controls [52]. No significant difference was observed between the disease and control group in PGP 9.5-positive nerve fibers, visualized by immunohistochemistry [52]. Using western blotting as a quantitative method to detect the neural markers, all three markers were expressed in endometrium from both endometriosis cases and controls (PGP 9.5: $P = 0.0991$, VR I: $P = 0.0621$, NGFp75: $P = 0.2586$) [52].

In another study, no statistical difference was observed in endometrial nerve fiber density, determined by PGP 9.5 staining, between women with ($n = 47$) and without endometriosis ($n = 21$) [53]. This study, however, was marked by several methodological drawbacks. Firstly, threshold for endometrial biopsy quality was low (one low-power field of well-oriented endometrial mucosa sample perceived to be sufficient to being classified as "satisfactory"). Secondly, the exact endometrial nerve fiber density was not mentioned, since data were classified as positive or negative depending on the presence or absence of nerve fibers [53]. This study highlighted that methodological factors such as the method of endometrial biopsy sampling and image analysis might influence the consistency of results for this semi-invasive diagnostic test [53]. Taking into account the uneven distribution of the nerve fibers in a biopsy, reliable results may require inspection of more than one section per biopsy [45]. Furthermore, the whole surface of an endometrial section should ideally be examined [49] as opposed to counting endometrial nerve fibers in randomly chosen fields [45]. Additionally, it is crucial that background staining during immunohistochemistry is reduced as much as possible, which can be challenging. In a research context, results should be analyzed by an experienced pathologist. While it is essential to refine methodology, it is equally important to select and phenotype the study population. All cases in the endometriosis group should have laparoscopically confirmed endometriosis, preferably with histological confirmation of the presence of endometrial glands and stroma in the lesions [49]. In some of the studies, this criterion was not met, as only in a part of the cases histological confirmation of endometriosis was available [45, 47]. Further, according to the modified QUADAS (Quality Assessment of Diagnostic Accuracy Studies) criteria [19], detailed information should be available regarding the demographics such as disease stage and cycle phase [49]. Study patients ideally have not received hormonal medication 3 months prior to surgery, because systemic exposure to hormonal medication might reduce the presence of nerve fibers in eutopic endometrium [43]. However, this medication-free period was as short as 1 month in one study [50] and could have been even shorter in another study stating that patients were not on medication only at the time of laparoscopy [45]. Additionally, one study included three patient groups (one on current hormonal therapy ($n = 11$), one without hormonal therapy ($n = 44$), and a group with unknown status ($n = 13$)) and found an overall poor sensitivity for the test that was independent of the treatment status [53]. This lack of significance might have been due to the low sample size in each group. The control group should be equally well characterized and should have absence of endometriosis confirmed by laparoscopy

(QUADAS criteria [19]). Included controls were only described in detail in a number of studies [43, 44]. They consisted of women undergoing tubal sterilization, assessment prior to tubal reanastomosis or investigation of infertility [43] and women with uterine fibroids, uterine prolapse, abdominal adhesions, and abnormal menstrual bleeding [44]. Two studies included only controls with a normal pelvis [49, 50]. Pain characteristics should be comparable in case and control groups, although this did not always seem to be the case. In the double-blind study by Al-Jefout, patients with pain symptoms were present in 87.5 % of the endometriosis cases, but only in 45.7 % of controls [47]. This could influence the results as previous studies have postulated a link between pain and nerve fiber ingrowth in ovarian or deep infiltrating endometriosis [54, 55]. Interestingly, the association between pain and the presence of nerve fibers in endometrium exists in women with other gynecological disorders such as adenomyosis or uterine fibroids, suggesting that the presence of nerve fibers is linked to the diagnosis of pelvic pain rather than to the occurrence of endometriosis [20, 56].

Implemented statistics were comparable in most studies with the use of univariate analysis such as the Mann–Whitney *U*-test as a nonparametric test to compare two groups [43, 44, 47] and the Kruskal–Wallis chi-square test for the comparison of multiple groups [47]. The Kolmogorov–Smirnov test [48] was used by one group to determine normality, before performing a student *t*-test or related nonparametric test to evaluate nerve fibers [48]. The use of the Kolmogorov–Smirnov test is discouraged, because of its poor performance in assessing normality [57]. Other groups mentioned using the student *t*-test, but did not state whether they had verified a normal data distribution first [50, 53]. Advanced multivariate statistical analysis was only performed in one study by Bokor and coworkers, using multivariate logistic regression and leave-one-out cross-validation (LOO-CV) analysis with least-squares support vector machines (LS-SVM) modeling [49].

In conclusion, it can be stated that the determination of nerve fiber density in the endometrium as a diagnostic test for endometriosis is a promising prospect. However, the techniques and study populations should be randomized and further validation with larger patient groups should be performed before this test can be used in the clinic. Up to now, none of the studies evaluating nerve fibers in endometrial biopsies have reached phase III of biomarker development. To make progress in this field, there is a need for well-designed phase II and III studies. Validation should be carried out in a patient population experiencing pain/infertility with a 30 % prevalence of endometriosis.

20.2.2 MicroRNAs and Endometriosis

Since endometriosis is a multifactorial and polygenic disease, aberrant expression of microRNA (miRNA) has been proposed as a potential pathogenic mechanism [20, 58]. Essentially, miRNAs are short (~22 nucleotides) single-stranded noncoding RNAs with the capacity to regulate gene expression at a posttranscriptional level through translational repression or messenger RNA (mRNA) degradation [59]. One miRNA may regulate the expression of several hundreds of mRNAs [60]. Diagnostic use of miRNA signatures has been proposed for various diseases, such as cancer, cardiovascular diseases, rheumatic diseases, and neurological disorders [61]. In cancer, miRNAs perform better than mRNAs to classify poorly differentiated tumors [62].

20.2.2.1 Endometrium

Between eutopic endometrium and endometriotic lesions, differential expression of a number of miRNAs has been shown and some of their mRNA targets, as predicted by in silico algorithms, have previously been identified as dysregulated in endometriosis [63–66]. A number of cellular events involved in the development of endometriotic lesions has been linked to miRNA dysfunction, such as hypoxic injury, inflammation, tissue repair, disrupted cell cycling, extracellular matrix remodeling, angiogenesis, cellular movement, and DNA methylation [65–68].

More importantly, differences in miRNA expression between eutopic endometrium of endometriosis patients and controls have been found, providing a potential role for miRNAs as biomarkers or therapeutic tools in endometriosis [20]. In a study conducted by Toloubeydokhti et al., miR-17-5p, miR-23a, miR-23b, and miR-542-3p were upregulated in eutopic endometrium ($n=5$) of patients with endometriosis, compared with controls ($n=5$) [69]. These miRNAs have previously been linked to cancer [70]. The predicted downstream targets were known to be involved in endometriosis (steroidogenic acute regulatory protein (StAR), aromatase, and COX-2) and were confirmed to be upregulated, using RT-PCR [69]. However, an independent research group found reduced expression of miR-23a and miR-23b in eutopic endometrium of endometriosis cases compared with disease-free controls [71]. This reduction in miRNA expression correlated with a 2.26-fold increase ($P=0.041$) in steroidogenic factor 1 (SF-1) expression [71]. In another study, endometrial miR-9 and miR-34 were significantly reduced in patients with moderate/severe endometriosis ($n=4$) compared with controls with uterine leiomyomata ($n=3$) [72]. Their targets were predicted to enhance the proliferative capacity of the endometrium [72]. In another study, an increased miR-21 expression throughout the menstrual cycle was reported to allow distinction between severe and mild endometriosis (controls: $n=12$, mild endometriosis: $n=19$, severe endometriosis: $n=44$) and associated with a downregulation of tumor suppressor genes such as *PTEN* [73]. In another study, it was found that miR135a/b expression was significantly upregulated in eutopic endometrium of endometriosis patients ($n=32$) compared with controls ($n=50$) in the proliferative phase (miR135a and miR135b) and the secretory phase (miR135b) [74]. This upregulation of miR135a/b was marked by a downregulation of HOX10 mRNA and protein (a regulator of endometrial receptivity) which was reversible by the addition of miR-135a/b inhibitors [74]. In yet another paper, the downregulation of miR-126 was observed in ectopic endometrium ($n=16$) and in eutopic endometrium ($n=31$) from women with endometriosis ($n = 31$) when compared with controls ($n = 27$) [75]. This downregulation of miRNA was inversely correlated with the expression of *Crk*, an oncogene [75].

20.2.2.2 Peripheral Blood

Recently, several studies of miRNA in peripheral blood have been performed in the context of endometriosis [76–78]. One study, investigating circulating miRNAs in plasma, showed a significant downregulation of miR-17-5p ($p = 0.011$), miR-20a ($p = 0.0020$), and miR-22 ($p = 0.0002$) in women with endometriosis ($n = 23$) compared with women without endometriosis ($n = 23$) [78]. Receiver operating characteristic (ROC) curve analysis permitted the calculation of the area under the curve (AUC) (0.74, 0.79, and 0.85 for miR-17-5p, miR-20a, and miR-22, respectively) after which a cutoff value could be set to determine sensitivity (70.0, 60.0, 90.0 % for miR-17-5p, miR-20a, and miR-22, respectively) and specificity (70.0, 90.0, 80.0 % for miR-17-5p, miR-20a, and miR-22, respectively) to differentiate between women with and without endometriosis [78]. Combined assessment of the three miRNAs resulted in an AUC of 0.90 [78]. Additionally, another study showed that discrimination was possible between plasma of healthy controls ($n = 20$) and endometriosis patients ($n = 33$) with 88 % sensitivity and 60 % specificity (AUC = 0.90), based on the assessment of miR-16, miR-191, and miR-195 which were all highly expressed in endometriosis [77]. Endometriosis and endometriosis-associated ovarian cancer (EAOC) ($n = 14$) could be distinguished from each other through a combination of miR-21, miR-362-5p, and miR-1274a with 57 % sensitivity and 91 % specificity and an AUC of 0.92. Distinction of endometriosis and serous ovarian cancer (SOC) ($n = 21$) was possible with 90 % sensitivity and 73 % specificity (AUC 0.88), based on the assessment of miR-362-5p, miR-628-3p, and miR-1915 [77]. A trend of elevated plasma miRNA expression compared with healthy controls was found in endometriosis cases and even more so in EAOC cases. This suggests that endometriosis might be a precursor stage of EAOC and the possibility for miRNA signatures to act as disease progression markers [77].

In serum of patients with endometriosis ($n = 60$) and controls ($n = 25$) the combination of miR-199a, miR-122, miR-145*, and miR-542-3p could predict endometriosis with 93.22 % sensitivity and 96.00 % specificity (AUC = 0.994) [76].

Currently, there is no agreement on which circulating miRNA can be used for data normalization. One group selected *U6* as a normalization control because of its use as internal control in other studies [76]. However, other investigators preferred miR-16 as endogenous control because it is more stable and less variable in circulation than other miRNAs [78]. Yet another research group used miR-132 for data normalization, as they found this miRNA to be homogeneously expressed across all samples [77].

It is also important to distinguish the presence of miRNAs in either plasma or serum. Although higher miRNA concentrations were observed in plasma than in serum in one study [79], this was not confirmed in another study [80]. This discrepancy might have been due to pre-analytical variability concerning blood tube type or differences in sample-processing protocols [79]. Conversely, other studies have shown an increased concentration of miRNAs in serum samples when compared to plasma samples of the same patient, although they conclude that plasma might be the sample of choice because miRNAs that are released during the coagulation process in serum samples may interfere with the true miRNA profile [81].

Interestingly, miRNAs are exceptionally stable in plasma, serum, and tissue samples, making them excellent candidates for biomarker research [80]. Possibly miRNA is protected from RNases in blood by being packaged in vesicles or bound to RNA-binding proteins [82].

Despite the potential advantages of a miRNA-based blood test for endometriosis, some possible pitfalls should be taken into consideration. It should be noted that apart from their best known function as transcriptional repressor, miRNAs can act as translational activators [83]. Therefore the relationship between miRNA and target mRNA is not necessarily an inverse one [72]. Additionally, in most miRNA studies, specific mRNA targets are often not experimentally verified, but only predicted by various computational algorithms [65, 72]. Beside the influence of the choice of mathematical algorithm, one mRNA can be the target of multiple miRNAs that might not all be altered, rendering validation in an in vitro setup essential to determine the effect of the dysregulation of the miRNA of interest [65, 72].

Since miRNA patterns change under the influence of reproductive hormones and are thus altered in different phases of the menstrual cycle [84], an adequate control group should be chosen, preferably without any other illness as this could also influence the miRNA profile [78].

The discrepancies observed in different miRNA results can be explained by differences in patient selection, microarray protocol, and choice of housekeeping genes for data normalization. Therefore a standardized methodological approach needs to be determined and controls and patients need to be selected according to the QUADAS criteria. The rationale for implementing next-generation sequencing is that a larger amount of miRNAs can be examined, without being dependent on the availability of probes [66]. Exceptionally important is the role of advanced statistical methodology in studies where many variables are compared. Therefore, all data should be controlled for multiple testing [85].

In conclusion, miRNAs are interesting subjects in the further development of biomarker research, although more extensive research in a larger population and validation in independent test sets should be conducted with full awareness of methodological issues and the complexity of miRNA mechanisms.

20.3 Conclusions

Despite its gradual progress, the biomarker research field still faces the challenge of successfully developing a clinically approved biomarker assay for endometriosis [20]. Up to now, no semi- or noninvasive diagnostic test exists for endometriosis [19]. Most studies so far have included limited numbers of patients, limited assessment of different cycle phases and endometriosis stages, limited number of biomarkers analyzed, limited statistical analysis (mostly univariate statistical analysis only), and the lack of validation in an independent test set of patients [20].

In the past, collaborations between research centers have been limited and standard operating procedures (SOPs) are different among centers [20]. Most biomarker studies remain at the level of phase I, the preclinical discovery phase, as reviewed by May et al. [19, 42]. Only a few biomarkers make it to phase II, the preclinical assay development and validation [39, 47, 86].

To develop a diagnostic test for endometriosis, semi-invasive techniques utilizing endometrial biopsies have been explored [87]. An increased amount of small unmyelinated nerve fibers in the functional layer of eutopic endometrium of endometriosis patients has been reported [45, 49, 88]. However, prospective validation of this method in a blinded fashion is needed in a larger patient population, using a standardized biopsy sampling technique and standard immunohistochemical and statistical methods. Validation should be carried out in a patient population experiencing pain/infertility with a 30 % prevalence of endometriosis.

At present, neither a single biomarker nor a panel of biomarkers measurable in peripheral blood has been validated as a noninvasive test for endometriosis [19], although panels with reasonable specificity and sensitivity have recently been published [39]. Panels of biomarkers that have been proposed as diagnostic tests in phase I and II trials should be validated in prospective phase III studies [20]. In this phase, diagnostic accuracy of the proposed panel needs to be confirmed in an independent test population with infertility/pain scheduled for surgery [20]. The predicted outcome should be compared with the actual presence of endometriosis. Future studies should also focus on the large and clinically relevant population of endometriosis patients using hormonal medication, which is underrepresented in published biomarker discovery studies.

In order to improve the specificity and sensitivity of previously proposed diagnostic models, several choices are possible: using advanced protein technology to discover new and unknown biomarkers, combining a blood test with a semi-invasive test, or adding clinical factors to a model.

Advanced protein technologies such as antibody-based large-scale protein arrays, allowing concurrent detection of up to 1,000 proteins, might be required to improve the diagnostic power of a noninvasive blood test for endometriosis. Antibody-based microarrays have already been applied in biomarker screening for cancer research [89]. Combined assessment of a blood sample and an endometrial biopsy is another option to increase the power of a diagnostic test. A study has been published, combining a noninvasive test measuring IL-6 serum levels with a semi-invasive test for the presence of nerve fibers [50]. Despite the high sensitivity and specificity obtained by this method, it might not be suitable for clinical use due to the need for two interventions (blood and endometrial biopsy sampling). Additionally, the diagnostic accuracy of a test might be enhanced by the incorporation of clinical factors into a non- or semi-invasive test. A diagnostic method published by Nnoaham et al. predicted any-stage endometriosis poorly, but stages III and IV accurately [40]. The most predictive factors for the presence of endometriosis were menstrual dyschezia and a history of benign ovarian cysts [40].

While genomics, transcriptomics, and proteomics have already been covered extensively in endometriosis research, metabolomics is an underdeveloped field with only one study published up to date [90]. More extensive research in this topic should clarify whether the alteration of the metabolomic profile in the blood of women with endometriosis could serve as a diagnostic test for endometriosis. Another field of interest could be stem cell markers and endometriosis. Stem progenitor cells may serve as early markers and also detect recurrence [91]. The endometrium contains endometrial/stem progenitor cells that have been reported to be present in the peritoneal cavity in women that have retrograde menstruation [91]. Positive immunostaining for stem cell markers such as CD9, CD34, c-Kit, Oct-4, and Musashi-1 was detected in isolated epithelial and stromal cells in eutopic and ectopic endometrium [92]. The expression of stemness-related markers suggested that endometriosis arises as a clonal proliferation with the putative involvement of stem cells (2). The limitation of this study was the small sample size [20].

In conclusion, biomarker research will have to proceed from the discovery phase to the validation phase, focusing on successfully conducting phase III and IV trials [20]. To achieve phase III biomarker validation in both semi- and noninvasive testing, independent patient populations should be investigated, preferably with a realistic prevalence of endometriosis (30 % in women with infertility and 30–50 % in women with pelvic pain) [20]. According to one of the QUADAS criteria, patient characterization regarding cycle phase and endometriosis stage should be clearly stated and the control group should be standardized [19, 20]. Patients should have laparoscopically confirmed presence or absence (for controls) of endometriosis [19]. The different stages and clinical classifications of endometriosis should be taken into account in further research, treating peritoneal, ovarian, and rectovaginal septum endometriosis as different entities [93, 94]. Because of the different types (superficial, deep, cyst) and location of endometriosis, it is possible that a different subset of biomarkers may be required for the diagnosis of different stages of endometriosis [16], i.e., women with peritoneal endometriosis may have different markers when compared to those with rectovaginal endometriosis [19, 20]. This requires more genomic analysis of the different lesion types and different locations.

Statistical approaches should be multivariate, instead of the univariate approaches used in many studies now, and the involvement of biostatisticians is crucial to extract a diagnostic test from raw data [20]. Standardized protocols for sample collection, processing, and storage along with reporting uniform clinical information are crucial to compare results between studies and to enable a multicenter biobanking approach [16, 95]. Collaborations are essential to obtain the large sample sizes that are required for the statistical power of validation studies [16].

References

1. Giudice LC, Kao LC. Endometriosis. Lancet. 2004;364(9447):1789–99.
2. Eskenazi B, Warner ML. Epidemiology of endometriosis. Obstet Gynecol Clin North Am. 1997;24(2):235–58.
3. Stilley JA, Birt JA, Sharpe-Timms KL. Cellular and molecular basis for endometriosis-associated infertility. Cell Tissue Res. 2012;349(3):849–62.
4. Asante A, Taylor RN. Endometriosis: the role of neuroangiogenesis. Annu Rev Physiol. 2011;73:163–82.
5. Fauconnier A, Chapron C. Endometriosis and pelvic pain: epidemiological evidence of the relationship and implications. Hum Reprod Update. 2005;11(6):595–606.
6. Giudice LC. Clinical practice. Endometriosis. N Engl J Med. 2010;362(25):2389–98.
7. Anaf V, Simon P, El Nakadi I, Fayt I, Buxant F, Simonart T, Peny MO, Noel JC. Relationship between endometriotic foci and nerves in rectovaginal endometriotic nodules. Hum Reprod. 2000;15(8):1744–50.
8. Tokushige N, Markham R, Russell P, Fraser IS. Nerve fibres in peritoneal endometriosis. Hum Reprod. 2006;21(11):3001–7.
9. Mechsner S, Schwarz J, Thode J, Loddenkemper C, Salomon DS, Ebert AD. Growth-associated protein 43-positive sensory nerve fibers accompanied by immature vessels are located in or near peritoneal endometriotic lesions. Fertil Steril. 2007;88(3):581–7.
10. Revised American Society for Reproductive Medicine classification of endometriosis: 1996. Fertil Steril. 1997;67(5):817–21
11. Brosens I, Puttemans P, Campo R, Gordts S, Kinkel K. Diagnosis of endometriosis: pelvic endoscopy and imaging techniques. Best Pract Res Clin Obstet Gynaecol. 2004;18 (2):285–303.
12. Sinaii N, Plumb K, Cotton L, Lambert A, Kennedy S, Zondervan K, Stratton P. Differences in characteristics among 1,000 women with endometriosis based on extent of disease. Fertil Steril. 2008;89(3):538–45.
13. Fraser IS. Recognising, understanding and managing endometriosis. J Hum Reprod Sci. 2008;1(2):56–64.
14. Olive DL, Pritts EA. Treatment of endometriosis. N Engl J Med. 2001;345(4):266–75.
15. Kennedy S, Bergqvist A, Chapron C, D'Hooghe T, Dunselman G, Greb R, Hummelshoj L, Prentice A, Saridogan E. ESHRE guideline for the diagnosis and treatment of endometriosis. Hum Reprod. 2005;20(10):2698–704.
16. Rogers PA, D'Hooghe TM, Fazleabas A, Gargett CE, Giudice LC, Montgomery GW, Rombauts L, Salamonsen LA, Zondervan KT. Priorities for endometriosis research: recommendations from an international consensus workshop. Reprod Sci. 2009;16(4):335–46.
17. Olive DL, Lindheim SR, Pritts EA. New medical treatments for endometriosis. Best Pract Res Clin Obstet Gynaecol. 2004;18(2):319–28.
18. D'Hooghe TM, Mihalyi AM, Simsa P, Kyama CK, Peeraer K, De Loecker P, Meeuwis L, Segal L, Meuleman C. Why we need a noninvasive diagnostic test for minimal to mild endometriosis with a high sensitivity. Gynecol Obstet Invest. 2006;62(3):136–8.
19. May KE, Conduit-Hulbert SA, Villar J, Kirtley S, Kennedy SH, Becker CM. Peripheral biomarkers of endometriosis: a systematic review. Hum Reprod Update. 2010;16(6):651–74.

20. Fassbender A, Vodolazkaia A, Saunders P, Lebovic D, Waelkens E, De Moor B, D'Hooghe T. Biomarkers of endometriosis. Fertil Steril. 2013;99(4):1135–45.
21. Evers JL, Van Steirteghem AC. All that glistens is not gold. Hum Reprod. 2009; 24(12):2972–3.
22. Meuleman C, Vandenabeele B, Fieuws S, Spiessens C, Timmerman D, D'Hooghe T. High prevalence of endometriosis in infertile women with normal ovulation and normospermic partners. Fertil Steril. 2009;92(1):68–74.
23. D'Hooghe TM, Debrock S, Hill JA, Meuleman C. Endometriosis and subfertility: is the relationship resolved? Semin Reprod Med. 2003;21(2):243–54.
24. Rogers PA, D'Hooghe TM, Fazleabas A, Giudice LC, Montgomery GW, Petraglia F, Taylor RN. Defining future directions for endometriosis research: workshop report from the 2011 World Congress of Endometriosis in Montpellier, France. Reprod Sci. 2013;20(5):483–99.
25. D'Hooghe T, Vodolazkaia A, Kyama C, Mwenda JM, Simoens S. Health economics of endometriosis. In: Rombauts L, Tsaltas J, Maher P, Healy D, editors. Endometriosis. 1st ed. Malden: Blackwell; 2008. p. 1–16.
26. Othman Eel D, Hornung D, Al-Hendy A. Biomarkers of endometriosis. Expert Opin Med Diagn. 2008;2(7):741–52.
27. Kalu E, Sumar N, Giannopoulos T, Patel P, Croucher C, Sherriff E, Bansal A. Cytokine profiles in serum and peritoneal fluid from infertile women with and without endometriosis. J Obstet Gynaecol Res. 2007;33(4):490–5.
28. Socolov R, Butureanu S, Angioni S, Sindilar A, Boiculese L, Cozma L, Socolov D. The value of serological markers in the diagnosis and prognosis of endometriosis: a prospective case–control study. Eur J Obstet Gynecol Reprod Biol. 2011;154(2):215–7.
29. Darai E, Detchev R, Hugol D, Quang NT. Serum and cyst fluid levels of interleukin (IL) -6, IL-8 and tumour necrosis factor-alpha in women with endometriomas and benign and malignant cystic ovarian tumours. Hum Reprod. 2003;18(8):1681–5.
30. Othman EEDR, Homung D, Salem HT, Khalifa EA, El-Metwally TH, Al-Hendy A. Serum cytokines as biomarkers for nonsurgical prediction of endometriosis. Eur J Obstet Gynecol Reprod Biol. 2008;137(2):240–6.
31. Bedaiwy MA, Falcone T, Sharma RK, Goldberg JM, Attaran M, Nelson DR, Agarwal A. Prediction of endometriosis with serum and peritoneal fluid markers: a prospective controlled trial. Hum Reprod. 2002;17(2):426–31.
32. Ohata Y, Harada T, Miyakoda H, Taniguchi F, Iwabe T, Terakawa N. Serum interleukin-8 levels are elevated in patients with ovarian endometrioma. Fertil Steril. 2008;90(4):994–9.
33. Pizzo A, Salmeri FM, Ardita FV, Sofo V, Tripepi M, Marsico S. Behaviour of cytokine levels in serum and peritoneal fluid of women with endometriosis. Gynecol Obstet Invest. 2002; 54(2):82–7.
34. Xavier P, Belo L, Beires J, Rebelo I, Martinez-de-Oliveira J, Lunet N, Barros H. Serum levels of VEGF and TNF-alpha and their association with C-reactive protein in patients with endometriosis. Arch Gynecol Obstet. 2006;273(4):227–31.
35. Gagne D, Rivard M, Page M, Lepine M, Platon C, Shazand K, Hugo P, Gosselin D. Development of a nonsurgical diagnostic tool for endometriosis based on the detection of endometrial leukocyte subsets and serum CA-125 levels. Fertil Steril. 2003;80(4):876–85.
36. Seeber B, Sammel MD, Fan X, Gerton GL, Shaunik A, Chittams J, Barnhart KT. Panel of markers can accurately predict endometriosis in a subset of patients. Fertil Steril. 2008; 89(5):1073–81.
37. Mihalyi A, Gevaert O, Kyama CM, Simsa P, Pochet N, De Smet F, De Moor B, Meuleman C, Billen J, Blanckaert N, Vodolazkaia A, Fulop V, D'Hooghe TM. Non-invasive diagnosis of endometriosis based on a combined analysis of six plasma biomarkers. Hum Reprod. 2010; 25(3):654–64.
38. Somigliana E, Vigano P, Tirelli AS, Felicetta I, Torresani E, Vignali M, Di Blasio AM. Use of the concomitant serum dosage of CA 125, CA 19–9 and interleukin-6 to detect the presence of

endometriosis. Results from a series of reproductive age women undergoing laparoscopic surgery for benign gynaecological conditions. Hum Reprod. 2004;19(8):1871–6.
39. Vodolazkaia A, El-Aalamat Y, Popovic D, Mihalyi A, Bossuyt X, Kyama CM, Fassbender A, Bokor A, Schols D, Huskens D, Meuleman C, Peeraer K, Tomassetti C, Gevaert O, Waelkens E, Kasran A, De Moor B, D'Hooghe TM. Evaluation of a panel of 28 biomarkers for the non-invasive diagnosis of endometriosis. Hum Reprod. 2012;27(9):2698–711.
40. Nnoaham KE, Hummelshoj L, Kennedy SH, Jenkinson C, Zondervan KT. World Endometriosis Research Foundation Women's Health Symptom Survey C Developing symptom-based predictive models of endometriosis as a clinical screening tool: results from a multicenter study. Fertil Steril. 2012;98(3):692–701. e695.
41. Surinova S, Schiess R, Huttenhain R, Cerciello F, Wollscheid B, Aebersold R. On the development of plasma protein biomarkers. J Proteome Res. 2011;10(1):5–16.
42. May KE, Villar J, Kirtley S, Kennedy SH, Becker CM. Endometrial alterations in endometriosis: a systematic review of putative biomarkers. Hum Reprod Update. 2011;17(5):637–53.
43. Tokushige N, Markham R, Russell P, Fraser IS. High density of small nerve fibres in the functional layer of the endometrium in women with endometriosis. Hum Reprod. 2006; 21(3):782–7.
44. Tokushige N, Markham R, Russell P, Fraser IS. Different types of small nerve fibers in eutopic endometrium and myometrium in women with endometriosis. Fertil Steril. 2007; 88(4):795–803.
45. Al-Jefout M, Andreadis N, Tokushige N, Markham R, Fraser I. A pilot study to evaluate the relative efficacy of endometrial biopsy and full curettage in making a diagnosis of endometriosis by the detection of endometrial nerve fibers. Am J Obstet Gynecol. 2007;197(6):578. e571-4.
46. Shams G. Comparison of pipelle de cornier with conventional dilation and curettage in terms of patients' acceptability. J Postgrad Med Inst. 2012;26(4):418–21.
47. Al-Jefout M, Dezarnaulds G, Cooper M, Tokushige N, Luscombe GM, Markham R, Fraser IS. Diagnosis of endometriosis by detection of nerve fibres in an endometrial biopsy: a double blind study. Hum Reprod. 2009;24(12):3019–24.
48. Aghaey Meibody F, Mehdizadeh Kashi A, Zare Mirzaie A, Ghajarie Bani Amam M, Shariati Behbahani A, Zolali B, Najafi L. Diagnosis of endometrial nerve fibers in women with endometriosis. Arch Gynecol Obstet. 2011;284(5):1157–62.
49. Bokor A, Kyama CM, Vercruysse L, Fassbender A, Gevaert O, Vodolazkaia A, De Moor B, Fulop V, D'Hooghe T. Density of small diameter sensory nerve fibres in endometrium: a semi-invasive diagnostic test for minimal to mild endometriosis. Hum Reprod. 2009;24(12): 3025–32.
50. Elgafor El Sharkwy IA. Combination of non-invasive and semi-invasive tests for diagnosis of minimal to mild endometriosis. Arch Gynecol Obstet. 2013;288(4):793–7.
51. Liutkeviciene R, Bumbuliene Z, Zakareviciene J. Density of nerve fibres in eutopic endometrium in women with endometriosis. Central Eur J Med. 2013;8(2):141–5.
52. Newman TA, Bailey JL, Stocker LJ, Woo YL, Macklon NS, Cheong YC. Expression of neuronal markers in the endometrium of women with and those without endometriosis. Hum Reprod. 2013;28(9):2502–10.
53. Leslie C, Ma T, McElhinney B, Leake R, Stewart CJ. Is the detection of endometrial nerve fibers useful in the diagnosis of endometriosis? Int J Gynecol Pathol. 2013;32(2):149–55.
54. Wang G, Tokushige N, Markham R, Fraser IS. Rich innervation of deep infiltrating endometriosis. Hum Reprod. 2009;24(4):827–34.
55. Zhang X, Yao H, Huang X, Lu B, Xu H, Zhou C. Nerve fibres in ovarian endometriotic lesions in women with ovarian endometriosis. Hum Reprod. 2010;25(2):392–7.
56. Zhang X, Lu B, Huang X, Xu H, Zhou C, Lin J. Innervation of endometrium and myometrium in women with painful adenomyosis and uterine fibroids. Fertil Steril. 2010;94(2):730–7.
57. D'Agostino R. Tests for normal distribution. In: Goodness-of-fit techniques, (1986)

58. D'Agostino R. Tests for normal distribution. In: Goodness-of-fit techniques, volume 68 of van Statistics: a series of textbooks and monographs. CRC; 1986. p. 576. ISBN: 0824774876, 9780824774875.
59. Bartel DP. MicroRNAs: genomics, biogenesis, mechanism, and function. Cell. 2004;116(2): 281–97.
60. Baek D, Villen J, Shin C, Camargo FD, Gygi SP, Bartel DP. The impact of microRNAs on protein output. Nature. 2008;455(7209):64–71.
61. de Planell-Saguer M, Rodicio MC. Analytical aspects of microRNA in diagnostics: a review. Anal Chim Acta. 2011;699(2):134–52.
62. Lu J, Getz G, Miska EA, Alvarez-Saavedra E, Lamb J, Peck D, Sweet-Cordero A, Ebert BL, Mak RH, Ferrando AA, Downing JR, Jacks T, Horvitz HR, Golub TR. MicroRNA expression profiles classify human cancers. Nature. 2005;435(7043):834–8.
63. Pan Q, Luo X, Toloubeydokhti T, Chegini N. The expression profile of micro-RNA in endometrium and endometriosis and the influence of ovarian steroids on their expression. Mol Hum Reprod. 2007;13(11):797–806.
64. Ohlsson Teague EM, Van der Hoek KH, Van der Hoek MB, Perry N, Wagaarachchi P, Robertson SA, Print CG, Hull LM. MicroRNA-regulated pathways associated with endometriosis. Mol Endocrinol. 2009;23(2):265–75.
65. Filigheddu N, Gregnanin I, Porporato PE, Surico D, Perego B, Galli L, Patrignani C, Graziani A, Surico N. Differential expression of microRNAs between eutopic and ectopic endometrium in ovarian endometriosis. J Biomed Biotechnol. 2010;2010:369549.
66. Hawkins SM, Creighton CJ, Han DY, Zariff A, Anderson ML, Gunaratne PH, Matzuk MM. Functional microRNA involved in endometriosis. Mol Endocrinol. 2011;25(5):821–32.
67. Teague EM, Print CG, Hull ML. The role of microRNAs in endometriosis and associated reproductive conditions. Hum Reprod Update. 2010;16(2):142–65.
68. Ramon LA, Braza-Boils A, Gilabert-Estelles J, Gilabert J, Espana F, Chirivella M, Estelles A. MicroRNAs expression in endometriosis and their relation to angiogenic factors. Hum Reprod. 2011;26(5):1082–90.
69. Toloubeydokhti T, Pan Q, Luo X, Bukulmez O, Chegini N. The expression and ovarian steroid regulation of endometrial micro-RNAs. Reprod Sci. 2008;15(10):993–1001.
70. Meng F, Henson R, Lang M, Wehbe H, Maheshwari S, Mendell JT, Jiang J, Schmittgen TD, Patel T. Involvement of human micro-RNA in growth and response to chemotherapy in human cholangiocarcinoma cell lines. Gastroenterology. 2006;130(7):2113–29.
71. Shen L, Yang S, Huang W, Xu W, Wang Q, Song Y, Liu Y. MicroRNA23a and MicroRNA23b deregulation derepresses SF-1 and upregulates estrogen signaling in ovarian endometriosis. J Clin Endocrinol Metab. 2013;98(4):1575–82.
72. Burney RO, Hamilton AE, Aghajanova L, Vo KC, Nezhat CN, Lessey BA, Giudice LC. MicroRNA expression profiling of eutopic secretory endometrium in women with versus without endometriosis. Mol Hum Reprod. 2009;15(10):625–31.
73. Aghajanova L, Giudice LC. Molecular evidence for differences in endometrium in severe versus mild endometriosis. Reprod Sci. 2011;18(3):229–51.
74. Petracco R, Grechukhina O, Popkhadze S, Massasa E, Zhou Y, Taylor HS. MicroRNA 135 regulates HOXA10 expression in endometriosis. J Clin Endocrinol Metab. 2011;96(12): E1925–33.
75. Liu S, Gao S, Wang XY, Wang DB. Expression of miR-126 and Crk in endometriosis: miR-126 may affect the progression of endometriosis by regulating Crk expression. Arch Gynecol Obstet. 2012;285(4):1065–72.
76. Wang WT, Zhao YN, Han BW, Hong SJ, Chen YQ. Circulating microRNAs identified in a genome-wide serum microRNA expression analysis as noninvasive biomarkers for endometriosis. J Clin Endocrinol Metab. 2013;98(1):281–9.
77. Suryawanshi S, Vlad AM, Lin HM, Mantia-Smaldone G, Laskey R, Lee M, Lin Y, Donnellan N, Klein-Patel M, Lee T, Mansuria S, Elishaev E, Budiu R, Edwards RP, Huang X. Plasma

microRNAs as novel biomarkers for endometriosis and endometriosis-associated ovarian cancer. Clin Cancer Res. 2013;19(5):1213–24.
78. Jia SZ, Yang Y, Lang J, Sun P, Leng J. Plasma miR-17-5p, miR-20a and miR-22 are down-regulated in women with endometriosis. Hum Reprod. 2013;28(2):322–30.
79. McDonald JS, Milosevic D, Reddi HV, Grebe SK, Algeciras-Schimnich A. Analysis of circulating microRNA: preanalytical and analytical challenges. Clin Chem. 2011;57(6): 833–40.
80. Mitchell PS, Parkin RK, Kroh EM, Fritz BR, Wyman SK, Pogosova-Agadjanyan EL, Peterson A, Noteboom J, O'Briant KC, Allen A, Lin DW, Urban N, Drescher CW, Knudsen BS, Stirewalt DL, Gentleman R, Vessella RL, Nelson PS, Martin DB, Tewari M. Circulating microRNAs as stable blood-based markers for cancer detection. Proc Natl Acad Sci U S A. 2008;105(30):10513–8.
81. Wang K, Yuan Y, Cho JH, McClarty S, Baxter D, Galas DJ. Comparing the MicroRNA spectrum between serum and plasma. PLoS One. 2012;7(7):e41561.
82. Etheridge A, Lee I, Hood L, Galas D, Wang K. Extracellular microRNA: a new source of biomarkers. Mutat Res. 2011;717(1–2):85–90.
83. Vasudevan S, Tong Y, Steitz JA. Switching from repression to activation: microRNAs can up-regulate translation. Science. 2007;318(5858):1931–4.
84. Kuokkanen S, Chen B, Ojalvo L, Benard L, Santoro N, Pollard JW. Genomic profiling of microRNAs and messenger RNAs reveals hormonal regulation in microRNA expression in human endometrium. Biol Reprod. 2010;82(4):791–801.
85. Streiner DL, Norman GR. Correction for multiple testing: is there a resolution? Chest. 2011;140(1):16–8.
86. Gajbhiye R, Sonawani A, Khan S, Suryawanshi A, Kadam S, Warty N, Raut V, Khole V. Identification and validation of novel serum markers for early diagnosis of endometriosis. Hum Reprod. 2012;27(2):408–17.
87. Kyama CM, Mihalyi A, Gevaert O, Waelkens E, Simsa P, Van de Plas R, Meuleman C, De Moor B, D'Hooghe TM. Evaluation of endometrial biomarkers for semi-invasive diagnosis of endometriosis. Fertil Steril. 2011;95(4):1338–43. e1331–3.
88. Medina MG, Lebovic DI. Endometriosis-associated nerve fibers and pain. Acta Obstet Gynecol Scand. 2009;88(9):968–75.
89. Liu T, Xue R, Dong L, Wu H, Zhang D, Shen X. Rapid determination of serological cytokine biomarkers for hepatitis B virus-related hepatocellular carcinoma using antibody microarrays. Acta Biochim Biophys Sin (Shanghai). 2011;43(1):45–51.
90. Dutta M, Joshi M, Srivastava S, Lodh I, Chakravarty B, Chaudhury K. A metabonomics approach as a means for identification of potential biomarkers for early diagnosis of endometriosis. Mol Biosyst. 2012;8(12):3281–7.
91. Verit F. Biomarkers of endometriosis-letter to the editor. Fertil Steril, 2013
92. Verit FF, Cetin O. Biomarkers of endometriosis. Fertil Steril. 2013;100(4):e19.
93. McKinnon B, Bersinger NA, Wotzkow C, Mueller MD. Endometriosis-associated nerve fibers, peritoneal fluid cytokine concentrations, and pain in endometriotic lesions from different locations. Fertil Steril. 2012;97(2):373–80.
94. Nisolle M, Donnez J. Peritoneal endometriosis, ovarian endometriosis, and adenomyotic nodules of the rectovaginal septum are three different entities. Fertil Steril. 1997;68(4): 585–96.
95. Gion M, Fabricio AS. New frontiers in tumor marker studies: from biobanking to collaboration in translational research. Int J Biol Markers. 2011;26(2):73–4.

Chapter 21
Classification of Endometriosis

Hans-Rudolf Tinneberg, Frank Tuttlies, Eniko Berkes, Gabriele Anja Krombach, Andreas Hackethal, Lutz Konrad, and Frank Oehmke

Abstract As endometriosis is a chronic disease which debilitates women of reproductive age and has a negative impact on work force and quality of life in general, a disease classification would help to estimate the extent of impact on various aspects.

The most common classification has been established by the American Fertility Society and finally revised as American Society of Reproductive Medicine Classification. It is based on a laparoscopic evaluation and scoring and stages from I to IV can be applied, reflecting the extent of disease.

Since this rASRM classification does not clearly reflect a prognosis for infertility patients, the endometriosis fertility index (EFI) was developed, which is eased on the rASRM classification, but in addition includes predicted ovarian and tubal function and historical parameters.

Since these two scoring algorithms do not consider deep infiltrating endometriosis, a classification, the Enzian classification was developed according to the TNM classification for cancer. It describes the extent of disease within three different pelvic compartments classified into three sizes.

The development of MRI led to an accurate preoperative mapping of respective endometriotic lesions and enabled an MRI-based radiological classification system

H.-R. Tinneberg (✉) • E. Berkes • L. Konrad • F. Oehmke
Direktor der Frauenkilnik, Department of Obstetrics and Gynaecology,
University of Giessen and Marburg, Klinikstraße 33, 35385 Gießen, Germany
e-mail: Hans-Rudolf.Tinneberg@gyn.med.uni-giessen.de

F. Tuttlies
Department of Obstetrics and Gynaecology, Public Hospital Villach, Villach, Austria

G.A. Krombach
Department of Radiology, University of Giessen, Gießen, Germany

A. Hackethal
Queensland Centre of Gynaecological Cancer, Royal Brisbane and Women's Hospital, Brisbane, Australia

T. Harada (ed.), *Endometriosis: Pathogenesis and Treatment*,
DOI 10.1007/978-4-431-54421-0_21, © Springer Japan 2014

(MARIE) that reflects both the localisation of endometriosis and concomitant reproductive function.

Up to date no classification exists that concludes all aspects of the disease, the pathophysiology, localisation, progression, pain and infertility, treatment, prognosis and recurrence.

Keywords Adhesions • Classification • Deep infiltrating endometriosis • Pain • Sterility

21.1 Introduction

Since the first descriptions of endometriosis by Lockyer et al. in 1918 [1] and Sampson et al. in 1921 [2] it became necessary to classify the disease with the aim to include histological differentiation as well as differentiation according to location and severity of the disease. Ideally, a classification has a common language that specifies the diagnosis, thereby allowing a standardisation of disease assessment. Furthermore, it enables research, as well as the clinical community to compare findings.

The early classification systems were based on the anatomical localisation of the disease and its similarity to malignancy. The classification systems before 1973 described mainly the anatomical distribution of endometriosis and did not correlate with the clinical outcome; thus they have not received widespread clinical acceptance. The Acosta classification [3] was the first one where a direct relationship could be established with different stages of the disease and clinical pregnancy rates. As a further development, the staging system of Kistner [4] tried to reflect the natural progression of the disease with moving from early peritoneal implants to ovarian and fallopian tube-ovarian involvement and dissemination within the pelvis. One of the most precise and detailed classification systems was the Buttram classification [5], which, however, has not received widespread acceptance. Table 21.1 gives an overview of the most common classification systems, which have been made since 1918.

An ideal classification would require that a consensus be reached over empirically as well as scientifically based data that are comprehensive for all cases. Terms would need to be defined unambiguously, and anatomic lesions, extent of disease, severity of pain, impact on fertility and organ function within the pelvis as well as social impact would need a simple translation into a verbal description. Founding variables would need to be recognised and the risk of complications should be indicated. Finally the ideal classification would also guide the treatment and estimate risk for recurrence.

To date, we are far from having an ideal endometriosis classification.

In this chapter we are introducing and analysing the currently used classification systems.

Table 21.1 The most important historical classification systems of endometriosis

Year	Classification system	Characteristics
1918	Lockyer [1]	First descriptions of the disease
1921	Sampson [2]	
1949	Wicks and Larson [6]	Grade I: The wall of the cavity is lined by large bloated phagocytic cells containing blood pigment and cellular debris, most abundant on the inner side of the wall Grade II: The epithelium remains and the individual epithelial cells appear atrophic. The stroma is partially or completely replaced by bloated phagocytic cells Grade III: Epithelium and stroma are both present. Neither the epithelium nor the stroma appears to be materially influenced by the cyclic hormonal situation of the ovary Grade IV: The lesion contains endometrium resembling that seen at some stage of the menstrual cycle as found in the uterus. Glands are always present and are supported by an abundant endometrial stroma
1951	Huffman [7]	Stage I a. Limited to uterosacral ligaments and/or b. Limited to ovaries and/or c. Superficial peritoneal implants Stage II a. Extensive involvement of one ovary, with lesser involvement of second ovary and/or b. Superficial implants both ovaries and/or c. Superficial bowel implants and/or d. Infiltrating lesions of uterus and uterosacral ligaments Stage III a. Extensively infiltrating both ovaries and/or b. Bilateral ovarian endometriotic cysts and/or c. Deeply invading rectovaginal lesions and/or d. Infiltrating nonobstructing bowel implants Stage IV a. Vesical invasion and/or b. Intestinal invasion, obstructive and/or c. Ureteral involvement
1954	Sturgies and Call [8]	Stage I: Early development Stage II: Active development Stage III: Endometrial inactivity (postmenopause)
1962	Riva [9]	Staging categories are defined according to the cumulative count of pelvic structures involved and surrounding adhesions. The first scale which tries to define who might benefit from the therapy
1966	Beecham [10]	Stage I: Scattered, small (1–2 mm) spots anywhere in the pelvis at laparotomy Stage II: Uterosacral ligaments, broad ligaments, cervix and ovaries are, collectively or individually, fixed, tender, nodular and slightly enlarged

(continued)

Table 21.1 (continued)

Year	Classification system	Characteristics
		Stage III: The same as stage II, with ovaries at least twice normal size; uterosacral ligaments, rectum and adnexa are confluent and the cul-de-sac is obliterated
		Stage IV: Massive involvement, internal pelvic viscera cannot be clearly distinguished by palpation
		Stages II–IV may be used to describe either the palpable finding at the physical examination or the palpable-visual findings at operation
1973	Acosta [3]	Mild
		1. Scattered, fresh lesions (i.e. implants not associated with scarring or retraction of the peritoneum) in the anterior or posterior cul-de-sac or pelvic peritoneum
		2. Rare surface implant on ovary, with no endometrioma, without surface scarring and retraction, and without periovarian adhesions
		3. No peritubular adhesions
		Moderate
		1. Endometriosis involving one or both ovaries, with several surface lesions, with scarring and retraction, or small endometriomas
		2. Minimal periovarian adhesions associated with ovarian lesions described
		3. Minimal peritubular adhesions associated with ovarian lesions described
		4. Superficial implants in the anterior/posterior cul-de-sac with scarring and retraction. Some adhesions, but not sigmoid invasion
		Severe
		1. Endometriosis involving one or both ovaries with endometrioma $>2 \times 2$cm (usually both)
		2. One or both ovaries bound down by adhesions associated with endometriosis, with or without tubal adhesions to ovaries
		3. One or both tubes bound down or obstructed by endometriosis; associated adhesions or lesions
		4. Obliteration of the cul-de-sac from adhesions or lesions associated with endometriosis
		5. Thickening of the uterosacral ligaments and cul-de-sac lesions from invasive endometriosis with obliteration of the cul-de-sac
		6. Significant bowel or urinary tract involvement
1977	Kistner [4]	Stage I: Areas of endometriosis are present on the posterior pelvic peritoneum (cul-de-sac, uterosacral ligaments) or on the surface of the broad ligaments but do not exceed 5 mm in diameter. Avascular adhesions may involve the tubes, but the fimbriae are free. The ovaries may show a few avascular adhesions, but there is no ovarian fixation. The surfaces of the bowel and the appendix are normal
		Stage IIA: Areas of endometriosis are present on the posterior pelvic peritoneum (cul-de-sac, uterosacral ligaments) and the broad ligaments but do not exceed 5 mm in diameter. Avascular adhesions may involve the tubes, but the fimbriae are free. Ovarian involvement has been subclassified as follows: *IIA-1*, endometrial cyst or surface is 5 cm or less; *IIA-2*, endometrial cyst or surface is

(continued)

Table 21.1 (continued)

Year	Classification system	Characteristics
		over 5 cm; *IIA-3*, ruptured endometrioma, the bowel and the appendix are normal
		Stage IIB: The posterior leaf of the broad ligament is covered by adherent ovarian tissue. The tubes present adhesions not removable by endoscopic procedures. The fimbriae are free. The ovaries are fixed to the broad ligament and show areas of endometriosis over 5 mm in diameter. The cul-de-sac presents multiple implants, but there is no adherent bowel nor is the uterus in fixed position. The bowel and the appendix are normal
		Stage III: The posterior leaf of the broad ligament may be covered by adherent tube or ovary. The tubal fimbriae are covered by adhesions. The ovaries are adherent to the broad ligament, and tube may or may not show surface endometriosis or endometriomas. The cul-de-sac shows multiple areas of endometriosis, but there is no evidence of adherent bowel or uterine fixation. The bowel and the appendix are normal
		Stage IV: Endometriosis involves the bladder serosa, and the uterus is in fixed, third-degree retroversion. The cul-de-sac is covered by adherent bowel or is obliterated by the fixed uterus. The bowel is adherent to the cul-de-sac, uterosacral ligaments or uterine corpus. The appendix may be involved by the endometriotic process
1974	Mitchell and Farber [11]	Similar staging system to that used in gynaecological malignancies with stage V for malignant transformation
1979	Buttram [5]	Stage I (Peritoneum)
		A. No peritoneal involvement
		B. Scattered superficial surface endometrial implants on the pelvic peritoneum (anterior or posterior cul-de-sac, uterosacral ligaments or the broad ligaments), which do not exceed 5 mm in diameter. Neither tubal nor ovarian involvement
		C. Same as for B, but invasive endometriosis or plaques or endometrial implants >5 mm in diameter. Fine, filmy adhesion may be present that may be lysed without great danger of resultant adhesions
		Stage II (Ovarian): 1, right; 2, left; 3, bilateral
		A. No ovarian involvement
		B. Superficial surface endometrial implants of ovary of <5 mm in diameter, which can be removed by scraping or fulguration without great danger of resultant adhesions. Fine, filmy adhesions may be present and lysed without great danger of resultant adhesions
		C. Invasive endometriosis (plaques or endometrioma) >5 mm but <2 cm that requires surgical removal. Fine, filmy adhesion may be present, which may be lysed without great danger of resultant adhesions
		D. Invasive endometriosis >2 cm that requires surgical removal or a ruptured endometrioma of any size. Fine, filmy adhesion may be present, which may be lysed without great danger of resultant adhesions
		E. B, C or D with sufficient dense adhesions to fix ovary to adjacent tissue (usually posterior leaf of broad ligament)

(continued)

Table 21.1 (continued)

Year	Classification system	Characteristics
		Stage III (Tubal): 1, right; 2, left; 3, bilateral
		A. No tubal involvement
		B. Superficial endometrial implants on tube that do not exceed 5 mm in diameter and can be removed by craping or fulguration without great danger of resultant adhesions. Fine, filmy adhesions may be present, which may be lysed without great danger of resultant adhesions
		C. Invasive endometriosis (plaques or endometrioma) >5 mm but <2 cm that requires surgical removal. Fine, filmy adhesions may be present, which may be lysed without great danger of resultant adhesions
		D. Tube involved with adhesions that distort tubal anatomy and/or limit tubal movement. Fimbriae are free and tube is patent. C may be present
		E. Fimbriae are covered by adhesions or distal end of tube is occluded. B, C or D may be present
		Stage IV (Cul-de-sac)
		A. Neither B nor C is present
		B. Invasive endometriosis of bladder or colon
		C. Posterior cul-de-sac obliterated and/or uterus fixed and retroverted. Bowel or adnexa may be adherent to cul-de-sac area. B is usually present

21.2 Classification of Superficial Endometriosis

21.2.1 The rASRM Classification

None of the classifications before 1978 have been widely accepted in the clinical practice, which motivated the American Fertility Society (AFS) to form a panel and introduce a new classification that has been published in 1979 [12]. The first revision was published in 1985 [13] and appeared in its final version in 1996 when the society had changed its name into American Society of Reproductive Medicine [14].

Even though it is called a classification, it rather is a scoresheet, where the peritoneum, the ovaries, the tubes and the cul-de-sac are listed (Fig. 21.1).

The size and depth of lesion corresponds to points, which by analogy are also assigned for adhesions on the ovaries and fallopian tubes as well as points for partial or complete obliteration of the cul-de-sac. A schematic drawing is provided where the localisation of lesions and adhesions can be drafted. The summing up of all points yields in a score, which then allows classifying the endometriosis into four grades of severity: stage I (minimal endometriosis: 1–5 points), stage II (mild endometriosis: 6–15 points), stage III (moderate endometriosis: 16–40 points) and

AMERICAN SOCIETY FOR REPRODUCTIVE MEDICINE
REVISED CLASSIFICATION OF ENDOMETRIOSIS

Patient's Name ________________ Date________

Stage I (Minimal) - 1-5
Stage II (Mild) - 6-15
Stage III (Moderate) - 16-40
Stage IV (Severe) - >40
Total________

Laparoscopy________ Laparotomy________ Photography________
Recommended Treatment________________

Prognosis________

PERITONEUM	ENDOMETRIOSIS	<1cm	1-3cm	>3cm
	Superficial	1	2	4
	Deep	2	4	6
OVARY	R Superficial	1	2	4
	Deep	4	16	20
	L Superficial	1	2	4
	Deep	4	16	20

POSTERIOR CULDESAC OBLITERATION	Partial	Complete
	4	40

	ADHESIONS	<1/3 Enclosure	1/3-2/3 Enclosure	>2/3 Enclosure
OVARY	R Filmy	1	2	4
	Dense	4	8	16
	L Filmy	1	2	4
	Dense	4	8	16
TUBE	R Filmy	1	2	4
	Dense	4*	8*	16
	L Filmy	1	2	4
	Dense	4*	8*	16

*If the fimbriated end of the fallopian tube is completely enclosed, change the point assignment to 16.

Denote appearance of superficial implant types as red [(R), red, red-pink, flamelike, vesicular blobs, clear vesicles], white [(W), opacifications, peritoneal defects, yellow-brown], or black [(B) black, hemosiderin deposits, blue]. Denote percent of total described as R___%, W___% and B___%. Total should equal 100%.

Additional Endometriosis: ________________

Associated Pathology: ________________

To Be Used with Normal Tubes and Ovaries

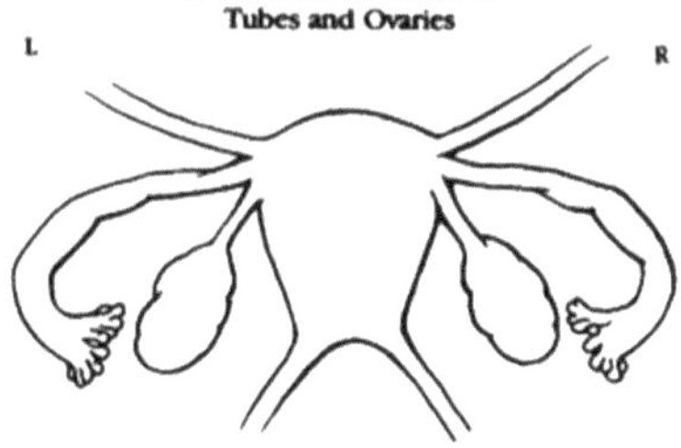

To Be Used with Abnormal Tubes and/or Ovaries

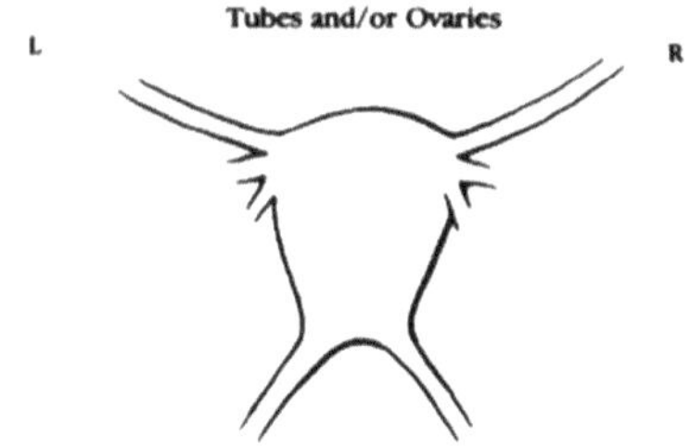

Fig. 21.1 The revised American Society for Reproductive Medicine classification of endometriosis. With permission from Elsevier (Fertility and Sterility, Licence number: 3184950406638)

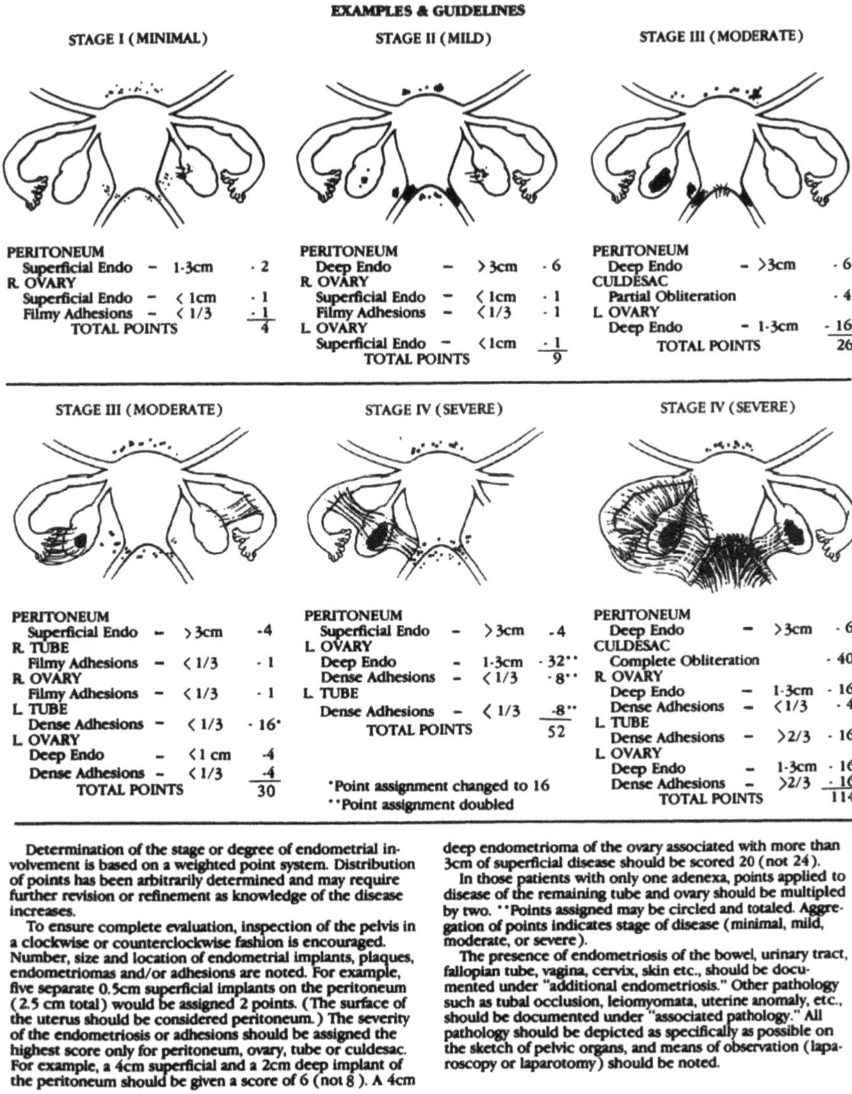

EXAMPLES & GUIDELINES

STAGE I (MINIMAL)

PERITONEUM
Superficial Endo - 1-3cm - 2
R. OVARY
Superficial Endo - < 1cm - 1
Filmy Adhesions - < 1/3 - 1
TOTAL POINTS 4

STAGE II (MILD)

PERITONEUM
Deep Endo - > 3cm - 6
R. OVARY
Superficial Endo - < 1cm - 1
Filmy Adhesions - < 1/3 - 1
L. OVARY
Superficial Endo - < 1cm - 1
TOTAL POINTS 9

STAGE III (MODERATE)

PERITONEUM
Deep Endo - >3cm - 6
CULDESAC
Partial Obliteration - 4
L. OVARY
Deep Endo - 1-3cm - 16
TOTAL POINTS 26

STAGE III (MODERATE)

PERITONEUM
Superficial Endo - > 3cm -4
R. TUBE
Filmy Adhesions - < 1/3 - 1
R. OVARY
Filmy Adhesions - < 1/3 - 1
L. TUBE
Dense Adhesions - < 1/3 - 16*
L. OVARY
Deep Endo - < 1 cm -4
Dense Adhesions - < 1/3 -4
TOTAL POINTS 30

STAGE IV (SEVERE)

PERITONEUM
Superficial Endo - > 3cm - 4
L. OVARY
Deep Endo - 1-3cm - 32**
Dense Adhesions - < 1/3 - 8**
L. TUBE
Dense Adhesions - < 1/3 - 8**
TOTAL POINTS 52

*Point assignment changed to 16
**Point assignment doubled

STAGE IV (SEVERE)

PERITONEUM
Deep Endo - > 3cm - 6
CULDESAC
Complete Obliteration - 40
R. OVARY
Deep Endo - 1-3cm - 16
Dense Adhesions - < 1/3 - 4
L. TUBE
Dense Adhesions - >2/3 - 16
L. OVARY
Deep Endo - 1-3cm - 16
Dense Adhesions - >2/3 - 16
TOTAL POINTS 114

Determination of the stage or degree of endometrial involvement is based on a weighted point system. Distribution of points has been arbitrarily determined and may require further revision or refinement as knowledge of the disease increases.

To ensure complete evaluation, inspection of the pelvis in a clockwise or counterclockwise fashion is encouraged. Number, size and location of endometrial implants, plaques, endometriomas and/or adhesions are noted. For example, five separate 0.5cm superficial implants on the peritoneum (2.5 cm total) would be assigned 2 points. (The surface of the uterus should be considered peritoneum.) The severity of the endometriosis or adhesions should be assigned the highest score only for peritoneum, ovary, tube or culdesac. For example, a 4cm superficial and a 2cm deep implant of the peritoneum should be given a score of 6 (not 8). A 4cm deep endometrioma of the ovary associated with more than 3cm of superficial disease should be scored 20 (not 24).

In those patients with only one adenexa, points applied to disease of the remaining tube and ovary should be multipled by two. **Points assigned may be circled and totaled. Aggregation of points indicates stage of disease (minimal, mild, moderate, or severe).

The presence of endometriosis of the bowel, urinary tract, fallopian tube, vagina, cervix, skin etc., should be documented under "additional endometriosis." Other pathology such as tubal occlusion, leiomyomata, uterine anomaly, etc., should be documented under "associated pathology." All pathology should be depicted as specifically as possible on the sketch of pelvic organs, and means of observation (laparoscopy or laparotomy) should be noted.

Fig. 21.1 (continued)

stage IV (severe endometriosis >40 points). In order to exemplify the different stages of the disease, examples are given which show the mode of scoring and the summing up of points.

The rASRM classification is currently the best known and the most widely used system for clinical and scientific applications throughout the world. Especially with examples given, it is easy to use and the four stages of severity can easily be understood by health professionals as well as by patients.

Unfortunately, this staging system involves a major potential of observer errors and has to be regarded as an arbitrary scoring system. Its reproducibility is limited and it fails to consider the different morphological lesion types (e.g. black or dark bluish lesions, red spots, white opacification, red-flame-like lesions, yellowish patches), as it has been described by Mettler et al. [15]. With respect to correlation to clinical symptoms Vercellini [16] reported a poor correlation between the extent of the disease and pelvic pain and Fujishita [17] a poor correlation between the extent of the disease and infertility. In particular the rASRM classification does not take into account the involvement of reputable structures which in essence means that deep infiltrating endometriosis (DIE) as the most impacting endometriosis is not represented.

Despite the disadvantages of the rASRM classification for classifying endometriosis, it is still widely used as the most popular endometriosis scoring system. It is easy to apply and publications can compare stages of severity.

21.2.2 The Endometriosis Fertility Index

The most widely used rASRM and Enzian scores (see below) describe properly the anatomical distribution of the respective superficial and deep infiltrating endometriotic lesions and concomitant adhesions, but are not eligible to provide information about the clinical outcome, the pain reduction and the reproductive performance after surgery.

In 2010 Adamson and Pasta analysing the clinical characteristics and reproductive results after surgical intervention of 569 infertile endometriosis patients in the USA in a prospective study, proposed a new staging system, the endometriosis fertility index (EFI) [18]. EFI predicts pregnancy rates in patients with surgically scored endometriosis who attempt non-ART conception. EFI could be regarded as a specifically further developed form of the rASRM classification, focusing on the reproductive outcome, and is not intended to assess the pain symptoms or predict the pain-reducing effect of the surgery.

The EFI score is based on three "surgical factors" and on one "history factor" that are presented in Fig. 21.2.

In the first step the least function (LF) score at conclusion of surgery is defined. LF reflects the predicted function of the fallopian tubes, the fimbriae and the ovaries, each scored from 0 to 4, depending on absent or nonfunctional state, severe dysfunction, moderate dysfunction, mild dysfunction and normal state. Table 21.2 represents the description of least function terms.

The better the function the higher the score. Scores are added and give the least function score. The LF score is completed with the categorised and valued rASRM lesion score as well as the rASRM total score.

The historical factors contribute to age, duration of infertility and history of prior pregnancies. The lower the age, the lower the duration of infertility, and the higher the number of previous pregnancies, the higher the historical score (Fig. 21.2).

ENDOMETRIOSIS FERTILITY INDEX (EFI) SURGERY FORM

LEAST FUNCTION (LF) SCORE AT CONCLUSION OF SURGERY

Score	Description		Left	Right
4 =	Normal	Fallopian Tube	☐	☐
3 =	Mild Dysfunction			
2 =	Moderate Dysfunction	Fimbria	☐	☐
1 =	Severe Dysfunction			
0 =	Absent or Nonfunctional	Ovary	☐	☐

To calculate the LF score, add together the lowest score for the left side and the lowest score for the right side. If an ovary is absent on one side, the LF score is obtained by doubling the lowest score on the side with the ovary.

Lowest Score ☐ Left + ☐ Right = ☐ LF Score

ENDOMETRIOSIS FERTILITY INDEX (EFI)

Historical Factors			Surgical Factors		
Factor	**Description**	**Points**	**Factor**	**Description**	**Points**
Age			LF Score ☐		
	If age is ≤ 35 years	2		If LF Score = 7 to 8 (high score)	3
	If age is 36 to 39 years	1		If LF Score = 4 to 6 (moderate score)	2
	If age is ≥ 40 years	0		If LF Score = 1 to 3 (low score)	0
Years Infertile			AFS Endometriosis Score		
	If years infertile is ≤ 3	2		If AFS Endometriosis Lesion Score is < 16	1
	If years infertile is > 3	0		If AFS Endometriosis Lesion Score is ≥ 16	0
Prior Pregnancy			AFS Total Score		
	If there is a history of a prior pregnancy	1		If AFS total score is < 71	1
	If there is no history of prior pregnancy	0		If AFS total score is ≥ 71	0
Total Historical Factors			**Total Surgical Factors**		

EFI = TOTAL HISTORICAL FACTORS + TOTAL SURGICAL FACTORS: ☐ Historical + ☐ Surgical = ☐ EFI Score

ESTIMATED PERCENT PREGNANT BY EFI SCORE

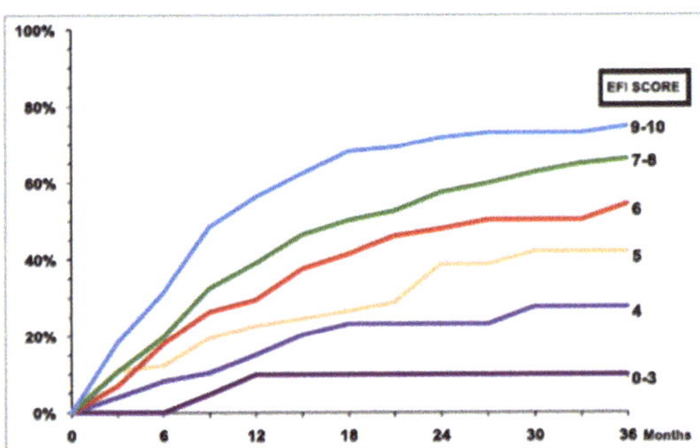

Fig. 21.2 Endometriosis fertility index (EFI). With permission from Elsevier (Fertility and Sterility, licence number: 3184941294427)

The total historical as well as the total surgical scores sum up to a score ranging between 0 and 10, with 0 representing the poorest and 10 the best prognosis. A coloured graph shows the respective estimated percentage of pregnancy likelihood depending on time after surgery and EFI score.

Table 21.2 Least function terms after Adamson and Pasta [18]

Structure	Dysfunction	Description
Tube	Mild	Slight injury to serosa of the fallopian tube
	Moderate	Moderate injury to serosa or muscularis of the fallopian tube; moderate limitation in mobility
	Severe	Fallopian tube fibrosis or mild/moderate salpingitis isthmica nodosa; severe limitation in mobility
	Nonfunctional	Complete tubal obstruction, extensive fibrosis or salpingitis isthmica nodosa
Fimbria	Mild	Slight injury to fimbria with minimal scarring
	Moderate	Moderate injury to fimbria, with moderate scarring, moderate loss of fimbrial architecture and minimal intrafimbrial fibrosis
	Severe	Severe injury to fimbria, with severe scarring, severe loss of fimbrial architecture and moderate intrafimbrial fibrosis
	Nonfunctional	Severe injury to fimbria, with extensive scarring, complete loss of fimbrial architecture, complete tubal occlusion or hydrosalpinx
Ovary	Mild	Normal or almost normal ovarian size; minimal or mild injury to ovarian serosa
	Moderate	Ovarian size reduced by one-third or more; moderate injury to ovarian surface
	Severe	Ovarian size reduced by two-thirds or more; severe injury to ovarian surface
	Nonfunctional	Ovary absent or completely encased in adhesions

Besides introducing the new EFI score, Adamson has prospectively validated and proven the effectiveness of the new scoring system analysing the predicted and actual reproductive results of 222 North American surgically treated endometriosis patients [18]. Three further external studies, performed in China, France and Belgium, have validated as well the clinical usefulness of the EFI score. In the study of Wei et al., 350 infertile patients were studied retrospectively. Within 3 years after surgery the cumulative pregnancy rates with EFI scores 8, 9 and 10 were 62.5, 69.8 and 81.1 % and with EFI scores 5, 6 and 7, 49.8, 43.9 and 41.6 % respectively, in accordance with the estimated pregnancy rates [19]. A French study of Yacoub et al. investigated in a retrospective study 132 infertile endometriosis patients and found that EFI showed a significant association between the severity of endometriosis, infertility and postoperative cumulative birth rates. However, the rASRM score fall short to predict pregnancies. The authors suggested that the EFI should be the main component in the choice of the postoperative ART management [20].

A further study performed in a Belgian population with 233 infertile endometriosis patients has also validated the effectiveness of the EFI and found the LF score the most important contributor to the total EFI score among all the other variables [21]. The authors concluded that the EFI classification system is a useful tool in counselling infertile endometriosis patients about their reproductive chances after surgery.

21.3 Classification of Deep Infiltrating Endometriosis

Several approaches have been published in the literature to classify deep infiltrating endometriosis (http://www.endometriose-sef.de) [22–24]. The intention of Chapron et al. was to propose a classification based on where the DIE lesions are located. The deep infiltrating lesions have been divided into two major compartments, anterior (DIE of the bladder) and posterior compartment (DIE of the sacrouterine ligaments, the vagina and intestines) and a subsequent operative procedure has been defined [22]. Another descriptive classification system of Koninckx tried to reflect all the possible manifestation and severity of endometriosis, classifying the so-called subtle, typical, cystic, deep and adenomyotic lesions [23]. In the meantime the group of German-speaking gynaecologist has developed a classification system, called Enzian, with the intention to describe deep infiltrating lesions in those compartments where the appropriate surgical removal can be performed.

21.3.1 The Enzian Classification

In 2005 Tuttlies et al. [24] published the Enzian classification, which has been revised in 2010 and 2011. The latest version was published in 2012 at the homepage of the SEF ("Stiftung für Endometriose-Forschung") (http://www.endometriose-sef.de).

The Enzian classification is exclusively devoted to describe deep infiltrating endometriosis and is supposed to be used additionally with the rASRM classification. Enzian is not an acronym or abbreviation for endometriosis issues but refers to a beautiful blue-coloured flower and also to the name of a hotel in the Alpes, where a group of Austrian and German experts since 2002 annually meet under the patronage of the SEF in order to discuss endometriosis-related problems.

The development of this classification followed in the early versions the master model of the TNM classification for cervical cancer inspired by the fact that deep infiltrating endometriosis shows significant characteristics of a malignant tumour, like crossing organ boundaries and likely infiltrating adjacent structures like bladder, ureter or intestines.

When comparing the rASRM classification, which has been established over decades, with the Enzian classification, the list of common sites demonstrates only little overlapping. The Enzian classification was designed to describe exclusively deep infiltrating endometriosis, which means that it is limited to a special, but challenging, clinically relevant situation. The Enzian classification is based on different topographic areas following a surgical way of separation of involved anatomic structures.

There are two main subclasses introduced to describe the clinical presentation of deep infiltrating endometriosis. On the one hand there is a group of three topographic relevant compartments in the posterior pelvis and on the other hand there

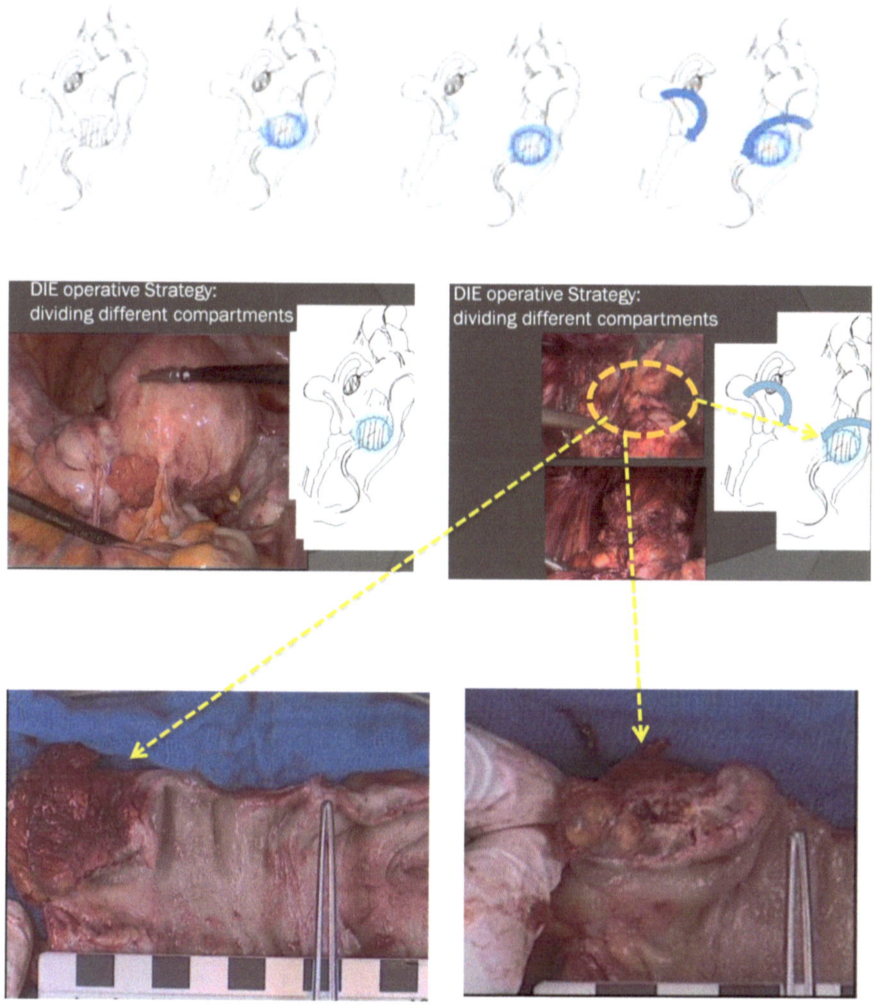

Fig. 21.3 Example for surgical route for successful separation of compartments A and C. Segmental rectum resection of two transmural infiltrative endometriotic lesions of 4 and 2 cm, respectively, Enzian C3 FI Sigma

is a group of different typical endometriotic infiltrations in distant organ sites. The three pelvic compartments of the Enzian classification describe the topographic anatomy of the pelvis. Successful and secure performance of surgical procedures is based on the initial separation and demonstration of the relevant anatomic structures which are involved (Fig. 21.3); in other words, the anatomical compartments for the Enzian classification follow the surgical procedure lining up the structures that are equally involved in typical presentation of typical DIE. Radical surgery for the management of DIE depends on initial reconstruction of the anatomy.

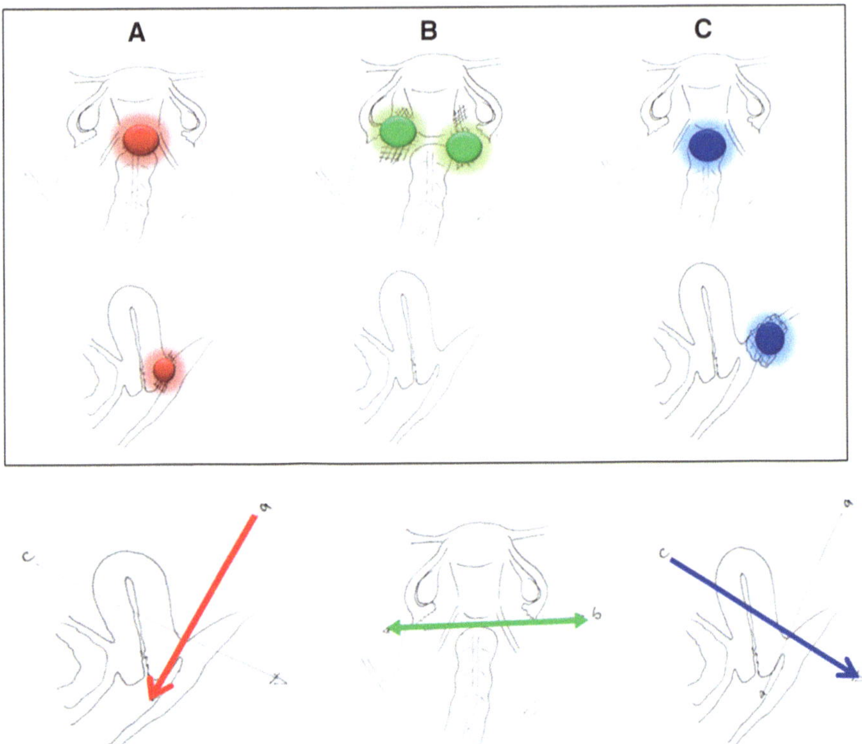

Fig. 21.4 The Enzian compartments *A*, *B* and *C*

The three posterior pelvic compartments were entitled “A, B and C” (Fig. 21.4) and embrace the pelvic manifestation of deep infiltrating endometriosis including the rectovaginal space, the vagina, the rectum and also the sacrouterine ligament with the pelvic sidewall.

The second group with the capital letter F (“far”) was designed to add important information about the location of infiltrative endometriosis, which is not directly involved to the pelvic site or distant from the cardinal posterior compartments of the pelvis as described above. Only important and typical presentations of DIE are listed, such as infiltration of the bladder, intrinsic ureter endometriosis, adenomyosis as infiltration of the uterus and distant bowel infiltration.

Compartment A (signed with red colour) includes the rectovaginal space from the pouch of Douglas along a longitudinal direction downwards to the vagina. Compartment B (signed with green colour) follows a horizontal line divided in a left and a right part starting from the sacrouterine ligament; further lateral obstructions like the external ureter compression as well as the involvement of the cardinal ligament up to the pelvic sidewall are included. Involvement of the splanchnic nerves may also be an important issue in extended pelvic sidewall infiltration. Compartment C (signed with blue colour) describes the dimension of rectal

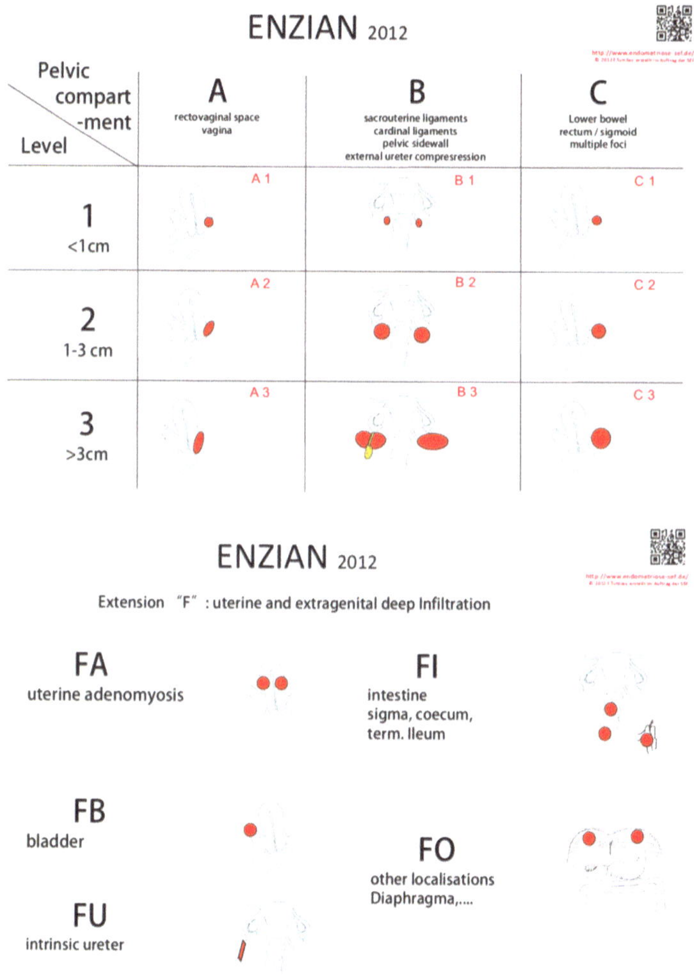

Fig. 21.5 The Enzian classification system

infiltration with respect to histological confirmation of muscular layer infiltration as an indispensable prerequisite.

Multiple bowel infiltrations are summarised under the description Enzian “FI” (far intestine) with a topographic information, for example, “FI Sigma” or “FI terminal ileum”.

The three pelvic compartments A, B and C are subjected to a consistent metric level system; 1 indicates that the lesions are less than 1 cm, 2 indicates between 1 and 3 cm and 3 over 3 cm (Fig. 21.5). The metric system classifies the dimension of the infiltration in each compartment.

The presence of adenomyosis is classified as FA (far adenomyosis), the transmural infiltration of the bladder wall as FB (far bladder) and the very rare presentation of intrinsic ureter endometriosis as FU (far ureter). The latter has to be distinguished from the more common extrinsic obstruction of the ureter, which would appear in the B3 group of the Enzian classification.

The Enzian classification of DIE is expressed as a multiple string code of the involved compartments starting with the initial Enzian letters. The involved compartments A, B and C are added with the appropriate metric level 1, 2 or 3, followed by the F subgroup. The complexity of the disease can be easily expressed by using an abstract code summarising the involved anatomical structures. The description of the more complex disease will result in an accordingly longer string.

An example of string may look like the following: *Enzian: A2, B3, C3, FA, FB, FI Sigma*, which means deep infiltrating endometriosis of the vagina 1–3 cm, ureter compression on one side by extrinsic endometriosis with dilatation of the urinating system above the obstruction, bowel infiltration of the rectum more than 3 cm, additional adenomyosis, infiltration of the bladder wall and bowel infiltration in the sigma.

With reference to the rASRM score peritoneal superficial endometriosis or the involvement of the fallopian tube-ovarian unit had been excluded from the Enzian scoring system and fertility aspects should be scored using the endometriosis fertility index (EFI). It is the distinguished purpose of the Enzian classification to describe the topographic manifestation of DIE and the size and extent of organ destruction; it is an easy-to-use system following an empiric pathway essential for a successful radical surgery.

21.4 Magnetic Resonance Imaging of Endometriosis (MARIE): Classification

Of uppermost importance for the imaging of patients suffering from deep infiltrating endometriosis is the detection and description of all manifestations of endometriosis in order to provide a reliable roadmap for surgical and conservative therapy. MRI has been established for diagnostic and pretherapeutic imaging of patients suspected to suffer from endometriosis [25]. Inherent to the method in contrast to ultrasound, clinical examination or laparoscopy, which offers only a limited field of view, spaces of the pelvis are equally accessible. For complete diagnostic evaluation of all pelvic spaces including the rectum, retrocervical space and vaginal fornices, careful preparation of the patient is indispensable [26]. For most scanning protocols 50 mL aqueous gel (ultrasound gel) is administered intravaginally (for distension of the vaginal cavity, assessment of the retrocervical area and vaginal fornices) and 150–200 mL water is administered into the rectum to obtain distension and increase contrast between bowel wall and lumen. Scopolamine-*N*-butyl bromide is intravenously injected immediately prior to MRI in order to reduce bowel movements and contractions of the uterus [27]. The bladder should be filled moderately, rendering the evaluation of the bladder wall possible. A reliable possibility to obtain moderate filling of the bladder is to ask patients not to empty the bladder one hour prior to scanning.

T2-weighted images in axial, sagittal and coronal orientation obtained with high resolution are crucial for the delineation of endometriotic lesions. T1-weighted 3D sequences with fat suppression are obtained prior and after intravenous injection of a gadolinium chelate contrast medium. On T1-weighted images obtained prior to the administration of contrast medium methaemoglobin appears with high signal intensity (bright). Methaemoglobin will be present in endometriosis 3 days up to 4 weeks after bleeding. Thereafter it is degraded into hemosiderin, which has low signal intensity on T1-weighted MR images. Fibrous components of endometriomas appear with low signal intensity on T2-weighted images and may enhance after the injection of contrast medium, depending on the size of the extracellular space in the lesions. Inflammatory lesions are also dark on T2-weighted images but strongly enhance after the injection of contrast medium on T1-weighted sequences. Endometriomas which do not contain predominantly blood or degraded blood components appear dark on T2-weighted sequences [25].

The involvement of the different anatomical structures in the pelvis has an unequal impact regarding fertility, physiologic function and required operative technique. Consequently a classification system for MRI should take these differences into account, and weighting of endometriotic lesions in different locations should be different regarding fertility and physiologic function (Table 21.3) [28]. In order to completely assess all present lesions, the compartments of the pelvis must be assessed in a systematic order. A structured report of a comprehensive MR scan for the detection of endometriosis should start with the description of site of lesions in the respective compartments, size of the lesion and structures involved. In the anterior compartment the bladder, vesicouterine pouch and vesicovaginal septum can be affected. The urethra is only rarely involved. Endometriosis of the anterior compartment usually does not cause infertility. Thus weighting regarding infertility is low (Table 21.3). On the other hand, the involvement of the urethra or bladder requires technically demanding operative strategies, so that weighting factor for structure is relatively high. The middle compartment contains the vagina, uterus, ovaries and uterine ligaments. The middle compartment is the most common site of endometriomas and the involvement of its structures often leads to infertility. This is mirrored in high scores regarding fertility for the respective anatomical structures of the middle compartment.

The rectovaginal pouch, uterosacral ligaments, posterior vaginal fornix and rectum are located in the posterior compartment. Most endometriotic lesions are located in the cul-de-sac [27]. The rectosigmoid is the most commonly affected part of the bowel. The involvement of the bowel requires technical demanding operation strategies and has a high impact on function, while fertility is rarely affected. Adhesions on the other hand might overlap the compartments and potentially have a high impact on fertility, depending on the structures involved.

For performing the MARIE classification, the three compartments are systematically assessed for endometriosis, lesion location is described and the size of

Table 21.3 Scoring system for MARIE classification

	≤1	1–2 cm	>2 cm
Anterior compartment			
Bladder	2 s	3 s	4 s
Vesicouterine pouch	0.5 s	1 s	1.5 s
Vesicovaginal septum	1 s	1.5 s	2 s
Urethra	3 s	4 s	5 s
Middle compartment			
Ovary (unilateral)	1 f	2 f	3 f
Ovaries bilateral, second side (value must be added to that of the first side)	3 f	4 f	5 f
Fallopian tube (unilateral)	4 f	4.5 f	5 f
Fallopian tubes, bilateral, second side (value must be added to that of first side)	7 f	8 f	9 f
Uterus (surface)	0.5 f	1 f	1.5 f
Vagina	0.5 s	1 s	1.5 s
Posterior compartment			
Rectovaginal septum	0.5 s	1 s	1.5 s
Cul-de-sac	1 s	2 s	3 s
Cul-de-sac and rectum	2 s	3 s	4 s
Rectum/sigmoid	3 s	4 s	5 s
Uterosacral ligament unilateral	1/0.5 s/f	2/1 s/f	3/1.5 s/f
Uterosacral ligament bilateral	1.5/1 s/f	2.5/1.5 s/f	3.5/2 s/f
Other			
Adhesions between bowel and ovaries/fallopian tubes	3/4 s/f	4/5 s/f	5/6 s/f
Adhesions between both ovaries	1/4 s/f	1.5/5 s/f	2/6 s/f
Adhesions between bowel and uterus	2/2 s/f	2.5/2.5 s/f	3/3 s/f
Adhesions without involvement of uterus, ovaries and fallopian tubes	2.5 s	3 s	3.5 s
Lesions outside the compartment of the pelvis but in pelvic region, except subcutaneous	2 s	3 s	4 s
Subcutaneous lesions, fascia not penetrated	0.5 s	1 s	1.5 s
Sciatic nerve	3 s	4 s	5 s
	Points	Class fertility	Class structures
MARIE classification			
	0.5–2	MARIE 1 f	MARIE 1 s
	2.5–6.5	MARIE 2 f	MARIE 2 s
	>7	MARIE 3 f	MARIE 3 s

lesions is measured. Points are added separately for *f* (fertility) and *s* (structures) according to Table 21.3 (Fig. 21.6 represents an example of MRI classification of a 28-year-old patient with deep infiltrating endometriosis). In cases of bilateral involvement (i.e. ovaries or fallopian tubes), first the more severely affected side is rated followed by the side with the smaller lesion. According to Table 21.3 MARIE classification for *f* and *e* values is assigned following the scheme MARIE × f × s.

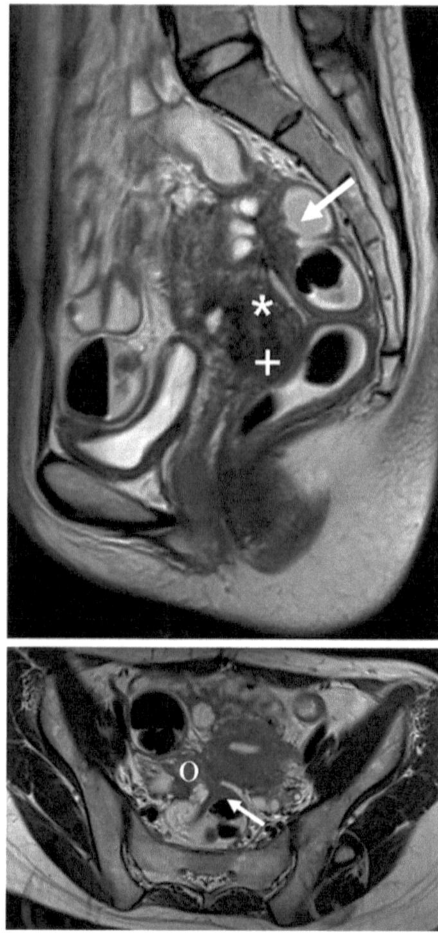

Fig. 21.6 Sagittal and axial T2-weighted images of a 28-year-old patient with deep infiltrating endometriosis. Lesions of both ovaries (right ovary diameter 3 cm, score 3f, left ovary 2 cm, score 4f), adhesion between right ovary and rectum with a diameter of 1.5 cm (score 4 s, 5f) lesion of the spatium rectovaginale (diameter 2 cm, score 1 s) and cul-de-sac (diameter 4 cm, score 3 s) are present (scores summing up to 12 f 8 s), resulting in MARIE 3 f 3 s

21.5 Discussion

Even though many classifications as well as scoring systems have been proposed since the first mentioning of endometriosis as a disease entity, no widespread agreement on a classification for endometriosis is obtained. This review describes four examples in more detail. The rASRM classification differentiates endometriosis in minimal, mild, moderate and severe stages and provides a score that includes superficial endometriotic implants as well as adhesions. The assignment of points according to the clinical situation was not developed on the basis of empirical data, but based on theoretical background and estimations. In case of a superficial non-infiltrating endometriosis, which is only manifested on the peritoneal surface, this scoring system including a graph makes a lot of sense; however, any sub- and retroperitoneal deep infiltrating manifestation is not considered with the rASRM classification. The most commonly used classification system to describe deep infiltrating endometriosis is the Enzian string code, which is used additionally to the rASRM. In addition to the rASRM and Enzian classification Hackethal et al. [29] showed that even in stage 1 endometriosis (rASRM classification) 25 % of those patients were suffering from deep infiltrating endometriosis. Even though this is in accordance with the initial aim of the rASRM classification omitting DIE can lead to a marked misjudgement of the impact of the disease and necessary treatment [30]. Since the EFI is a specific further development of the rASRM classification, DIE with no peritoneal, ovarian or tubal infiltration would not have been reflected in the EFI score; however it could be responsible for infertility. This would apply to DIE of the rectovaginal space as well as adenomyosis. However, only limited data are available on the impact of such manifestations of DIE on fertility. Therefore, the EFI will likely not be suitable to fully reflect the impact of different locations and manifestations of endometriosis on fertility. It is probably because of this reason that EFI gives major importance on historical factors as it is very well known that the duration of infertility, age of a patient and prior history of pregnancies are extremely strong predictors.

Haas et al. [31] compared the rASRM classification with the Enzian classification. They clearly concluded that the Enzian classification is a clear supplement to the rASRM classification with regard to the description of the manifestations of DIE. They found an overlapping of description, especially in peritoneal disease of the pouch of Douglas or cul-de-sac, which could be repetitive in the Enzian classification as well as in rASRM classification.

The development of a radiological classification system is extremely useful in the preparation of the surgical procedure and counselling patients preoperatively about the required surgical steps. It has to be kept in mind that endometriosis surgery is almost never easy and straightforward. A presurgical adequate classification of disease can potentially improve patients' outcome by the organisation of multidisciplinary surgical teams or referral of patients to specialised surgical endometriosis centres.

Unfortunately there is no ideal classification of endometriosis at the moment that would be able to reflect all the aspects of endometriosis, the pathogenesis, anatomical distribution, clinical manifestation, progression and recurrence. The way to define the perfect classification system is long and lots of basic research as well as well-conducted clinical trials in a large multicentre set-up are needed to better understand the clinical nature of the disease and develop a classification system, which encompass all these aspects.

References

1. Lockyer C. Fibroids and allied tumors (Myoma and Adenomyoma): their pathology, clinical features and surgical treatment. London: Macmillan; 1918.
2. Sampson JA. Perforating hemorrhagic (chocolate) cysts of the ovary. Arch Surg. 1921;3:254–323.
3. Acosta AA, Buttram VC, Besch PK, Malinak LR, Franklin RR, Vanderheyden JD. A proposed classification of pelvic endometriosis. Obstet Gynecol. 1973;42:19–25.

4. Kistner RW, Siegler AM, Behrman SJ. Suggested classification for endometriosis: relationship to infertility. Fertil Steril. 1977;28:1008–10.
5. Buttram VC. An expanded classification of endometriosis. Fertil Steril. 1978;30:240–2.
6. Wicks MJ, Larson CP. Histologic criteria for evaluating endometriosis. Northwest Med. 1949;48:611–3.
7. Huffman JW. External endometriosis. Am J Obstet Gynecol. 1951;62:1243–52.
8. Sturgis SH, Call BJ. Endometriosis peritonei—relationship of pain to functional activity. Am J Obstet Gynecol. 1954;68:1421–31.
9. Riva HL, Kawasaki DM, Messinger AJ. Further experience with norethynodrel in treatment of endometriosis. Obstet Gynecol. 1962;19:111–7.
10. Beecham CT. Classification of endometriosis [editorial]. Obstet Gynecol. 1966;28:437.
11. Mitchell GW, Farber M. Medical versus surgical management of endometriosis. In: Reid DE, Christian CD, editors. Controversy in obstetrics and gynecology, vol. 2. Philadelphia: WB Saunders; 1974. p. 631–6.
12. American Fertility Society. Classification of endometriosis. Fertil Steril. 1979;32:631–4.
13. American Fertility Society. Revised American Fertility Society Classification: 1985. Fertil Steril. 1985;43:351–2.
14. Revised American society of reproductive medicine classification of endometriosis: 1996. Fertil Steril. 1996;67:817–21.
15. Mettler L, Schollmeyer T, Lehmann-Willenbrock E, Schüppler U, Schmutzler A, Ahukla D, et al. Accuracy of laparoscopic diagnosis of endometriosis. JSLS. 2003;7:15–8.
16. Vercellini P, Fedele L, Aimi G, De Giorgi O, Consonni D, Crosignani PG. Reproductive performance, pain recurrence and disease relapse after conservative surgical treatment for endometriosis: the predictive value of the current classification system. Hum Reprod. 2006;21:2679–85.
17. Fujishita A, Khan KN, Masuzaki H, Ishimaru T. Influence of pelvic endometriosis and ovarian endometrioma on fertility. Gynecol Obstet Invest. 2002;53:40–5.
18. Adamson GD, Pasta DJ. Endometriosis fertility index: the new, validated endometriosis staging system. Fertil Steril. 2010;94:1609–15.
19. Wei DM, Yu Q, Sun AJ, Tian QJ, Chen R, Deng CY, et al. Relationship between endometriosis fertility index and pregnancies after laparoscopic surgery in endometriosis-associated infertility. Zhonghua Fu Chan Ke Za Zhi. 2011;46:806–8.
20. Yacoub A, Ferdinus C, Mourtialon P, Girod S, M-N Huot, Douvier S, et al. Is Endometriosis Fertility Index a good tool to predict pregnancy in patients with surgically documented endometriosis followed by ART treatment? World Congress of Endometriosis, Montpellier, France. Clinical Free Oral Communication S#10-2. 7 September 2011.
21. Thomasetti C, Geysenbergh B, Meuleman C, Timmerman D, Fieuws S, D'Hooghe T. External validation of the endometriosis fertility index (EFI) staging system for predicting non-ART pregnancy after endometriosis surgery. Hum Reprod. 2013;28:1280–8.
22. Chapron C, Fauconnier A, Vieira M, Barakat H, Dousset B, Pansini V, et al. Anatomical distribution of deeply infiltrating endometriosis: surgical implications and proposition for a classification. Hum Reprod. 2003;18:157–61.
23. Koninckx PR, Ussia A, Adamyan L, Wattiez A. An endometriosis classification, designed to be validated. Gynecol Surg. 2011;8:1–6.
24. Tuttlies F, Keckstein J, Ulrich U, Possover M, Schweppe KW, Wustlich M, et al. ENZIAN-Score, a classification of deep infiltrating endometriosis. Zentralbl Gynakol. 2005;127:275–81.
25. Coutinho A, Bittencourt LK, Pires CE, et al. MR imaging in deep pelvic endometriosis: a pictorial assay. Radiographics. 2011;31:549–67.
26. Loubeyre P, Petignat P, Jacob S, Egger JF, Dubuisson JB, Wenger JM. Anatomic distribution of posterior deeply infiltrating endometriosis on MRI after vaginal and rectal gel opacification. Am J Radiol. 2009;192:1625–31.

27. Bazot M, Lafont C, Rouzier R, Roseau G, Thomassin-Naggara I, Daraï E. Diagnostic accuracy of physical examination, transvaginal sonography, rectal endoscopic sonography and magnetic resonance imaging to diagnose deep infiltrating endometriosis. Fertil Steril. 2009;6:1825–33.
28. Krombach G, Oehmke F, Schneider C, Tinneberg H. Magnetic resonance imaging of endometriosis (MARIE) classification. Radiology. Submitted
29. Hackethal A, Luck C, Konrad L, Muenstedt K, Tinneberg HR, Oehmke F. Deep infiltrating endometriosis is frequent in all stages of endometriosis and the depth of infiltration influences surgical parameters proportionally. J Endometriosis. 2012;2:205–2012.
30. Tuttlies F, Keckstein J, Ulrich U, Possover M, Schweppe KW, Wustlich M, et al. ENZIAN-Klassifikation zur Diskussion gestellt: Eine neue differenzierte Klassifikation der tief infiltrierenden Endometriose. J Gynäkol Endokrinol. 2008;18:7–13.
31. Haas D, Chvatal R, Habelsberger A, Wurm P, Schimetta W, Oppelt P. Comparison of revised American fertility Society and ENZIAN staging: a critical evaluation of classifications of endometriosis on the basis of our patient population. Fertil Steril. 2011;95:1574–8.

Chapter 22
The Association of Endometriosis with Ovarian Cancer: A Critical Review of Epidemiological Data

Sun-Wei Guo

Abstract Although endometriosis is well recognized as a benign gynecologic condition, its association with ovarian cancer has frequently been reported. Many review papers on this topic have been published, yet there seems to be no consensus as to whether or not endometriosis is a precursor of ovarian cancer and whether or not any actions should be taken based on our current knowledge on the endometriosis-ovarian cancer association. In this chapter, I shall critically review epidemiological and clinical prevalence data for and against the link, point out the challenges in proving the causal link, and, in the end, sketch some ways to solve this problem. I shall provide a tutorial review of epidemiological studies, measures of effect size, and confounding and point out the connection between the prevalence data and the relative risk estimate. Funnel plots are used to examine the asymmetry of risk estimates, in which the risk estimates such as OR are plotted on a logarithmic scale against the inverse of their corresponding measures of precision. Areas in need of further research are also outlined.

Keywords Association • Case-control studies • Endometriosis • Epidemiology • Ovarian cancer

22.1 Introduction

Although endometriosis is well recognized as a benign gynecologic condition, its association with ovarian cancer has often been reported and mentioned in literature. A PubMed search with the keyword, endometriosis, yielded a total of 19,621

S.-W. Guo, M.Med., Ph.D. (✉)
Shanghai OB/GYN Hospital, Fudan University, 419 Fangxie Road, Shanghai 200011, China

Department of Biochemistry, Shanghai College of Medicine, Fudan University, Shanghai, China
e-mail: hoxa10@gmail.com

T. Harada (ed.), *Endometriosis: Pathogenesis and Treatment*,
DOI 10.1007/978-4-431-54421-0_22, © Springer Japan 2014

papers. Using the combination of "endometriosis" and "ovarian cancer," it turned up 2,544 papers or 13.0 % of the total literature on endometriosis. In contrast, 3,722 (19.0 %), 3,542 (18.0 %), and 515 (2.6 %) papers were on endometriosis and infertility, endometriosis and pain, and endometriosis and inflammation, respectively (accessed June 18, 2013). Many review papers on this topic have been published, yet there is no consensus as to whether or not endometriosis is a precursor of ovarian cancer [1]. While many scientists sit on the fences, some investigators think that the ovarian endometriomas "could be viewed as a neoplastic process," considering the malignant transformation of endometriosis as rather obvious [2]. Other investigators are more cautious, arguing that, among the nine criteria of causality, proposed by Hill [3], many are still unfulfilled [4].

However, a Lancet Oncology paper, published early last year, seemed to tip the balance of this debate towards the conclusion that endometriosis is a precursor of ovarian cancer. From a pooled analysis with primary data from 13 case-control studies, Pearce et al. reported that women with self-reported endometriosis were associated with a significantly increased risk of clear cell (odds ratio (OR) = 3.05), low-grade serous (OR = 2.11), and endometrioid invasive (OR = 2.04), but not high-grade serous invasive ovarian cancer [5]. The authors of that paper concluded that "we will develop a risk stratification model that combines genetic and epidemiological risk to better stratify women into high-risk, intermediate-risk, and low-risk categories, allowing better individualization of prevention and early detection approaches such as risk-reduction surgery and screening." The lead author, Dr. Celeste Leigh Pearce, was even more optimistic, stating, in a journal news release, that "This breakthrough could lead to better identification of women at increased risk of ovarian cancer and could provide a basis for increased cancer surveillance of the relevant population, allowing better individualization of prevention and early detection approaches such as risk-reduction surgery and screening" (http://health.usnews.com/health-news/news/articles/2012/02/22/endometriosis-could-raise-risk-of-3-ovarian-cancers, accessed January 15, 2013). In other words, endometriosis is indeed a precursor of ovarian cancer and, as such, certain measures should be taken accordingly.

Ovarian cancer is by far the most lethal malignancy of the female reproductive system. Over 90 % of ovarian cancers arise from the surface epithelium [6]. Despite advances in radical surgery and chemotherapy, the overall survival has changed very little in the last 30 years [7]. With the advent of molecular biology, a great deal of efforts have been focused on early detection, yet this attempt often brings with roller-coaster experience and consequently it has so far not resulted in any tangible survival benefit to the patients. Faced with such an abject failure, it is important to identify the precursor(s) of ovarian cancer, even for some specific histotypes.

With this in perspective, it is perhaps understandable as why there have been so much attention on the endometriosis-ovarian cancer link. However, how solid is the evidence for this link? Would the evidence, gathered so far, warrant any actionable measures such as that suggested by Dr. Pearce? These are simple yet weighty issues that are worth careful examination.

In this chapter, I shall critically review the evidence in support of the link, point out the challenges in proving the causal link, and, in the end, sketch some ways to solve this problem. Due to space limitation, I shall restrict my attention to epidemiological and clinical data. While there is a growing body of literature documenting shared molecular aberrations between endometriosis and ovarian cancer, suffice to say that, due to the nature of these studies, many such aberrations are indicative of association, only suggestive for a causal link, simply because the temporality of the link is difficult to prove.

22.2 Methods

A systematic and comprehensive search of PubMed was performed for all studies published up to June 18, 2013, using the following combination of search terms of "endometriosis," "ovarian cancer," "epidemiology," and "association." The studies had to report epigenetic aberrations in endometriosis. The search was limited to publications written in English.

For each retrieved case-control studies, the OR and its 95 % confidence interval (CI) and the standard error (SE) of the log OR were extracted. The choice of log OR was simply due to the fact that, in contrast to the OR, its SE is unaffected by the magnitude of the log OR. For cohort studies, the standardized incidence ratio (SIR), rate ratio (RR), or hazard ratio (HR) and their SEs were extracted.

Funnel plots were used to examine asymmetry, in which the risk estimates such as OR were plotted on a logarithmic scale against the inverse of their corresponding standard errors, a measure of precision [8]. If bias is absent, small studies will have ORs that are widely scattered but symmetric about the OR estimates provided by larger, more precise studies. In this case, the plot would resemble an inverted funnel with the tip pointing roughly towards the true log OR. If publication bias is present, the plot will be asymmetric because some negative studies are not published

All computations were made with R statistics software system version 3.0.9 [9]. The statistical routine *rmeta* was used.

22.3 The Role of the Funding Source

The sponsor of the study had no role in study design, data collection, data analysis, data interpretation, or writing of this report.

22.4 Evidence from Clinical Series

22.4.1 Early Criteria

As early as 1925, Sampson proposed histopathological criteria for inferring that the malignancy arose from endometriosis, or the causal relationship between endometriosis and malignancy: (1) clear evidence of endometriosis close to the tumor ("proximity"); (2) the carcinoma must be seen to arise in endometriosis and not to be invading it from other sources ("arising from endometriosis"); and (3) presence of tissue resembling endometrial stroma surrounding characteristic glands ("endometrial stroma plus glands") [10]. Scott later added one more criterion: the demonstration of a histology-proven transition from benign endometriosis to cancer ("transition") [11].

Clearly, these criteria are all based on histological evidence, which, in turn, are based on tissue samples taken from patients. While the "proximity" and "endometrial stroma plus glands" criteria may be relatively easy to establish, the inference of "arising from endometriosis" and "transition" has, by necessity, to be based on a single snapshot, in contrast to serial observations, of the histological images or morphologic features during a presumably long period of tumorigenesis and, as such, can be challenging to establish. It is no wonder that these criteria, considered to be stringent, are rarely fulfilled [1, 12].

The morphologic data can tell us something, but only to a certain extent. For example, ovarian cancer was once regarded as a single disease since by morphology the tumor seemingly originated from ovary but now a dualistic model of carcinogenesis of ovarian cancer based on distinctive clinicopathologic and molecular genetic features seems to have replaced the older view [7, 13]. Also, just by morphology or histological data, it would be very difficult to find that there are 4 main subtypes of breast cancer caused by different subsets of genetic and epigenetic abnormalities [14]. In addition, since the choice of tissue sections entails certain degree of selection, it may be susceptible to attribution error, especially when the pathologists are inexperienced.

22.4.2 Prevalence Data: An Intimate Connection with the Odds Ratio

About a dozen reports on the prevalence of endometriosis in women with ovarian cancer have been published. If we denote the prevalence of endometriosis (E) as $P(E)$, the prevalence of women with both endometriosis and ovarian cancer (O) (often called endometriosis-associated ovarian cancer or EAOC) as $P(E, O)$, and the proportion of E among women with O as the conditional probability $P(E/O)$, then we can denote the relative risk of having O in women with E vs. women without E ($\overline{E}$) as $\mathrm{RR} = P(O|E)/P(O|\overline{E})$, that is, the relative risk of having O when a woman has E vs. woman who does not. This is the quantity that most, if not all, epidemiological studies attempt to estimate. Here, the age dependency is often ignored for ease of exposition.

Since both $P(O/E)$ and $P(O|\overline{E})$ are small (because the lifetime risk of developing O is about 1 % or 0.01 and even lower for some specific histotypes of ovarian cancers), $1 - P(O|E) \approx 1 - P(O|\overline{E}) \approx 1$,

$$\mathrm{RR} = \frac{P(O|E)}{P(O|\overline{E})} \approx \frac{\frac{P(O|E)}{1-P(O|E)}}{\frac{P(O|\overline{E})}{1-P(O|\overline{E})}} = \mathrm{OR}$$

That is, when ovarian cancer is rare (indeed it is), the OR obtained from case-control studies is merely an approximation to RR.

By Bayes' theorem and after some simple algebra, it is easy to see that $\mathrm{RR} = P(E/O)[1-P(E)]/(P(E)/[1-P(E/O)])$. That is, the true RR depends only on the prevalence of endometriosis (which we have a fairly good idea) and the prevalence of endometriosis among women with ovarian cancer (which can be estimated from data, at least in theory). Note that this RR does not depend on the prevalence of O. Hence we can calculate RR even for some specific histotypes of ovarian cancer, such as clear cell or endometrioid ovarian cancers. It is noted that RR can be expressed in a more revealing form, as $\mathrm{RR} = r_O/r$, where $r_O = P(E/O)/[1-P(E/O)]$, the odds of having endometriosis given that the woman has O, and $r = P(E)/[1-P(E)]$, the odds of having endometriosis in the general population.

22.4.3 Prevalence Data from Published Studies

The prevalence data extracted from 13 studies reporting the prevalence of endometriosis in women with ovarian cancers, along with the estimated RR using either the 10 % prevalence for endometriosis or the 5 % for ovarian endometriomas, are listed in Table 22.1. It can be seen that there are enormous variations in the reported prevalence, and, consequently, the RR estimates also vary greatly from study to study. It should be noted that the reported prevalence of endometriosis in women with ovarian cancer is likely to be an underestimate of $P(E/O)$, since some endometriotic lesions may not have been found by the surgeon who performed the operation, or pathologists who performed histologic examination may not have found any lesion which might still exist. On the other hand, $P(E/O)$ is prone to be overestimated if one is single-mindedly trying to find all cases of ovarian cancer-associated endometriosis while dismissing or discarding cases with ovarian cancer but no endometriosis, consciously or otherwise. Anyhow, it can be seen from Table 22.1 that some RR estimates based on the reported prevalence still deviate greatly from the OR estimates reported from case-control studies, especially for clear cell and endometrioid histotypes. In fact, all, except one, OR

Table 22.1 Prevalence of endometriosis in women with ovarian cancers and the estimated relative risk of developing ovarian cancer in women with endometriosis vs. women without

ID	Author	Year of publication	Overall: Prevalence (%)	Overall: RR ($P=10$ %)	Overall: RR ($P=5$ %)	Clear cell and endometrioid: Prevalence (%)	Clear cell and endometrioid: RR ($P=10$ %)	Clear cell and endometrioid: RR ($P=5$ %)	Remark
A71	Aure et al. [15]	1971	4.2 (35/831)	0.39	0.83	12.5 (34/271)	1.29	2.71	
K72	Kurman et al. [16]	1972	NR	–	–	10.2 (5/49)	1.02	2.16	
R79	Russell [17]	1979	11.3 (46/407)	1.15	2.42	34.3 (36/105)	4.70	9.92	
B89	Brescia et al. [18]	1989	NR	–	–	18.4 (14/76)	2.03	4.28	
V93	Vercellini et al. [19]	1993	11.1 (52/466)	1.12	2.37	25.0 (38/152)	3.00	6.33	
C96	De La Cuesta et al.	1996	NR	–	–	40.0 (16/40)	6.00	12.67	
J97	Jimbo et al. [20]	1997	14.5 (25/172)	1.53	3.22	35.6 (16/45)	4.96	10.50	
F97	Fukunaga et al. [21]	1997	24.1 (54/224)	2.86	6.03	49.4 (40/81)	8.79	18.55	
O00	Ogawa et al. [22]	2000	29.1 (37/127)	3.69	7.80	66.0 (33/50)	17.47	36.88	
V00	Vercellini et al. [23]	2000	43.5 (91/209)	6.93	14.63	60.7 (54/89)	13.90	29.35	Only unilateral cancer and left-sided lesions were considered
O03	Oral et al. [24]	2003	7.7 (14/182)	0.75	1.59	26.3 (5/19)	3.21	6.79	
D11	Dzatic-Smiljkovic et al. [25]	2011	11.0 (23/210)	1.11	2.35	33.3 (19/57)	4.49	9.49	
K12	Kondi-Pafiti et al. [26]	2012	5.9 (1/17)	0.56	1.19	0.0 (0/16)	0.00	0.00	

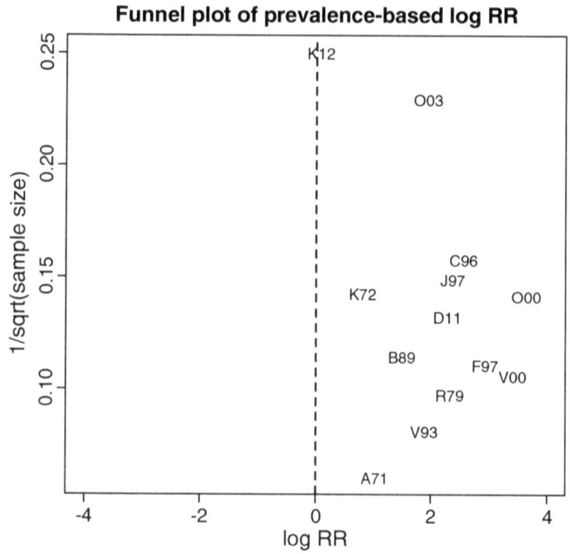

Fig. 22.1 Funnel plot for the 13 log-transformed prevalence-based RRs, using data extracted from Table 22.1 and assuming a 5 % prevalence of endometriosis in the general population. The *dashed line* represents RR = 1. The alphabet-numeric combinations are the IDs shown in Table 22.1, and each ID represents one study. Note that for study K12, a Bayes estimate for binomial distribution assuming a non-informative prior (uniform distribution) was used, since otherwise the data would yield a RR of 0

estimates are pretty large. It is unclear as to whether some seemingly high prevalence estimates are genuine or a result of ascertainment bias, population idiosyncrasy, or chance events.

Based on all published prevalence estimates listed in Table 22.1, one can get a pooled estimate of prevalence for all histotypes of ovarian cancer weighted by the sample size, which is 12.9 %, yielding an RR estimate of 1.33 if a prevalence of 10 % is assumed, or 2.81 if a prevalence of 5 % is assumed. For clear cell and endometrioid ovarian cancers, the pooled estimate of prevalence is 28.0 % and the corresponding RR estimates are 3.51 and 7.40, respectively, depending on the endometriosis prevalence.

Note that, since $RR = r_O/r$, where $r_O = P(E/O)/[1-P(E/O)]$ and $r = P(E)/[1-P(E)]$, r is a constant when $P(E)$ is assumed to be a fixed number (say, 5 %); hence we can calculate the standard error of log RR, which is equivalent to the standard error of log r_O, or $\log[P(E/O)]-\log[1-P(E/O)]$. By delta method, it is easy to see that the standard error of log RR is inversely proportional to the squared root of the sample size n. Hence, we can plot the log RR listed in Table 22.1 against the squared root of the sample size n reported in the study (Fig. 22.1).

It is interesting to see from Fig. 22.1 that when the estimated log RRs were plotted against the squared root of the sample size of the study, the seemingly large RRs seen in Table 22.1, when all placed in the funnel plot in Fig. 22.1, seem to gravitate to a point close to 1, but perhaps slightly greater than 1.

22.5 Epidemiological Evidence

22.5.1 Cohort Studies

In a typical cohort study, two cohorts or two groups of people, one with and one without a particular attribute (in our case, women with or without endometriosis), are identified and followed up longitudinally. The incidence of a particular event—quite often, disease (ovarian cancer, in our case)—in the two groups is evaluated and compared. In this way, whether having the particular attribute (exposure) would increase or decrease the incidence can be investigated.

Due to constraint in time and resources, cohort studies are seldom conducted concurrently or truly prospectively. Instead, many cohort studies are conducted retrospectively. In the latter case, the cohorts are identified and assembled in the past based on archived records. In this case, the occurrence of the event of interest is often retrieved from the records as well. While retrospective cohort studies require much less resources and time, their major disadvantage is their exclusive reliance on available information, sometimes the subjects' own memory. Consequently, the quality of exposure or disease data can be compromised (e.g., recall bias).

In epidemiology, the outcome is frequently a disease. One common outcome measure in cohort studies is incidence, or the risk of developing certain disease within a specified period of time given no occurrence prior to that time period. It can be expressed either in cumulative incidence (incidence proportion) or incidence rate with a denominator (called incidence density rate or person-time incidence rate). In analytical epidemiology, one measure that is used very frequently is the standardized incidence ratio (SIR), which is a ratio or percentage quantifying the increase or decrease in incidence of a study cohort with reference to the general population.

While the SIR provides a succinct measure of the change from the incidence from the reference population or cohort, it becomes a bit cumbersome when there are some confounding factors that need to be controlled for, especially in retrospective cohort studies. In these circumstances, the rate ratio (RR, also called ratio of incidence densities) or hazard rate (HR) would be more convenient, and their use would render the use of some sophisticated statistical models such as the Cox regression model possible, facilitating elaborate statistical analysis. The RR gives the ratio of the event rate in the cohort of interest (say, women with endometriosis) vs. that in the reference group after adjustment for other known confounders. Both SIR and RR provide a measure of causality (or, rather, association, especially for retrospective cohort studies) between exposures and outcomes.

So far, seven cohort studies, with varying qualities, on endometriosis-ovarian cancer link can be identified (Table 22.2). Some of them were population-based and prospective studies, and others were hospital-based or retrospective cohort studies. These studies yielded either SIR or RR estimates, along with 95 % confidence intervals (CIs) (Table 22.2).

Table 22.2 Published cohort studies reporting ovarian cancer risk in women with endometriosis

ID	Author	Year of publication	Cohort size	Length of follow-up	# of cases	SIR or RR	S.E.	95 % CI
B97	Brinton et al. [27]	1997	20,686	11.4	29	1.92	0.38	1.3–2.8
O02	Olson et al. [28]	2002	1,392	13	13	0.78*	0.74	0.25–2.44
B04	Brinton et al. [29]	2004	1,919	18.8	13	1.26*	0.29	0.6–2.6
B05	Brinton et al. [30]	2005	2,491	NA	50	1.69*	0.09	1.27–2.25
M06	Melin et al. [31]	2006	66,187	12.7	122	1.43	0.133	1.19–1.71
M07	Melin et al. [32]	2007	63,630	13.4	134	1.37	0.12	1.14–1.62
K07	Kobayashi et al. [33]	2007	6,398	12.8	46	8.95	2.85	4.12–15.3
A10	Aris [34]	2010	2,854	10	333	1.6*	0.10	1.12–2.09
S12N	Stewart et al. [35]	2012				3.11* (for nulliparous women)	0.52	1.13–8.57
S12P						1.52* (for parous women)	0.76	0.43–6.75

SIR standard incidence ratio, *RR* rate ratio, *SE* standard error, *CI* confidence interval
*"SIR or RR" column are RR estimates

From these SIRs and their CIs, their standard errors (SEs) can be easily calculated. Since all the RRs were calculated based on logistic or Poisson regression models after adjusting for possible confounding factors, the SE of the log-transformed RR can be calculated based on RRs and their CIs.

In evaluating risk estimates—be it SIR, RR, or OR if from case-control studies—from various studies, funnel plots are often employed [36]. In funnel plots, risk estimates, such as RRs or log RRs, are placed on the horizontal axis against some measure of study size or precision, such as their standard errors, on the vertical axis. The funnel plot is so named because of its shape: in the absence of selection biases (such as publication bias and bias in inclusion criteria), true heterogeneity (i.e., size of effect differs according to study size), and data irregularities (such as poor methodological design of small studies, inadequate analysis, and fraud), studies of large or small sample sizes should be more or less symmetrically scattered around the true log RR. Hence the plot should have the shape of a funnel with wide opening on the top (due to sampling variability), with the tip of the funnel pointing to the bottom and centering on the true log RR [36]. The choice of log OR instead of OR is due to the fact that the standard error of RR is related with the odds

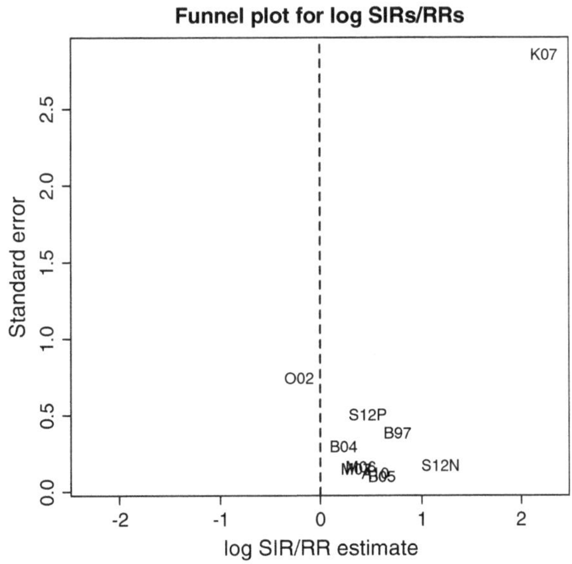

Fig. 22.2 Funnel plot for the 9 log-transformed SIRs/RRs, using data extracted from Table 22.2. The *dashed line* represents SIR = 1 or RR = 1. The alphabet-numeric combinations are the IDs shown in Table 22.2, and each ID represents one study

ratio, while the standard error of log OR is purely a function of sample sizes in different exposure-disease status combinations. The use of log OR also renders ORs that are greater than 1 or less than 1 symmetric about 1 (=0 on the log scale).

When plotting the 9 log-transformed SIRs/RRs against their SEs in a funnel plot (Fig. 22.2), two features can be noted. First, the plot looks like an asymmetric funnel, with its tip gravitating towards somewhere near log SIR or log RR = 0, i.e., SIR = 1 or RR = 1. Since there is no indication of bias in inclusion criteria or heterogeneity, this suggests that there may be a publication bias towards favoring positive studies and higher estimates of odds ratios may well be a chance variation. In addition, the plot seems to suggest that the true SIR or RR is near 1.

Second, the SIR estimate, K07 in the plot, provided by Kobayashi et al. [33] is situated at the rim of the funnel, suggesting that while it gave a larger SIR estimate, it is not a precise estimate.

The paper by Aris [34] gave $P(E) = 0.107$ and $P(E|O) = 0.14$, yielding RR = 1.36 as discussed above. This is very close to the RR estimate of 1.6 reported by the paper.

22.5.2 An Overview on Case-Control Studies

Case-control studies are an alternative to cohort studies for investigating the association between exposure (in our case, having endometriosis) and disease (ovarian cancer). The basic questions for such studies are the degree of association between risk for disease and the factor(s) under investigation, the extent to which the observed association may result from bias, confounding, and/or chance, and the extent to which they may be described as causal [37]. A case-control study compares cases (in our case, women with ovarian cancer) and controls (women without ovarian cancer, say) with respect to their exposure (or lack thereof) or levels of exposure to a suspecting risk factor (in our case, having endometriosis). When the risk factor at hand is a dichotomous variable, such as having endometriosis or not, the outcome measure is typically the odds of exposure in cases as compared with that in controls, or OR. When the occurrence of disease is rare, such as ovarian cancer, the OR estimated from case-control studies becomes an acceptable approximation to the relative risk. Case-control studies can be a powerful tool in the investigation of exposure-disease relationship when both the disease and the exposure are rare. A prime example is the uncovering of the relationship between in utero exposure to diethylstilbestrol (DES) and vaginal adenocarcinomas in the daughters [38]. That study was based on just eight cases, each with four matched controls. Seven out of eight cases had been exposed to DES in utero, but in contrast none of the 32 controls had.

As with SIR or RR used in cohort studies, the OR or relative risk (RR) used in case-control studies is the measure of association between disease and exposure. However, the association could be causal but also could be merely a correlation. For women with endometriosis (E), or with ovarian cancer (O), the association between E and O could be due to a variety of scenarios. Figure 22.3 shows several scenarios in which E and O can be found to be associated. Scenario a is the case where factor X has a causal relationship with both E and O. E and O are associated simply because of the presence of the common risk factor X, which may or may not be measured in a study. It should be noted that E and O share at least one common risk factor, that is, the incessant ovulation/menstruation. Incessant ovulation or unopposed estrogen exposure is a known major risk factor for ovarian cancer [39]. Similarly, incessant menstruation is a known major and consistently identified risk factor for endometriosis [40]. Figure 22.4 shows two numerical examples, perhaps somewhat extreme but nonetheless not unusual cases. In example a, failure to control for the confounding factor gives rise to spurious results. It is interesting to point out that, while the OR for the O-E association in each stratum of factor X is 1, the OR for the association with pooled levels of the factor is $1.35 > 1$. Of course, the failure to control for confounders can also go to the other direction, in which the pooled OR can be smaller than ORs in each stratum (example b).

In Fig. 22.3, scenario b shows the case in which both factors X and E represent the same underlying cause for O, such as the case when X and E represent different aspects of the same factor. Scenario c is the case where E leads to X, which, in turn, has a causal relationship with O. In the case of E-O association, it is possible that the diagnosis of endometriosis may result in the use of danazol, an androgenic agent, which could increase the risk of O in light of the "androgen hypothesis" of ovarian cancer [41, 42]. In other words, it could be the exposure to an androgenic agent, once a popular therapeutic for endometriosis, that increases the risk of ovarian cancer, not the endometriosis itself. Scenario d is the case in which E-O has a causal relationship.

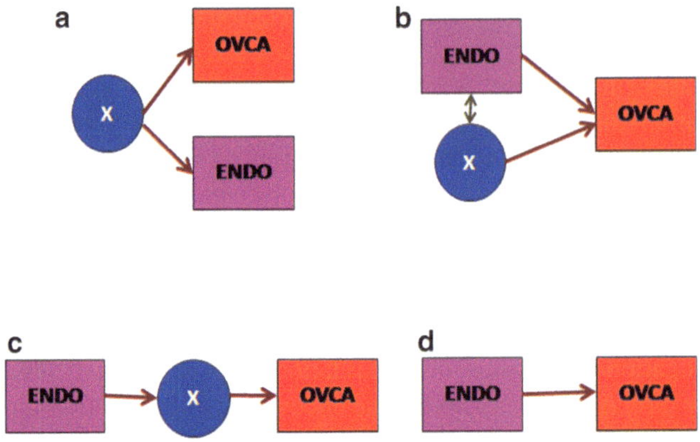

Fig. 22.3 Diagrams showing 4 different scenarios in which *E* and *O* can be found associated

a

	Factor X + Exposure E +	Factor X + Exposure E −	Factor X - Exposure E +	Factor X - Exposure E −	Pooled levels of Factor X Exposure E +	Pooled levels of Factor X Exposure E −
Case	60	50	5	6	65	56
Control	6	5	50	60	56	65
OR	1		1		1.35	

b

	Factor X + Exposure E +	Factor X + Exposure E −	Factor X - Exposure E +	Factor X - Exposure E −	Pooled levels of Factor X Exposure E +	Pooled levels of Factor X Exposure E −
Case	100	100	90	10	190	110
Control	10	90	100	100	110	190
OR	9.0		9.0		2.98	

Fig. 22.4 Two hypothetical examples showing that failure to control for confounding can lead to spurious results. (**a**) Artificially inflated OR; (**b**) underestimated OR

It should be noted that factor *X* in scenario a is considered a confounding factor. Confounding is the distortion of a disease/exposure association brought about by the association of other factors with both disease (*O*) and exposure (*E*) [37].

The magnitude of OR is a measure of the strength of association, or the effect size. In general, when an OR is large, say greater than 10, the association is likely to be genuine. For example, the relative risk of having cervical cancer in women with HPV positivity vs. negativity is about 1000. Depending on the number of daily cigarettes consumed, the OR for smoking-lung cancer association ranges from 7 to about 27. The OR for the association between the DES exposure and vaginal cancer is about 40. In contract, for an association with an OR < 2, it is likely that the OR estimate could be a result of confounding or bias and needs to be scrutinized rigorously even though the association could also be genuine [43].

22.5.3 Case-Control Studies

Eleven case-control studies can be identified (Table 22.3). As expected, these studies vary in the types of ovarian cancer and the selection of controls (women with endometriosis or endometriomas, or infertility). Note that the last study listed in Table 22.3 is somewhat different from the rest, since both cases and controls had endometriosis, but the risk (protective) factor of interest was whether or not the subject had all visible endometriotic lesions removed [53]. Regardless, the forest plot revealed that the pooled (raw) OR estimate is 1.54 (95 % CI = 1.43–1.66, excluding the last study; Fig. 22.5), suggesting that overall, the OR value is moderate. In addition, there is little heterogeneity ($p = 0.47$ for heterogeneity test).

As with the SIR/RR estimates, the funnel plot of the log ORs from the ten studies indicates that the plot also looks like an asymmetric funnel, with its tip pointing towards somewhere near log OR = 0, i.e., OR = 1 (Fig. 22.6). Since there is no indication of bias in inclusion criteria or heterogeneity, this suggests that there may be a publication bias towards favoring positive studies and higher estimates of odds ratios may well be a chance variation. In addition, the plot seems to suggest that the true OR is quite moderate.

The study by Melin et al. [53] is of particular interest since, unlike other case-control studies, it examined the effect of surgical treatment on the endometriosis-ovarian cancer association. By linkage to the National Swedish Cancer Register, it identified all women diagnosed with epithelial ovarian cancer at least 1 year after the endometriosis diagnosis (cases). Two controls per case with no ovarian cancer before the date of cancer diagnosis of the case were randomly selected from the study base and matched for the year of birth. It found an OR of 0.30 (95 % CI = 0.12–0.74) for women who received a complete removal of all visible endometriosis. That is, for a woman with endometriosis, her risk of developing ovarian cancer could be cut by 70 % if she had all visible endometriotic lesions removed. It is worth noting that so far no other case-control studies have taken surgical completeness into consideration, since the study by Melin et al. strongly suggests this can be a protective factor.

22.5.4 Other Considerations

The control for shared risk (and/or protective) factors between E and O appears to be a big challenge in sorting out the relationship between E and O association. Besides the scenario depicted in Fig. 22.4a, it is known that E and O share some other common risk/protective factors, for example, the use of oral

Table 22.3 Published case-control studies reporting ovarian cancer risk in women with endometriosis

ID	Author	Year of publication	# of cases	# of controls	# case w/ endo	# controls w/ endo	Adjusted OR (95%CI)	Remark
N00	Ness et al. [44]	2000	764	1,364	66	85	1.7 (1.2–2.4)	
N02	Ness et al. [45]	2002	3,678	5,268	51	39	1.73 (1.10–2.71)	Originally considered infertility as a possible risk factor but also looked at patients with infertility due to endometriosis
M04	Modugno et al. [46]	2004	2,089	2,943	177	184	1.32 (1.06–1.65)	This study also included some data from Ness et al. [44]
B04	Borgfeld et al. [47]	2004	27,050	81,254	81	181	1.34 (1.03–1.75)	
M08	Merritt et al. [48]	2008	1,555	1,500	124	87	1.31 (0.97–1.78)	
N08	Nagle et al. [49]	2008	87	1,450	13	87	3.0 (1.5–5.9)	For endometrioid and clear cell ovarian cancers
R08	Rossing et al. [50]	2008	585	1,293	64	94	1.6 (1.1–2.3)	For invasive ovarian cancer
W09	Wu et al. [51]	2009	604	679	51	37	1.66 (1.01–2.75)	
P12	Pearce et al. [5]	2012	7,911	13,226	738	818	1.46 (1.31–1.63)	Invasive clear cell and endometrioid ovarian cancers
M13	Merritt et al. [52]	2013	358	2,100	51	165	1.92 (1.36–2.71)	Low-grade serous, endometrioid/mixed, mucinous and clear cell
E13	Melin et al. [53]	2013	197	402	52	201	0.30 (0.12–0.74)	All cases and controls had endometriosis. The factor of interest was whether or not the subject had a radical extirpation of all visible endometriosis

OR odds ratio, *SE* standard error, *CI* confidence interval, # numbers, *endo* endometriosis, *w/* with

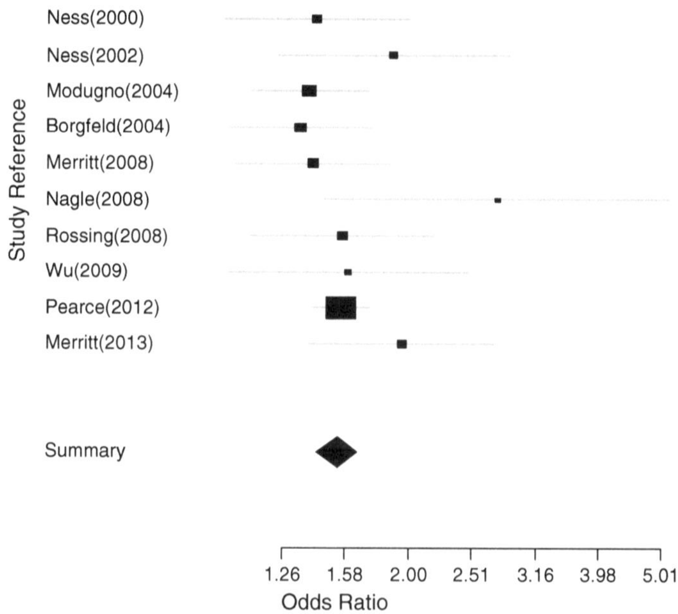

Fig. 22.5 Forest plot summarizing the results from 10 case-control studies using data from Table 22.3

Fig. 22.6 Funnel plot for the log ORs, using data extracted from Table 22.3. The *dashed line* represents OR = 1. The alphabet-numeric combinations are the IDs shown in Table 22.3, and each ID represents one study

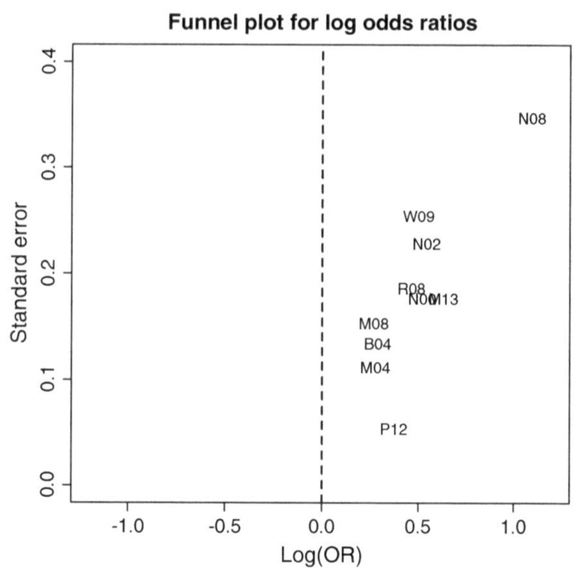

contraceptives (OC) and age at menarche. These factors are very likely to be causally associated with both *E* and *O*, effectively making them confounding factors when assessing the *E-O* association in case-control studies. However, while some studies did control for OC use, few, if any, controlled for the number of ovulations/menstrual cycles.

While the mean age at onset of ovarian cancer is about 56 years [4], the onset of endometriosis occurs mostly and typically during women's reproductive age. This has been taken as a support for temporality requirement in the Hill's 9 criteria of causality [4]. Indeed, the reported mean age of EAOC cases is often significantly younger than ovarian cancer patients without endometriosis but older than women with endometriosis alone [34].

However, the case-control studies published so far have not demonstrated a clear, graded temporal relationship between endometriosis and ovarian cancer. Most epithelial tumors take a latent period of at least 15 years to develop [4]. If endometriosis is a precursor of certain types of ovarian cancer, then it should take a certain latent period, likely to be shorter than 15 years, for ovarian cancer to develop. Consequently, one would see that after excluding some cases with endometriosis, say, $\leq$3 years of interval between the diagnosis of endometriosis and of ovarian cancer, the OR would go up since this would effectively remove many "noisy" cases which would dilute the association signal. Unfortunately, we actually see the opposite from the study by Pearce et al. [5]. Figure 22.7 is a graphical rendition of its sensitivity analysis (Table 4 in [5]). One can see that once the cases who had at least 3, 5, or 10 years of interval between the diagnosis of endometriosis and of ovarian cancer were removed, the OR estimate goes down considerably.

22.6 Should Any Action Be Taken?

Given the somewhat consistent but rather moderate increase in OR, some investigators believe that ovarian cancer originates from endometriosis, at least for clear cell carcinoma and endometrioid adenocarcinoma [54]; hence, screening, laboratory, and imaging evaluation should be "recommended for early detection of malignant disorders in women with endometriosis" [55]. Some even show that patients with EAOC actually had a more favorable prognosis [56–58]. However, other studies do not find such evidence [59, 60].

Due to the low incidence of ovarian cancer and the rather moderate increase in risk, extreme caution needs to be exercised when conveying the message to the public and also in the context of screening. For clear cell ovarian cancer, the prevalence is reported to be 13 per 100,000 women (Surveillance Epidemiology and End Results: http://seer.cancer.gov/statfacts/html/ovary.html, accessed January 17, 2013). Assuming, perhaps too optimistically, that a screening test exists that is 99 % sensitive and 99 % specific. Even with this rosy scenario, the corresponding positive predictive value is a disappointing 3.7 %. In other words,

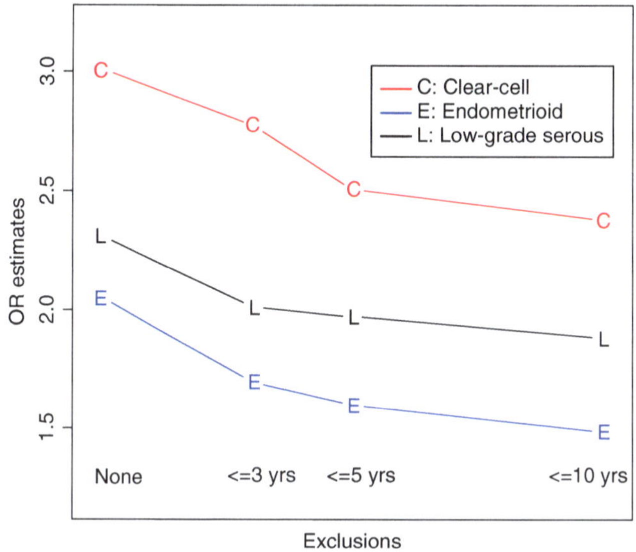

Fig. 22.7 A graphical rendition of the sensitivity analysis for the association of endometriosis and risk of invasive ovarian cancer based on timing (time interval) of diagnosis between the two diseases, as reported by Pearce et al. [5] (their Table 4). When patients with the time interval less than or equal to 3 years, 5 years, and 10 years are excluded, the decrease in the OR estimate is seen

out of 100 women who have tested positive, fully 96 would have a false positive result and be likely to be subjected to invasive procedures. Therefore, given the low incidence and also the moderate increase in OR, it is perhaps premature to talk about screening.

22.7 Conclusion

From the funnel plots for the SIR/RRs reported from cohort studies and the ORs from case-control studies, it seems that there may be a publication bias towards favoring positive studies. In addition, the plots seem to suggest that the true effect size is very moderate. Yet the vast discrepancy between RRs estimated from prevalence of endometriosis in women with ovarian cancer and ORs reported from published case-control studies is puzzling. Since the prevalence is likely an underestimate, the true RR is likely to be higher, which would highlight the discrepancy even more. It is unclear as to what factors contributed to the discrepancy. Have all epidemiological studies published so far underestimated the effect size due to failure to control for some, yet to be identified, confounders or certain biases of unknown sources? Or have many studies reporting the prevalence of endometriosis in ovarian cancer somehow overreported, perhaps unwittingly, because of ascertainment or selection bias and population idiosyncrasy or have simply fallen into the trap of attribution error? There is no answer as of now, and to address these questions would warrant more studies.

While the presence of ovarian endometriomas may generate a pro-inflammatory microenvironment that may be conducive to the development of ovarian cancer, it is noted that most, if not all, diseases, especially those associated with pain, have signs of inflammation. Even obesity has signs of inflammation. What is unclear is how the pro-inflammatory milieu in endometriosis per se leads to ovarian cancer. It is also unclear as to whether the peritoneal or vagino-rectal deep infiltrating endometriosis would also increase the risk of ovarian cancer more than that of other gynecological cancers. Moreover, the failure in providing or adjustment for information on treatment in many published epidemiological studies raises the question as to whether a surgery or drug treatment can actually reduce the risk of ovarian cancer. It also raises the question as to whether the use of danazol, an androgenic agent and once a popular therapeutics, could increase the risk of ovarian cancer. Finally, due to the nature of case-control studies, it cannot rule out that both endometriosis and ovarian cancer (especially clear cell or endometrioid type) may simply share some common risk and/or protective factors—such as the "incessant menstruation" and OC use, or yet to be identified—so that an elevated OR is still an association, but the relationship is by no means causal.

The finding reported by Melin et al. [53] that the risk of developing ovarian cancer in women with endometriosis could be cut by 70 % if they had all visible endometriotic lesions removed is particularly interesting. So far almost all other case-control studies published failed to control the effect of surgical treatment on the endometriosis-ovarian cancer association, even though the diagnosis of endometriosis is usually established by laparoscopic visualization of lesions, which is almost always followed by surgical removal of the lesions. Of course, some subtypes of endometriotic lesions, such as deep infiltrating endometriosis, can be challenging to remove completely. But does this mean that those women who had a complete removal of all their visible lesions are those who had less severe endometriosis? How does this surgical completeness or radicality interact with the extensiveness or severity of endometriosis and impact the risk of developing ovarian cancer? There are no data to answer these questions.

While younger age at diagnosis of endometriosis compared to that of ovarian cancer is often taken as a proof of temporality in the causal link, many epidemiological studies have not clearly demonstrated a temporal relationship between endometriosis and ovarian cancer. Since it is now well documented that, similar to cancer, endometriotic lesions are monoclonal in origin [61], one way to prove the temporal relationship, perhaps once for all, and to provide a convincing proof that some histotypes of ovarian cancer originate from endometriosis is to reconstruct a phylogenetic trees delineating the relationship between endometriotic lesions and ovarian cancer based on molecular clock. A proof-of-concept study demonstrating the utility of the molecular clock in reconstructing the geological relationship among pieces of endometrial fragments demonstrates that the phylogenetic approach is feasible using today's genetic technology [62].

In summary, while published clinical and epidemiological studies strongly implicated the risk, though moderate, of developing certain histotypes of ovarian cancer in women with endometriosis, many stones are still left unturned. Future studies need to determine whether the association is causal with a clear temporal relationship or merely association due to exposure to shared risk factors. Given the moderate association, it is perhaps premature to institute any actionable measures as of now. Future studies also need to resolve an apparent discrepancy in estimated effect size between the clinical data and epidemiological data and to further delineate the molecular pathways linking endometriosis and ovarian cancer. Care should be taken to avoid making "just-so" stories.

Acknowledgment I would like to thank Professor Paolo Vercellini for stimulating the discussion when preparing for this chapter. This research was supported in part by grant 81270676 from the National Science Foundation of China and financial support from Fudan University and the Shanghai Key Laboratory of Female Reproductive Endocrine-Related Diseases.

Conflict of Interest Statement. None declared.

References

1. Sayasneh A, Tsivos D, Crawford R. Endometriosis and ovarian cancer: a systematic review. ISRN Obstet Gynecol. 2011;2011:140310. doi:10.5402/2011/140310.
2. Kobayashi H, Kajiwara H, Kanayama S, Yamada Y, Furukawa N, Noguchi T, Haruta S, Yoshida S, Sakata M, Sado T, Oi H. Molecular pathogenesis of endometriosis-associated clear cell carcinoma of the ovary (review). Oncol Rep. 2009;22(2):233–40.
3. Hill AB. The environment and disease: association or causation? Proc R Soc Med. 1965;58:295–300.
4. Vigano P, Somigliana E, Parazzini F, Vercellini P. Bias versus causality: interpreting recent evidence of association between endometriosis and ovarian cancer. Fertil Steril. 2007;88 (3):588–93.
5. Pearce CL, Templeman C, Rossing MA, Lee A, Near AM, Webb PM, Nagle CM, Doherty JA, Cushing-Haugen KL, Wicklund KG, Chang-Claude J, Hein R, Lurie G, Wilkens LR, Carney ME, Goodman MT, Moysich K, Kjaer SK, Hogdall E, Jensen A, Goode EL, Fridley BL, Larson MC, Schildkraut JM, Palmieri RT, Cramer DW, Terry KL, Vitonis AF, Titus LJ, Ziogas A, Brewster W, Anton-Culver H, Gentry-Maharaj A, Ramus SJ, Anderson AR, Brueggmann D, Fasching PA, Gayther SA, Huntsman DG, Menon U, Ness RB, Pike MC, Risch H, Wu AH, Berchuck A. Association between endometriosis and risk of histological subtypes of ovarian cancer: a pooled analysis of case-control studies. Lancet Oncol. 2012;13 (4):385–94.
6. Godwin AK, Testa JR, Hamilton TC. The biology of ovarian cancer development. Cancer. 1993;71(2 Suppl):530–6.
7. Vaughan S, Coward JI, Bast Jr RC, Berchuck A, Berek JS, Brenton JD, Coukos G, Crum CC, Drapkin R, Etemadmoghadam D, Friedlander M, Gabra H, Kaye SB, Lord CJ, Lengyel E, Levine DA, McNeish IA, Menon U, Mills GB, Nephew KP, Oza AM, Sood AK, Stronach EA, Walczak H, Bowtell DD, Balkwill FR. Rethinking ovarian cancer: recommendations for improving outcomes. Nat Rev Cancer. 2011;11(10):719–25. doi:10.1038/nrc3144.
8. Light R, Pilleman DB. Summing up. The science of reviewing research. Cambridge: Harvard University Press; 1984.

9. Team RDC. R: A language and environment for statistical computing. R Foundation for Statistical Computing, Vienna; 2009 (ISBN 3-900051-07-0, http://www.R-project.org.).
10. Sampson JA. Endometrial carcinoma of the ovary arising in endometrial tissue in that organ. Arch Surg. 1925;10(1–72).
11. Scott RB. Malignant changes in endometriosis. Obstet Gynecol. 1953;2(3):283–9.
12. Somigliana E, Vigano P, Parazzini F, Stoppelli S, Giambattista E, Vercellini P. Association between endometriosis and cancer: a comprehensive review and a critical analysis of clinical and epidemiological evidence. Gynecol Oncol. 2006;101(2):331–41.
13. Kurman RJ, Shih Ie M. Molecular pathogenesis and extraovarian origin of epithelial ovarian cancer–shifting the paradigm. Hum Pathol. 2011;42(7):918–31.
14. Network TCGA. Comprehensive molecular portraits of human breast tumours. Nature. 2012;490(7418):61–70.
15. Aure JC, Hoeg K, Kolstad P. Carcinoma of the ovary and endometriosis. Acta Obstet Gynecol Scand. 1971;50(1):63–7.
16. Kurman RJ, Craig JM. Endometrioid and clear cell carcinoma of the ovary. Cancer. 1972;29 (6):1653–64.
17. Russell P. The pathological assessment of ovarian neoplasms. I: Introduction to the common 'epithelial' tumours and analysis of benign 'epithelial' tumours. Pathology. 1979;11(1):5–26.
18. Brescia RJ, Dubin N, Demopoulos RI. Endometrioid and clear cell carcinoma of the ovary. Factors affecting survival. Int J Gynecol Pathol. 1989;8(2):132–8.
19. Vercellini P, Parazzini F, Bolis G, Carinelli S, Dindelli M, Vendola N, Luchini L, Crosignani PG. Endometriosis and ovarian cancer. Am J Obstet Gynecol. 1993;169(1):181–2.
20. Jimbo H, Yoshikawa H, Onda T, Yasugi T, Sakamoto A, Taketani Y. Prevalence of ovarian endometriosis in epithelial ovarian cancer. Int J Gynaecol Obstet. 1997;59(3):245–50.
21. Fukunaga M, Nomura K, Ishikawa E, Ushigome S. Ovarian atypical endometriosis: its close association with malignant epithelial tumours. Histopathology. 1997;30(3):249–55.
22. Ogawa S, Kaku T, Amada S, Kobayashi H, Hirakawa T, Ariyoshi K, Kamura T, Nakano H. Ovarian endometriosis associated with ovarian carcinoma: a clinicopathological and immunohistochemical study. Gynecol Oncol. 2000;77(2):298–304.
23. Vercellini P, Scarfone G, Bolis G, Stellato G, Carinelli S, Crosignani PG. Site of origin of epithelial ovarian cancer: the endometriosis connection. BJOG. 2000;107(9):1155–7.
24. Oral E, Ilvan S, Tustas E, Korbeyli B, Bese T, Demirkiran F, Arvas M, Kosebay D. Prevalence of endometriosis in malignant epithelial ovary tumours. Eur J Obstet Gynecol Reprod Biol. 2003;109(1):97–101.
25. Dzatic-Smiljkovic O, Vasiljevic M, Djukic M, Vugdelic R, Vugdelic J. Frequency of ovarian endometriosis in epithelial ovarian cancer patients. Clin Exp Obstet Gynecol. 2011;38(4):394–8.
26. Kondi-Pafiti A, Papakonstantinou E, Iavazzo C, Grigoriadis C, Salakos N, Gregoriou O. Clinicopathological characteristics of ovarian carcinomas associated with endometriosis. Arch Gynecol Obstet. 2012;285(2):479–83.
27. Brinton LA, Gridley G, Persson I, Baron J, Bergqvist A. Cancer risk after a hospital discharge diagnosis of endometriosis. Am J Obstet Gynecol. 1997;176(3):572–9.
28. Olson JE, Cerhan JR, Janney CA, Anderson KE, Vachon CM, Sellers TA. Postmenopausal cancer risk after self-reported endometriosis diagnosis in the Iowa Women's Health Study. Cancer. 2002;94(5):1612–8.
29. Brinton LA, Lamb EJ, Moghissi KS, Scoccia B, Althuis MD, Mabie JE, Westhoff CL. Ovarian cancer risk associated with varying causes of infertility. Fertil Steril. 2004;82(2):405–14.
30. Brinton LA, Sakoda LC, Sherman ME, Frederiksen K, Kjaer SK, Graubard BI, Olsen JH, Mellemkjaer L. Relationship of benign gynecologic diseases to subsequent risk of ovarian and uterine tumors. Cancer Epidemiol Biomarkers Prev. 2005;14(12):2929–35.
31. Melin A, Sparen P, Persson I, Bergqvist A. Endometriosis and the risk of cancer with special emphasis on ovarian cancer. Hum Reprod. 2006;21(5):1237–42.

32. Murta EF, Nomelini RS, Ferreira FA, Lima MA. Ovarian clear cell carcinoma associated with endometriosis: a case report with immunohistochemical study. Eur J Gynaecol Oncol. 2007;28 (5):403–5.
33. Kobayashi H, Sumimoto K, Moniwa N, Imai M, Takakura K, Kuromaki T, Morioka E, Arisawa K, Terao T. Risk of developing ovarian cancer among women with ovarian endometrioma: a cohort study in Shizuoka, Japan. Int J Gynecol Cancer. 2007;17(1):37–43.
34. Aris A. Endometriosis-associated ovarian cancer: a ten-year cohort study of women living in the Estrie Region of Quebec, Canada. J Ovarian Res. 2010;3:2.
35. Stewart LM, Holman CD, Aboagye-Sarfo P, Finn JC, Preen DB, Hart R. In vitro fertilization, endometriosis, nulliparity and ovarian cancer risk. Gynecol Oncol. 2013;128:260–4
36. Sterne JAC, Egger M, Smith GD. Investigating and dealing with publication and other biases. In: Egger M, Smith GD, Altman DG, editors. Systematic reviews in Health Care: meta-analysis in context. London: BMJ Books; 2001. p. 189–208.
37. Breslow NE, Day NE. Statistical methods in cancer research. vol. 1: The analysis of case-control studies. Lyon: IARC Scientific Publications No. 32. International Agency for Research on Cancer; 1980.
38. Herbst AL, Ulfelder H, Poskanzer DC. Adenocarcinoma of the vagina. Association of maternal stilbestrol therapy with tumor appearance in young women. N Engl J Med. 1971;284 (15):878–81. doi:10.1056/NEJM197104222841604.
39. Casagrande JT, Louie EW, Pike MC, Roy S, Ross RK, Henderson BE. "Incessant ovulation" and ovarian cancer. Lancet. 1979;2(8135):170–3.
40. Vercellini P, Crosignani P, Somigliana E, Vigano P, Buggio L, Bolis G, Fedele L. The 'incessant menstruation' hypothesis: a mechanistic ovarian cancer model with implications for prevention. Hum Reprod. 2011;26(9):2262–73.
41. Risch HA. Hormonal etiology of epithelial ovarian cancer, with a hypothesis concerning the role of androgens and progesterone. J Natl Cancer Inst. 1998;90(23):1774–86.
42. Cottreau CM, Ness RB, Modugno F, Allen GO, Goodman MT. Endometriosis and its treatment with danazol or lupron in relation to ovarian cancer. Clin Cancer Res. 2003;9(14):5142–4.
43. Rothman KJ, Poole C. A strengthening programme for weak associations. Int J Epidemiol. 1988;17(4):955–9.
44. Ness RB, Grisso JA, Cottreau C, Klapper J, Vergona R, Wheeler JE, Morgan M, Schlesselman JJ. Factors related to inflammation of the ovarian epithelium and risk of ovarian cancer. Epidemiology. 2000;11(2):111–7.
45. Ness RB, Cramer DW, Goodman MT, Kjaer SK, Mallin K, Mosgaard BJ, Purdie DM, Risch HA, Vergona R, Wu AH. Infertility, fertility drugs, and ovarian cancer: a pooled analysis of case-control studies. Am J Epidemiol. 2002;155(3):217–24.
46. Modugno F, Ness RB, Allen GO, Schildkraut JM, Davis FG, Goodman MT. Oral contraceptive use, reproductive history, and risk of epithelial ovarian cancer in women with and without endometriosis. Am J Obstet Gynecol. 2004;191(3):733–40.
47. Borgfeldt C, Andolf E. Cancer risk after hospital discharge diagnosis of benign ovarian cysts and endometriosis. Acta Obstet Gynecol Scand. 2004;83(4):395–400.
48. Merritt MA, Green AC, Nagle CM, Webb PM. Talcum powder, chronic pelvic inflammation and NSAIDs in relation to risk of epithelial ovarian cancer. Int J Cancer. 2008;122(1):170–6. doi:10.1002/ijc.23017.
49. Nagle CM, Olsen CM, Webb PM, Jordan SJ, Whiteman DC, Green AC. Endometrioid and clear cell ovarian cancers: a comparative analysis of risk factors. Eur J Cancer. 2008;44 (16):2477–84.
50. Rossing MA, Cushing-Haugen KL, Wicklund KG, Doherty JA, Weiss NS. Risk of epithelial ovarian cancer in relation to benign ovarian conditions and ovarian surgery. Cancer Causes Control. 2008;19(10):1357–64.
51. Wu AH, Pearce CL, Tseng CC, Templeman C, Pike MC. Markers of inflammation and risk of ovarian cancer in Los Angeles County. Int J Cancer. 2009;124(6):1409–15.

52. Merritt MA, De Pari M, Vitonis AF, Titus LJ, Cramer DW, Terry KL. Reproductive characteristics in relation to ovarian cancer risk by histologic pathways. Hum Reprod. 28(5):1406–17.
53. Melin AS, Lundholm C, Malki N, Swahn ML, Sparen P, Bergqvist A. Hormonal and surgical treatments for endometriosis and risk of epithelial ovarian cancer. Acta Obstet Gynecol Scand. 2013;92(5):546–54. doi:10.1111/aogs.12123.
54. Kuhn E, Kurman RJ, Shih IM. Ovarian cancer is an imported disease: fact or fiction? Curr Obstet Gynecol Rep. 2012;1(1):1–9.
55. Baldi A, Campioni M, Signorile PG. Endometriosis: pathogenesis, diagnosis, therapy and association with cancer (review). Oncol Rep. 2008;19(4):843–6.
56. Erzen M, Rakar S, Klancnik B, Syrjanen K. Endometriosis-associated ovarian carcinoma (EAOC): an entity distinct from other ovarian carcinomas as suggested by a nested case-control study. Gynecol Oncol. 2001;83(1):100–8.
57. Wang S, Qiu L, Lang JH, Shen K, Huang HF, Pan LY, Wu M, Yang JX, Guo LN. Prognostic analysis of endometrioid epithelial ovarian cancer with or without endometriosis: a 12-year cohort study of Chinese patients. Am J Obstet Gynecol. 2013;209:241.
58. Melin A, Lundholm C, Malki N, Swahn ML, Sparen P, Bergqvist A. Endometriosis as a prognostic factor for cancer survival. Int J Cancer. 2011;129(4):948–55. doi:10.1002/ijc.25718.
59. Cuff J, Longacre TA. Endometriosis does not confer improved prognosis in ovarian carcinoma of uniform cell type. Am J Surg Pathol. 2012;36(5):688–95.
60. Noli S, Cipriani S, Scarfone G, Villa A, Grossi E, Monti E, Vercellini P, Parazzini F. Long term survival of ovarian endometriosis associated clear cell and endometrioid ovarian cancers. Int J Gynecol Cancer. 2013.
61. Wu Y, Basir Z, Kajdacsy-Balla A, Strawn E, Macias V, Montgomery K, Guo SW. Resolution of clonal origins for endometriotic lesions using laser capture microdissection and the human androgen receptor (HUMARA) assay. Fertil Steril. 2003;79 Suppl 1:710–7.
62. Wu Y, Guo SW. Reconstructing cellular lineages in endometrial cells. Fertil Steril. 2008;89(2):481–4. doi:10.1016/j.fertnstert.2007.03.028.

Chapter 23
Surgical Management of Endometriosis

Imari Deura and Tasuku Harada

Abstract Endometriosis, a common disease affecting about 10 % of women of reproductive age, causes pelvic pain and infertility. Pelvic endometriosis is histologically categorized into peritoneal superficial endometriosis, ovarian endometrioma, and deep infiltrating endometriosis (DIE). Surgical treatment for endometriosis aims to relieve symptoms and preserve fertility, in most cases by restoring anatomy, by lysing adhesions, and by removing endometriotic lesions. Laparoscopic surgery, which is the standard surgical procedure for endometriosis, reduces pelvic pain and improves fertility by means of excision and ablation of endometriotic lesions. Managing endometriomas in women who wish to conceive is controversial because two main risks may occur after conservative surgery: recurrence of the disease and significant reduction in ovarian reserve. Surgical treatment for endometriosis should be tailored to the individual according to clinical presentation and personal wishes. In this chapter, we describe laparoscopic conservative surgery for pelvic endometriosis, particularly for ovarian endometrioma.

Keywords Cystectomy • Infertility • Laparoscopic surgery • Ovarian endometrioma • Ovarian reserve

23.1 Surgical Approach for Endometriosis

Laparoscopy compared with laparotomy is considered the gold standard surgical treatment for endometriosis, especially when endometriomas are present. The two approaches do not differ in terms of pain relief, fertility outcome, and risk of recurrence [1–4]. One randomized controlled trial (RCT) revealed that laparoscopic

I. Deura (✉) • T. Harada
Department of Obstetrics and Gynecology, Tottori University
School of Medicine, Yonago, Japan
e-mail: imari@med.tottori-u.ac.jp

T. Harada (ed.), *Endometriosis: Pathogenesis and Treatment*,
DOI 10.1007/978-4-431-54421-0_23, © Springer Japan 2014

surgery for endometriomas was associated with less pain after surgery, shorter hospital stay, and faster recovery compared with laparotomy and that the complication rate and operative time were similar in the two approaches [5]. A meta-analysis of 27 RCTs comparing the outcome of laparoscopic surgery and laparotomy for benign gynecologic pathologies also showed that the two approaches exposed patients equally to complications [6]. These results suggest that laparoscopic surgery, minimum invasive technique, is feasible and safe as well as laparotomy and that it should be used as a first-line choice in conservative surgery for endometriosis.

23.2 Surgical Treatment for Endometriosis-Associated Pain

Endometriosis is present in approximately 70 % of patients with pelvic pain [7]. Endometriotic lesions and adhesions are clearly associated with pain symptoms, which include dysmenorrhea, non-menstrual chronic pelvic pain, dyspareunia, and dyschezia. These symptoms significantly affect the quality of life of women of reproductive age. Lesions and adhesions are included in several scoring systems, for example, the commonly used revised American Fertility Society (rAFS) classification, which describes the severity of endometriosis, but not the severity of pain. The relationship between the stage or lesion type of endometriosis and severity of pelvic pain has been studied, but the results are inconsistent [8]. Severe pelvic pain is associated with DIE; however, the depth of endometriosis does not affect the stage of rAFS classification. This may be one reason that this scoring system failed to show severity of pain.

Endometriosis can be treated either medically or surgically. Surgery allows visual diagnosis and is usually used when medical treatment fails or produces unacceptable side effects or when conception is desired. The aim of surgical treatment is to restore anatomy by dividing adhesions and removing visible endometriotic lesions, thus relieving pain. Endometriosis often develops in women of reproductive age; therefore, laparoscopic surgery commonly needs to preserve fertility.

The RCT reported by Sutton et al. showed that laparoscopic laser ablation resulted in statistically significant pain relief at 6 months after surgery in women with minimal to moderate endometriosis compared with diagnostic laparoscopy [9]. A follow-up study of Sutton's RCT demonstrated that pain relief after laparoscopic laser ablation continued at 1 year in 90 % of those who initially responded [10]. Abbott et al. performed a randomized, placebo-controlled trial of patients with minimal to severe endometriosis, comparing laparoscopic excision with placebo, and found that 80 % of the excision group had reduced pain and improved quality of life by 6 months compared with only 32 % in the placebo group. Surprisingly, diagnostic laparoscopy was associated with a 20 % placebo response rate [11]. A meta-analysis consisting of five RCTs also demonstrated an advantage in using laparoscopic surgery for pelvic pain associated with endometriosis compared with diagnostic laparoscopy alone [12]. The two RCTs reported that 20–38 % of patients had no improvement in symptoms after operative laparoscopy [9, 11], implying that surgical treatment alone for endometriosis-associated pain has limitations.

Which of the laparoscopic surgical modalities is most effective for pain relief in endometriosis is inconclusive. Healey et al. showed no difference in pain relief between laparoscopic ablation and excision at 12 months after surgery for patients with minimal to severe endometriosis [13]. A similar result was reported in another study of minimal to mild endometriosis [14].

Several surgical procedures to interrupt pelvic nerve pathways have been performed to reduce pelvic pain caused by endometriosis, such as uterine nerve ablation, presacral neurectomy, uterosacral ligament resection, and so on. However, there is insufficient evidence of pain relief to recommend their use [15, 16].

23.3 Surgical Treatment for Endometriosis-Associated Infertility

Endometriosis is present in 20–68 % of subfertile women [17]. Severe endometriosis may impair fertility due to anatomical distortion caused by adhesions. However, endometriosis is associated with infertility even in the early stages without adhesions. The exact mechanism by which endometriosis interferes with fertility is not fully understood, and therefore the strategy for treatment is controversial. Medical treatment that suppresses ovarian function has no effect to improve fertility in women with endometriosis and should not be offered to patients wishing to conceive [18]. Adamson et al. demonstrated that surgical treatment was superior to medical treatment regarding the pregnancy rate of infertile women with minimal and mild endometriosis [19]. Whether surgical treatment or artificial reproductive technique should be performed first has been debated.

Endometriosis is treated surgically by lysing adhesions and excising or ablating endometriotic lesions.

A meta-analysis consisting of two RCTs demonstrated that laparoscopic surgery, including excision and ablation with adhesiolysis, improves fertility in patients with minimal and mild endometriosis compared with diagnostic laparoscopy alone [20]. There seems to be a negative correlation between the stage of endometriosis and the spontaneous cumulative pregnancy rate after surgical excision of endometriosis. No evidence recommends choosing laparoscopic surgery first for patients with moderate or severe endometriosis complaining of infertility alone [21].

23.4 Ovarian Endometrioma

23.4.1 Surgery for Endometrioma

Ovarian endometrioma, also known as chocolate cyst, is a form of endometriosis located on the ovaries. Between 17 and 44 % of patients with endometriosis have endometriomas [22–24]. Endometriosis by itself does not always cause endometriosis-related symptoms. No consensus has been reached on the definitive intervention for endometrioma, particularly in infertile women.

Surgical treatment is usually recommended for large symptomatic endometrioma, and the indication for surgery also depends on the risks of rupture, infection, torsion of the ovary, and malignant formation. Laparoscopic surgery is the gold standard for endometrioma [5], but which is the best modality of conservative surgery remains controversial. Drainage of endometriomas alone is not recommended because of the high recurrence rate [25]. Two main modalities are used: ablation of the cyst wall and cyst excision, also called cystectomy. Laparoscopic cystectomy has been considered a first-line choice of surgical treatment. A meta-analysis demonstrated that laparoscopic cystectomy for endometriomas larger than 3 cm in diameter increased spontaneous conception in subfertile women with less recurrence of pain symptoms and fewer endometriomas compared with ablation alone. Ovarian response to gonadotrophin stimulation after surgery was similar between the two modalities despite concerns over the more damaging effect of cystectomy on ovarian reserve [26].

23.4.2 ART and Endometrioma

Endometrioma may interfere with the outcome of artificial reproductive technology (ART). ART cycles of women with endometriomas have several problems, including difficulty monitoring ovarian response by ultrasound, poor ovarian response to controlled ovarian stimulation (COH), and infection after oocyte pick up [27–29]. Gupta et al. showed decreased ovarian response to COH with in vitro fertilization (IVF) cycles of patients with endometriomas compared with controls [30], which implies a decline of ovarian reserve due to endometrioma itself.

Endometriomas larger than 3 cm are generally treated surgically before ART, but surgery may actually decrease the success of ART due to damaged ovarian reserve. Demirol et al. evaluated the outcome of intracytoplasmic sperm injection (ICSI) in patients with prior cystectomy for endometrioma between 3 and 6 cm in diameter compared with ICSI alone. Cystectomy resulted in longer COH, higher FSH requirement, and lower mature oocyte number, but fertilization, pregnancy, and implantation rates did not differ [31]. Two meta-analyses concluded that surgical treatment of endometriomas prior to ART did not improve reproductive outcome [32, 33].

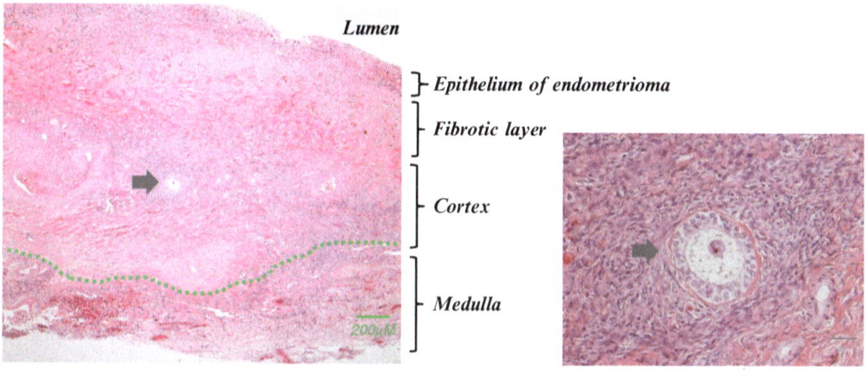

Fig. 23.1 Normal ovarian tissue adjacent to the cyst wall of endometrioma. The tissue specimen of the stripped cyst wall of endometrioma contains normal ovarian tissue. *Arrows* ovarian follicle

23.4.3 Ovarian Reserve and Endometrioma

The pathogenesis of endometrioma is controversial. Endometrioma is generally believed to result initially from a deposit of endometrium that passed through the fallopian tube causing adherence of the ovary to the pelvic peritoneum and progressive vagination of the ovary [34–36]. Considering that endometrioma is a pseudocyst, cyst excision may involve removing some ovarian tissue [37]. One concern over performing cystectomy for endometrioma is that it may damage ovarian reserve when normal ovarian cortex is removed and thermal coagulation is used for hemostasis, resulting in the loss of follicles (Fig. 23.1).

Ovarian reserve is defined as the total ovarian follicle pool including primordial and growing follicles [38]. Serum anti-Mullerian hormone (AMH) is the most useful, reliable, and sensitive marker of ovarian reserve compared with other known serum markers [39]. AMH is stable throughout the menstrual cycle and sensitive to decline in ovarian reserve with aging and is not affected by the use of hormones [40]. Serum AMH correlates to antral follicle count (AFC) measured by ultrasound, which is also a reliable marker of ovarian reserve [41].

A meta-analysis of eight prospective cohort studies to investigate the effect of cystectomy for endometrioma on ovarian reserve as determined by serum AMH level found that serum concentration of AMH significantly decreased after surgery [42]. Multivariate analyses showed that the risk factors associated with reduction of serum AMH after cystectomy were as follows: bilateral endometriomas, presurgical serum AMH level, and the presence of normal ovarian tissue in the enucleated cyst [43–45]. Var et al. compared postsurgical ovarian reserve determined by AFC between laparoscopic cystectomy and ablation for bilateral endometriomas. AFC was significantly decreased in cystectomized ovaries compared with ablated ovaries [46]. One surgical modality used as an alternative to cystectomy, a three-step procedure proposed by Donnez et al., involves drainage of the cyst during laparoscopy, GnRH agonist treatments, and then laser vaporization of the remains during a second laparoscopy [47]. Ovarian reserve, determined by AMH and AFC, was less diminished after the three-step procedure for endometrioma compared with cystectomy [48, 49]. Donnez et al. also proposed a combined technique consisting of excision of a large part of the endometrioma and laser vaporization of the remaining 10–20 % of the cyst wall close to the hilus. AFC after the combined technique was similar to that of women without endometriosis or contralateral normal ovaries [50]. Use of electrosurgical coagulation to achieve hemostasis after stripping the endometrioma may amplify damage to ovarian reserve. Why ovarian reserve declines after cystectomy is not precisely understood, but it may relate to the methods used for hemostasis, including suturing the ovaries and bipolar coagulation [51, 52]. Details of the studies evaluating ovarian reserve before and after cystectomy are shown in Table 23.1 [53–57].

We know that laparoscopic cystectomy for endometrioma has a negative impact on ovarian reserve, but we should take into account that the presence of endometrioma per se is also associated with a decrease in ovarian reserve [58].

23.4.4 Recurrence of Endometrioma

The recurrence of endometrioma after conservative surgery is a serious problem. Postoperative recurrence rates vary between 6 and 78 % after 2–5 years, depending on the surgical modality and the length of postoperative time [59–66]. Details of the studies evaluating the recurrence rates of endometriomas after surgery are shown in Table 23.2. Long-term follow-up is necessary to assess endometrioma recurrence after surgery. The risk factors for recurrent endometrioma are often varied, and the rAFS staging system is not predictive of recurrence [67, 68].

Cochrane study comparing the recurrence of endometriomas and pain symptoms after surgery showed that cystectomy is more advantageous than ablation [26]. Carmona et al. found an earlier recurrence of endometriomas at 5 years of follow-up after ablation compared with cystectomy [69].

Repeated surgery for recurrent endometriomas is not recommended. The probability of conception after secondary surgery is almost half that after a primary surgery. The repetitive damage to the ovaries should be avoided to preserve the already reduced reproductive potential.

Curing endometriosis by conservative surgery alone is difficult, and studies have shown that postoperative medical treatment can only delay the recurrence of endometrioma [70]. However, a recent report showed that treating with long-term oral contraceptives decreases the recurrence of endometrioma.

The patients should be informed of the risk of postoperative recurrence, and long-term adjuvant treatment to suppress ovulation suggested until pregnancy is desired.

Table 23.1 Ovarian reserve before and after cystectomy

Study	Design	Sample size	Follow-up (month)	Variable	Outcome		*P* value
					Preoperative	Postoperative	
Tsolakidis 2009 [49]	RCT	10	10	AMH	3.9 ± 1.3	2.9 ± 0.6	0.002
Pados 2010 [48]	RCT	10	12	AFC	2.0 ± 1.3	2.4 ± 0.8	NS
Biacchiardi 2011 [53]	Prospective cohort	43	9	AMH	3.0 ± 0.4	1.3 ± 0.3	<0.001
Celik 2012 [45]	Prospective cohort	65	6	AMH	1.8 ± 1.7	0.7 ± 0.8	<0.001
Ercan 2010 [54]	Prospective cohort	64	1	AMH	1.6 ± 1.1	1.4 ± 1.2	NS
Ercan 2011 [55]	Prospective cohort	36	3	AMH	2.0 ± 0.4	1.95 ± 0.6	NS
Kitajima 2011 [44]	Prospective cohort	19	3	AMH	4.3 ± 3.0	3.0 ± 2.5	NA
Hirokawa 2011 [45]	Prospective cohort	38	1	AMH	3.9 ± 2.5	2.1 ± 1.6	<0.001
Hwu 2011 [56]	Prospective cohort	31	3	AMH	3.9 ± 0.4	2.01 ± 0.2	<0.01
Lee 2010 [57]	Prospective cohort	13	3	AMH	4.7 ± 2.5	3.3 ± 2.1	<0.05
Uncu 2013 [58]	Prospective cohort	30	6	AMH	2.8 ± 2.2	1.8 ± 1.3	0.02
Var 2011 [46]	RCT	48	6	AFC	5.6 ± 1.1	3.67 ± 1.3	0.001

Note: Values are mean ± SD. AMH levels are reported in nanograms per milliliter. $P < 0.05$ was statistically significant
RCT randomized controlled trial, *AMH* anti-Mullerian hormone, *AFC* antral follicle counts, *NS* not statistically significant, *NA* not available

Table 23.2 Recurrence rate of endometrioma after cystectomy or ablation

Study	Design	Sample size	Follow-up (year)	Recurrence rate Cystectomy (%)	Ablation (%)	*P* value
Alborzi 2004 [59]	RCT	100	2	17.3	31.3	0.16
Beretta 1998 [60]	RCT	64	2	6.2	18.8	NS
Busacca 1999 [61]	Retrospective follow-up	366	4	11.7		NA
Carmona 2011 [69]	RCT	74	5	22.2	36.8	0.2
Fedele 2006 [62]	Descriptive	305	5	18.9		NA
Hart 2011 [26]	Meta-analysis	164	2	13.1	26.3	<0.05
Hemmings 1998 [63]	Retrospective	103	3	8.0	12.0	NS
Kikuchi 2006 [64]	Retrospective	315	3	27.0		NA
Koga 2006 [65]	Retrospective	224	2	30.4		NA
Saleh 1999 [66]	Retrospective	231	4	25.0	78.0	0.0003

Note: $P < 0.05$ was statistically significant. *RCT* randomized clinical trial, *NS* not statistically significant, *NA* not available

23.5 Laparoscopic Techniques for Endometriosis

Laparoscopic conservative surgery for endometriosis aims to restore anatomy by means of adhesiolysis and by destructing endometriotic lesions. Advanced technical skills and systematic surgical procedures are required to prevent damage to adjacent organs, particularly in cases with an obliterated cul-de-sac.

Peritoneal endometriosis can be destructed by excision or ablation, the latter being commonly used. Symptom relief after surgery does not differ between excision and ablation [71]. Bipolar coagulation and vaporization with CO_2 laser or plasma energy are often used as ablation techniques. Laser vaporization penetrates tissue at a shallow depth, which is useful to avoid deep thermal tissue damage.

Delicate manipulation of forceps is needed to dissect pelvic adhesions. There are two types of adhesions in endometriosis, filmy adhesions and dense adhesions with fibrotic tissue. Filmy adhesions can be dissected bluntly, while dense adhesions require sharp dissection. A contralateral traction should be applied with the proper instruments (e.g., a uterine manipulator). Dissection techniques are used to lyse adhesions surrounding the ovaries, remove the ovarian cysts, and open the obliterated cul-de-sac.

To free adhesions surrounding the ovaries, contralateral traction should be applied (Fig. 23.2a). Fibrotic tissue can be dissected sharply using monopolar diathermy with pure cutting current. Sharp and blunt dissections are repeated alternatively until the whole length of the utero-ovarian ligament is visible. The cyst is almost always ruptured during this procedure.

The procedures for ovarian cystectomy are followed. The content of the cyst is aspirated. The ovarian incision obtained by cyst rupture is enlarged (Fig. 23.2b). The cleavage plane between the cyst wall and the ovarian tissue should be adequately identified (Fig. 23.2c). The cyst wall is bluntly stripped from ovarian tissue

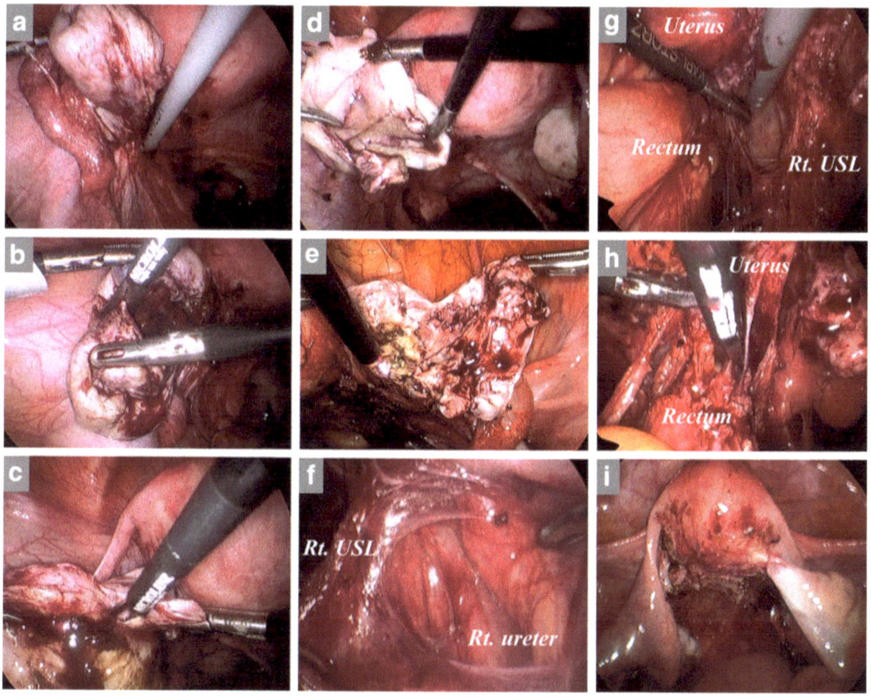

Fig. 23.2 Laparoscopic techniques for endometriosis. (**a**) The adhesion surrounding the left ovary is freed. (**b**) The ovarian incision obtained by cyst rupture is enlarged. (**c**) The cleavage plane between the cyst wall and normal ovarian tissue is adequately identified. (**d**) The cyst wall is bluntly stripped from normal ovarian tissue. (**e**) Laser vaporization is applied to the cyst wall close to the left ovarian hilus. (**f**) The spaces outside the right uterosacral ligament are opened and the right ureter is separated from the right uterosacral ligaments. *Rt. USL* the right uterosacral ligament. (**g**) The space inside the right uterosacral ligament is opened and the rectum is separated from the right uterosacral ligaments. The right uterosacral ligament. (**h**) Sharp dissection using the scissors is applied between the uterus and the rectum. (**i**) The obliterated cul-de-sac is opened

with atraumatic forceps and scissors applying a contralateral traction (Fig. 23.2d). The boundary between the cyst wall and the ovarian tissue should be exposed constantly. After removal of the cyst wall, hemostasis is achieved with the pinpoint bipolar coagulation of bleeding sites on the ovary. The combined technique is sometimes used for patients with bilateral or multiple endometriomas [50] (Fig. 23.2e). The vasopressin injection technique may be useful to decrease bleeding after stripping the endometrioma [72], but an inadequate cleavage plane resulting from hydrodissection may cause the removal of normal ovarian tissue.

The procedures to open an obliterated cul-de-sac are followed. First, the bilateral ureters are identified. The spaces outside the bilateral uterosacral ligament are opened and the ureters are separated from the uterosacral ligaments (Fig. 23.2f). After separation of the ureters, the spaces inside the uterosacral ligaments are opened and the rectum is separated from the uterosacral ligaments (Fig. 23.2g).

The adhesion between the rectum and the uterine cervix can be dissected bluntly with a contralateral traction when the adhesion is not dense. Sharp dissection is needed to dissect dense adhesions with fibrotic tissue. Monopolar diathermy with pure cutting current can dissect dense adhesions surrounding the rectum. Sharp dissection using the scissors should be used to avoid thermal injury of the rectum (Fig. 23.2h). After these procedures to open the obliterated cul-de-sac, it is possible to remove the DIE lesions of the uterosacral ligaments and the rectovaginal septum (Fig. 23.2i).

23.6 Conclusions

Surgical candidates might include the following patients with endometriosis: those with severe pain symptoms, large ovarian endometriomas, and infertility caused by minimal and mild endometriosis.

Surgery for endometriosis has an important role in relieving pain symptoms and improving fertility by lysing adhesions and removing lesions. However, the optimal procedure is as yet undetermined because of several controversial issues: the recurrence of disease and ovarian reserve decline after conservative surgery. Complete cure of endometriosis is not currently possible by surgery alone, particularly the conservative procedure. Surgical treatment of endometriosis should be tailored to the individual according to clinical presentation and personal wishes, and combined treatment with medical treatment or ART after surgery is needed. We cannot deal with all patients with endometriosis in the same way.

References

1. Catalano GF, Marana R, Caruana P, Muzzi L, Mancuso S. Laparoscopic versus microsurgery by laparotomy for excision of ovarian cysts in patients with moderate or severe endometriosis. J Am Assoc Gynecol Laparosc. 1996;3:267–70.
2. Adamson GD, Subak LL, Pasta DJ, Hurd SJ, von Franque O, Rodrigues BD. Comparison of CO_2 laser laparoscopy with laparotomy for treatment of endometriomata. Fertil Steril. 1992;57:965–73.
3. Bateman BG, Kolp LA, Mills S. Endoscopic versus laparotomy management of endometriomas. Fertil Steril. 1994;62:690–5.
4. Milingos S, Loutradis D, Kallipolitis G, Laiapi A, Drakakis P, Antsaklis A, et al. Comparison of laparoscopy with laparotomy for the treatment of extensive endometriosis with large endometriomata. J Gynecol Surg. 1999;15:131–6.
5. Mais V, Ajossa S, Guerriero S, Piras B, Floris M, Palomba M, et al. Laparoscopic management of endometriomas: a randomized trial versus laparotomy. J Gynecol Surg. 1996;12:41–6.
6. Chapron C, Fauconnier A, Goffinet F, Breart G, Dubuisson JB. Laparoscopic surgery is not inherently dangerous for patients with benign gynaecological pathologies. Hum Reprod. 2002;17:1334–42.
7. Practice Committee of the American Society for Reproductive Medicine. Treatment of pelvic pain associated with endometriosis. Fertil Steril. 2008;90(5):S260–9.

8. Vercellini P, Fedele L, Aimi G, Pietropaolo G, Consonni D, Crosignani PG. Association between endometriosis stage, lesion type, patients characteristics and severity of pelvic pain symptoms: a multivariate analysis of over 1000 patients. Hum Reprod. 2007;22(1):266–71.
9. Sutton CJ, Ewen SP, Whitelaw N, Haines P. Prospective, randomized, double-blind, controlled trial of laser laparoscopy in the treatment of pelvic pain associated with minimal, mild, and moderate endometriosis. Fertil Steril. 1994;62(4):696–700.
10. Sutton CJ, Pooley AS, Ewen SP, Haines P. Follow-up report on a randomized controlled trial of laser laparoscopy in the treatment of pelvic pain associated with minimal to moderate endometriosis. Fertil Steril. 1997;68(6):1070–4.
11. Abbott J, Hawe J, Hunter D, Holmes M, Finn P, Garry R. Laparoscopic excision of endometriosis: a randomized, placebo-controlled trial. Fertil Steril. 2004;82(4):878–84.
12. Jacobson TZ, Duffy JMN, Barlow D, Koninckx PR, Garry R. Laparoscopic surgery for pelvic pain associated with endometriosis. Cochrane Database Syst Rev. 2009;4, CD001300.
13. Healey M, Ang WC, Cheng C. Surgical treatment of endometriosis: a prospective randomized double-blinded trial comparing excision and ablation. Fertil Steril. 2010;94(7):2536–40.
14. Wright J, Loftfallah H, Jones K, Lovell D. A randomized trial of excision versus ablation for mild endometriosis. Fertil Steril. 2005;83:1830–6.
15. Proctor M, Larthe P, Farquhar C, Khan K, Johnson N. Surgical interruption of pelvic nerve pathway for primary and secondary dysmenorrhoea. Cochrane Database Syst Rev. 2006;3, CD002119.
16. Vercellini P, Aimi G, Busacca M, Apolone G, Uglietti A, Crosignari PG. Laparoscopic uterosacral ligament resection for dysmenorrheal associated randomized, controlled trial. Fertil Steril. 2003;80(2):310–9.
17. Marcoux S, Maheux R, Berube S, the Canadian Collaborative Group on Endometriosis. Laparoscopic surgery in infertile women with minimal or mild endometriosis. New Eng J Med. 1997;337(4):217–22.
18. Hughes E, Brown J, Collins JJ, Farquhar C, Fedorkow DM, Vanderkerchove P. Ovulation suppression for endometriosis. Cochrane Database Syst Rev. 2007;3, CD000155.
19. Adamson GD, Pasta DJ. Surgical treatment of endometriosis-associated infertility: meta-analysis compared with survival analysis. Am J Obstet Gynecol. 1994;171(6):1488–504.
20. Jacobson TZ, Barlow DH, Konincks PR, Olive D, Farquhar C. Laparoscopic surgery for subfertility with endometriosis. Cochrane Database Syst Rev. 2010;1, CD001398.
21. Kennedy S, Bergqvist A, Chapron C, D'Hooghe T, Dunselman G, Greb R, et al. ESHRE guideline for the diagnosis and treatment of endometriosis. Hum Reprod. 2005;20(10):2698–704.
22. Jenkins S, Olive DL, Haney AF. Endometriosis: pathogenetic implications of the anatomic distribution. Obstet Gynecol. 1986;67:335–8.
23. Guruppo Italiano per lo studio dell'endometriosi. Prevalence and anatomical distribution of endometriosis in women with selected gynaecological conditions: results from a multicentric Italian study. Hum Reprod. 1994;9:1158–62.
24. Redwine DB. Ovarian endometriosis: a marker for more extensive pelvic and intestinal disease. Fertil Steril. 1999;72:310–5.
25. Donnez J, Nisolle M, Gillerot S, Anaf V, Clercks-Braun F, Casanas-Roux F. Ovarian endometrial cysts: the role of gonadotropin-releasing hormone agonist and/or drainage. Fertil Steril. 1994;62:63–6.
26. Hart RJ, Hickey M, Maouris P, Buckett W. Excisional surgery versus ablative surgery for ovarian endometriomata. Cochrane Database Syst Rev. 2008;2, CD004992.
27. Matson PL, Yovich JL. Treatment of infertility associated with endometriosis by in vitro fertilization. Fertil Steril. 1986;46:432–4.
28. Oehninger S, Acosta AA, Kreiner D, Muasher SJ, Jones Jr HW, Rosenwaks Z. In vitro fertilization and embryo transfer (IVF/embryo transfer): an established and successful therapy for endometriosis. J In Vitro Fert Embryo Transf. 1988;5:249–56.

29. Pellicer A, Oliveria N, Ruiz A, Remohi J, Simon C. Exploring the mechanism(s) of endometriosis-related infertility: an analysis of embryo development and implantation in assisted reproduction. Hum Reprod. 1995;10:91–7.
30. Gupta S, Agarwal A, Agarwal R, Loret de Mola JR. Impact of ovarian endometrioma on assisted reproduction outcomes. Reprod Biomed Online. 2006;13(3):349–60.
31. Demirol A, Guven S, Baykal C, Gurgan T. The effect of ovarian cystectomy of endometriosis on ART outcome. Reprod Biomed Online. 2006;12(5):639–43.
32. Tsoumpou I, Kyrgiou M, Gelbaya TA, Nardo LG. The effect of surgical treatment for endometrioma on in vitro fertilization outcomes: a systematic review and meta-analysis. Fertil Steril. 2009;92:75–87.
33. Benchop L, Farquhar C, van der Poel N, Heineman MJ. Interventions for women with endometrioma prior to assisted reproductive technology. Cochrane Database Syst Rev. 2010;11, CD008570.
34. Sampson JA. Peritoneal endometriosis due to the menstrual dissemination of endometrial tissue into the peritoneal cavity. Am J Obstet Gynecol. 1927;14:422–69.
35. Brosens IA, Puttemans PJ, Deprest J. The endoscopic localization of endometrial implants in the ovarian chocolate cyst. Fertil Steril. 1994;61:1034–8.
36. Hughesdon PE. The structure of endometrial cysts of the ovary. Obstet Gynecol. 1957;44:481–7.
37. Vercellini P, Chapron C, De GIorgi O, Consonni D, Frontino G, Crosignani PG. Coagulation or excision of ovarian endometriomata? Am J Obstet Gynecol. 2003;188:606–10.
38. Durlinger AL, Visser JA, Themmen AP. Regulation of ovarian function: the role of anti-Mullerian hormone. Reproduction. 2002;124:601–9.
39. van Rooij IA, Broekmans FJ, te Velde ER, Fauser BC, Bancsi LF, de Jong FH, et al. Serum anti-Mullerian hormone levels: a novel measure of ovarian reserve. Hum Reprod. 2002;17 (12):3065–71.
40. Seifer DB, Maclaughlin DT. Mullerian Inhibiting Substance is an ovarian growth factor of emerging clinical significance. Fertil Steril. 2007;88:539–46.
41. Fanchin R, Sconauer LM, Righini C, Guibourdenche J, Frydman R, Taieb J. Serum anti-Mullerian hormone is more strongly related to ovarian follicular status than serum inhibin B, Estradiol, FSH and LH on day 3. Hum Reprod. 2003;18:323–7.
42. Raffi F, Metwally M, Amer S. The impact of excision of ovarian endometrioma on ovarian reserve: a systematic review and meta-analysis. J Clin Endocrinol Metab. 2012;97(9):3146–54.
43. Hirokawa W, Iwase A, Goto M, Takikawa S, Nagatomo Y, Nakahara T, et al. The post-operative decline in serum anti-Mullerian hormone correlates with the bilaterality and severity of endometrioma. Hum Reprod. 2011;26:904–10.
44. Kitajima M, Khan KN, Hiraki K, Inoue T, Fujishita A, Masuzaki H. Changes in serum anti-Mullerian hormone levels may predict damage to residual normal ovarian tissue after laparoscopic surgery for women with ovarian endometrioma. Fertil Steril. 2011;95:2589–91.
45. Celik HG, Dogan E, Okyay E, Ulukus C, Saatli B, Uysal S, et al. Effect of laparoscopic excision of endometriomas on ovarian reserve: serial changes in the serum antimullerian hormone levels. Fertil Steril. 2012;97:1472–8.
46. Var T, Batioglu S, Tonguc E, Kahyaoglu I. The effect of laparoscopic ovarian cystectomy versus coagulation in bilateral endometriomas on ovarian reserve as determined by antral follicle count and ovarian volume: a prospective randomized study. Fertil Steril. 2011;95:2247–50.
47. Donnez J, Nisolle M, Gillet N, Smets M, Bassil S, Casanas-Roux F. Large ovarian endometriomas. Hum Reprod. 1996;11:641–6.
48. Pados G, Tsolakidis D, Assimakopoulos E, Athanatos D, Tarlatzis B. Sonographic changes after laparoscopic cystectomy compared with three-stage management in patients with ovarian endometriomas: a prospective randomized study. Hum Reprod. 2010;25(3):672–7.
49. Tsolakidis D, Pados G, Valilis D, Athanatos D, Tsalikis T, Giannakou A, et al. The impact on ovarian reserve after laparoscopic ovarian cystectomy versus three-stage management in patients with endometriomas: a prospective randomized study. Fertil Steril. 2010;94(1):71–7.

50. Donnez J, Lousse JC, Jadoul P, Donnez O, Squifflet J. Laparoscopic management of endometriomas using a combined technique of excisional (cystectomy) and ablative surgery. Fertil Steril. 2010;94:28–32.
51. Ferrero S, Venturini PL, Gillott DJ, Remorgida V, Leone Roberti Maggiore U. Hemostasis by bipolar coagulation versus suture after surgical stripping of bilateral ovarian endometriomas: a randomized controlled trial. J Minim Invasive Gynecol. 2012;9(6):722–30.
52. Coric M, Barisic D, Pavicic D, Karadza M, Banovic M. Electrocoagulation versus suture after laparoscopic stripping of ovarian endometriomas assessed by antral follicle count; preliminary results of randomized clinical trial. Arch Gynecol Obstet. 2011;283:373–8.
53. Biacchiardi CP, Piane LG, Camanni M, Delterro F, Delpiano EM, Marchino GL, et al. Laparoscopic stripping of endometriomas negatively affects ovarian follicular reserve even if performed by experienced surgeons. Reprod Biomed Online. 2011;23:740–6.
54. Ercan CM, Sakinci M, Duru NK, Alanbay I, Karashin KE, Baser I. Antimullerian hormone levels after laparoscopic endometrioma stripping surgery. Gynecol Endocrinol. 2010;26:468–72.
55. Ercan CM, Duru NK, Karasahin KE, Coksuer H, Dede M, Baser I. Ultrasonographic evaluation and anti-Mullerian hormone levels after laparoscopic stripping of unilateral endometriomas. Eur J Obstet Gynecol. 2011;158:2080–4.
56. Hwu YM, Wu FS, Li SH, Sun FJ, Lin MH, Lee RK. The impact of endometrioma and laparoscopic cystectomy on serum anti-Mullerian hormone levels. Reprod Biol Endocrinol. 2011;9:80.
57. Lee DY, Younf Kim N, Jae Kim M, Yoon BK, Choi D. Effects of laparoscopic surgery on serum anti-Mullerian hormone levels in reproductive-aged women with endometrioma. Gynecol Endocrinol. 2011;27:733–6.
58. Uncu G, Kasapoglu I, Ozerkan K, Seyhan A, Yilmaztepe AO, Ata B. Prospective assessment of the impact of endometriomas and their removal on ovarian reserve and determinants of the rate of decline in ovarian reserve. Hum Reprod. 2013;28:2140–5.
59. Alborzi S, Momtahan M, Parsanezhad ME, Dehbashi S, Zolghadri J, Alborzi S. A prospective, randomized study comparing laparoscopic ovarian cystectomy versus fenestration and coagulation in patients with endometriomas. Fertil Steril. 2004;82(6):1633–7.
60. Beretta P, Franchi M, Ghezzi F, Busacca M, Zupi E, Bolis P. Randomized clinical trial of two laparoscopic treatments of endometriomas: cystectomy versus drainage and coagulation. Fertil Steril. 1998;70:1176–80.
61. Busacca M, Marana R, Caruana P, Candiani M, Muzzi L, Calia C, et al. Recurrence of endometrioma after laparoscopic excision. Am J Obstet Gynecol. 1999;180:519–23.
62. Fedele L, Bianchi S, Zanconato G, Berlanda N, Raffaelli R, Fontana E. Laparoscopic excision of recurrent endometriomas: long-term outcome and comparison with primary surgery. Fertil Steril. 2006;85:694–9.
63. Hemmings R, Bissonnette F, Bouzayen R. Results of laparoscopic treatments of ovarian endometriomas: laparoscopic ovarian fenestration and coagulation. Fertil Steril. 1998;70:527–9.
64. Kikuchi I, Takeuchi H, Kitade M, Shimanuki H, Kumakiri J, Kinoshita K. Recurrence rate of endometriomas following a laparoscopic cystectomy. Acta Obstet Gynecol. 2006;85:1120–4.
65. Koga K, Takemura Y, Osuga Y, Yoshino O, Hirota Y, Hirata T, et al. Recurrence of ovarian endometrioma after laparoscopic excision. Hum Reprod. 2006;21:2171–4.
66. Saleh A, Tulandi T. Reoperation after laparoscopic treatment of ovarian endometriomas by excision and by fenestration. Fertil Steril. 1999;72:322–4.
67. Roberts CP, Rock JA. The current staging system for endometriosis: does it help? Obstet Gynecol Clin North Am. 2003;30:115–32.
68. Vercellini P, Fedele L, Aimi G, De Giorgi O, Consonni D, Crosignani PG. Reproductive performance, pain recurrence and disease relapse after conservative surgical treatment for endometriosis: the predictive value of the current classification system. Hum Reprod. 2006;21:2679–85.

69. Carmona F, Martínez-Zamora MA, Rabanal A, Martínez-Román S, Balasch J. Ovarian cystectomy versus laser vaporization in the treatment of ovarian endometriomas: a randomized clinical trial with a five-year follow-up. Fertil Steril. 2011;96(1):251–4.
70. Vercellini P, Somigliana E, Vigano P, De Matteis S, Barbara G, Fedele L. The effect of second-line surgery on reproductive performance of women with recurrent endometriosis: a systematic review. Acta Obstet Gynecol Scand. 2009;88:1074–82.
71. Muzii L, Marana R, Caruana P, Catalano GF, Margutti F, Panici PB. Postoperative administration of monophasic combined oral contraceptives after laparoscopic treatment of ovarian endometriomas: a prospective, randomized trial. Am J Obstet Gynecol. 2000;183:588–92.
72. Saeki A, Matsumoto T, Ikuma K, Tanase Y, Inaba F, Oku H, et al. The vasopressin injection technique for laparoscopic excision of ovarian endometrioma: as technique to reduce the use of coagulation. J Minim Invasive Gynecol. 2010;17(2):176–9.

Chapter 24
Systematic Laparoscopic Surgery for Complete Obliteration of the Cul-de-sac

Yoshiaki Ota, Masaaki Andou, Keiko Ebisawa, Kazuko Fujiwara, Tomonori Hada, Hiroyuki Kanao, and Ikuko Ota

Abstract Endometriosis has been reported as a major cause of pelvic pain. Most notably, deep infiltrating endometriosis is a very active disease that occurs in 20 % of women with endometriosis. We have been actively dissecting deep infiltrating diseased areas within the sacral ligaments around the uterus in order to improve dysmenorrhea and chronic pelvic pain caused by deep infiltrating endometriosis. Laparoscopic surgery is an ideal option to treat deep infiltrating endometriosis involving complete cul-de-sac obliteration due to its minimal invasiveness and ability to achieve an appropriate depth of surgical field. It is important to prevent pain recurrence by providing systematic surgery and removing the deep infiltrating endometriosis safely and widely. To reduce recurrence, it is ideal to provide postoperative education to maintain the effect of surgery.

Keywords Complete cul-de-sac obliteration • Deep infiltrating endometriosis (DIE) • Laparoscopic surgery

24.1 Introduction

Endometriosis occurs in 6–10 % of women of reproductive age [1]. There are three histological classifications: peritoneal endometriosis, endometrioma, and deep infiltrating endometriosis [2]. Treatment is largely divided into either surgical or pharmacological intervention.

Y. Ota (✉) • M. Andou • K. Ebisawa • K. Fujiwara • T. Hada • H. Kanao
Department of Obstetrics and Gynecology, Kurashiki Medical Center, Kurashiki, Japan
e-mail: yoshimon@cj8.so-net.ne.jp

I. Ota
Department of Obstetrics and Gynecology, Kurashiki Heisei Hospital, Kurashiki, Japan

T. Harada (ed.), *Endometriosis: Pathogenesis and Treatment*,
DOI 10.1007/978-4-431-54421-0_24, © Springer Japan 2014

In pharmacological intervention, recently, it has become a trend to use either low-dose estrogen–progestin (LEP) or dienogest but neither option is practical for women who are preparing to conceive.

On the other hand, the surgical option is expected to provide early pain relief.

Endometriosis has been reported as a major cause of pelvic pain. Most notably, deep infiltrating endometriosis is a very active disease that occurs in 20 % of women with endometriosis and is strongly associated with pelvic pain [3, 4].

Furthermore, deep infiltrating endometriosis is not only a cause of infertility, but also may lead to functional impairments of retroperitoneal organs by causing compartment pressure and constriction.

We have been actively dissecting deep infiltrating diseased areas within the sacral ligaments around the uterus in order to improve dysmenorrhea and chronic pelvic pain caused by deep infiltrating endometriosis.

It is important to prevent possible residual diseases and ureteral and rectal injury when considering cases specifically involving complete cul-de-sac obliteration.

Laparoscopic surgery is an ideal option to treat deep infiltrating endometriosis involving complete cul-de-sac obliteration due to its minimal invasiveness and ability to achieve an appropriate depth of surgical field.

In this article, focusing on deep infiltrating endometriosis with complete cul-de-sac obliteration, we report our surgical methods and results.

24.2 Subjects

Between January 2008 and July 2012, we performed 622 laparoscopic surgical resections of endometriosis in patients of childbearing age. Among them, those with and without deep infiltrating endometriosis (DIE) numbered 369 and 253, respectively. Therefore, 60 % of cases had DIE (Fig. 24.1). We divided our cohort into four groups, as follows: 372 (age: 33.91 ± 5.75) cases without postoperative pharmacological treatment, 123 (age: 31.60 ± 5.70) cases with postoperative low-dose estrogen–progestins (LEP), 35 (age: 30.94 ± 5.97) cases with postoperative treatment with 1 mg of dienogest, and 92 (age: 33.32 ± 6.23) cases of postoperative treatment with 2 mg of dienogest (Table 24.1).

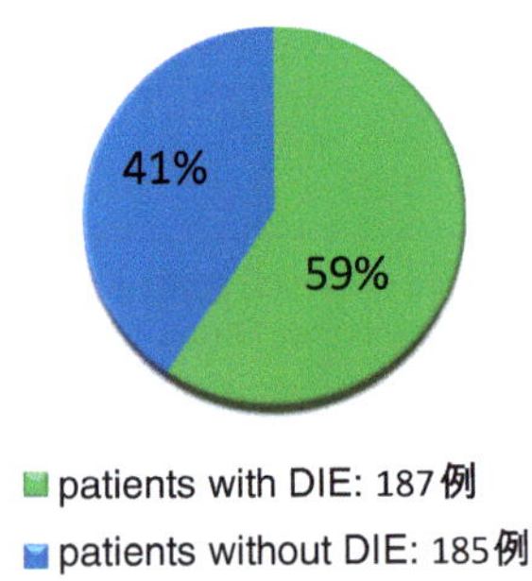

Fig. 24.1 Sixty percent of cases had deep infiltrating endometriosis

Table 24.1 Between January 2008 and July 2012, we performed 622 laparoscopic surgical resections of endometriosis in patients of childbearing age

	No postoperative pharmacotherapy ($n = 372$)	COC treatment ($n = 123$)	Dienogest treatment 1 mg/day ($n = 35$)	Dienogest treatment 2 mg/day ($n = 92$)	*P*-value
Age (years)	33.91 ± 5.75	31.60 ± 5.70	30.94 ± 5.97	33.32 ± 6.23	0.01
Presence of deep infiltrating endometriosis					
–	185	48	8	12	0.01
+	187	75	27	80	
Beecham classification					
Stage I	16	1	1	1	0.08
Stage II	209	65	14	26	
Stage III	60	21	7	17	
Stage IV	87	36	13	48	
Laterality of endometriotic cysts					
–	31	5	2	10	0.075
+					
Monolateral	196	76	17	40	
Bilateral	145	42	15	43	

24.3 Surgical Methods: Excision of Cul-de-sac Obliteration and DIE Method

Firstly, in the case of complete cul-de-sac obliteration, deep infiltrating endometriosis is distributed around the uterosacral ligament.

Deep infiltrating endometriosis is attached to the rectum and urinary tubes.

Therefore, when removing the deep infiltrating endometriosis, it is important to separate the rectum and urinary tube from the diseased area in order to prevent tissue damage and avoid leaving residual diseases.

Therefore, we have been dissecting interstitial spaces between deep infiltrating endometriosis and the urinary tube which center around the uterosacral ligament.

This interstitial space is Okabayashi's pararectal space, and we have termed the outside of the uterosacral ligament "the lateral pararectal space, LPRS."

Furthermore, we refer to the interstitial space between the rectum and lateral pararectal space as "the median pararectal space, MPRS" (Fig. 24.2).

24.3.1 Method to Separate Ureter

In most cases, deep infiltrating endometriosis is distributed around the uterosacral ligament and cervix uteri, and almost all cases involve adhesion of the lower urinary tube to the outer side of the uterosacral ligament.

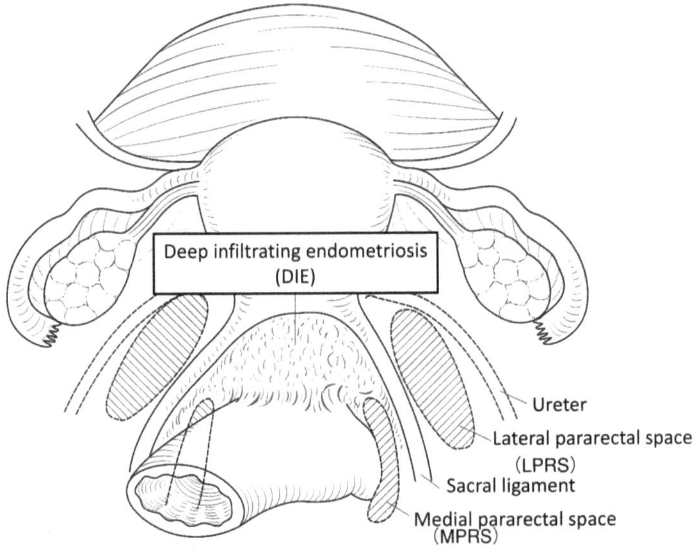

Fig. 24.2 Anatomy of cul-de-sac obliteration. "The lateral pararectal space" is consistent with the outside of the uterosacral ligament. "The medial pararectal space" is consistent with the interstitial space between the rectum and lateral pararectal space

Especially, adhesion occurs between the uterosacral ligament and either the urinary tube or rectum, and the urinary tube may be unpredictably shifted; therefore, identifying and separating the urinary tube first may facilitate a safe operation.

In cases of cul-de-sac obliteration, we identify the urinary tube where it crosses the common iliac artery and trace it down as far as possible.

We locate and unfold the posterior side of the broad ligament of the uterus, and identify the urinary tube.

Next, we open the LPRS which consists of the internal aspect of the urinary tube and extraluminal space of the uterosacral ligament.

This leads to separation of the urinary tube from the deep infiltrating endometriosis centered around the uterosacral ligament (Fig. 24.3).

24.3.2 *Method to Obliterate Complete Cul-de-sac Adhesion*

In the case of complete cul-de-sac adhesion, the strongest adhesion is at the posterior uterine cervix and anterior aspect of the rectum.

When the direction of the rectum is not clear, it is possible to cause rectal damage while dissecting between the posterior uterine cervix and anterior aspect of the rectum.

Therefore, we have been approaching from the lateral rectal side.

We dissect the lateral rectal fossa from the rectum and then deeply obliterate the space outside the lateral rectal fossa.

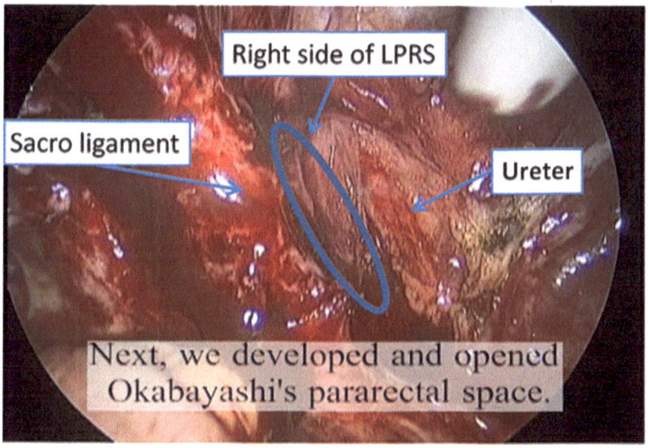

Fig. 24.3 LPRS lateral pararectal space. Developing on the right side of the LPRS. The ureter was separated from the sacral ligament

This space is the MPRS described earlier. Then, we proceed to dissect the MPRS further anterior toward the posterior part of the vagina.

This leads to complete separation of the deep infiltrating endometriosis centered around the uterosacral ligament and rectum.

Furthermore, it has become possible to laterally identify part of the anterior aspect of the rectum.

In this way, dissecting from the lateral side leads to gradual identification of the rectal outline.

Approaching the right and left lateral sides leads to identification of the remaining strongest point of adhesion between the posterior uterus and anterior rectum.

At this step, since we have clearly outlined the anterior aspect of the rectum, it is safe to proceed with dissecting the center part of the rectum.

Dissection of the remaining center part of the rectum leads to separation of the cul-de-sac obliteration (Fig. 24.4).

24.3.3 *Method of Deep Infiltrating Endometriosis Excision*

Firstly, disseminate the LPRS to separate the ureter and deep infiltrating endometriosis centered around the uterosacral ligament. Then, by disseminating the MPRS to separate the rectum, deep infiltrating endometriosis will be isolated, attaching to the posterior aspect of the uterus in the shape of an upside-down U.

This isolated deep infiltrating endometriosis will be removed from the posterior side of the uterus without injuring the deep uterine vein.

Since the urinary tube and rectum have been isolated, it is possible to further separate the diseased area systematically (Fig. 24.5).

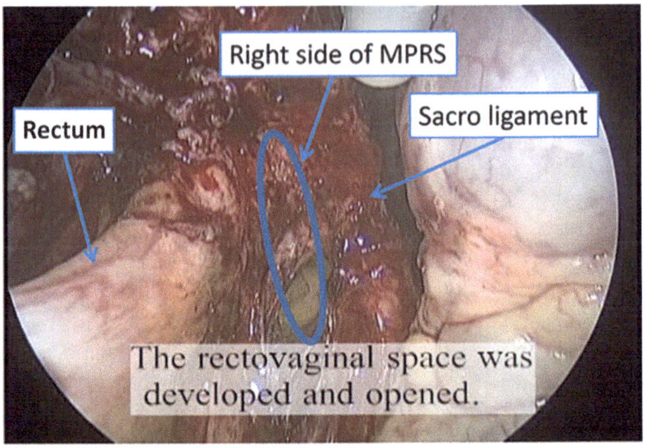

Fig. 24.4 MPRS medial pararectal space. Developing on the right side of the MPRS. The rectum was separated from the side of the sacral ligament

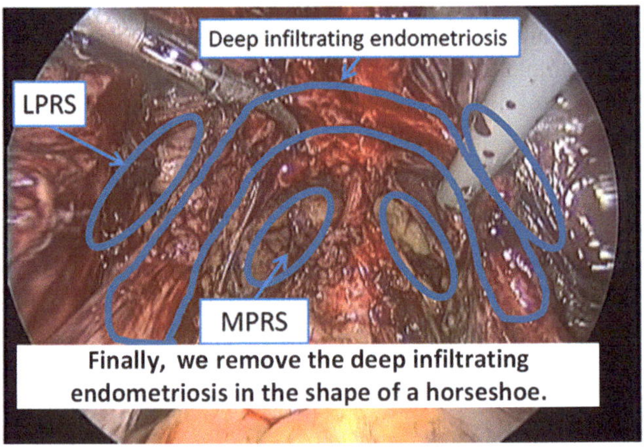

Fig. 24.5 Isolation of DIE in the shape of a horseshoe. The LPRS and MPRS should be developed to isolate DIE from the lateral pararectal space. It is shaped like a horseshoe

24.3.4 Checking Damage After Excision of Cul-de-sac Obliteration

As described earlier, it is important to check for rectal damage after disseminating the MPRS and removing the cul-de-sac obliteration.

Firstly, we perform digital rectal examination by extending the dissected area, and confirm that damage is not present laparoscopically.

Then, we perform a leak test. The leak test is performed by pumping 50–100 mL of air into the rectum using a large soft catheter (Figs. 24.6 and 24.7).

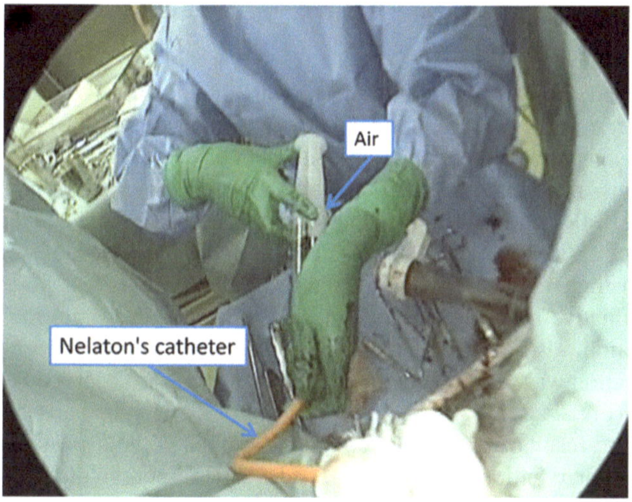

Fig. 24.6 Air leak test. To check for rectal injury, the air leak test is important. Nelaton's catheter was inserted into the anus and 50 mL of air was pumped into the rectum using a syringe

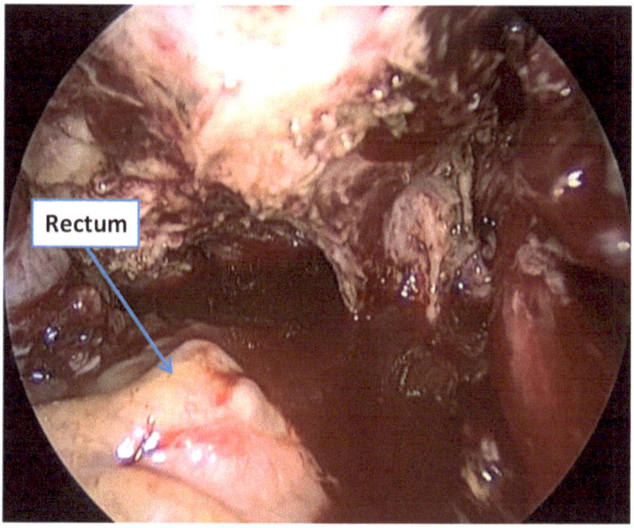

Fig. 24.7 Air leak test. Checking air leak from the rectum using a laparoscope from the inter-abdominal side. Sometimes, pin hole rectal injury occurred in the pararectal area. If rectal injury is overlooked, it will cause serious postoperative complications

24.4 Surgical Outcome

Three hundred and seventy-two subjects who did not receive pharmacological treatment after surgery were divided into two groups: 187 cases with surgical resection of deep infiltrating endometriosis, and 185 cases without deep infiltrating endometriosis. We defined recurrence of chocolate cyst of 2 cm or larger by either ultrasound or MRI, and recurrence of pelvic pain as a VAS score equal to or greater than the score assessed prior to the operation. The cumulative risk of recurrence was calculated using the Kaplan–Meier method, and the log-rank test was performed.

The cumulative risk of recurrence in the group with deep infiltrating endometriosis resection was 6 % at 3 years postoperatively, while that of those who did not require resection was 10 %. No significant difference was observed between these two groups (Fig. 24.8).

Since these results were compared among groups without postoperative pharmacological intervention, they indicate adequate resection of deep infiltrating endometriosis and pain control. Therefore, these results show that our operating method of systematic resection of deep infiltrating endometriosis is effective.

On the other hand, recurrence of chocolate cyst at 4 years postoperatively was 30 % in both groups (Fig. 24.9).

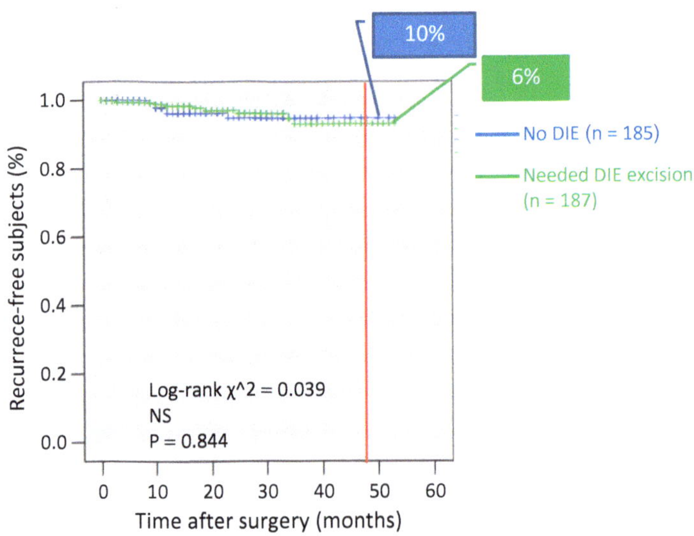

Fig. 24.8 The effect on pain of systematic DIE and endometrioma excision. Comparison of the recurrence rate of pain in the presence/absence of deep infiltrating endometriosis (372 women receiving no medical therapy after surgery). The recurrence rate of pain was 10 % after surgery at 4 years. There was no the significant difference between the No DIE group and Needed DIE excision group for 4 years. Systematic DIE excision mostly controlled pain recurrence for 4 years

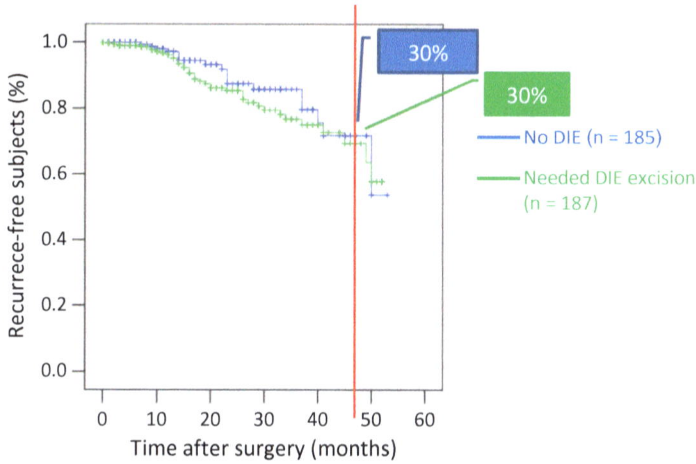

Fig. 24.9 The effect on endometrioma recurrence of systematic DIE and endometrioma excision. Comparison of recurrence rate of endometrioma by the presence/absence of deep endometriosis (372 women who received no medical therapy after surgery). The recurrence rate of endometrioma was 30 % at 3 years. There was no significant difference between the No DIE group and Needed DIE excision group for 4 years. One reason is that surgery is often incomplete to maintain the ovarian reserve. Endometrioma will recur in 30 % after surgery within 4 years

24.5 Discussion

Treatment for endometriosis is largely divided into two types: surgical intervention and pharmacological treatment.

Recently, it has become a trend to use pharmacological treatment with either low-dose estrogen–progestin (LEP) or dienogest, but neither option is practical for women who are preparing to conceive.

On the other hand, surgery provides rapid pain relief, but, among surgical methods, the biggest setback of fertility – preserving surgery has been the high recurrence rate. It has been reported that the recurrence rate at 2 to 5 years postoperatively of the chocolate cyst was 12 to 30 % [5–10], while the recurrence rate of pain was 10–49 % [5, 8, 11, 12].

Also, it has been clearly reported that deep infiltrating endometriosis has an association with strong pelvic pain, and in those with disease around the uterosacral ligament, the odds ratio of chronic pelvic pain was 2.1, while the odds ratio of dyspareunia was 2.0 [2]. Therefore, we have completely removed deep infiltrating endometriosis and optimized surgery to prevent ureteral and rectal injury.

Specifically, in cases with complete cul-de-sac obliteration, we performed LPRS and MPRS to systemically separate the urinary tube and rectum from deep infiltrating endometriosis.

With this method, the 4-year postoperative pain recurrence rate was similar in both groups, that is, almost 15 % for both patients with or without deep infiltrating endometriosis.

These results are from the study of cases without postoperative pharmacological intervention and, therefore, our systematic resection was considered effective for pain control at 4 years postoperatively.

On the other hand, the cumulative risk of recurrence of ovarian chocolate cyst was 30 % at 4 years postoperatively. Recurrence of pain was considered to be the recurrence of deep infiltrating endometriosis, and the recurrence rate of ovarian chocolate cyst was 3 to 5 times higher than that of deep infiltrating endometriosis.

The ovarian reserve needs to be considered in cases of ovarian chocolate cyst surgery; however, it is possible to enucleate large fields in the case of deep infiltrating endometriosis. The recurrence rate may be associated with differences in both operative backgrounds. Therefore, it is important to prevent pain recurrence by providing systematic surgery and removing the deep infiltrating endometriosis safely and widely. On the other hand, in cases of ovarian chocolate cyst, we provide surgery while considering the ovarian reserve. In terms of recurrence, as Vercellini and others reported that recurrence can be reduced to 37 % at 3 years postoperatively by providing combined oral contraceptives (COCs), we think that it is optimal to provide combined oral contraceptives (COCs) postoperatively [13].

24.6 Conclusion

In cases of deep infiltrating endometriosis with complete cul-de-sac obliteration, it is ideal to provide systematic enucleation to avoid rectal and urinary tube damage with the LPRS and MPRS in order to prevent pain recurrence.

References

1. Giudice LC, Kao LC. Endometriosis. Lancet. 2004;364:1789–99.
2. Chapron C. Ovarian endometrioma: severe pelvic pain is associated with deeply infiltrating endometriosis. Hum Reprod. 2012;27(3):702–11.
3. Vercellini P. Endometriosis: what a pain it is. Semin Reprod Endocrinol. 1997;15(3):251–61.
4. Chapron C. Operative management of deep endometriosis infiltrating the uterosacral ligaments. J Am Assoc Gynecol Laparosc. 1999;6(1):31–7.
5. Busaca M. Recurrence of ovarian endometrioma after laparoscopic excision. Am J Obstet Gynecol. 1999;180:519–23.
6. Saleh A. Reoperation after laparoscopic treatment of ovarian endometriomas by excision and by fenestration. Fertil Steril. 1999;72:322–4.
7. Ghezzi F. Recurrence of endometriosis and anatomical location of the primary lesion. Fertil Steril. 2001;75:136–40.
8. Jones KD. Recurrence of chocolate cysts after laparoscopic ablation. J Am Assoc Gynecol Laparosc. 2002;9:315–20.

9. Vercellini P. Coagulation or excision of ovarian endometriomas? Am J Obstet Gynecol. 2003;188:606–10.
10. Koga K. Recurrence of ovarian endometrioma after laparoscopic excision. Hum Reprod. 2006;21:2171–4.
11. Vercellini P. Association between endometriosis stage, lesion type, patient characteristics and severity of pelvic pain symptoms: a multivariate analysis of over 1000 patients. Hum Reprod. 2007;22:266–71.
12. Liu X. Patterns of and risk factors for recurrence in women with ovarian endometriomas. Obstet Gynecol. 2007;109(6):1411–20.
13. Vercellini P. Postoperative oral contraceptive exposure and risk of endometrioma recurrence. Am J Obstet Gynecol. 2008;198:504. e1–504e5.

Chapter 25
Prevention of Recurrence After Surgery

Yutaka Osuga, Yuri Takemura, Masashi Takamura, and Kaori Koga

Abstract Recurrence of ovarian endometrioma after excision imposes profound encumbrance on the suffered women, with increasing pain, subfertility/infertility, and a risk of ovarian cancer. Postoperative recurrence is relatively common, the rate ranging from 11 to 32 % in 1–5 years. To date, a number of risk factors for the recurrence have been reported, i.e., younger age, larger cysts, high rASRM scores, previous medical treatment, previous surgery for endometriosis, and short-term postoperative medical treatment. In contrast, postoperative pregnancy reduces the risk. Several biomarkers are suggested to predict the recurrence but not yet validated in clinical practice. Postoperative OC use for a long period has been demonstrated to reduce the recurrence remarkably. Postoperative GnRH analogue use is also effective for the reduction of the recurrence. There still remain some issues on the duration and the drugs most suitable for the prevention.

Keywords Endometrioma • Oral contraceptive • Recurrence • Surgery

25.1 Introduction

Endometriosis is a disease defined as the presence of endometrium-like lesions outside the uterus. Although the exact etiology has not yet been determined, it is widely accepted that endometrial cells in the retrograde menstruation attach, invade, and grow in the peritoneum to cause the disease. It occurs in women of reproductive age and deteriorates the quality of life of the affected women by inducing infertility/subfertility and intractable pain. Treatment of the disease is mainly conducted with drugs and/or surgery. A mainstream of medical treatment is

Y. Osuga (✉) • Y. Takemura • M. Takamura • K. Koga
Department of Obstetrics and Gynecology, School of Medicine, the University of Tokyo, Japan, 7-3-1 Hongo Bunkyo, Tokyo 113-8655, Japan
e-mail: yutakaos-tky@umin.ac.jp

T. Harada (ed.), *Endometriosis: Pathogenesis and Treatment*,
DOI 10.1007/978-4-431-54421-0_25, © Springer Japan 2014

hormonal treatment. However, hormonal drugs cannot be used for those who want to conceive since the drugs inhibit ovulation. In addition, some pain symptoms are occasionally resistant to medical treatment. Likewise, hormonal drugs are often not effective to eradicate developed lesions, such as endometrioma. On the other hand, surgical treatment is appropriate for removing developed lesions and often effective to mitigate drug-resistant pain. Widespread use of laparoscopic surgery makes it less invasive to treat endometriosis by surgery.

Surgical treatment for endometriosis, while having relatively effective outcome in the short term, has a problem in the long period after surgery. Hysterectomy with bilateral oophorectomy is radical enough to cure endometriosis, but the procedure is not acceptable for patients who want to maintain fertility. For these patients, excision of endometriosis lesions (conservative surgery) is a method of choice. This treatment often entails recurrence both in symptoms and in histology. Recently, the concern is gaining traction because more and more women need conservative surgery due to increasing tendency to childbearing in late reproductive ages.

This problem, however, is not so new. An incipient report that examined the recurrence after conservative surgery, while performed by open surgery in those days, indicated several noticeable findings. The authors followed 423 patients treated with conservative surgery and found 13.5 and 40.3 % cumulative recurrence rates in 3 and 5 years, respectively [1]. They found that severity of disease was not predictive of recurrence and pregnancy delayed recurrence.

There are a number of reports also in the era of laparoscopic surgery. When we read these papers, we notice the complexity of the problems regarding "recurrence." Some papers examine recurrence of pain, while others examine recurrence of endometriosis lesions detected by laparoscopy or imaging. Some papers study recurrence of endometriosis in general while others study recurrence of a specific type of endometriosis, e.g., peritoneal lesion, ovarian endometrioma, and deep endometriosis at the cul-de-sac. The operation methods are either not uniform, including excision of the cyst (cystectomy) and coagulation or vaporization using electric devises or lasers. In this chapter, we focus on the recurrence of endometrioma, which can be easily detected by transvaginal ultrasound, after laparoscopic excision.

25.2 Recurrence of Endometrioma After Laparoscopic Excision

25.2.1 Recurrence Rate

Postoperative recurrence rate for endometrioma ranges from 11 to 32 % in 1–5 years [2–11]. The variation partly comes from the difference of the definition of recurrence; some define it by the presence of ovarian cysts greater than 3 cm [5, 10] while others define it by the size at least 2 cm [6, 8]. Instinctively, the time after surgery is related to the recurrence rate. However, unless patients are regularly followed up, as often with the case of asymptomatic patients, it is difficult to accurately quantify the time of recurrence. It is thus not obvious in which time period the patient is most susceptible to recurrence, or whether there is a specific period of time after which a patient is less likely to develop recurrence. According to Evers et al. the recurrence rate during the first 5 years gradually increases [12]. This might imply that endometriosis will eventually reappear in all patients who underwent complete removal of the lesions. In accordance with this notion, a longitudinal study by Liu et al. showed that the recurrence rates continued to increase with time, 7.8, 17.7, and 32.3 % at 1, 2, and 3 years, respectively [10]. In contrast, Kikuchi et al. drew a cumulative recurrence rate curve and demonstrated that the cumulative rate reaches a plateau at around 48 months after surgery [6]. Further studies with longer follow-up are needed to settle the issue.

Whether the recurrence of endometrioma occurs by de novo or the relapse of residual endometrioma is poorly understood as well as the origin of endometrioma per se. To address the issue, the recurrence rate was studied with analysis of the side in which endometrioma recurred, supposing that recurrence in the contralateral ovary should be de novo. Exacoustos et al. analyzed 62 patients with recurrent endometrioma and found that 12 patients had recurrence on the counter-lateral untreated ovary [13]. Kikuchi et al. also analyzed 26 cases with recurrence after hemilateral surgery and found that 11 cases had recurrence on the counter-lateral untreated ovary [6]. These findings suggest that the recurrence of endometrioma is not totally dependent on the presence of the residual endometrioma but in part on de novo occurrence. Of course, it cannot be denied that a lesion on the contralateral ovary undetected by the initial laparoscopy may have progressed after surgery. Although the difference between de novo and relapse is critical for optimal management of this disorder, it is impossible at the moment to discriminate clearly the origin by just looking at and following up the patents and the lesions. Further ingenious studies seem to be necessary to resolve the issue. Collectively, there is no doubt that the recurrence of endometrioma after laparoscopic excision is a common and serious problem, although the actual recurrence rate varies among studies.

25.2.2 *Risk Factor and Biomarker of Recurrence*

Since endometriosis has characteristics of a chronic disease, it would be useful if doctors are able to estimate the probability of recurrence before surgery. To this end, a number of studies have been conducted analyzing various factors which might associate with recurrence. We retrospectively studied a total of 224 patients who had undergone laparoscopic cystectomy of endometrioma [8]. The patients had a minimum of 2 years of postoperative follow-up after laparoscopic cystectomy. Recurrence was defined as the presence of endometrioma more than 2 cm in size, detected by ultrasonography within 2 years of surgery. We assumed that

Table 25.1 Univariate and logistic regression analysis of factors related to the recurrence of ovarian endometrioma

	Univariate analysis	Logistic regression analysis	
Factors	*P* values	*P* values	Odds ratio (95 % confidence interval)
Age (years)	NS		
Infertility	NS		
Pain	NS		
Presence of uterine myoma	NS		
Presence of adenomyosis	NS		
Previous medical treatment of endometriosis	<0.05	<0.01	2.324 (1.232–4.383)
Previous surgery of ovarian endometrioma	NS		
Multiple cysts	NS		
Largest cyst diameter (cm)	<0.05	<0.05	1.182 (1.004–1.391)
Bilateral involvement	NS		
Coexistence of deep endometriosis	NS	NS	0.456 (0.198–1.052)
Revised ASRM score	NS	NS	1.010 (1.000–1.021)
Postoperative medical treatment	NS		
Postoperative pregnancy	<0.05	<0.05	0.292 (0.028–0.317)

ASRM American Society for Reproductive Medicine [8]

14 variables (age, presence of infertility, pain, uterine myoma, adenomyosis, previous medical treatment of endometriosis, previous surgery for ovarian endometriosis, single or multiple cysts, the size of the largest cyst at laparoscopy, unilateral or bilateral involvement, coexistence of deep endometriosis, revised American Society for Reproductive Medicine (ASRM) score, postoperative medical treatment, and postoperative pregnancy) might associate with the recurrence and evaluated these variables to assess their independent effects on the recurrence using logistic regression analysis. As a result, the overall rate of recurrence was 30.4 % (68/224). Significant factors that were independently associated with higher recurrence were previous medical treatment of endometriosis [odds ratio (OR) = 2.324, 95 % confidence interval (95 % CI) = 1.232–4.383, $P = 0.0092$) and larger diameter of the largest cyst (OR = 1.182, 95 % CI = 1.004–1.391, $P = 0.0442$). As shown in Table 25.1, postoperative pregnancy was associated with lower recurrence (OR = 0.292, 95 % CI = 0.028–0.317, $P = 0.0181$). It seems intuitively reasonable that the larger cyst associates with the higher recurrence rate. In contrast, it appears to be difficult to construe the association between previous medical treatment and the higher recurrence risk. The finding may be explained by two possible mechanisms. The first is that the medication may mask endometriotic lesions and allow them to escape from removal at operations. Because more than half of the women who were categorized into previous medical treatment group had continued their medication until the time of operation, it may be possible that the medication might yield latent lesions that remain and recur after the operation. The

other possible reason for a negative impact of medical treatment on endometrioma recurrence is that hormonal-suppressive therapy may alter some genomic characteristics of endometriotic lesions. As for malignant transformation of endometriosis, it is proposed that hormonal ablative treatments may cause negative selection, suppress the normal, eukaryotic cells more than aneuploid cells bearing chromosomal aberrations, and increase the rate of dyskaryotic cells in the endometriotic implants [14]. We conjecture that "negative selection" may also contribute to the recurrence of disease, making the lesion more active, progressive, and liable to recurrence. The association of postoperative pregnancy and lower rate of recurrence is an interesting finding but needs careful interpretation. A possible scenario is that subsequent pregnancy may have a protective effect on endometrioma recurrence. An absence of retrograde menstruation and formation of corpora lutea [15], both of which are known to cause endometriosis, and persistent exposure to progesterone are thought to contribute to the protective effect of pregnancy. Conversely, those who tended not to recur had more probability to be pregnant given that endometriosis causes infertility/subfertility.

Several risk factors have been reported by others. In general, the more advanced the endometriosis, the more the disease recurs. Larger cysts [8] and high rASRM scores [6, 7, 10, 16, 17] are reported to be risk factors for recurrence. Factors that may correlate with the severity of endometriosis such as previous medical treatment [8, 10], previous surgery for endometriosis [3, 17], and short-term postoperative medical treatment [9] are also identified as risk factors. Younger age at surgery is reported as a risk factor by two studies [6, 10]. A younger age at surgery would correlate with a younger age at onset and possibly a disease type that is more aggressive and prone to recurrence than the endometrioma associated with an older age of onset.

A few researches are trying to find out biomarkers for recurrence of ovarian endometriomas. Increased expression of progesterone receptor isoform B, nuclear factor kappa-B, SLIT/ROBO1, and cyclooxygenase-2 are shown to be associated with higher risk of recurrence [18–20]. However, whether they are practically useful in predicting the recurrence awaits further studies.

25.2.3 Postoperative Medical Managements to Prevent Recurrence

Until recently, postoperative medical treatment that prevents recurrence has not been developed successfully. In the face of the fact that postoperative pregnancy decreases the risk of recurrence, as described above, we came up with the idea if postoperative oral contraceptives might decrease recurrence. We thus conducted a before and after study on postoperative OC treatment. In 2005, our clinic introduced the "OC recommendation," that is, at the time of the operation, we provided each patient with information about OC and the known possible benefits and risks and let

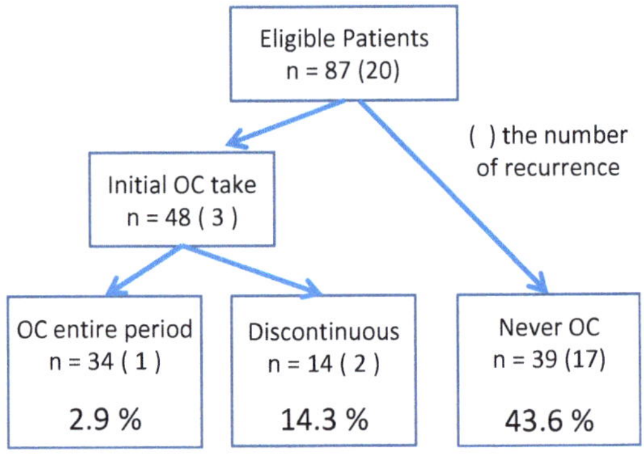

Fig. 25.1 Recurrence after laparoscopic excision of endometrioma. Flowchart of the patients who underwent laparoscopic excision of endometrioma after May 2005, for the retrospective cohort study. A total of 87 patients were followed up for 24 months. Of the 87 patients, 48 started to take OCs, but 39 did not. Of the 48 patients who had started OC, 34 continued OC for the entire study period (24 months), whereas 14 discontinued

the patient decide whether or not to take OC. Women who chose to take OC were given a cyclic (21 days pills/7 days no pill), monophasic OC containing ethinyl estradiol (0.035 mg) and norethisterone (1.0 mg) (Ortho-M 21®, Mochida, Tokyo, Japan), in the first menstrual cycle after laparoscopy. We then conducted a historical study to compare the 2-year recurrence rate before and after the introduction of the "OC recommendation." The overall recurrence rate in patients who underwent laparoscopy after the introduction of the "OC recommendation" was significantly lower than that in patients who received laparoscopy before the introduction (18.6 versus 33.1 %, relative risk 0.56, 95 % CI 0.32–0.97, $P < 0.05$) [21]. Figure 25.1 depicts the recurrence rate in those who used OC which was significantly lower than others (non-OC users plus those who quit OC) (2.9 versus 35.8 %, relative risk 0.08, 95 % CI 0.01–0.48, $P < 0.001$) [21]. This study indicated that postoperative OC use reduces the risk of ovarian endometrioma after laparoscopic excision.

In addition to our study, there have been several studies that evaluate the role of postoperative OC on the recurrence of endometrioma. In contrast to the classical report showing OC had no effect on disease recurrence when used for up to 6 months [22], all studies that tested postoperative OC for 2 years or more demonstrated protective effect of OC on recurrence [11, 21, 23]. The different outcomes between short-term and long-term studies indicate that the duration of treatment with OC affects recurrence. Indeed, Vercellini et al. compared cumulative recurrence according to the duration of postoperative OC use and found that women who used OC for less than 12 months were at higher risk of recurrence than women using OC for 12 months or more [11].

GnRH analogue also has an effect to mitigate recurrence. Jee et al. analyzed the influence of postoperative GnRH analogue according to the duration of the treatment and found that a 6-month treatment had a beneficial impact compared with a 3- and 4-month treatment and expectant management, although the differences did not reach statistical significance [24]. In another report, patients who received 3–6 months of GnRH analogue therapy alone and patients who received OC after GnRH analogue were compared. As a result, recurrent endometrioma after 60 months was significantly lower in OC plus GnRH analogue group than in GnRH analogue alone group (6.1 versus 43.3 %) [25]. It seems that GnRH analogue treatment longer than 6 months reduces the recurrence, and additional OC treatment may maintain the effect. However, the benefit of GnRH analogue should be weighed against the risk of adverse effects associated with estrogen deprivation.

25.3 Summary

Postoperative recurrence of endometrioma is a common event and prevention of the recurrence is needed to manage women with endometriosis successfully for a long period. Thanks to recent extensive studies, it has been established that long-term administration of OC after surgery is safe and tolerable and recommended for those who do not want to conceive immediately after the surgery. However, there still remain some issues regarding what kind of drugs are most suitable and how long the drug should be used. Further studies are warranted to improve strategies to prevent the recurrence.

References

1. Wheeler JM, Malinak LR. Recurrent endometriosis: incidence, management, and prognosis. Am J Obstet Gynecol. 1983;146(3):247–53.
2. Busacca M, Chiaffarino F, Candiani M, Vignali M, Bertulessi C, Oggioni G, Parazzini F. Determinants of long-term clinically detected recurrence rates of deep, ovarian, and pelvic endometriosis. Am J Obstet Gynecol. 2006;195(2):426–32.
3. Busacca M, Marana R, Caruana P, Candiani M, Muzii L, Calia C, Bianchi S. Recurrence of ovarian endometrioma after laparoscopic excision. Am J Obstet Gynecol. 1999;180(3):519–23.
4. Ghezzi F, Beretta P, Franchi M, Parissis M, Bolis P. Recurrence of ovarian endometriosis and anatomical location of the primary lesion. Fertil Steril. 2001;75(1):136–40.
5. Alborzi S, Momtahan M, Parsanezhad ME, Dehbashi S, Zolghadri J, Alborzi S. A prospective, randomized study comparing laparoscopic ovarian cystectomy versus fenestration and coagulation in patients with endometriomas. Fertil Steril. 2004;82(6):1633–7.
6. Kikuchi I, Takeuchi H, Kitade M, Shimanuki H, Kumakiri J, Kinoshita K. Recurrence rate of endometriomas following a laparoscopic cystectomy. Acta Obstet Gynecol Scand. 2006;85(9):1120–4.
7. Parazzini F, Bertulessi C, Pasini A, Rosati M, Di Stefano F, Shonauer S, Vicino M, Aguzzoli L, Trossarelli GF, Massobrio M, Bracco G, Perino A, Moroni S, Beretta P. Determinants of short term recurrence rate of endometriosis. Eur J Obstet Gynecol Reprod Biol. 2005;121(2):216–9.

8. Koga K, Takemura Y, Osuga Y, Yoshino O, Hirota Y, Hirata T, Morimoto C, Harada M, Yano T, Taketani Y. Recurrence of ovarian endometrioma after laparoscopic excision. Hum Reprod. 2006;21(8):2171–4.
9. Vercellini P, Fedele L, Aimi G, De Giorgi O, Consonni D, Crosignani PG. Reproductive performance, pain recurrence and disease relapse after conservative surgical treatment for endometriosis: the predictive value of the current classification system. Hum Reprod. 2006;21 (10):2679–85.
10. Liu X, Yuan L, Shen F, Zhu Z, Jiang H, Guo SW. Patterns of and risk factors for recurrence in women with ovarian endometriomas. Obstet Gynecol. 2007;109(6):1411–20.
11. Vercellini P, Somigliana E, Daguati R, Vigano P, Meroni F, Crosignani PG. Postoperative oral contraceptive exposure and risk of endometrioma recurrence. Am J Obstet Gynecol. 2008;198 (5):504.e1–5.
12. Evers JL, Dunselman GA, Land JA, Bouckaert PX. Is there a solution for recurrent endometriosis? Br J Clin Pract Suppl. 1991;72:45–50. discussion 51-43.
13. Exacoustos C, Zupi E, Amadio A, Amoroso C, Szabolcs B, Romanini ME, Arduini D. Recurrence of endometriomas after laparoscopic removal: sonographic and clinical follow-up and indication for second surgery. J Minim Invasive Gynecol. 2006;13(4):281–8. doi:10.1016/j.jmig.2006.03.002.
14. Blumenfeld Z. Hormonal suppressive therapy for endometriosis may not improve patient health. Fertil Steril. 2004;81(3):487–92.
15. Vercellini P, Somigliana E, Vigano P, Abbiati A, Barbara G, Fedele L. 'Blood On The Tracks' from corpora lutea to endometriomas. BJOG. 2009;116(3):366–71.
16. Busacca M, Bianchi S, Agnoli B, Candiani M, Calia C, De Marinis S, Vignali M. Follow-up of laparoscopic treatment of stage III-IV endometriosis. J Am Assoc Gynecol Laparosc. 1999;6 (1):55–8.
17. Porpora MG, Pallante D, Ferro A, Crisafi B, Bellati F, Benedetti Panici P. Pain and ovarian endometrioma recurrence after laparoscopic treatment of endometriosis: a long-term prospective study. Fertil Steril. 2010;93(3):716–21.
18. Shen F, Liu X, Geng JG, Guo SW. Increased immunoreactivity to SLIT/ROBO1 in ovarian endometriomas: a likely constituent biomarker for recurrence. Am J Pathol. 2009;175 (2):479–88.
19. Shen F, Wang Y, Lu Y, Yuan L, Liu X, Guo S-W. Immunoreactivity of progesterone receptor isoform B and nuclear factor kappa-B as biomarkers for recurrence of ovarian endometriomas. Am J Obstet Gynecol. 2008;199(5):486.e1–486.e10.
20. Yuan L, Shen F, Lu Y, Liu X, Guo S-W. Cyclooxygenase-2 overexpression in ovarian endometriomas is associated with higher risk of recurrence. Fertil Steril. 2009;91 (4, Suppl):1303–6.
21. Takamura M, Koga K, Osuga Y, Takemura Y, Hamasaki K, Hirota Y, Yoshino O, Taketani Y. Post-operative oral contraceptive use reduces the risk of ovarian endometrioma recurrence after laparoscopic excision. Hum Reprod. 2009;24(12):3042–8.
22. Muzii L, Marana R, Caruana P, Catalano GF, Margutti F, Panici PB. Postoperative administration of monophasic combined oral contraceptives after laparoscopic treatment of ovarian endometriomas: A prospective, randomized trial. Am J Obstet Gynecol. 2000;183(3):588–92.
23. Seracchioli R, Mabrouk M, Frascà C, Manuzzi L, Montanari G, Keramyda A, Venturoli S. Long-term cyclic and continuous oral contraceptive therapy and endometrioma recurrence: a randomized controlled trial. Fertil Steril. 2010;93(1):52–6.
24. Jee BC, Lee JY, Suh CS, Kim SH, Choi YM, Moon SY. Impact of GnRH agonist treatment on recurrence of ovarian endometriomas after conservative laparoscopic surgery. Fertil Steril. 2009;91(1):40–5.
25. Lee D-Y, Bae D-S, Yoon B-K, Choi D. Post-operative cyclic oral contraceptive use after gonadotrophin-releasing hormone agonist treatment effectively prevents endometrioma recurrence. Hum Reprod. 2010;25(12):3050–4.

Chapter 26
Ovarian Reserve in Patients with Endometriosis

Michio Kitajima and Hideaki Masuzaki

Abstract The number of follicles present in human ovaries is finite. Ovarian reserve is currently defined as the number and quality of the follicles left in the ovary at any given time. As several novel tests for ovarian reserve, such as anti-Müllerian hormone (AMH) and antral follicle count (AFC), are widely introduced into gynecological practice recently, the knowledge on the physiology of follicular development and mechanism of maintenance of ovarian reserve are rapidly accumulating. Diminished ovarian reserve is a major concern in women with endometriosis-associated infertility. Cystectomy for endometriomas could negatively impact on postoperative ovarian reserve. Some women who had surgery for endometriomas suffer from poor ovarian response, which is directly linked to treatment results in infertility care. In addition, endometriomas themselves may be a cause of diminished ovarian reserve. Chronic inflammation in the local pelvic environment may affect the status of the dormant follicle in the ovarian cortex. Determination of ovarian reserve may serve as an important role in the management of reproductive health issues in women with endometriosis.

Keywords Anti-Müllerian hormone (AMH) • Antral follicle count (AFC) • Endometrioma • Endometriosis • Ovarian reserve

---

M. Kitajima (✉) • H. Masuzaki
Department of Obstetrics and Gynecology, Graduate School of Biomedical Sciences, Nagasaki University, Nagasaki, Japan
e-mail: m-kita@nagasaki-u.ac.jp

T. Harada (ed.), *Endometriosis: Pathogenesis and Treatment*,
DOI 10.1007/978-4-431-54421-0_26, © Springer Japan 2014

26.1 Ovarian Reserve Testing in Women with Endometriosis

26.1.1 Physiological Basis of Ovarian Reserve Testing

The human ovary contains limited numbers of primordial follicles. These dormant follicles are activated and also demised incessantly from fetus to the age of menopause. Loss of nongrowing follicles in women's ovary is age dependent. Age-related declining curve of ovarian reserve resembles decline of women's fecundability along with age [1]. However, there are substantial variations in the decline of reproductive capacity with age [2]. These variations may be defined in part by several confounding variables. Indeed, Wallace et al. [3] showed that the estimated number of nongrowing follicle present in the ovaries gets wider variation after the age of 25 years, which indicates that factors other than age (e.g., smoking, BMI, parity, stress, systemic disease, etc.) become more important in determining the rate at which nongrowing follicles are lost through atresia.

Ovarian reserve is currently defined as the number and quality of the follicles left in the ovary at any given time [4]. The number of remaining primordial follicles in the ovary may define the number of follicular pool to be selected [3]. The size of follicular pool is closely related to selectable follicular cohort in stimulation cycles. Thus, women with decreased ovarian reserve will not be able to produce sufficient multiple follicular growth in IVF treatment, which is a major determinant of treatment success [5]. Response to gonadotropin may represent the size of the cohort of FSH-sensitive follicles in the ovaries and is directly related to the magnitude of ovarian reserve.

However, since not all the women with infertility receive ovulation induction and as individual ovarian reserve may show wide variation, tests of ovarian reserve to identify each reproductive potential may be valuable in particular clinical situations. In ART settings, testing ovarian reserve before initiation of treatment cycle may be useful in tailoring stimulation protocol. Ovarian reserve testing may also be useful to predict women's age at menopause. On the other hand, the markers of ovarian reserve can be used to evaluate surgical damage to normal ovarian tissue when one attempts to perform fertility sparing surgery for several indications including endometriosis. These tests may also be used to evaluate the effects of pharmaceutical chemicals, anticancer drugs, and hormonal agents on ovarian reserve.

26.1.2 The Varieties of Tests for Ovarian Reserve Determination

There are several clinical tests to estimate ovarian reserve [4]. However, it is still unclear that these tests can measure quality and quantity of remaining primordial follicles in ovaries precisely [4, 6]. Counting all the follicles present in serial sections of whole ovary by histological analysis after oophorectomy may be a direct way to evaluate remaining primordial follicles in ovaries, but it cannot be applicable to reproductive aged women. Since follicles in the ovarian cortex may not distribute homogenously, a biopsied small sample of the ovarian cortex may not always represent remaining primordial follicles [7, 8]. Considering its invasiveness and in the context of ovarian reserve testing, ovarian biopsy may not serve as a useful test to estimate ovarian reserve [9].

Classically, serum FSH and estradiol (E2) levels in the early follicular phase (i.e., cycle day 2–4) had long been utilized as markers for ovarian reserve. Inhibin-B is also reported as a serum marker for ovarian reserve. Stimulation test using clomiphene citrate, gonadotropin, or GnRH agonist had been reported. Alternatively, ultrasonographic determination of antral follicle count (AFC) in the early follicular phase and ovarian volume may serve as surrogate markers for ovarian reserve instead of blood sampling [10, 11]. Although various markers and tests of ovarian reserve had been reported, the clinical value of testing for basal FSH and inhibin-B value is limited [4, 12]. Ultrasonographic markers, such as AFC and ovarian volume, correlate well with age-related decline of ovarian reserve. However, it is difficult to assess the exact number of antral follicles and ovarian volume of the cystic ovary, such as endometrioma, before cystectomy [13].

26.1.3 AMH: A Novel Marker for Ovarian Reserve

Recently, serum anti-Müllerian hormone (AMH) levels had got wide popularity to predict ovarian responsiveness in ART settings. AMH is a dimeric glycoprotein, belongs to the transforming growth factor-β family, and is produced solely by the granulosa cells of the recruited follicles until they become sensitive to FSH [14, 15]. The serum level of AMH declines with age, is menstrual cycle independent, and is unaffected by gonadotropin or GnRH agonist administration [16]. In addition, it is very sensitive to changes in ovarian reserve with advancing age and correlates well with antral follicle count [17]. Therefore, measurements of serum AMH may be superior to other markers of ovarian reserve, given its reliability and convenience, to indicate the number of growing follicles and estimate ovarian follicular reserve. However, although compromised response to controlled ovarian stimulation can be diagnosed, decreased AMH may not always be an absolute determinant of women's fecundability. For example, women with undetectable serum AMH value occasionally become pregnant [18]. As these limitations may be due to threshold of the present assay system, development of more sensitive detection method may bring about further understanding of the relationship between ovarian reserve testing by AMH and ovarian functions.

26.1.4 *Role of Ovarian Reserve Tests in Women with Endometriosis*

Infertility is the main concern of women with endometriosis. The cause of infertility in endometriosis is multifactorial and pathogenesis of endometriosis-associated infertility remains uncertain [19]. The ovary is one of the frequent anatomical locations in which endometriosis may develop. Although it is still controversial, diminished ovarian reserve after surgical intervention to ovarian endometriosis had been a large clinical concern in infertility care [20]. In addition, ovarian function may be distorted by the disease itself [21]. On the other hand, some reports argued that endometriosis is a significant confounding variable that affects the age of menopause [22, 23]. In this view, endometriosis and its associated events through women's reproductive life span, such as chronic inflammation, infertility, and repeated pelvic surgery, may bring about considerable effects on ovarian functions. Diminished ovarian reserve may be a key element of endometriosis-associated infertility and possible confounders in health issue in women with endometriosis at late reproductive stage. Therefore, accurate estimation of ovarian reserve in women with endometriosis may serve an important clinical role.

26.2 Surgery for Endometriosis and Ovarian Reserve

26.2.1 *Influence of Cystectomy for Endometrioma on Ovarian Reserve*

26.2.1.1 Ovarian Response After Cystectomy for Endometrioma

Laparoscopic cystectomy for endometrioma is common and seems to be feasible in terms of postoperative fecundability and recurrence rate compared with that of fenestration and coagulation of the cyst wall [24, 25]. However, the safety of this technique with respect to residual ovarian damage has been questioned [20]. On the other hand, there had been conflicting reports on ovarian response to ovulation induction in infertile women with previous surgical excision of endometrioma [26–29]. Under gonadotropin stimulation, the damage by surgery may be masked. Even skilled hands show excellent results, cystectomy for endometrioma may cause unavoidable risk of surgical injury to residual normal ovarian tissue [30]. This may cause loss of ovarian follicles in women who were operated on for endometrioma [31, 32]. According to a recent report, absence of follicular growth was observed in 13 % of operated ovaries, although this event never occurred in the contralateral gonad [33].

26.2.1.2 Effects of Cystectomy for Endometrioma on Serum AMH Levels

We previously demonstrated that serum AMH levels significantly decreased in women with endometrioma compared to that of women with other benign ovarian cyst after unilateral laparoscopic cystectomy [34]. Interestingly, postsurgical changes in serum AMH levels were significantly more prominent in women with normal ovarian tissue found in dissected cyst wall. In addition, multivariate analysis with several confounding variables revealed that type of the cyst (endometrioma) and presence of normal ovarian tissue in dissected specimen were significantly associated with postsurgical decline in serum AMH levels. However, when we analyzed the model with these two variables together, the statistical significance for the type of the cyst was lost. In other words, proper surgery avoiding damage to surrounding normal ovarian tissue may not result in overt loss of ovarian reserve compared to similar surgery applied to other normal benign ovarian cyst. Meta-analysis and systematic review of literatures evaluating the impact of surgery for endometriomas on ovarian reserve as determined by serum AMH showed a statistically significant decrease in serum AMH concentration after ovarian cystectomy [35, 36]. Studies utilizing several tests of ovarian reserve other than AMH, such as AFC and inhibin-B, also showed negative impact of cystectomy for endometriomas on ovarian reserve [37–39].

26.2.1.3 Time Course Change of Marker for Ovarian Reserve After Cystectomy for Endometrioma

Recently, several authors reported time course change in serum AMH value postsurgery up to 1 year. Sugita et al. [40] analyzed the pattern of sequential changes in the serum AMH levels within 1 year after cystectomy for endometriomas. Although serum AMH levels decreased in almost all cases immediately (at 1 month) after surgery, they found that 51 % of patients showed partial recovery of AMH levels at 1 year after surgery, and in these women, the number of follicles removed by surgery was significantly more compared to that of women who showed persistent decrease in AMH value at 1 year after surgery. Celik et al. [41] also reported serial change in postsurgical AMH levels and its associations with other clinicopathological factors. They found that serum AMH decreased significantly at the sixth month (61 %) postoperatively. The FSH level increased significantly at the sixth week but returned to normal at the sixth month. The AFC increased significantly at the sixth week and at the sixth month. These results may indicate that the acute decrease in the serum AMH levels caused by surgical removal of the ovarian cortex may result in alterations of selectable follicular cohort, which may affect the values of several ovarian reserve markers after ovarian cystectomy.

26.2.2 *Influence of Other Surgical Techniques for Endometrioma on Ovarian Reserve*

Surgical technique other than cystectomy, such as laser ablations or electrocoagulations of the cyst wall, may show different effects on ovarian reserve after surgery. Even the decreases in AFC and ovarian volume were found for both coagulation and cystectomy, but the decrease was statistically significantly more frequent in cystectomized ovaries than in coagulated ovaries. Also, in the in vitro fertilization cycles, the ovarian response to ovulation induction was statistically significantly reduced in cystectomized ovaries as compared with coagulated ovaries [42]. When compared with plasma energy ablation, cystectomy is responsible for a statistically significant decrease in ovarian volume and a statistically significant reduction in AFC. This data should be taken into account in therapeutic decision-making concerning women attempting pregnancy, especially where there are other risk factors for postoperative ovarian failure [43]. Three-stage laparoscopic management with CO_2 laser and GnRH analogs showed favorable results compared to cystectomy in terms of postsurgical serum AMH levels and echographic parameters for ovarian reserve [44, 45]. Combined technique with CO_2 laser vaporization and stripping of the cyst wall with postsurgical GnRHa therapy did not compromise postsurgical ovarian volume and AFC [46]. These results may indicate that selection of surgical technique may improve postoperative reduction of ovarian reserve. The overall efficacy of each surgical technique for endometriomas may be judged by postoperative fecundability including maintenance of ovarian reserve as well as recurrence rate and symptom improvement. Some reports argued associations between recurrence and postsurgical ovarian reserve as they found higher ovarian responsiveness in gonads that developed recurrent endometriomas [47].

26.3 Ovarian Reserve in Women with Endometriosis Did Not Undergo Ovarian Surgery

26.3.1 *The Effects of Unoperated Endometrioma on Ovarian Reserve*

The effects of endometriosis on ovarian reserve are largely contributed by surgical intervention to ovarian endometriosis. However, even women with endometriosis before surgical interventions or women with endometriosis without ovarian involvement may show diminished ovarian reserve. Endometriomas themselves could be linked to reduced ovarian reserve, and damage to normal ovarian tissue may precede surgery. In IVF patients with unilateral ovarian lesion, the presence of ovarian endometriomas is associated with a reduced responsiveness to gonadotropins comparing to those of contralateral intact gonads. This deleterious effect was more evident in women with larger and multiple lesion, and in those who were more responsive to ovarian hyperstimulation [48]. However, another study showed that the presence of an endometrioma does not markedly affect responsiveness to hyperstimulation [49]. By the determination of serum AMH levels, the presence of ovarian endometriomas is associated with a significant reduction in ovarian reserve. In addition, bilateral endometrioma exerts a more profound negative impact on ovarian reserve than unilateral endometrioma, regardless of either conservative or surgical intervention [50]. On the other hand, the rate of spontaneous ovulations significantly decreased in the ovaries with endometriomas [51]. As ovulation induction may compensate decreased ovarian function in ovaries with endometriomas, the presence of endometriomas per se may deteriorate ovarian reserve.

We recently demonstrated decreased follicular density, associated fibrosis, and deterioration of normal structure of ovarian cortex in ovaries that are affected by endometriomas [21]. By serial histological analysis, microscopic endometriotic foci on the surface of ovarian cortex were found and they showed extensive hemorrhage conjoined with infiltration of inflammatory cells and fibrosis [21]. In addition, the size of primordial follicles is significantly smaller and increased recruitment and atresia of early follicles were evidenced in the cortex of affected ovaries. These results may support endometriomas themselves that are the cause of diminished ovarian reserve in women with endometriosis. Deterioration of ovarian reserve may precede surgery and destructive surgery may exacerbate their reproductive potential further.

26.3.2 The Effects of Non-ovarian Endometriosis on Ovarian Reserve

Endometriosis that develops in other anatomical sites besides the ovary, such as pelvic peritoneal implants and rectovaginal nodules, is a common feature of endometriosis, and their pathogenesis may be different from ovarian endometriomas [52]. Presence of deep infiltrating endometriosis in addition to ovarian endometriomas negatively affects ovarian reserve in terms of antral follicle count and number of oocytes retrieved [53]. In infertile patients with minimal/mild endometriosis, although serum FSH did not show any difference compared to control women without endometriosis, decreased serum AMH levels were significantly lower [54]. However, other investigators reported that peritoneal endometriosis and ovarian endometriomas per se do not result in lower AMH levels. AMH levels are decreased in women with previous endometrioma surgery independently of the presence of current endometriomas [55]. Several confounding variables affecting ovarian reserve such as severity of intrapelvic inflammation and adhesion should be taken into account in women with and without ovarian involvement.

26.4 Summary and Perspective

Endometriosis can be regarded as a chronic disease that requires long-term medical or surgical management through women's reproductive life span. Cystectomy for endometrioma may cause significant detrimental effects on ovarian reserve. In addition, inflammation provoked by endometriosis may affect the homeostasis of dormant follicles in the ovarian cortex. Development and selection of surgical methods and search for suitable medical treatment to minimize the damage to normal ovarian tissue in women with endometriosis are urgently expected [56]. Further research may be warranted to determine the mechanism of diminished ovarian reserve in women with endometriosis.

References

1. Faddy MJ, Gosden RG, Gougeon A, Richardson SJ, Nelson JF. Accelerated disappearance of ovarian follicles in mid-life: implications for forecasting menopause. Hum Reprod. 1992;7:1342–6.
2. te Velde ER, Pearson PL. The variability of female reproductive ageing. Hum Reprod Update. 2002;8:141–54.
3. Wallace WH, Kelsey TW. Human ovarian reserve from conception to the menopause. PLoS One. 2010;5:e8772.
4. Broekmans FJ, Kwee J, Hendriks DJ, Mol BW, Lambalk CB. A systematic review of tests predicting ovarian reserve and IVF outcome. Hum Reprod Update. 2006;12:685–718.
5. Sunkara SK, Rittenberg V, Raine-Fenning N, Bhattacharya S, Zamora J, Coomarasamy A. Association between the number of eggs and live birth in IVF treatment: an analysis of 400 135 treatment cycles. Hum Reprod. 2011;26:1768–74.
6. Bukman A, Heineman MJ. Ovarian reserve testing and the use of prognostic models in patients with subfertility. Hum Reprod Update. 2001;7:581–90.
7. Qu J, Godin PA, Nisolle M, Donnez J. Distribution and epidermal growth factor receptor expression of primordial follicles in human ovarian tissue before and after cryopreservation. Hum Reprod. 2000;15:302–10.
8. Schmidt KL, Byskov AG, Nyboe Andersen A, Müller J, Yding AC. Density and distribution of primordial follicles in single pieces of cortex from 21 patients and in individual pieces of cortex from three entire human ovaries. Hum Reprod. 2003;18:1158–64.
9. Kwok R, Johnson NP. Ovarian biopsy has no role as a routine diagnostic test of ovarian reserve: a systematic review. Reprod Biomed Online. 2012;24:492–5.
10. Scheffer GJ, Broekmans FJ, Dorland M, Habbema JD, Looman CW, te Velde ER. Antral follicle counts by transvaginal ultrasonography are related to age in women with proven natural fertility. Fertil Steril. 1999;72:845–51.
11. Wallace WH, Kelsey TW. Ovarian reserve and reproductive age may be determined from measurement of ovarian volume by transvaginal sonography. Hum Reprod. 2004;19:1612–7.
12. Bancsi LF, Broekmans FJ, Mol BW, Habbena JD, te Velde ER. Performance of basal follicle-stimulating hormone in the prediction of poor ovarian response and failure to become pregnant after in vitro fertilization: a meta-analysis. Fertil Steril. 2003;79:1091–100.
13. Maheswari A, Fowler P, Bhattacharya S. Assessment of ovarian reserve—should we perform tests of ovarian reserve routinely? Hum Reprod. 2006;21:2729–35.

14. van Rooij IA, Broekmans FJ, te Velde ER, Fauser BC, Bancsi LF, de Jong FH, Themmen AP. Serum anti-Müllerian hormone levels: a novel measure of ovarian reserve. Hum Reprod. 2002;17:3065–71.
15. Visser JA, Themmen AP. Anti-Mullerian hormone and folliculogenesis. Mol Cell Endocrinol. 2005;234:81–6.
16. Seifer DB, MacLaughlin DT. Mullerian inhibiting substance is an ovarian growth factor of emerging clinical significance. Fertil Steril. 2007;88:539–46.
17. Hansen KR, Hodnett GM, Knowlton N, Craig LB. Correlation of ovarian reserve tests with histologically determined primordial follicle number. Fertil Steril. 2011;95:170–5.
18. Weghofer A, Dietrich W, Barad DH, Gleicher N. Live birth chances in women with extremely low-serum anti-Mullerian hormone levels. Hum Reprod. 2011;26:1905–9.
19. Ozkan S, Murk W, Arici A. Endometriosis and infertility: epidemiology and evidence-based treatments. Ann N Y Acad Sci. 2008;1127:92–100.
20. Busacca M, Vignali M. Endometrioma excision and ovarian reserve: a dangerous relation. J Minim Invasive Gynecol. 2009;16:142–8.
21. Kitajima M, Defrère S, Dolmans MM, Colette S, Squifflet J, Van Langendonckt A, Donnez J. Endometriomas as a possible cause of reduced ovarian reserve in women with endometriosis. Fertil Steril. 2011;96:685–91.
22. Yasui T, Hayashi K, Mizunuma H, Kubota T, Aso T, Matsumura Y, Lee JS, Suzuki S. Association of endometriosis-related infertility with age at menopause. Maturitas. 2011;69:279–83.
23. Pokoradi AJ, Iversen L, Hannaford PC. Factors associated with age of onset and type of menopause in a cohort of UK women. Am J Obstet Gynecol. 2011;205:34.e1–13.
24. Canis M, Mage G, Pouly JL, Wattiez A, Manhes H, Bruhat MA. Laparoscopic diagnosis of adnexal cystic masses: a 12-year experience with long-term follow-up. Obstet Gynecol. 1994;83:707–12.
25. Alborzi S, Momtahan M, Parsanezhad ME, Dehbashi S, Zolghadri J, Alborzi S. A prospective randomized study comparing laparoscopic ovarian cystectomy versus fenestration and coagulation in patients with endometriomas. Fertil Steril. 2004;82:1633–7.
26. Loh FH, Tan AT, Kumar J, Ng SC. Ovarian response after laparoscopic ovarian cystectomy for endometriotic cysts in 132 monitored cycles. Fertil Steril. 1999;72:316–21.
27. Ho HY, Lee RK, Hwu YM, Lin MH, Su JT, Tsai YC. Poor response to ovaries with endometrioma previously treated with cystectomy to controlled ovarian hyperstimulation. J Assist Reprod Genet. 2002;19:507–11.
28. Somigliana E, Ragni G, Benedetti F, Borroni R, Vegetti W, Crosignani PG. Does laparoscopic excision of endometriotic ovarian cysts significantly affect ovarian reserve? Insights from IVF cycles. Hum Reprod. 2003;18:2450–3.
29. Ragni G, Somigliana E, Benedetti F, Paffoni A, Vegetti W, Restelli L, Crosignani PG. Damage to ovarian reserve associated with laparoscopic excision of endometriomas: a quantitative rather than a qualitative injury. Am J Obstet Gynecol. 2005;193:1908–14.
30. Biacchiardi CP, Piane LD, Camanni M, Deltetto F, Delpiano EM, Marchino GL, Gennarelli G, Revelli A. Laparoscopic stripping of endometriomas negatively affects ovarian follicular reserve even if performed by experienced surgeons. Reprod Biomed Online. 2011;23:740–6.
31. Muzii L, Bellati F, Bianchi A, Palaia I, Manci N, Zullo MA, et al. Laparoscopic stripping of endometriomas: a randomized trial on different surgical techniques. Part II: pathological results. Hum Reprod. 2005;20:1987–92.
32. Dilek U, Pata O, Tataroglu C, Aban M, Dilek S. Excision of endometriotic cyst wall may cause loss of functional ovarian tissue. Fertil Steril. 2006;85:758–60.
33. Benaglia L, Somigliana E, Vighi V, Ragni G, Vercellini P, Fedele L. Rate of severe ovarian damage following surgery for endometriomas. Hum Reprod. 2010;25:678–82.
34. Kitajima M, Khan KN, Hiraki K, Inoue T, Fujishita A, Masuzaki H. Changes in serum anti-Müllerian hormone levels may predict damage to residual normal ovarian tissue after laparoscopic surgery for women with ovarian endometrioma. Fertil Steril. 2011;95:2589–91. e1.

35. Raffi F, Metwally M, Amer S. The impact of excision of ovarian endometrioma on ovarian reserve: a systematic review and meta-analysis. J Clin Endocrinol Metab. 2012;97:3146–54.
36. Somigliana E, Berlanda N, Benaglia L, Viganò P, Vercellini P, Fedele L. Surgical excision of endometriomas and ovarian reserve: a systematic review on serum antimüllerian hormone level modifications. Fertil Steril. 2012;98:1531–8.
37. Almog B, Sheizaf B, Shalom-Paz E, Shehata F, Al-Talib A, Tulandi T. Effects of excision of ovarian endometrioma on the antral follicle count and collected oocytes for in vitro fertilization. Fertil Steril. 2010;94:2340–2.
38. Ercan CM, Duru NK, Karasahin KE, Coksuer H, Dede M, Baser I. Ultrasonographic evaluation and anti-mullerian hormone levels after laparoscopic stripping of unilateral endometriomas. Eur J Obstet Gynecol Reprod Biol. 2011;158:280–4.
39. Coric M, Goluza T, Juras J. Inhibin B for assessment of ovarian reserve after laparoscopic treatment of ovarian endometriomas. Int J Gynaecol Obstet. 2012;116:169–70.
40. Sugita A, Iwase A, Goto M, Nakahara T, Nakamura T, Kondo M, Osuka S, Mori M, Saito A, Kikkawa F. One-year follow-up of serum antimüllerian hormone levels in patients with cystectomy: are different sequential changes due to different mechanisms causing damage to the ovarian reserve? Fertil Steril. 2013;100:516–22.e3.
41. Celik HG, Dogan E, Okyay E, Ulukus C, Saatli B, Uysal S, Koyuncuoglu M. Effect of laparoscopic excision of endometriomas on ovarian reserve: serial changes in the serum antimüllerian hormone levels. Fertil Steril. 2012;97:1472–8.
42. Var T, Batioglu S, Tonguc E, Kahyaoglu I. The effect of laparoscopic ovarian cystectomy versus coagulation in bilateral endometriomas on ovarian reserve as determined by antral follicle count and ovarian volume: a prospective randomized study. Fertil Steril. 2011;95:2247–50.
43. Roman H, Auber M, Mokdad C, Martin C, Diguet A, Marpeau L, Bourdel N. Ovarian endometrioma ablation using plasma energy versus cystectomy: a step toward better preservation of the ovarian parenchyma in women wishing to conceive. Fertil Steril. 2011;96:1396–400.
44. Pados G, Tsolakidis D, Assimakopoulos E, Athanatos D, Tarlatzis B. Sonographic changes after laparoscopic cystectomy compared with three-stage management in patients with ovarian endometriomas: a prospective randomized study. Hum Reprod. 2010;25:672–7.
45. Tsolakidis D, Pados G, Vavilis D, Athanatos D, Tsalikis T, Giannakou A, Tarlatzis BC. The impact on ovarian reserve after laparoscopic ovarian cystectomy versus three-stage management in patients with endometriomas: a prospective randomized study. Fertil Steril. 2010;94:71–7.
46. Donnez J, Lousse JC, Jadoul P, Donnez O, Squifflet J. Laparoscopic management of endometriomas using a combined technique of excisional (cystectomy) and ablative surgery. Fertil Steril. 2010;94:28–32.
47. Somigliana E, Benaglia L, Vercellini P, Paffoni A, Ragni G, Fedele L. Recurrent endometrioma and ovarian reserve: biological connection or surgical paradox? Am J Obstet Gynecol. 2011;204:529.e1-5.
48. Somigliana E, Infantino M, Benedetti F, Arnoldi M, Calanna G, Ragni G. The presence of ovarian endometriomas is associated with a reduced responsiveness to gonadotropins. Fertil Steril. 2006;86:192–6.
49. Benaglia L, Pasin R, Somigliana E, Vercellini P, Ragni G, Fedele L. Unoperated ovarian endometriomas and responsiveness to hyperstimulation. Hum Reprod. 2011;26:1356–61.
50. Hwu YM, Wu FS, Li SH, Sun FJ, Lin MH, Lee RK. The impact of endometrioma and laparoscopic cystectomy on serum anti-Müllerian hormone levels. Reprod Biol Endocrinol. 2011;9:80.
51. Benaglia L, Somigliana E, Vercellini P, Abbiati A, Ragni G, Fedele L. Endometriotic ovarian cysts negatively affect the rate of spontaneous ovulation. Hum Reprod. 2009;24:2183–6.
52. Nisolle M, Donnez J. Peritoneal endometriosis, ovarian endometriosis, and adenomyotic nodules of the rectovaginal septum are three different entities. Fertil Steril. 1997;68:585–96.

53. Papaleo E, Ottolina J, Viganò P, Brigante C, Marsiglio E, De Michele F, Candiani M. Deep pelvic endometriosis negatively affects ovarian reserve and the number of oocytes retrieved for in vitro fertilization. Acta Obstet Gynecol Scand. 2011;90:878–84.
54. Lemos NA, Arbo E, Scalco R, Weiler E, Rosa V, Cunha-Filho JS. Decreased anti-Müllerian hormone and altered ovarian follicular cohort in infertile patients with mild/minimal endometriosis. Fertil Steril. 2008;89:1064–8.
55. Streuli I, de Ziegler D, Gayet V, Santulli P, Bijaoui G, de Mouzon J, Chapron C. In women with endometriosis anti-Müllerian hormone levels are decreased only in those with previous endometrioma surgery. Hum Reprod. 2012;27:3294–303.
56. Jadoul P, Kitajima M, Donnez O, Squifflet J, Donnez J. Surgical treatment of ovarian endometriomas: state of the art? Fertil Steril. 2012;98:556–63.

Chapter 27
Infertility Treatment of Endometriosis Patients

Kaori Koga, Osamu Yoshino, Yasushi Hirota, Tetsuya Hirata, Miyuki Harada, and Yutaka Osuga

Abstract Endometriosis is common in infertile patients, but infertility treatment of endometriosis patients is controversial and varied. This article summarizes evidence concerning infertility treatment of endometriosis patients. Endometriosis impairs fertility by causing both anatomical and biochemical distortion in female reproductive system. Medical treatment of endometriosis does not improve fertility, whereas there is some evidence that surgery for mild endometriosis does. There is conflicting evidence regarding removal of endometriomas due to the potential impact on ovarian reserve. Assisted reproductive technology (ART) improves pregnancy rates, although the pregnancy rates are lower than for women without endometriosis. Some women with infertility and endometriosis may benefit from a combination of medical treatment, ART, and surgery. The decision about whether to undergo laparoscopy or superovulation (SO) with intrauterine insemination (IUI) or pursue ART will depend on a variety of factors such as the patient's age and symptoms, other infertility factors, risk of surgery, the presence of endometrioma, and ovarian reserve.

Keywords Assisted reproductive technology (ART) • Endometriosis • Infertility • Laparoscopy

27.1 Introduction

Management of infertility with endometriosis raises a number of complex clinical questions. This article will review the current literature regarding endometriosis-associated infertility including its pathophysiology and treatment.

K. Koga (✉) • Y. Hirota • T. Hirata • M. Harada • Y. Osuga
Obstetrics and Gynecology, The University of Tokyo, Tokyo, Japan
e-mail: kawotan-tky@umin.ac.jp

O. Yoshino
Obstetrics and Gynecology, University of Toyama, Toyama, Japan

T. Harada (ed.), *Endometriosis: Pathogenesis and Treatment*,
DOI 10.1007/978-4-431-54421-0_27,

27.1.1 Epidemiology of Endometriosis and Infertility

The fecundity rate in normal couples is in the range of 15–20 % per month and decreases with age of the female partner [1]. In contrast, in women with untreated endometriosis, monthly fecundability is 2–10 % [2]. Early studies suggested that 25–50 % of infertile women have endometriosis and that 30–50 % of women with endometriosis are infertile [3]. Other reports have confirmed that infertile women are 6 to 8 times more likely to have endometriosis than fertile women [4].

27.1.2 Mechanisms by Which Endometriosis Adversely Impacts Fertility

Endometriosis impacts fertility in both mechanical and biochemical manners. Mechanically, pelvic adhesions accompanied with endometriosis cause anatomical distortions and these impair oocyte release from the ovary or inhibit ovum pickup or transport by fallopian tubes. Adhesions may also cause abnormal myometrial contractions and impair fertilization and embryo transport [5]. Biochemically, endometriosis is known to alter peritoneal immune environment, endocrine status, and oocyte/embryo quality. Many studies demonstrated that peritoneal fluid even in mild endometriosis contains increased concentrations of prostaglandins, proteases, and inflammatory cytokines such as IL-1, IL-6, and TNFα [6] and these alterations may have adverse effects on oocyte, sperm, embryo, and fallopian tube functions. It has also been proposed that women with endometriosis may have endocrine and ovulatory disorders, including luteinized unruptured follicle syndrome, luteal phase dysfunctions, abnormal follicular growth, and premature as well as multiple luteinizing hormone (LH) surges [7]. In addition, abnormalities of oocyte and embryo quality have been described in women with endometriosis. In oocyte donation cycles, when donor oocytes from women with endometriosis are transferred into women without endometriosis, implantation rates are lower, suggesting that the embryo quality is reduced in women with endometriosis [8]. At the same time, newer research identifies alternations in gene expression and genetic defects in the endometrium of women with endometriosis [9, 10]. Taken together, it seems to be multifactorial, involving mechanical and biochemical mechanisms by which endometriosis causes infertility, and this indicates that controlling of this disease may improve fertility.

27.2 Expectant Management

Women with mid-moderate endometriosis are able to conceive without any medical or surgical intervention, although the fecundability is significantly lower compared with women without endometriosis. Multiple studies evaluating patients with endometriosis who undergo expectant management report their fecundity rate to be around 2.40–3.0 per 100 person-months [11, 12]. Therefore, the option of expectant management is not unreasonable for patients with mid-moderate disease, especially for young patients. In contrast, in women with more severe disease, pregnancy rates are much lower [13], and expectant management in those with severe disease is only delaying the start of effective treatment.

27.3 Medical Treatment

Medications used for controlling endometriosis are hormonal medications including combined oral contraceptives (OC), progestins, danazol, and gonadotropin-releasing hormone agonist (GnRHa). Although these medications may help reduce pain, they have shown no benefit in the management of endometriosis-associated infertility. A large meta-analysis of 23 trials including more than 3,000 women demonstrated that there was no difference in pregnancy or live birth rates with preceding ovulation suppression with OC, progestins, or danazol in subfertile women with endometriosis (odds ratio (OR) = 1.02, 95 % confidence interval (CI), 0.70–1.52, $P = 0.082$) [14]. Not only was there no benefit from ovulation suppression, but it also delayed the patient from conceiving while taking the suppressive agents. Therefore, medical therapy should be discouraged in patients with endometriosis who wish to conceive [13].

27.4 Surgical Treatment

Surgery for endometriosis can be both diagnostic and therapeutic. Surgical treatment of endometriosis aims to remove macroscopic endometriosis and restore normal pelvic anatomy, as well as normal pelvic immunological and hormonal environment. Surgery, however, may not be able to completely reverse the chronic inflammatory state or repair severe anatomical distortion and might even negatively affect fertility by for instance reducing ovarian function. It is therefore important to weigh up the benefits and the harm when measuring the effect of surgery.

27.4.1 Mild Endometriosis

The Canadian Collaborative Group on Endometriosis conducted a RCT with 341 women to determine whether laparoscopic surgery enhanced fecundity in infertile women with minimal or mild endometriosis. They found that either resection or ablation of minimal and mild endometriosis significantly enhanced fecundity in infertile women compared with diagnostic laparoscopy alone (cumulative probability of pregnancy 30.7 % and 17.7 %, $P = 0.006$) [11]. However, another RCT of 101 women with minimal to mild endometriosis demonstrated no difference in live birth rates between women who underwent laparoscopic treatment of endometriosis by ablation or resection compared with diagnostic laparoscopy alone (19.6 % and 22.2 %, OR = 0.75, 95 % CI, 0.30–1.85) [15]. Subsequently, a Cochrane review concluded that in infertile patients with early-stage endometriosis, surgical treatment, compared with diagnostic laparoscopy alone, had significant benefits in clinical pregnancy and in ongoing pregnancy after 20 weeks (OR = 1.66, 95 % CI, 1.09–2.51 and OR = 1.94, 95 % CI, 1.09–2.51, respectively) [16, 17].

These studies suggest that there may be a role for laparoscopic surgery of mild-to-moderate disease to improve fertility. However, it should be kept in mind that overall pregnancy rate in these studies remains still very low. The overall absolute difference is 8.6 % in favor of laparoscopic surgery [18], and this means that the number of women who needed to undergo laparoscopic surgery for one additional clinical pregnancy is approximately 12. Thus, although there is objective evidence that surgery is better than no treatment, surgery may not always be the best treatment to improve fertility.

27.4.2 Severe Endometriosis

There are few RCT studying the effects of surgery on fecundity in advanced-staged diseases, and thus, there is insufficient evidence to recommended surgery for the treatment of infertility in severe disease. Our previous study analyzed pregnancy outcome in 186 infertile women for a follow-up period of 18 months after laparoscopy and found that the pregnancy rate for women with minimal/mild endometriosis appeared to be the highest, followed by the non-endometriosis group and the moderate/severe endometriosis group (45.1, 33.8, and 27.6 %, respectively) [19, 20]. Accordingly, the benefit of laparoscopic surgery in increasing fecundity seems high in mild endometriosis but limited in severe endometriosis, and alternative therapies should be considered for those with severe endometriosis.

27.4.3 Ovarian Endometrioma

A 2008 Cochrane review examined the current literature regarding laparoscopic ablation versus excision of endometriomas and found that the excision of the cyst was associated with a subsequent increased spontaneous pregnancy rate in women who had documented prior subfertility (OR = 5.21, 95 % CI, 2.04–13.29) [21]. This review also identified an RCT which demonstrated an increased ovarian follicular response to gonadotropin in those who underwent excisional surgery compared with ablative surgery [21]. These and other observational studies suggest that, in women with stage III/IV endometriosis who have no other identifiable infertility factors, surgery may increase fertility [22]; however, one may be aware of a possible adverse consequence, the loss of viable ovarian cortex [23]. After the first infertility operation, additional surgery for recurrent endometriosis has only rarely increased fecundity, and these patients may be better treated by assisted reproductive technology (ART) [24].

27.4.4 Deep Endometriosis

Vercellini et al. conducted a nonrandomized study of 105 women comparing surgery with expectant management. They found no difference in a 12-month probability of conception (20.5 % in surgical group and 34.7 % in expectant $P=0.12$) [25]. A large prospective cohort study of 500 women treated with laparoscopic rectal shaving of endometriotic lesions found that 57 % of women wishing to conceive had conceived naturally in a mean follow-up of 3.1 years [26]. A nonrandomized study by Stepinewska et al. looked at the effect of removing bowel endometriosis and found that women who had a colorectal segmental resection for bowel endometriosis had a higher monthly fecundity rate (MFR) than women with bowel disease left unexcised (MFR 2.3 % in resection of bowel disease and 0.84 % in bowel disease left $P=0.03$) [27]. However, the complication rate in the bowel resection was considerably high. Therefore, surgery should be conducted only when the benefit overweighs the complication risk. For instance, deep endometriosis is always accompanied with severe pain requiring ovulation suppression, but when a patient wishes to conceive, she should discontinue hormonal treatments. Therefore, surgery for deep endometriosis should be primarily aimed for reducing pain and in turn allowing patients to conceive and should not be performed only for the aim of improving fertility.

27.5 Superovulation (SO) and Intrauterine Insemination (IUI)

In a crossover RCT among patients with unexplained infertility or surgically corrected endometriosis, the pregnancy rate per cycle was significantly higher with four cycles of clomiphene citrate/IUI than with four cycles of timed intercourse (9.5 % vs. 3.3 %, respectively) [24]. An RCT among 49 women with stage I/II endometriosis and infertility compared three cycles of gonadotropin/IUI with 6 months of expectant management and found that the pregnancy rate per cycle was 0.15 % in the gonadotropin/IUI group and 0.045 % in the untreated group ($P<0.05$) [28]. Another study reported increased fecundity with gonadotropin therapy compared to no treatment (7.3 % vs. 2.8 %, respectively) in women with infertility and minimal/mild endometriosis [29, 30]. A much larger study by Tummon et al. randomized 103 patients (311 cycles) and found that the cumulative live birth rates was fivefold higher following SO/IUI (OR = 5.6, 95 % CI, 1.8–17.4) [30]. Nevertheless, there is strong evidence from a large number of observational studies that the outcomes following SO/IUI in women with endometriosis are more unfavorable compared with women with other etiologies. The largest of these studies analyzed 14,968 cycles in 3,371 couples and found that women with endometriosis had a 30 % lower chance of achieving pregnancy than women without endometriosis (adjusted OR = 0.71, 95 % CI, 0.54–0.92) [31]. Collectively, there is evidence to support SO/IUI in women with endometriosis, especially with mild, surgically corrected endometriosis; however, the benefit is still lower than in infertile women without endometriosis. It is also important to mention that SO with clomiphene or gonadotropin may potentially enhance the progress of endometriosis and thus in turn may negatively impact on the long-term fecundity.

27.6 Assisted Reproductive Technology (ART)

In vitro fertilization (IVF) is currently the most effective treatment of endometriosis-associated infertility, although the presence of endometriosis seems to adversely affect IVF results.

27.6.1 ART and Endometriosis

Barnhart et al. performed a meta-analysis of 22 observational studies and concluded that women with endometriosis have poorer IVF outcomes than women with tubal infertility (OR = 0.56, 95 % CI, 0.44–0.70) [32]. In addition, women with more severe disease had worse outcomes than women with minimal/mild disease (OR = 0.60, 95 % CI, 0.42–0.87) [32]. This same study also showed that there were significant decreases in fertilization and implantation rates and in the number of oocyte retrieved in patients with endometriosis [32]. While endometriosis may affect IVF results, IVF maximizes cycle fecundability for those with endometriosis, especially in those with distortion of pelvic anatomy due to moderate or severe disease. In one RCT, a subgroup of 21 women with endometriosis and infertility had IVF ($n = 15$) or expectant management ($n = 6$). None of the women in the expectant management group became pregnant compared to five of the 15 women who received IVF (33 %) [33]. These findings suggest that woman with endometriosis, especially with severe condition, should be encouraged to undergo ART, although at the same time she should be informed that the success rate of ART is lower than that in women with other infertility factors.

Table 27.1 Pros and cons of expectant and surgical management of endometriomas prior to ART

Expectant	Surgery
Pros	
Avoid surgery	Exclusive malignancy
Lower FSH doses	Relieve pain
Increased E2	Reduce the risk of cyst complications (e.g., rupture)
Increased follicles	Facilitate access to oocyte retrieval
Cons	
Pain	Risk of damage of normal ovarian tissue
No histological diagnosis	Reduced number of oocytes collected
Risk of pelvic infection following oocyte retrieval	Risks of surgical complication

27.6.2 *Surgical Treatment Prior to ART*

27.6.2.1 Ovarian Endometrioma

The benefit of surgical treatment of endometriomas prior to IVF is still controversial. There are no randomized trials comparing laparoscopic excision to expectant management before IVF/intracytoplasmic sperm injection (ICSI) cycles. One systematic review found that surgery (aspiration or cystectomy) versus expectant management showed no evidence of a benefit for clinical pregnancy with either technique [34]. Another meta-analysis of five nonrandomized trials found that excision of an endometrioma is no better than no treatment prior to IVF [35]. These findings suggest that surgery for endometrioma prior to scheduled IVF/ICSI does not improve the result of ART.

However, there are possible benefits of surgical treatment for endometrioma prior to ART, including prevention of possible ruptured endometrioma, facilitation of oocyte retrieval, detection of occult malignancy [36], avoidance of contamination of follicular fluid with endometrioma content, and prevention of progression of endometriosis and these benefits should be taken into account when surgery is considered. On the contrary, clinicians should be also aware of the disadvantages of surgery including surgical trauma, surgical complications, economic costs, and, most importantly, the potential of decreasing ovarian response [37, 38]. There is evidence that ovarian surgery reduces the number of oocytes retrieved, reduces peak estradiol levels, and increases total FSH requirement [38, 39]. A prospective study also demonstrated that ovarian surgery led to complete ovarian failure in the operated ovary in 13 % of the cases [40]. Therefore, a removal of an endometrioma is not warranted for infertility alone, and clinicians balance the benefits and the risk when considering surgery prior to ART. The pros and cons of the management of endometriomas prior to ART are summarized in Table 27.1.

27.6.2.2 Deep Endometriosis

A nonrandomized prospective cohort study of 179 women with deep infiltrating endometriosis and infertility examined the impact of surgery prior to IVF versus IVF alone. The pregnancy rate in the surgery group following IVF was 41 %, and the no surgery group was 24 % ($P = 0.004$) suggesting a benefit to removing deep disease prior to IVF [41]. However, surgery for deep endometriosis is a major surgery with inherent morbidity and thus, decision to perform surgery must be made on an individual basis with extensive counseling.

27.6.3 Medical Treatment Prior to ART

Multiple studies have shown that prolonged GnRHa treatment before IVF may improve fertility rates in advanced endometriosis [42–44]. A Cochrane review summarized the findings of these three RCTs, which collectively comprised 165 women with infertility and severe endometriosis. The pretreatment with GnRHa significantly increased the clinical pregnancy and the live birth rates compared with no pretreatment (OR = 4.28, 95 % CI, 2.00–9.15 and OR = 9.19, 95 % CI, 1.08–78.22, respectively). Proposed mechanisms are via increased retrieved oocytes, higher implantation rates, and reduced preclinical abortions [45, 46]. Similar to GnRHa, the use of OC has been shown to improve outcomes. De Ziegler et al. conducted a nonrandomized comparison and suggested that ART outcomes following 6–8 weeks of OC in women with endometriosis are comparable with the outcomes of age-matched controls without endometriosis [47]. Regarding patients with endometriomas, the effectiveness of GnRHa and OC is rather controversial. A Cochran review in 2010 concluded that administration of GnRHa does not significantly affect the clinical pregnancy rate when given before ART in patients with endometriomas, despite the pretreatment improved ovarian response and increased the number of mature oocytes aspirated. In contrast, the study by De Ziegler et al. showed improvement using pre-ART continuous OC therapy for 6–8 weeks even in those with endometriomas. Collectively, it seems that medical treatment for endometriosis seems to benefit on ART outcomes; however, one should also be aware that the medical treatment delays the commencement of ART, and this may also impact the outcome of ART especially in patients with advanced age.

27.7 Conclusions

Given the abovementioned non-RCT and RCT evidences, the Japanese Society of Obstetrics and Gynecology (JSOG) published a guideline and recommendations for the management of women with endometriosis (Fig. 27.1) (JSOG) [48].

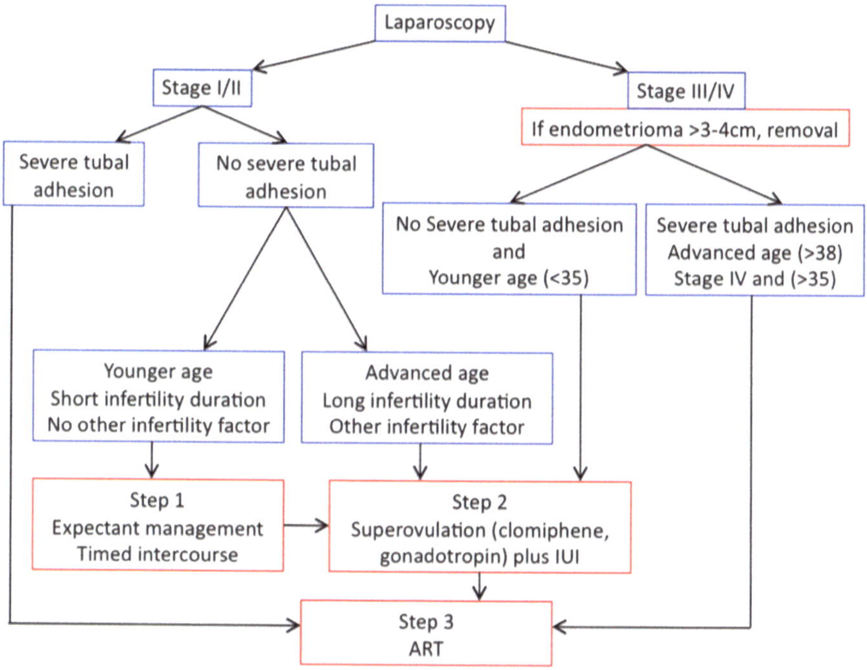

Fig. 27.1 Algorism for management of infertile patents with endometriosis published by the Japanese Society of Obstetrics and Gynecology (JSOG)

For infertile women with suspected endometriosis, laparoscopy is recommended. If laparoscopy is performed, ablation or excision of visible endometriosis should be considered. Expectant management after laparoscopy is an option for younger women.

For infertile women with stage I/II endometriosis, factors such as the women's age, duration of infertility, and other infertility factors must be taken into consideration. When laparoscopy is undergone, ablation or excision of visible endometriosis should be performed. Expectant management or timed intercourse is an option for women in younger age (age < 30) and shorter infertility period (<3 years) and no other infertility factor. If a woman does not conceive after 3–6 months of expectant management, SO with clomiphene or gonadotropin with IUI should be considered and if this also fails, step-up to ART is recommended. For women with advanced age (age > 30) or with longer infertility duration (>3 years) or with other infertility factor, physicians should not manage them expectantly, but consider starting SO with IUI immediately. For women with severe tubal adhesion, immediate ART is recommended.

For infertile women with stage III/IV endometriosis, adhesiolysis and removal of peritoneal lesion should be done at laparoscopy. If the endometrioma is large ($>$3–4 cm), removal should be performed to confirm the diagnosis histologically. Following the laparoscopy, the fecundity rate without assisted treatment is very

Table 27.2 International guidelines on surgical treatment of endometriosis-associated infertility

	Recommendation			
Clinical condition	ESHRE 2005 [49]	ASRM 2012 [18]	RCOG 2006 [50]	JSOG 2010 [48]
Minimal/mild endometriosis (stage I–II disease)	Limited benefit: surgery recommended	Small benefit: surgery recommended	Demonstrated benefit: surgery recommended	Small benefit: surgery recommended
Moderate/severe endometriosis (stage III–IV disease)	Possible but unproven benefit: surgery recommended	Possible benefit: surgery recommended	Possible benefit: recommendation uncertain	Possible benefit: surgery recommended though still controversial
Postoperative adjuvant treatment	No benefit: not recommended	No benefit: not recommended	No benefit: not recommended	No recommendation
Surgery before IVF	Recommended if endometrioma $\geq$4 cm	Doubtful benefit: no recommendation	Recommended if endometrioma $\geq$4 cm	Recommended if endometrioma >3 – 4 cm
Recurrent endometriosis	No recommendation	Second-line surgery not recommended	No recommendation	Second-line surgery not recommended

low, thus discouraging expectant management. ART should be considered if 6–8 cycles of SO and IUI failed in younger (age < 37) women or immediately after laparoscopy in women with advanced age (age > 38). Table 27.2 summarizes the international guidelines on surgical treatment of endometriosis-associated infertility [18, 48, 49, 50].

In any stage and condition of endometriosis, female age is the most important factor in designing therapy. After age 35, there is a significant decrease in fecundity. In addition, fecundity may be decreased due to the additive adverse effects of endometriosis progression as age increased. Consequently, in the older infertile women with endometriosis, a more aggressive therapeutic plan especially with ART may be reasonable. The patient with endometriosis should be informed that she may have a decreased success rate after ART compared to a woman undergoing ART for another indication, and the pregnancy rate will further decrease as her age advances.

In conclusion, the association between infertility and endometriosis is complex, and treatment alternatives for infertility with endometriosis have both risks and benefits. Complete and detailed information on these risks and benefits must be provided to infertile patients to allow unbiased choices among possible options.

References

1. Schwartz D, Mayaux MJ. Female fecundity as a function of age: results of artificial insemination in 2193 nulliparous women with azoospermic husbands. Federation CECOS. N Engl J Med. 1982;306(7):404–6. doi:10.1056/NEJM198202183060706.
2. Hughes EG, Fedorkow DM, Collins JA. A quantitative overview of controlled trials in endometriosis-associated infertility. Fertil Steril. 1993;59(5):963–70.
3. Counsellor V. Endometriosis. A clinical and surgical review. Am J Obstet Gynecol. 1938;36:877.
4. Verkauf BS. Incidence, symptoms, and signs of endometriosis in fertile and infertile women. J Fla Med Assoc. 1987;74(9):671–5.
5. Holoch KJ, Lessey BA. Endometriosis and infertility. Clin Obstet Gynecol. 2010;53 (2):429–38.
6. Koga K, Osuga Y, Taketani Y. Peritoneal environment in endometriosis. Nihon Rinsho. 2001;59 Suppl 1:48–56.
7. Schenken RS, Asch RH, Williams RF, Hodgen GD. Etiology of infertility in monkeys with endometriosis: luteinized unruptured follicles, luteal phase defects, pelvic adhesions, and spontaneous abortions. Fertil Steril. 1984;41(1):122–30.
8. Garrido N, Navarro J, Garcia-Velasco J, Remoh J, Pellice A, Simon C. The endometrium versus embryonic quality in endometriosis-related infertility. Hum Reprod Update. 2002;8 (1):95–103.
9. Giudice LC, Kao LC. Endometriosis. Lancet. 2004;364(9447):1789–99.
10. Lessey BA, Castelbaum AJ, Sawin SW, Buck CA, Schinnar R, Bilker W, Strom BL. Aberrant integrin expression in the endometrium of women with endometriosis. J Clin Endocrinol Metab. 1994;79(2):643–9.
11. Marcoux S, Maheux R, Berube S. Laparoscopic surgery in infertile women with minimal or mild endometriosis. Canadian Collaborative Group on Endometriosis. N Engl J Med. 1997;337(4):217–22.

12. Berube S, Marcoux S, Langevin M, Maheux R. Fecundity of infertile women with minimal or mild endometriosis and women with unexplained infertility. The Canadian Collaborative Group on Endometriosis. Fertil Steril. 1998;69(6):1034–41.
13. Ozkan S, Murk W, Arici A. Endometriosis and infertility: epidemiology and evidence-based treatments. Ann N Y Acad Sci. 2008;1127:92–100.
14. Hughes E, Brown J, Collins JJ, Farquhar C, Fedorkow DM, Vandekerckhove P. Ovulation suppression for endometriosis. Cochrane Database Syst Rev. 2007;3, CD000155.
15. Parazzini F. Ablation of lesions or no treatment in minimal-mild endometriosis in infertile women: a randomized trial. Gruppo Italiano per lo Studio dell'Endometriosi. Hum Reprod. 1999;14(5):1332–4.
16. Jacobson TZ, Duffy JM, Barlow D, Farquhar C, Koninckx PR, Olive D. Laparoscopic surgery for subfertility associated with endometriosis. Cochrane Database Syst Rev. 2010;1, CD001398.
17. Jacobson TZ, Barlow DH, Koninckx PR, Olive D, Farquhar C. Laparoscopic surgery for subfertility associated with endometriosis. Cochrane Database Syst Rev. 2002;4, CD001398.
18. Endometriosis and Infertility: A Committee Opinion. Fertil Steril. 2006;86(5 Suppl 1):S156–60.
19. Maruyama M, Osuga Y, Momoeda M, Yano T, Tsutsumi O, Taketani Y. Pregnancy rates after laparoscopic treatment. Differences related to tubal status and presence of endometriosis. J Reprod Med. 2000;45(2):89–93.
20. Osuga Y, Koga K, Tsutsumi O, Yano T, Maruyama M, Kugu K, Momoeda M, Taketani Y. Role of laparoscopy in the treatment of endometriosis-associated infertility. Gynecol Obstet Invest. 2002;53 Suppl 1:33–9.
21. Hart RJ, Hickey M, Maouris P, Buckett W. Excisional surgery versus ablative surgery for ovarian endometriomata. Cochrane Database Syst Rev. 2008;2, CD004992.
22. Schenken RS. Modern concepts of endometriosis. Classification and its consequences for therapy. J Reprod Med. 1998;43(3 Suppl):269–75.
23. Donnez J, Nisolle M, Gillet N, Smets M, Bassil S, Casanas-Roux F. Large ovarian endometriomas. Hum Reprod. 1996;11(3):641–6.
24. Deaton JL, Gibson M, Blackmer KM, Nakajima ST, Badger GJ, Brumsted JR. A randomized, controlled trial of clomiphene citrate and intrauterine insemination in couples with unexplained infertility or surgically corrected endometriosis. Fertil Steril. 1990;54(6):1083–8.
25. Vercellini P, Pietropaolo G, De Giorgi O, Daguati R, Pasin R, Crosignani PG. Reproductive performance in infertile women with rectovaginal endometriosis: is surgery worthwhile? Am J Obstet Gynecol. 2006;195(5):1303–10.
26. Donnez J, Squifflet J. Complications, pregnancy and recurrence in a prospective series of 500 patients operated on by the shaving technique for deep rectovaginal endometriotic nodules. Hum Reprod. 2010;25(8):1949–58.
27. Stepniewska A, Pomini P, Bruni F, Mereu L, Ruffo G, Ceccaroni M, Scioscia M, Guerriero M, Minelli L. Laparoscopic treatment of bowel endometriosis in infertile women. Hum Reprod. 2009;24(7):1619–25.
28. Fedele L, Bianchi S, Marchini M, Villa L, Brioschi D, Parazzini F. Superovulation with human menopausal gonadotropins in the treatment of infertility associated with minimal or mild endometriosis: a controlled randomized study. Fertil Steril. 1992;58(1):28–31.
29. Kemmann E, Ghazi D, Corsan G, Bohrer MK. Does ovulation stimulation improve fertility in women with minimal/mild endometriosis after laser laparoscopy? Int J Fertil Menopausal Stud. 1993;38(1):16–21.
30. Tummon IS, Asher LJ, Martin JS, Tulandi T. Randomized controlled trial of superovulation and insemination for infertility associated with minimal or mild endometriosis. Fertil Steril. 1997;68(1):8–12.
31. Steures P, van der Steeg JW, Mol BW, Eijkemans MJ, van der Veen F, Habbema JD, Hompes PG, Bossuyt PM, Verhoeve HR, van Kasteren YM, van Dop PA. Prediction of an ongoing pregnancy after intrauterine insemination. Fertil Steril. 2004;82(1):45–51. doi:10.1016/j.fertnstert.2003.12.028S0015028204006119 [pii].

32. Barnhart K, Dunsmoor-Su R, Coutifaris C. Effect of endometriosis on in vitro fertilization. Fertil Steril. 2002;77(6):1148–55.
33. Soliman S, Daya S, Collins J, Jarrell J. A randomized trial of in vitro fertilization versus conventional treatment for infertility. Fertil Steril. 1993;59(6):1239–44.
34. Benschop L, Farquhar C, van der Poel N, Heineman MJ. Interventions for women with endometrioma prior to assisted reproductive technology. Cochrane Database Syst Rev. 2010;11, CD008571.
35. Tsoumpou I, Kyrgiou M, Gelbaya TA, Nardo LG. The effect of surgical treatment for endometrioma on in vitro fertilization outcomes: a systematic review and meta-analysis. Fertil Steril. 2009;92(1):75–87.
36. Pearce CL, Templeman C, Rossing MA, Lee A, Near AM, Webb PM, Nagle CM, Doherty JA, Cushing-Haugen KL, Wicklund KG, Chang-Claude J, Hein R, Lurie G, Wilkens LR, Carney ME, Goodman MT, Moysich K, Kjaer SK, Hogdall E, Jensen A, Goode EL, Fridley BL, Larson MC, Schildkraut JM, Palmieri RT, Cramer DW, Terry KL, Vitonis AF, Titus LJ, Ziogas A, Brewster W, Anton-Culver H, Gentry-Maharaj A, Ramus SJ, Anderson AR, Brueggmann D, Fasching PA, Gayther SA, Huntsman DG, Menon U, Ness RB, Pike MC, Risch H, Wu AH, Berchuck A. Association between endometriosis and risk of histological subtypes of ovarian cancer: a pooled analysis of case–control studies. Lancet Oncol. 2012;13 (4):385–94.
37. Somigliana E, Vercellini P, Vigano P, Ragni G, Crosignani PG. Should endometriomas be treated before IVF-ICSI cycles? Hum Reprod Update. 2006;12(1):57–64.
38. Almog B, Sheizaf B, Shalom-Paz E, Shehata F, Al-Talib A, Tulandi T. Effects of excision of ovarian endometrioma on the antral follicle count and collected oocytes for in vitro fertilization. Fertil Steril. 2011;94(6):2340–2.
39. Demirol A, Guven S, Baykal C, Gurgan T. Effect of endometrioma cystectomy on IVF outcome: a prospective randomized study. Reprod Biomed Online. 2006;12(5):639–43.
40. Benaglia L, Somigliana E, Vighi V, Ragni G, Vercellini P, Fedele L. Rate of severe ovarian damage following surgery for endometriomas. Hum Reprod. 2010;25(3):678–82.
41. Bianchi PH, Pereira RM, Zanatta A, Alegretti JR, Motta EL, Serafini PC. Extensive excision of deep infiltrative endometriosis before in vitro fertilization significantly improves pregnancy rates. J Minim Invasive Gynecol. 2009;16(2):174–80.
42. Guo YH, Lu N, Zhang Y, Su YC, Wang Y, Zhang YL, Sun YP. Comparative study on the pregnancy outcomes of in vitro fertilization-embryo transfer between long-acting gonadotropin-releasing hormone agonist combined with transvaginal ultrasound-guided cyst aspiration and long-acting gonadotropin-releasing hormone agonist alone. Contemp Clin Trials. 2012;33 (6):1206–10.
43. Ozkan S, Arici A. Advances in treatment options of endometriosis. Gynecol Obstet Invest. 2009;67(2):81–91.
44. Surrey ES, Voigt B, Fournet N, Judd HL. Prolonged gonadotropin-releasing hormone agonist treatment of symptomatic endometriosis: the role of cyclic sodium etidronate and low-dose norethindrone "add-back" therapy. Fertil Steril. 1995;63(4):747–55.
45. Surrey ES, Silverberg KM, Surrey MW, Schoolcraft WB. Effect of prolonged gonadotropin-releasing hormone agonist therapy on the outcome of in vitro fertilization-embryo transfer in patients with endometriosis. Fertil Steril. 2002;78(4):699–704.
46. Olivennes F, Feldberg D, Liu HC, Cohen J, Moy F, Rosenwaks Z. Endometriosis: a stage by stage analysis–the role of in vitro fertilization. Fertil Steril. 1995;64(2):392–8.
47. de Ziegler D, Gayet V, Aubriot FX, Fauque P, Streuli I, Wolf JP, de Mouzon J, Chapron C. Use of oral contraceptives in women with endometriosis before assisted reproduction treatment improves outcomes. Fertil Steril. 2010;94(7):2796–9.
48. The general rules for clinical management of endometriosis. Jpn Soc Obstet Gynecol. 2010:59–61.
49. Kennedy S, Bergqvist A, Chapron C, D'Hooghe T, Dunselman G, Greb R, Hummelshoj L, Prentice A, Saridogan E. ESHRE guideline for the diagnosis and treatment of endometriosis. Hum Reprod. 2005;20(10):2698–704. doi:10.1093/humrep/dei135.
50. The investigation and management of endometriosis. Guideline No. 24. London: RCOG; 2006.

Chapter 28
Pregnancy Complications Associated with Endometriosis

Ivo Brosens and Giuseppe Benagiano

Abstract An association between endometriosis and infertility has been confirmed by a large number of studies, although mechanisms are still debated. The availability of in vitro fertilization represented a major step forward in achieving pregnancy in women with endometriosis, although in both peritoneal and ovarian disease, there is an adverse effect on ovulation rates, markers of ovarian reserve, and response to ovarian stimulation. Results have improved using intracytoplasmic sperm injection.

When achieved, pregnancy may be complicated by spontaneous hemoperitoneum, a rare but potentially fatal event. Data on incidence of preeclampsia, small for gestational age (SGA), and preterm birth are not univocal. A large cohort study found an increased risk of preterm birth; another observed no evidence for an association between endometriosis and risk of pregnancy hypertension, or preeclampsia; a third found increased rates of both preterm birth and SGA. In pregnancies complicated by the presence of ovarian endometrioma no differences have been observed in late pregnancy and neonatal outcomes.

Endometriosis patients seem to be at an increased risk of placenta previa and postpartum hemorrhage. An association has been found also when pregnancy is achieved through in vitro fertilization, suggesting that events around the time of implantation may be responsible.

With regard to pathophysiology, the hypothesis has been proposed that defective spiral artery remodeling may be the cause of major obstetrical syndromes in endometriosis and adenomyosis and that endometrial and myometrial junctional zone (MJZ) abnormalities represent a risk factor for the vascular development of the placental bed.

I. Brosens, M.D. (✉)
Leuven Institute for Fertility and Embryology, Catholic University Leuven, Leuven, Belgium
e-mail: ivo.brosens@med.kuleuven.be

G. Benagiano, M.D.
Department of Gynecology, Obstetrics and Urology, Sapienza University, Rome, Italy

T. Harada (ed.), *Endometriosis: Pathogenesis and Treatment*,
DOI 10.1007/978-4-431-54421-0_28,

Available evidence supports the idea of a reversibility of MJZ changes by appropriate medication inducing a prolonged hypoestrogenic period.

Keywords Adenomyosis • Endometriosis • Obstetrical complications • Spontaneous hemoperitoneum

28.1 Introduction

A clinical association between endometriosis and infertility has been suspected for more than 60 years [1, 2] and confirmed by a large number of studies, although mechanisms are still debated [3, 4]. Indeed, a study conducted some time ago reported that between 30 and 50 % of women with endometriosis are infertile and the prevalence of endometriosis in women with infertility may be between 25 and 50 % [5]. Recently, an opinion by the American Society for Reproductive Medicine [5] confirmed such an association stating that "endometriosis typically present with pelvic pain, infertility, or an adnexal mass, and may require surgery."

Although decreased fertility in women with endometriosis is today well established, causes seem to be multifactorial, involving mechanical, molecular, genetic, and environmental ones [4–6].

In the event of severe disease causes are usually evident, since pelvic anatomy becomes distorted and, when this happens, mechanical factors, such as pelvic adhesions, may directly impair fertility disrupting oocyte release or pickup, altering sperm motility, disorganizing myometrial contractions, and impairing fertilization and tubal embryo transport [7].

In 2010, de Ziegler et al. [4] summarized possible mechanisms through which endometriosis may impair fertility at all stages. These include:

- Changes in the composition and characteristics of peritoneal fluid capable of affecting fertilization and associated with pelvic inflammation. As a result, sperm motility may be impaired and sperm capacitation inhibited; in addition, oocyte–sperm interactions may also be hindered, sperm binding to the *zona pellucida* decreased, and the acrosome reaction and sperm–oocyte fusion impaired.
- A direct effect of endometriosis on oocyte and embryo quality has been proposed, although there is no agreement on this point.
- In the presence of an ovarian endometrioma, the age-dependent decline in the number of ovarian follicles can occur earlier in life.
- The eutopic endometrium is altered in women with endometriosis and may become less receptive because of a local production of estradiol and of progesterone resistance.

In conclusion, endocrine and paracrine pathways in human endometriotic cells that are modulated by estrogens and progestogens, including chemotaxis and apoptosis, are perturbed in women with endometriosis, contributing to inflammatory responses. These phenomena promote adhesion formation and infertility [8].

The availability of in vitro fertilization (IVF) followed by embryo transfer (ET) has been considered as a major step forward in achieving pregnancy in women suffering from endometriosis. Unfortunately, it was soon found that in both peritoneal and ovarian diseases, there is an adverse effect on ovulation rates, markers of ovarian reserve, and response to ovarian stimulation [9]. In particular, the presence of an endometrioma can reduce ovarian reserve and decrease the number of oocytes retrieved [10, 11]; this effect has been attributed to endometriosis itself [10], although these findings are controversial [12–14].

In a recent Chinese cohort study, following surgery for endometrioma, the bFSH level was higher and the numbers of oocytes retrieved were lower [15]. It seems therefore that, on the one hand, cystectomy carries away ovarian follicles and, on the other, endometriosis itself seems to have a detrimental effect on ovarian follicles.

The latter hypothesis is substantiated by studies involving patients with peritoneal endometriosis: back in 2001, Hock et al. found that women with stage III/IV (rAFS) have a reduced ovarian reserve compared to women with stage I/II [16]. This observation is consistent with progressive loss of ovarian reserve in women with increasing stages of endometriosis, independent of age. As pointed out by Hauzman et al. [17], in patients with endometriosis, endometrial receptivity is also compromised; this is evidenced in oocyte donation cycles, where lower implantation rates can be observed in subjects without endometriosis if they receive an oocyte from a patient with endometriosis. Interestingly, oocytes donated by healthy subjects provide the patient with endometriosis similar chances to achieve pregnancy to women without the disease.

The solution proposed for women with endometriosis who wish to achieve pregnancy through IVF-ET is the use of intracytoplasmic sperm injection (ICSI). Indeed, a recent Norwegian study [18] found that, using ICSI and leaving aside patients with endometrioma, infertile women with various stages of endometriosis have the same success rates as patients with tubal factor. On the basis of their results these authors have urged the European Society of Human Reproduction and Embryology (ESHRE) to modify its recommendations.

Notwithstanding the abovementioned problems, a large number of women with endometriosis-associated infertility can today conceive following surgery and/or IVF-ET. This makes mandatory an evaluation of pregnancy and its outcome in women with endometriosis, given that recent epidemiological studies are drawing the attention to changes in the uterine environment in association with this condition. The cellular and molecular changes in the endometrium in association with endometriosis and adenomyosis have been reviewed by Benagiano et al. [19]. Changes in the inner myometrium, the so-called myometrial junction zone (JZ), have been observed since it became possible to diagnose adenomyosis by magnetic resonance (MR) imaging. These structural modifications were first described by Bazot et al. [20, 21] and Kunz et al. [22, 23]. However, endometriosis and adenomyosis are at present diagnosed, respectively, by laparoscopy and imaging techniques (MR and ultrasonography) and the two are not both routinely performed as complementary examinations when endometriosis or adenomyosis is diagnosed [24]. At any rate, in reviewing obstetrical complications in association with endometriosis, the presence of alteration in the myometrial JZ is of critical importance. Therefore, this review will also include studies on pregnancy complications in women with adenomyosis. After reviewing the obstetrical complications the underlying mechanisms in the endometrium and myometrial JZ will be discussed.

28.2 Spontaneous Hemoperitoneum in Pregnancy and Postpartum

28.2.1 *Rare, but Dramatic*

Pregnancy may have a beneficial effect on endometriotic implants, but carries an increased risk of spontaneous hemoperitoneum in pregnancy (SHiP), fortunately a rare event, but an important cause of maternal and fetal death [25]. A review of case reports suggests a major role of pelvic endometriosis in the pathogenesis of SHiP [26]. Even cases where no endometriosis is noted at the time of intervention may be caused by endometriosis, since peritoneal endometriotic implants undergo decidual changes in the first trimester of pregnancy, characterized by loss of pigmentation and fibrosis, which renders visual diagnosis more difficult [27]. If the lesion is not biopsied at the time of an emergency laparotomy, the diagnosis of endometriosis as a cause for SHiP will often be missed.

Massive spontaneous hemoperitoneum associated with mild endometriosis has also been described in the postpartum period and at the time of menstruation [28–30]. In addition, rupture of the sigmoid or appendix during late pregnancy in nulliparous women has been related to decidualization of endometriotic implants [31–33].

28.2.2 *Pathogenesis*

Invasiveness of severe endometriosis has been suggested as a reason for SHiP, but there is no apparent correlation between SHiP and stage of endometriosis. An alternative explanation is that SHiP results from involution of decidualized ectopic endometrium during pregnancy. In the differentiation of mesenchymal cells, decidualization represents "the point of no return"; after which the cellular integrity becomes inextricably dependent upon sustained progesterone signaling [34]. Falling progesterone levels not only reverse the decidual phenotype, but also induce the expression of a gene network that encodes for chemokines, proinflammatory cytokines, matrix metalloproteinases, and apoptotic factors, leading to influx of inflammatory cells, proteolytic breakdown of the extracellular matrix, cell death, and bleeding. Interestingly, emerging evidence suggests that endometriosis is associated with progesterone resistance, characterized by suboptimal expression of target genes [35]. Therefore, it is tempting to speculate that "functional" progesterone withdrawal triggers involution of the decidual phenotype of the ectopic endometrium surrounding distended parametrial veins, leading to peritoneal bleeding of unpredictable severity.

28.3 Obstetrical Complications Associated with Endometriosis

28.3.1 Preeclampsia, Small for Gestational Age (SGA), and Preterm Birth

In 2003, a matched case-control study of 137 pregnant patients with endometriosis, including IVF patients, found no difference in pregnancy outcome [36]. A few years later, a retrospective case-control study of infertile women with laparoscopy-confirmed endometriosis from the University of Ghent found a significantly lower incidence of preeclampsia and pregnancy-induced hypertension in women with endometriosis than in a control group of male-factor infertility (0.8 % versus 7.5 %, 95 % CI: 1.7–33.3) [37]. These studies set the stage for several other investigations evaluating the risk of obstetrical complications in women with endometriosis (Table 28.1).

A nationwide Swedish study including 1,442,675 singleton births between 1992 and 2006 reported in 13.090 singleton births among 8,922 women diagnosed with endometriosis, an increased risk of preterm birth irrespective of assisted reproduction technology (ART), antepartal bleeding/placental complications, preeclampsia, and Caesarean section. There was no association between endometriosis and SGA or stillbirth [38]. On the other hand, a population-based, longitudinal Australian

Table 28.1 Obstetrical complications of pregnancy after ART in women with endometriosis

	In comparison with	
Nature of complication	Naturally conceived	ART without endometriosis
Preterm birth	Increased (38, 40)[a]	
Preeclampsia	Increased (38)	
Antepartum hemorrhage	Increased (38)	
Caesarean section	Increased (38)	
Placenta previa	Increased (50)	Increased (50)
SGA birth	No increase (38)	
Stillbirth	No increase (38)	

[a]Increased only if endometrioma

study found in 3,239 women with endometriosis aged between 15 and 45 years no evidence for an association between endometriosis and subsequent risk of either pregnancy hypertension or preeclampsia, even after adjusting for age and gestational age [39]. A retrospective cohort study by Fernando et al. [40] found in 95 singletons ART babies from patients with ovarian endometriomas increased rates of preterm birth and SGA in comparison with community birth records and with other forms of endometriosis.

The association between endometriosis and preeclampsia remains controversial. Unfortunately, the epidemiological studies were not controlled for changes in the myometrial JZ that plays a critical role in the pathogenesis of pregnancy complications such as preeclampsia or SGA and to a lesser extent in preterm birth and preterm premature rupture of the membranes [41–43]. It should be noted that a case-control study of preterm delivery in patients with adenomyosis by Juang et al. [44] found an increased risk of both spontaneous preterm delivery and preterm premature rupture of the membranes. This finding underlines the interest to evaluate potential changes in the myometrial JZ in studies on obstetrical complications in women with endometriosis.

28.3.2 Presence of Ovarian Endometrioma During Pregnancy

Pregnancy complicated by ovarian endometrioma is a rare event [45]. Benaglia et al. [46] analyzed data from patients achieving singleton clinical pregnancies through IVF comparing the pregnancy outcome between 78 pregnant women with endometriomas at the time of IVF and 156 patients who achieved pregnancy through IVF without endometriomas. No differences were observed in late pregnancy and neonatal outcomes between the two groups. In particular, the rate of preterm birth and SGA was similar. However, the study included all hemorrhagic cysts from 1 cm persisting for 2 months. Garcia-Velasco and Somigliana [47] recommended proceeding directly to IVF to reduce time to pregnancy, to avoid potential surgical complications, and to limit patient costs. On the other hand, no attention is paid to the progressive vascular sclerosis in the endometrioma bed as demonstrated by the color Doppler sonographic studies of Qiu et al. [48] indicating that the delayed diagnosis and surgery are the main factors of follicular loss.

28.3.3 Placenta Previa and Postpartum Hemorrhage

ART has been suspected for some reason to increase the risk of obstetrical hemorrhages including placenta previa, a life-threatening complication of pregnancy. The retrospective cohort study by Healy et al. [49] compared the prevalence of antepartum hemorrhage, placenta previa, placental abruption, and primary postpartum hemorrhage in women with singleton births between 1991 and 2004. Endometriosis patients had more placenta previa (1.7; 1.2–2.4) and postpartum hemorrhage (1.3; 1.1–1.6) than those without endometriosis. The exploratory analysis of factors in the IVF/ICSI group, showing associations with fresh embryo transfers in stimulated cycles, endometriosis, and hormone treatments, suggested that events around the time of implantation may be responsible and that suboptimal endometrial function is the critical mechanism. Takemura et al. [50] confirmed by logistic regression analysis in a group of consecutive 318 pregnancies conceived by ART that the risk of placenta previa in relation of ten variables (maternal age, gravidity, parity, male or female fetus, previous abortion, previous Caesarean delivery, endometriosis, ovulatory disorder, tubal disease, and male infertility) is related to endometriosis (odds ratio = 15.1; 95 % CI = 7.6–500.0) and tubal disease (odds ratio = 4.4; 95 % CI = 1.1–26.3). According to the study of Sazonova et al. [51] blastocyst transfer increases the risk of placenta previa after IVF in singleton pregnancies.

In a recent retrospective study, Vercellini et al. [52] assessed pregnancy outcome in 419 women who achieved a first spontaneous singleton pregnancy after surgery for different types of endometriosis. The study found an incidence of placenta previa of 7.6 % in 150 women with rectovaginal lesions; 2.1 % in 69 with ovarian endometriomas plus peritoneal implants; and 2.4 % in 100 women with peritoneal implants only. No case of placenta previa was observed in 100 women with ovarian endometriomas only.

28.3.4 Pathophysiology of the Myometrial Junction Zone in Endometriosis

Endometriosis, a chronic inflammatory disorder, disrupts coordinated progesterone responses throughout the reproductive tract, including in the endometrium. This phenomenon is increasingly referred to as "progesterone resistance." Emerging evidence suggests that progesterone resistance in endometriosis is not just a consequence of perturbed progesterone signal transduction caused by chronic inflammation, but is associated with epigenetic chromatin changes that determine the intrinsic responsiveness of endometrial cells to differentiation cues [53]. Petraglia et al. [54] speculated that an exaggerated inflammatory reaction or the lack of a response can activate the inflammatory process in placental membranes and myometrium. An overlap of molecules and mechanisms may explain the evidence that preterm birth is a common outcome in pregnant patients with endometriosis. A correlation with preterm birth has been suggested for both endometriosis [38, 40] and adenomyosis [44].

In the human, the process of tissue remodeling in preparation of deep placentation starts in the secretory phase of the menstrual cycle. Successful pregnancy requires full transformation of the spiral arteries in the placental bed artery from their origin in the myometrial junction zone [55]. Recently Brosens et al. [56] discussed the hypothesis of defective spiral artery remodeling as a cause of major obstetrical syndromes in endometriosis and adenomyosis. The process is first characterized by an influx of specialized uterine natural killer cells and decidualization of the endometrial stroma and its vasculature; then, after implantation, the interstitial and endovascular trophoblast invasion begins. The final process results in transformation of the spiral arteries into large uteroplacental arteries in the endometrium and myometrial JZ. Kim et al. [42, 43] suggested that in the absence of an adequate decidual effect endovascular trophoblast cell invasion is arrested at the level of the endometrial–myometrial junction and failed to progress into the myometrial spiral arteries. This could explain the vascular resistance in preterm premature rupture of the membranes and preterm birth. Defective endovascular trophoblast invasion can also be secondary to absence of natural killer cells in the thickened myometrial JZ. It is generally accepted that natural killer cells, which are present around spiral arteries in the basal decidua, but not deeper in the myometrium, play a role in determining the depth of interstitial and endovascular trophoblast [57, 58].

The question then arises whether the endometrial and myometrial JZ abnormalities associated with endometriosis at the time of implantation represent a risk factor for the vascular development of the placental bed. Unfortunately, no studies have yet been performed on biopsies of the placental bed in women with endometriosis to investigate the pattern and extent of deep placentation decidualization. Despite the lack of histopathological investigations, clinical studies have reported an association between endometriosis and disorders such as preterm delivery that are associated with defective deep placentation.

28.4 Pituitary Downregulation and Pregnancy Outcome in Endometriosis and Adenomyosis

The vital question is whether the uterine microenvironment in endometriosis and adenomyosis can be improved by medical therapy and pregnancy rates in infertile patients enhanced.

Recently, Maubon et al. [59] investigated in a retrospective study the impact of the JZ structure on the likelihood of pregnancy after IVF-ET treatment and found that a pelvic MR scan showing a thickened uterine JZ represents a negative predictive factor for embryo implantation after IVF-ET.

Nakagawa et al. [60] suggested that treatment with a superagonist gonadotropin-releasing hormone analog (GnRHa) prior to IVF-ET could improve the implantation rate following IVF in infertile patients with endometriosis. The results of this study were confirmed in a retrospective study of 74 infertile patients with surgically proven endometriosis and adenomyosis who were treated with IVF-ET [61]. All patients were pretreated with long-term GnRHa prior to IVF-ET. The contemporary presence of adenomyosis had apparently no adverse effects on IVF-ET outcomes in women with endometriosis when pretreated with long-term pituitary downregulation. In a small case series Tremellen and Russell [62] described four women, who previously had undergone multiple unsuccessful IVF cycles because of failure of implantation of good quality embryos who had a coexisting uterine adenomyosis. The inactivation of adenomyosis by an ultra-long pituitary downregulation regime promptly resulted in successful pregnancy for all four women. Given that the majority of fertility clinics are now moving towards the more "patient-friendly" antagonist protocol, where patients are not placed in a hypoestrogen state before commencing ovarian stimulation, the question of whether adenomyosis has an impact on IVF success rates in GnRHa antagonist-stimulated IVF treatment needed to be examined. In a recent retrospective cohort study of 748 patients who underwent a screening transvaginal ultrasound to identify possible pelvic pathology before commencing their IVF treatment, Talluri and Tremellen [63] identified 213 patients who were eligible to be included in the adenomyosis study as they had no obvious underlying uterine or embryonic factors that could have interfered with successful implantation. The adenomyosis group had a viable clinical pregnancy rate of 23.6 compared with 44.6 in the non-adenomyosis group ($P = 0.017$). This is the first study to clearly describe an implantation problem in a relatively large cohort exclusively undergoing GnRHa antagonist cycles in women with ultrasound-diagnosed adenomyosis. Thus, available evidence supports the idea of a reversibility of myometrial JZ changes by appropriate medication inducing a prolonged hypoestrogenic period. More studies will be required to evaluate the beneficial effect of pituitary downregulation during the cycle of conception on deep placentation in women with adenomyosis and the potential of this treatment for the prevention of major obstetrical complications associated with defective deep placentation.

28.5 Conclusions

Subtle lesions and symptoms of endometriosis often disappear during pregnancy and postpartum. The shedding of decidualized tissue may cause bleeding and the differential diagnosis of spontaneous hemoperitoneum should be taken into account in pregnancy and postpartum, since both maternal and fetal outcomes can be dramatic.

The available data on the association between endometriosis and obstetrical complications are still controversial for several reasons. In the first place, studies are frequently based on laparoscopy for the diagnosis of endometriosis and fail to take into account myometrial JZ thickening or adenomyosis as a potential risk of obstetrical complications. Secondly, the diagnosis of the endometrioma is still based on laparoscopy and ultrasound, but fails to take into account the degree of vascular sclerosis and follicular loss, as demonstrated by the color Doppler flow sonographic studies of Qiu et al. [48]. Finally, the potential effect of prolonged hypoestrogenic treatment may modify risk factors at the time of conception. It is clear that, together with studies reporting an increased risk for preterm birth in women with endometriosis, physicians must be aware that close antenatal follow-up and early diagnosis of vascular complications are crucial.

References

1. McGoogan LS. Sterility and endometriosis. Arch Surg. 1949;59:437–44.
2. Kistner RW. Endometriosis and infertility. Clin Obstet Gynecol. 1959;2:877–89.
3. Carvalho LFP, Rossener R, Azeem A, Malvezzi H, Simões Abrão M, Agarwal A. From conception to birth: how endometriosis affects the development of each stage of reproductive life. Minerva Ginecol. 2013;65:181–98.
4. de Ziegler D, Borghese B, Chapron C. Endometriosis and infertility: pathophysiology and management. Lancet. 2010;376:730–8.
5. Verkauf BS. Incidence, symptoms, and signs of endometriosis in fertile and infertile women. J Fla Med Assoc. 1987;74(9):671–5.
6. Practice Committee of the American Society for Reproductive Medicine. Endometriosis and infertility: a committee opinion. Fertil Steril. 2012;98:591–8.
7. Macer ML, Taylor HS. Endometriosis and infertility. A review of the pathogenesis and treatment of endometriosis-associated infertility. Obstet Gynecol Clin North Am. 2012;39:535–49.
8. Reis FM, Petraglia F, Taylor RN. Endometriosis: hormone regulation and clinical consequences of chemotaxis and apoptosis. Hum Reprod Update. 2013;19:406–18.
9. Shah DK. Diminished ovarian reserve and endometriosis: insult upon injury. Semin Reprod Med. 2013;31:144–9.
10. Loh FH, Tan AT, Kumar J, Ng SC. Ovarian response after laparoscopic ovarian cystectomy for endometriotic cysts in 132 monitored cycles. Fertil Steril. 1999;72:316–21.
11. Horikawa T, Nakagawa K, Ohgi S, Kojima R, Nakashima A, Ito M, et al. The frequency of ovulation from the affected ovary decreases following laparoscopic cystectomy in infertile women with unilateral endometrioma during a natural cycle. J Assist Reprod Genet. 2008;25:239–44.
12. Tinkanen H, Kujansuu E. In vitro fertilization in patients with ovarian endometriomas. Acta Obstet Gynecol Scand. 2000;79:119–22.
13. Donnez J, Wyns C, Nisolle M. Does ovarian surgery for endometriomas impair the ovarian response to gonadotropin? Fertil Steril. 2001;76:662–5.
14. Demirol A, Guven S, Baykal C, Gurgan T. Effect of endometrioma cystectomy on IVF outcome: a prospective randomized study. Reprod Biomed Online. 2006;12:639–43.
15. Lin X-N, Wei M-L, Tong X-M, Xu W-H, Zhou F, Huang Q-X, Wen G-F, Zhang S-Y. Outcome of in vitro fertilization in endometriosis-associated infertility: a 5-year database cohort study. Chin Med J. 2012;125:2688–93.
16. Hock DL, Sharafi K, Dagostino L, Kemmann E, Seifer DB. Contribution of diminished ovarian reserve to hypofertility associated with endometriosis. J Reprod Med. 2001;46:7–10.
17. Hauzman EE, Garcia-Velasco JA, Pellicer A. Oocyte donation and endometriosis: what are the lessons? Semin Reprod Med. 2013;31:173–7.
18. Opøien HK, Fedorcsak P, Omland AK, Abyholm T, Bjercke S, Ertzeid G, Oldereid N, Mellembakken JR, Tanbo T. In vitro fertilization is a successful treatment in endometriosis-associated infertility. Fertil Steril. 2012;97:912–8.
19. Benagiano G. Brosens I, Habiba M. Structural and molecular features of the endomyometrium in endometriosis and adenomyosis. Hum Reprod Update. 2014;20(3):386–402.

20. Bazot M, Darai E, Hourani R, Thomassin I, Cortez A, Uzan S, Buy JN. Pelvic endometriosis: MR imaging for diagnosis and prediction of extension of disease. Radiology. 2004;232:379–89.
21. Bazot M, Fiori O, Darai E. Adenomyosis in endometriosis – prevalence and impact on fertility. Evidence from magnetic resonance imaging. Hum Reprod. 2006;21:1101–2. Author reply 1102–3.
22. Kunz G, Beil D, Huppert P, Noe M, Kissler S, Leyendecker G. Adenomyosis in endometriosis - Prevalence and impact on fertility. Evidence from magnetic resonance imaging. Hum Reprod. 2005;20:2309–16.
23. Kunz G, Herbertz M, Beil D, Huppert G, Leyendecker G. Adenomyosis as a disorder of the early and late human reproductive period. Reprod Biomed Online. 2007;15:681–5.
24. Benagiano G, Brosens I. Adenomyosis and Endometriosis have a common origin. J Obstet Gynaecol India. 2011;61:146–53.
25. Ginsburg KA, Valdes C, Schnider G. Spontaneous uteroovarian vessel rupture during pregnancy: three case reports and a review of the literature. Obstet Gynecol. 1987;69:474–6.
26. Brosens JJ, Parker MG, McIndoe A, Pijnenborg R, Brosens IA. A role for menstruation in preconditioning the uterus for successful pregnancy. Am J Obstet Gynecol. 2009;200:615.e1–615.e6.
27. Moen MH, Muus KM. Endometriosis in pregnant and nonpregnant women at tubal sterilization. Hum Reprod. 1991;6:699–702.
28. Fiadjoe P, Thomas-Phillips A, Reddy K. Massive haemoperitoneum due to uterine artery erosion by endometriosis and a review of the literature. Gynecol Surg. 2008;5:133–5.
29. O'Leary SM. Ectopic decidualization causing massive postpartum intraperitoneal hemorrhage. Obstet Gynecol. 2006;108:776–9.
30. Uri FI, Opaneye A. Haemoperitoneum due to cornual endometriosis after laparoscopic sterilisation. Br J Obstet Gynaecol. 1979;86:664–5.
31. Clement PB. Perforation of the sigmoid colon during pregnancy: a rare complication of endometriosis. Case report. Br J Obstet Gynaecol. 1977;84:548–50.
32. Gini PC, Chukudebelu WO, Onuigbo WI. Perforation of the appendix during pregnancy: a rare complication of endometriosis. Case report. Br J Obstet Gynaecol. 1981;88:456–8.
33. Loverro G, Cormio G, Greco P, Altomare D, Putignano G, Selvaggi L. Perforation of the sigmoid colon during pregnancy: a rare complication of endometriosis. J Gynecol Surg. 1999;15:155–7.
34. Brosens JJ, Gellersen B. Death or survival—progesterone-dependent cell fate decisions in the human endometrial stroma. J Mol Endocrinol. 2006;36:389–98.
35. Burney RO, Talbi S, Hamilton AE, Vo KC, Nyegaard M, Nezhat CR, et al. Gene expression analysis of endometrium reveals progesterone resistance and candidate susceptibility genes in women with endometriosis. Endocrinology. 2007;148:3814–26.
36. Kortelahti M, Anttila MA, Hippelainen MI, Heinonen ST. Obstetric outcome in women with endometriosis – a matched case-control study (2003). Gynecol Obstet Invest. 2003;56:207–12.
37. Brosens IA, De Sutter P, Hamerlynck T, Imeraj L, Yao Z, Cloke B, Brosens JJ, Dhont M. Endometriosis is associated with a decreased risk of pre-eclampsia. Hum Reprod. 2007;22:1725–9.
38. Stephansson O, Kieler H, Granath F, Falconer H. Endometriosis, assisted reproduction technology, and risk of adverse pregnancy outcome. Hum Reprod. 2009;24:2341–7.
39. Hadfield RM, Lain SJ, Raynes-Greenow CH, Morris JM, Roberts CL. Is there an association between endometriosis and the risk of pre-eclampsia? A population based study. Hum Reprod. 2009;24:2348–52.
40. Fernando S, Breheny S, Jaques AM, Halliday JL, Baker G, Healy D. Preterm birth, ovarian endometriomata, and assisted reproduction technologies. Fertil Steril. 2009;91:325–30.
41. Brosens I, Derwig I, Brosens J, Fusi L, Benagiano G, Pijnenborg R. The enigmatic uterine junctional zone: The missing link between reproductive disorders and major obstetrical disorders? Hum Reprod. 2010;25:569–74.
42. Kim YM, Chaiworapongsa T, Gomez R, Bujold E, Yoon BH, Rotmensch S, Thaler HT, Romero R, et al. Failure of physiologic transformation of the spiral arteries in the placental bed in preterm premature rupture of membranes. Am J Obstet Gynecol. 2002;187:1137–42.

43. Kim YM, Bujold E, Chaiworapongsa T, Gomez R, Yoon BH, Thaler HT, Rotmensch S, Romero R. Failure of physiologic transformation of the spiral arteries in patients with preterm labor and intact membranes. Am J Obstet Gynecol. 2003;189:1063–9.
44. Juang C-M, Chou P, Yen M-S, Twu N-F, Horng H-C, Hsu W-L. Adenomyosis and risk of preterm delivery. Br J Obstet Gynaecol. 2007;114:165–9.
45. Rossman F, D'Ablaing 3rd G, Marrs RP. Pregnancy complicated by ruptured endometrioma. Obstet Gynecol. 1983;62:519–21.
46. Benaglia L, Bermejo A, Somigliana E, Scarduelli C, Ragni G, Fedele L, Garcia-Velasco JA. Pregnancy outcome in women with endometriomas achieving pregnancy through IVF. Hum Reprod. 2012;27:1663–7.
47. Garcia-Velasco JA, Somigliana E. Management of endometriomas in women requiring IVF: to touch or not to touch. Hum Reprod. 2009;24:496–501.
48. Qiu JJ, Liu M-H, Zhang Z-X, Chen L-P, Yang Q-C. Transvaginal color Doppler sonography predicts ovarian interstitial fibrosis and microvascular injury in women with ovarian endometriotic cysts. Acta Obstet Gynecol Scand. 2012;91:605–12.
49. Healy DL, Breheny S, Halliday J, Jaques A, Rushford D, Garrett C, Talbot JM, Baker HWG. Prevalence and risk factors for obstetric haemorrhage in 6730 singleton births after assisted reproductive technology in Victoria Australia. Hum Reprod. 2010;25:265–74.
50. Takemura Y, Osuga Y, Fujimoto A, Oi N, Tsutsumi R, Koizumi M, Yano T, Taketani Y. Increased risk of placenta previa is associated with endometriosis and tubal factor infertility in assisted reproductive technology pregnancy. Gynecol Endocrinol. 2013;29:113–5.
51. Sazonova A, Kllen K, Thurin-Kjellberg A, Wennerholm U-B, Bergh C. Factors affecting obstetric outcome of singletons born after IVF. Hum Reprod. 2011;26:2878–86.
52. Vercellini P, Parazzini F, Pietropaolo G, Cipriani S, Frattaruolo MP, Fedele L. Pregnancy outcome in women with peritoneal, ovarian and rectovaginal endometriosis: A retrospective cohort study. Br J Obstet Gynaecol. 2012;119:1538–43.
53. Al-Sabbagh M, Lam EW-F, Brosens JJ. Mechanisms of endometrial progesterone resistance. Mol Cell Endocrinol. 2012;358:208–15.
54. Petraglia F, Arcuri F, de Ziegler D, Chapron C. Inflammation: a link between endometriosis and preterm birth. Fertil Steril. 2012;98:36–40.
55. Brosens IA, Robertson WB, Dixon HG. The role of the spiral arteries in the pathogenesis of preeclampsia. Obstet Gynecol Annu. 1972;1:177–91.
56. Brosens I, Pijnenborg R, Benagiano G. Defective myometrial spiral artery remodelling as a cause of major obstetrical syndromes in endometriosis and adenomyosis. Placenta. 2013;34:100–5.
57. King A, Hiby SE, Gardner L, Joseph S, Bowen JM, Verma S, et al. Recognition of trophoblast HLA class I molecules by decidual NK cell receptors e a review. Placenta. 2000;21(Suppl1): S81–5.
58. Wallace AE, Fraser R, Cartwright JE. Extravillous trophoblast and decidual natural killer cells: a remodelling partnership. Hum Reprod Update. 2012;18:458–71.
59. Maubon A, Faury A, Kapella M, Pouquet M, Piver P. Uterine junctional zone at magnetic resonance imaging: a predictor of in vitro fertilization implantation failure. J Obstet Gynaecol Res. 2010;36:611–8.
60. Nakagawa K, Yamano S, Nakasaka H, Komatsu J, Hinokio K, Aono T. Effectiveness of pre-treatment with gonadotropin-releasing hormone agonist to the patients with endometriosis in in vitro fertilization and embryo transfer. Jpn J Fertil Steril. 2000;45:1–6.
61. Mijatovic V, Florijn E, Halim N, Schats R, Hompes P. Adenomyosis has no adverse effects on IVF/ICSI outcomes in women with endometriosis treated with long-term pituitary down-regulation before IVF/ICSI. Eur J Obstet Gynecol Reprod Biol. 2010;151:62–5.
62. Tremellen K, Russell P. Adenomyosis is a potential cause of recurrent implantation failure during IVF treatment. Aust N Z J Obstet Gynaecol. 2011;51:280–3.
63. Thalluri V, Tremellen KP. Ultrasound diagnosed adenomyosis has a negative impact on successful implantation following GnRH antagonist IVF treatment. Hum Reprod. 2012;27:3487–92.

Chapter 29
Malignant Transformation of Endometriosis

Hiroshi Kobayashi

Abstract The association between endometriosis and epithelial ovarian cancer has been supported by years of epidemiologic research. Approximately 1.0 % of women with endometriosis may undergo malignant transformation. The malignant transformation is believed to progress in a stepwise fashion through an intermediary endometriotic lesion, atypical endometriosis. The greatest risk is associated with epithelial ovarian cancer of endometrioid and clear cell histology. Endometriosis and ovarian cancer may share a common pathogenic mechanism: hyperestrogenism, excess oxidative stress, and inflammation derived from repeated hemorrhage and iron, contributing to ovarian tumorigenesis. The iron-induced signals can contribute to carcinogenesis via three processes: step 1, by increasing oxidative stress, which facilitates the accumulation of somatic mutations, contributing to endometriosis-associated ovarian cancer initiation; step 2, by creating an estrogen-dependent microenvironment, supporting endometrioid adenocarcinoma progression; and step 3, by surviving stressful periods, thereby contributing to clear cell carcinoma progression. In conclusion, some endometriosis lesions may predispose to ovarian cancer, but future studies are needed to know the exact mechanisms of endometriosis-associated ovarian cancer.

Keywords Endometriosis • Inflammation • Iron • Ovarian cancer • Oxidative stress

H. Kobayashi, M.D., Ph.D. (✉)
Department of Obstetrics and Gynecology, Nara Medical University, 840 Shijo-cho, Kashihara 634-8522, Nara, Japan
e-mail: hirokoba@naramed-u.ac.jp

T. Harada (ed.), *Endometriosis: Pathogenesis and Treatment*,
DOI 10.1007/978-4-431-54421-0_29, © Springer Japan 2014

29.1 Introduction

Endometriosis is a benign hormone-dependent condition and a common gynecologic disorder, with an estimated frequency of approximately 10 % among women of reproductive age. This disease often results in a serious clinical problem because of its potential for adverse sequelae, including severe dysmenorrhea, chronic pelvic pain, infertility, and possibly developing ovarian cancer [1]. The exact etiology and pathogenesis of endometriosis have yet to be elucidated. It may mainly cause retrograde menstruation, implantation of menstrual tissue, and peritoneal metaplasia in a woman with an improper immune response and a genetic predisposition to developing endometriotic lesions. Thus, the pathogenesis of endometriosis is multifactorial, including the role of genetics, hormonal factors, environmental factors, and immune system.

The pathogenesis of endometriosis has been an area of active investigation, including retrograde menstruation theory, coelomic metaplasia theory, embryonic rest theory, lymphovascular metastasis theory, stem cell theory, and others [2]. Several studies exploring the differential expression of genes between autologous eutopic and ectopic endometrium from patients with endometriosis or between eutopic endometrium from women with or without endometriosis may provide a better understanding of the pathogenesis and pathophysiology of the disorder. The genome-wide profiling and pathway-based enrichment analysis revealed that genes related to cell cycle, growth factors, signal transduction, transcription factors, hormones, cytokines, chemokines and (pro)inflammation, proteases, cell adhesion and motility, stress response and detoxification, immune response, and metabolism were affected in the pathogenesis process of endometriosis [3–16].

Furthermore, it is generally assumed that histologically benign endometriotic lesions may be caused by the genetic defects that are permissive for malignant transformation. Studies have documented loss of heterozygosity and mutations of tumor suppressor genes in endometriosis (see Sect. 29.3). This disorder exhibits high genetic instability that is involved in the cell phenotype changes that take place during cancer progression [17]. Endometriosis shows a monoclonal pattern in origin, suggesting that individual glands of the lesion are derived from single precursor cells. Also, the genome-wide transcriptome of endometriosis does resemble that found in ovarian cancer.

29.2 Epidemiologic Research

Epithelial ovarian cancers have been classified into four major histologic subtypes: serous (~60 %), endometrioid (~10–20 %), clear cell (<10 %), and mucinous (<5 %). Serous, endometrioid, clear cell, and mucinous ovarian tumors histologically resemble the phenotypes of the fallopian tube, proliferative endometrium, gestational endometrium, and endocervix/gastrointestinal tract, respectively.

Comparing the profile of epithelial ovarian cancer between Japanese and Caucasians, clear cell carcinomas (27.6 vs. <10 %) are more common in Japan, possibly with fewer serous adenocarcinomas (40.7 vs. 60 %). One possibility is that the Japanese may exhibit a lower proportion of serous adenocarcinoma compared to the United States population. This may reflect a proportional change.

The investigators have focused on latest knowledge of the genetic and environmental factors affecting the development of epithelial ovarian cancer and outline future challenges in its pathogenesis research [18]. The time trend analyses of incidence between 1973 and 2005 in the United States exhibited a decline by 27 % in epithelial ovarian cancer incidence [19, 20]. The incidence trend of ovarian cancer in the United States is similar to the trends observed in most of the European countries. In contrast, an increase in epithelial ovarian cancer rates has been reported in Japan. It is generally accepted that oral contraceptive (OC) use reduces the risk of ovarian cancer and endometrial cancer. Although the exact reasons for the higher ovarian cancer incidence rates in Japan are unknown, the trends may be due to changes in risk factors, such as diet and environmental factors and the low prevalence of OC use (2–3 %) in Japan. Although some part of the pathogenesis has been unveiled, the complete events of genetic and epigenetic changes associated with epithelial ovarian cancer remain to be identified.

The association between endometriosis and malignant transformation has often been described in the medical literature. A literature search of MEDLINE (online PubMed database) was conducted for published articles from 1966 to October 2010 using the keywords endometriosis combined with malignant transformation [21]. The search revealed an increase in reports describing endometriosis-associated malignant transformation. Overall, more than 400 articles were included following a process of independent review of each article and six were graded as good quality [22–27]. Numerous epidemiologic studies have shown an association between endometriosis and ovarian cancer [28, 29]. Epidemiologic studies have shown an increased risk of epithelial ovarian cancer, especially endometrioid and clear cell histologies, among women with endometriosis. Brinton et al. examined the records of 20,686 women hospitalized with endometriosis between 1969 and 1983 [22]. Standardized incidence ratios (SIRs) of cancers were calculated to compare the cancer incidence of the study cohort with that of the general population. After adjustment for age, period, and comorbidities, the hazards ratio was 1.9 for the endometriosis group compared with the control group, indicating that this cohort had an increased overall risk of ovarian cancer. They also found further increases in ovarian cancer risk among women with long-standing histories of ovarian endometrioma (SIR, 4.2) [22]. The same group reported that patients with endometriosis had the risk (4.19-fold) compared with the general population if they presented with primary infertility [24].

There is one unique epidemiologic study in Japan, supporting the hypothesis that ovarian endometrioma increases the subsequent risk of developing ovarian cancer [30]. A cohort of 6,398 women with a clinically documented ovarian endometrioma enrolled between 1985 and 1995 in the prefecture-wide Shizuoka Cohort Study on Endometriosis and Ovarian Cancer Programme has prospectively analyzed, with follow-up through 2002. During follow-up of up to 17 years of the ovarian endometrioma cohort, 46 incident ovarian cancers were identified, yielding that the ovarian cancer risk was elevated significantly among women with ovarian endometrioma (SIR, 8.95). The elevated risk of developing ovarian cancer was mainly restricted to women with ovarian endometrioma diagnosed after age 40 (advancing age). Tumor size 9 cm or greater in diameter was an independent predictive factor of patients with development of ovarian cancer [31]. This analysis was restricted to those with a clinically diagnosed ovarian endometrioma. Therefore, it has been proposed that ovarian endometrioma has been identified as a possible risk factor for ovarian cancer.

Surveillance of endometriosis might result in a number of newly diagnosed cases of ovarian cancer [20]. It is generally accepted that the incidence of malignant transformations ranges between 0.7 and 1.0 % in women with endometriosis in Japan. Although this finding is consistent with the results of six studies that support a positive association between endometriosis and risk of ovarian cancer [22–27], Kobayashi's group found an SIR of 8.95, compared with other studies reporting SIR less than 5.0. These data provide novel and exciting possibilities. A number of factors contribute to the results including ethnic disparities and differences in genetic predisposition. A significantly increased risk may be found for Japanese. Ovarian endometrioma may have higher cancer risk than pelvic endometriosis. Ovarian cancer in Japan is a growing concern because long-term ovarian cancer trends in incidence show rising rates.

29.3 Ovarian Cancer Susceptibility Genes

Although the etiology and the ovarian carcinogenesis still need clarification, the link between ovarian carcinogenesis and (epi)genetic mutations is well established [18]. The investigators have utilized genome-wide gene expression analysis and association studies to identify a specific gene signature distinguishing ovarian cancer from controls and which served as a molecular signature for complicated histologies. Recent high-throughput whole genome or targeted sequencing studies have also identified numerous somatic mutations across the whole exome in a variety of neoplasms.

High-grade serous ovarian carcinomas develop rapidly without a definite precursor lesion. Multiple genetic and epigenetic changes are involved in the molecular pathogenesis of serous adenocarcinoma, for example, high-grade serous carcinomas are characterized by the tumor suppressor gene TP53 mutations. They also have germline or somatic loss-of-function mutations in BRCA1 or BRCA2 or promoter methylation of BRCA1. Mucinous adenocarcinoma most probably arises via an adenoma-borderline tumor-carcinoma sequence. KRAS mutation (up to 75 %) and lack of TP53 mutations are common in mucinous tumors. Mutations of Wnt/CTNNB1 (beta-catenin) are common in endometrioid adenocarcinoma. Loss-of-function mutations of PIK3CA (phosphatidylinositol-4,5-bisphosphate 3-kinase, catalytic subunit alpha)/PTEN (phosphatase and tensin homolog) are common in low-grade endometrioid carcinoma [18]. In contrast, high-grade endometrioid carcinomas harbored TP53 mutations and lacked CTNNB1, PIK3CA, or PTEN mutations [18]. Mutations of PIK3CA are observed most frequently in clear cell carcinoma. Recent studies implicated a tumor suppressor gene ARID1A (AT-rich interactive domain 1A (SWI-like)) as frequently disrupted in endometriosis-associated ovarian cancer and clear cell and endometrioid adenocarcinomas. ARID1A plays a role in chromatin remodeling, which leads to cell cycle arrest and cell death in the event of DNA damage. The loss-of-function mutations of ARID1A may result in susceptibility to carcinogenesis through a defect in the repair or replication of damaged DNA. All atypical endometriosis and 86 % of non-atypical endometriosis lost ARID1A expression. ARIDA expression was retained in areas of endometriosis from sites distant from the malignant lesion [32]. These data suggest that loss of ARID1A expression occurs as a very early event in the endometriosis-atypical endometriosis sequence [33]. In endometriosis-associated ovarian cancer, clear cell carcinomas harbor frequent mutations of ARID1A and PIK3CA genes and moderate mutations of PPP2R1A (protein phosphatase 2, regulatory subunit A, alpha) and KRAS [32, 33], while endometrioid cancer harbors mutations of PTEN, CTNNB1, and KRAS [34, 35]. The investigators failed to identify one potential driver mutation in endometriosis-associated ovarian cancer samples. The development of cancer takes place in a multi-step process during which cells acquire a series of mutations, including ARID1A, PPP2R1A, PIK3CA, PTEN, KRAS, or Wnt/CTNNB1. These mutations may be significant factor for endometriosis-associated ovarian carcinogenesis, but various questions have yet to be answered. This model postulates the existence of additional mutations that establish carcinogenesis after acquisition of these mutations. Future studies will represent the remarkable genetic research achievements in the pathogenesis of endometriosis-associated ovarian cancer.

29.4 Pathogenesis of Endometriosis-Associated Ovarian Cancer

Epidemiologic studies account for the fact that endometriosis has been associated with an increased risk of epithelial ovarian cancer. Genome-wide studies demonstrate that endometriosis shares several genetic characteristics with ovarian cancer. The same pathophysiology (immune alterations, excess oxidative stress and inflammation, estrogen excess, and steroid hormone interaction) orchestrates the progression of endometriosis and its transformation to ovarian cancer. These facts show that some endometriosis has been shown to undergo malignant transformation. Ovarian cancer precursor lesions are known to be atypical endometriosis, which was identified in ~50 % of these histologic subtypes. Many investigators agree that the potential of invasive epithelial malignancies arises in atypical endometriosis [36–38]. Malignant transformation of endometriosis is not a single entity; rather it is a term defining a group of histologically distinct tumors. Each histologic subtype is clinically and genetically unique. The malignant transformation of endometriosis is classified into three groups: (i) epithelial ovarian cancers (endometrioid adenocarcinoma and clear cell carcinoma), (ii) other Müllerian-type tumors, including Müllerian-type mucinous borderline tumor and serous borderline tumor, and (iii) sarcomas such as adenosarcoma and endometrial stromal sarcoma in the female pelvic cavity [21]. Epithelial ovarian cancer is a popular tumor of malignant transformation [39].

Genome-wide studies have facilitated the genetic basis of pathogenesis and pathophysiology of endometriosis and endometriosis-associated ovarian cancer owing to the advent of new network-based analysis methods. Several investigators identified the endometriosis susceptibility genes and pathways that may be potential pathophysiology of endometriosis progression [3–16]. The endometriosis susceptibility genes were grouped into pathways or networks based on functional annotation. Interestingly, current molecular studies have sought to link endometriosis with endometriosis-associated ovarian cancer through pathways or networks related to inflammation, oxidative stress, and hyperestrogenism [40].

29.5 Inflammation and Immunity

Previous epidemiologic observations suggest that a number of factors that suppress ovulation or menstruation, including gravidity, breast feeding, oral contraception, and gynecologic surgery including hysterectomy and tubal ligation, reduced the risk of ovarian cancer. Endometriosis, perineal talc use, and asbestos exposure increase the risk, while aspirin or NSAIDs use decreases the risk. Ovulation, endometriosis, and talc use may be associated with inflammatory responses of the ovarian surface epithelium and pelvic peritoneum, contributing to ovarian tissue remodeling, proliferation, and tumorigenesis. These risk factors support that persistent pelvic inflammation may play a role in ovarian cancer risk [41]. In general, chronic inflammation has been implicated in a variety of cancers, including gastric cancer (Helicobacter pylori infection), colorectal cancer (ulcerative colitis and Crohn's disease), lung cancer (tobacco smoking-associated chronic inflammation), malignant mesothelioma and lung cancer (asbestos exposure), hepatocellular carcinoma (hepatitis B and C infection), ovarian cancer (a long history of endometriosis), and others.

Recent advances in innate immunity illuminate the molecular mechanism underlying inflammation-induced carcinogenesis. Innate immunity is made possible by a network of pattern-recognition receptors (PRRs), which include the toll-like receptors (TLRs), Nod-like receptors (NLRs), RIG-like receptors (RLRs), and cytosolic DNA receptors. TLRs mediate interactions between environmental stimuli and innate immunity and trigger inflammatory signals. TLRs are involved in not only the host defense against microbial infections but also stimulation of tumor cell growth and carcinogenesis. Overexpression of PRRs in endometriosis stimulates chronic inflammation pathways, accelerates endometriosis proliferation, and subsequently causes carcinogenesis. Yamada et al. discussed the role of innate immunity in the pathogenesis of endometriosis-associated ovarian cancer, with respect to endogenous ligands, their PRRs, and their signaling pathways [42].

29.6 Oxidative Stress

Increased generation of reactive oxygen species (ROS) is implicated in the pathogenesis of a variety of human diseases, which include cancer, atherosclerosis, diabetes, neurodegenerative diseases, cardiovascular disease, and aging. Repetitive hemorrhage and the accumulation of heme and iron within endometriotic cysts and peritoneal cavity play a role in the development of ovarian cancer through the formation of ROS under a Fenton reaction [43, 44]. Excessive iron increases cancer risk by free radical-induced chromosomal instability. Persistent oxidative stress induced by endometriosis-dependent hemorrhage might be associated with carcinogenesis.

Recent studies have noted a set of genes that distinguished clear cell carcinoma from non-clear cell carcinoma and confirmed specific expression of a transcription factor, hepatocyte nuclear factor-1beta (HNF-1beta), in clear cell carcinoma, and genetic alteration may be involved in oxidative stress [45]. HNF-1beta is significantly upregulated in ovarian clear cell carcinoma and rarely expressed in non-clear cell carcinoma specimens [46]. Of the clear cell carcinoma susceptibility genes, 87 % are redox-related genes, including anti-oxidative and detoxification enzymes [45]. Forty-one percent of the genes upregulated in clear cell carcinoma samples are downstream targets of HNF-1beta [47]. HNF-1beta is thought to play a role in anti-apoptosis, detoxification, survival, cell cycle regulation, and glycogen synthesis. Sixty percent of the endometriosis cases also exhibited the overexpression of HNF-1beta [48]. Endometriosis has evolved adaptive mechanisms to cope with oxidative stress. Excess hemorrhage and iron can induce high levels of oxidative stress that may have deleterious effects on endometriotic cell growth. Endometriotic cells exhibit a higher production of HNF-1beta to detoxify ROS and survive under oxidative stress conditions. HNF-1beta also plays key roles in triggering DNA damage response without causing cell death and regulating timely cell cycle arrest. HNF-1beta upregulation is sufficient to accumulate the iron-induced genomic instability, which may be enhanced and accumulated with increasing cell passage. Genomic instability might be increased even further upon exposure to iron, ultimately resulting in carcinogenesis. Endometriotic cells have developed efficient ways to cope with oxidative stress and seemingly survive stressful periods by launching a minimal set of protection mechanisms and by temporarily bringing several key genes such as HNF-1beta. These data allow us to speculate that excess oxidative stress might be implicated in the development of endometriosis-associated clear cell carcinoma.

29.7 Estrogen

Endometriosis and endometrioid adenocarcinoma share a common hormonal mechanism. Hyperestrogenism is a common finding with development of estrogen-dependent lesions and is a significant risk factor for the development of cancer from endometriosis [49]. Endometrioid adenocarcinoma of the ovary and endometrium develops in the setting of excess endogenous and exogenous estrogen exposure. Estrogen drives cell proliferation and activates the PI3K and MAPK proliferative pathways, which are frequently dysregulated in cancer. Estrogen is supposed to participate in the early stages of endometrial tumorigenesis, through the accumulation of random genetic errors and increased telomerase activity. Genomic and nongenomic estrogen receptor (ER) signaling pathways play a role in the onset and development of tumors arising from or outside the reproductive system. Endometrioid adenocarcinoma of the ovary is predominantly positive for ER; however, the molecular link between estrogen and endometrial carcinogenesis remains poorly understood.

In contrast, clear cell carcinoma specifically exhibits negative ER expression and estrogen independency. The iron-mediated ROS oxidatively modifies genomic DNA and, subsequently, ER depletion may be observed, possibly through DNA methylation of the promoter region, histone deacetylation, heme and iron binding, chromatin remodeling, and ubiquitin ligase activity [50, 51]. ER is thought to be inactivated mainly through aberrant DNA methylation [52]. Loss of estrogen function may be a turning point in clear cell carcinoma progression and aggressiveness. Endometriosis-associated ovarian cancer has a dual pathway in carcinogenesis, estrogen-dependent ovarian carcinogenesis with an endometrioid morphology, and estrogen-independent, oxidative stress-dependent carcinogenesis with the clear cell morphology [53].

29.8 Conclusion

The endometriosis contains abundant iron due to repeated episodes of hemorrhage. Iron is a mutagenic and carcinogenic compound and causes oxidative stress due to generation of ROS. The iron-induced ROS signaling cascades can contribute to carcinogenesis via three major processes: step 1, by increasing oxidative stress, which facilitates the accumulation of somatic mutations and promotes DNA mutagenesis, histone modification, chromatin remodeling, and gene products activation/inactivation, thus contributing to endometriosis-associated ovarian cancer initiation; step 2, by creating a microenvironment that supports sustained growth, angiogenesis, migration, and invasion of cancer cells via estrogen-dependent mechanisms, thus supporting tumor progression of endometrioid adenocarcinoma; and step 3, by surviving stressful periods via temporarily HNF-1beta overexpression, thereby contributing to clear cell carcinoma progression (Fig. 29.1). The high

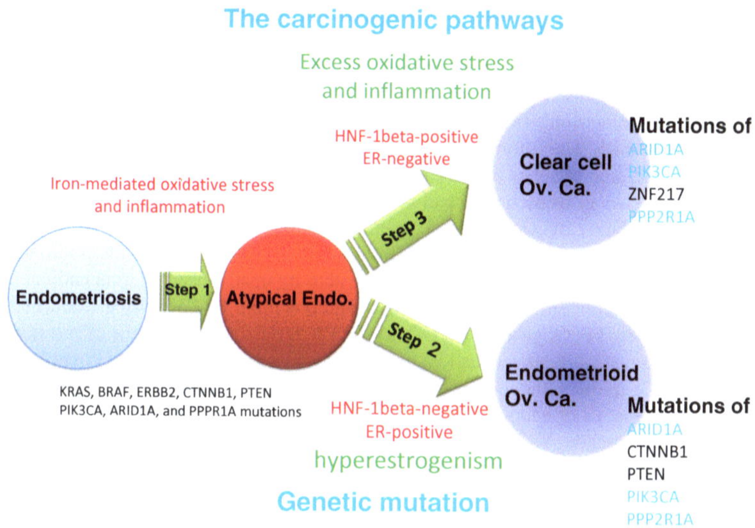

Fig. 29.1 The carcinogenic pathways. Endometriosis may contribute to carcinogenesis via three processes: step 1, by increasing oxidative stress, which facilitates the accumulation of somatic mutations, contributing to endometriosis-associated ovarian cancer initiation; step 2, by creating an estrogen-dependent microenvironment, supporting endometrioid adenocarcinoma progression; and step 3, by surviving stressful periods via temporarily HNF-1beta overexpression, thereby contributing to clear cell carcinoma progression

incidence of malignant transformation in high-risk women with endometriosis (advancing age and tumor size 9 cm or greater in diameter) further supports intensive targeted surveillance.

Acknowledgments Grant support: Supported by Grant-in-Aid for Scientific Research from the Ministry of Education, Science, and Culture of Japan to the Department of Obstetrics and Gynecology, Nara Medical University (H. Kobayashi).

Conflict of Interest The authors declare no conflict of interest.

References

1. Giudice LC, Kao LC. Endometriosis. Lancet. 2004;364:1789–99.
2. Figueira PG, Abrão MS, Krikun G, Taylor HS. Stem cells in endometrium and their role in the pathogenesis of endometriosis. Ann N Y Acad Sci. 2011;1221:10–7.
3. Arimoto T, Katagiri T, Oda K, Tsunoda T, Yasugi T, Osuga Y, Yoshikawa H, Nishii O, Yano T, Taketani Y, Nakamura Y. Genome-wide cDNA microarray analysis of gene-expression profiles involved in ovarian endometriosis. Int J Oncol. 2003;22:551–60.

4. Bischoff F, Simpson JL. Genetics of endometriosis: heritability and candidate genes. Best Pract Res Clin Obstet Gynaecol. 2004;18:219–32.
5. Hu WP, Tay SK, Zhao Y. Endometriosis-specific genes identified by real-time reverse transcription-polymerase chain reaction expression profiling of endometriosis versus autologous uterine endometrium. J Clin Endocrinol Metab. 2006;91:228–38.
6. Burney RO, Talbi S, Hamilton AE, Vo KC, Nyegaard M, Nezhat CR, Lessey BA, Giudice LC. Gene expression analysis of endometrium reveals progesterone resistance and candidate susceptibility genes in women with endometriosis. Endocrinology. 2007;148:3814–26.
7. Zafrakas M, Tarlatzis BC, Streichert T, Pournaropoulos F, Wölfle U, Smeets SJ, Wittek B, Grimbizis G, Brakenhoff RH, Pantel K, Bontis J, Günes C. Genome-wide microarray gene expression, array-CGH analysis, and telomerase activity in advanced ovarian endometriosis: a high degree of differentiation rather than malignant potential. Int J Mol Med. 2008;21:335–44.
8. Honda H, Barrueto FF, Gogusev J, Im DD, Morin PJ. Serial analysis of gene expression reveals differential expression between endometriosis and normal endometrium. Possible roles for AXL and SHC1 in the pathogenesis of endometriosis. Reprod Biol Endocrinol. 2008;6:59.
9. Guo SW. Epigenetics of endometriosis. Mol Hum Reprod. 2009;15:587–607.
10. Kobayashi H, Yamada Y, Kanayama S, Furukawa N, Noguchi T, Haruta S, Yoshida S, Sakata M, Sado T, Oi H. The role of iron in the pathogenesis of endometriosis. Gynecol Endocrinol. 2009;25:39–52.
11. Pelch KE, Schroder AL, Kimball PA, Sharpe-Timms KL, Davis JW, Nagel SC. Aberrant gene expression profile in a mouse model of endometriosis mirrors that observed in women. Fertil Steril. 2010;93:1615–27.
12. Borghese B, Barbaux S, Mondon F, Santulli P, Pierre G, Vinci G, Chapron C, Vaiman D. Research resource: genome-wide profiling of methylated promoters in endometriosis reveals a subtelomeric location of hypermethylation. Mol Endocrinol. 2010;24:1872–85.
13. Evian Annual Reproduction (EVAR) Workshop Group 2010, Fauser BC, Diedrich K, Bouchard P, Domínguez F, Matzuk M, Franks S, Hamamah S, Simón C, Devroey P, Ezcurra D, Howles CM. Contemporary genetic technologies and female reproduction. Hum Reprod Update. 2011;17:829–47.
14. Nasu K, Kawano Y, Tsukamoto Y, Takano M, Takai N, Li H, Furukawa Y, Abe W, Moriyama M, Narahara H. Aberrant DNA methylation status of endometriosis: epigenetics as the pathogenesis, biomarker and therapeutic target. J Obstet Gynaecol Res. 2011;37:683–95.
15. Borghese B, Santulli P, Héquet D, Pierre G, de Ziegler D, Vaiman D, Chapron C. Genetic polymorphisms of DNMT3L involved in hypermethylation of chromosomal ends are associated with greater risk of developing ovarian endometriosis. Am J Pathol. 2012;180:1781–6.
16. Wu Y, Strawn E, Basir Z, Halverson G, Guo SW. Promoter hypermethylation of progesterone receptor isoform B (PR-B) in endometriosis. Epigenetics. 2006;1:106–11.
17. Munksgaard PS, Blaakaer J. The association between endometriosis and ovarian cancer: a review of histological, genetic and molecular alterations. Gynecol Oncol. 2012;124:164–9.
18. Kurman RJ, Shih IM. Molecular pathogenesis and extraovarian origin of epithelial ovarian cancer–shifting the paradigm. Hum Pathol. 2011;42:918–31.
19. Goodman MT, Shvetsov YB. Incidence of ovarian, peritoneal, and fallopian tube carcinomas in the United States, 1995–2004. Cancer Epidemiol Biomarkers Prev. 2009;18:132–9.
20. Haruta S, Furukawa N, Yoshizawa Y, Tsunemi T, Nagai A, Kawaguchi R, Tanase Y, Yoshida S, Kobayashi H. Molecular genetics and epidemiology of epithelial ovarian cancer. Oncol Rep. 2011;26:1347–56.
21. Higashiura Y, Kajihara H, Shigetomi H, Kobayashi H. Identification of multiple pathways involved in the malignant transformation of endometriosis. Oncol Lett. 2012;4:3–9.
22. Brinton LA, Gridley G, Persson I, Baron J, Bergqvist A. Cancer risk after a hospital discharge diagnosis of endometriosis. Am J Obstet Gynecol. 1997;176:572–9.

23. Ness RB, Cramer DW, Goodman MT, Kjaer SK, Mallin K, Mosgaard BJ, Purdie DM, Risch HA, Vergona R, Wu AH. Infertility, fertility drugs, and ovarian cancer: a pooled analysis of case–control studies. Am J Epidemiol. 2002;155:217–24.
24. Brinton LA, Lamb EJ, Moghissi KS, Scoccia B, Althuis MD, Mabie JE, Westhoff CL. Ovarian cancer risk associated with varying causes of infertility. Fertil Steril. 2004;82:405–14.
25. Borgfeldt C, Andolf E. Cancer risk after hospital discharge diagnosis of benign ovarian cysts and endometriosis. Acta Obstet Gynecol Scand. 2004;83:395–400.
26. Ness RB. Endometriosis and ovarian cancer: thoughts on shared pathophysiology. Am J Obstet Gynecol. 2003;189:280–94.
27. Purdie DM, Bain CJ, Siskind V, Russell P, Hacker NF, Ward BG, Quinn MA, Green AC. Hormone replacement therapy and risk of epithelial ovarian cancer. Br J Cancer. 1999;81:559–63.
28. Somigliana E, Vigano' P, Parazzini F, Stoppelli S, Giambattista E, Vercellini P. Association between endometriosis and cancer: a comprehensive review and a critical analysis of clinical and epidemiological evidence. Gynecol Oncol. 2006;101(2):331–41.
29. Dinulescu DM, Ince TA, Quade BJ, Shafer SA, Crowley D, Jacks T. Role of K-ras and Pten in the development of mouse models of endometriosis and endometrioid ovarian cancer. Nat Med. 2005;11:63–70.
30. Kobayashi H, Sumimoto K, Moniwa N, Imai M, Takakura K, Kuromaki T, Morioka E, Arisawa K, Terao T. Risk of developing ovarian cancer among women with ovarian endometrioma: a cohort study in Shizuoka. Jpn Int J Gynecol Cancer. 2007;17:37–43.
31. Kobayashi H, Sumimoto K, Kitanaka T, Yamada Y, Sado T, Sakata M, Yoshida S, Kawaguchi R, Kanayama S, Shigetomi H, Haruta S, Tsuji Y, Ueda S, Terao T. Ovarian endometrioma–risks factors of ovarian cancer development. Eur J Obstet Gynecol Reprod Biol. 2008;138:187–93.
32. Wiegand KC, Shah SP, Al-Agha OM, Zhao Y, Tse K, Zeng T, Senz J, McConechy MK, Anglesio MS, Kalloger SE, Yang W, Heravi-Moussavi A, Giuliany R, Chow C, Fee J, Zayed A, Prentice L, Melnyk N, Turashvili G, Delaney AD, Madore J, Yip S, McPherson AW, Ha G, Bell L, Fereday S, Tam A, Galletta L, Tonin PN, Provencher D, Miller D, Jones SJ, Moore RA, Morin GB, Oloumi A, Boyd N, Aparicio SA, Shih IM, Mes-Masson AM, Bowtell DD, Hirst M, Gilks B, Marra MA, Huntsman DG. ARID1A mutations in endometriosis-associated ovarian carcinomas. N Engl J Med. 2010;363:1532–43.
33. Yamamoto S, Tsuda H, Takano M, Tamai S, Matsubara O. Loss of ARID1A protein expression occurs as an early event in ovarian clear-cell carcinoma development and frequently coexists with PIK3CA mutations. Mod Pathol. 2012;25:615–24.
34. Kolasa IK, Rembiszewska A, Janiec-Jankowska A, Dansonka-Mieszkowska A, Lewandowska AM, Konopka B, Kupryjańczyk J. PTEN mutation, expression and LOH at its locus in ovarian carcinomas. Relation to TP53, K-RAS and BRCA1 mutations. Gynecol Oncol. 2006;103:692–7.
35. Palacios J, Gamallo C. Mutations in the beta-catenin gene (CTNNB1) in endometrioid ovarian carcinomas. Cancer Res. 1998;58:1344–7.
36. Ogawa S, Kaku T, Amada S, Kobayashi H, Hirakawa T, Ariyoshi K, Kamura T, Nakano H. Ovarian endometriosis associated with ovarian carcinoma: a clinicopathological and immunohistochemical study. Gynecol Oncol. 2000;77:298–304.
37. Ballouk F, Ross JS, Wolf BC. Ovarian endometriotic cysts. An analysis of cytologic atypia and DNA ploidy patterns. Am J Clin Pathol. 1994;102:415–9.
38. Sato N, Tsunoda H, Nishida M, Morishita Y, Takimoto Y, Kubo T, Noguchi M. Loss of heterozygosity on 10q23.3 and mutation of the tumor suppressor gene PTEN in benign endometrial cyst of the ovary: possible sequence progression from benign endometrial cyst to endometrioid carcinoma and clear cell carcinoma of the ovary. Cancer Res. 2000;60:7052–6.

39. Brinton LA, Sakoda LC, Sherman ME, Frederiksen K, Kjaer SK, Graubard BI, Olsen JH, Mellemkjaer L. Relationship of benign gynecologic diseases to subsequent risk of ovarian and uterine tumors. Cancer Epidemiol Biomarkers Prev. 2005;14:2929–35.
40. Worley MJ, Welch WR, Berkowitz RS, Ng SW. Endometriosis-associated ovarian cancer: a review of pathogenesis. Int J Mol Sci. 2013;14:5367–79.
41. Ness RB, Grisso JA, Cottreau C, Klapper J, Vergona R, Wheeler JE, Morgan M, Schlesselman JJ. Factors related to inflammation of the ovarian epithelium and risk of ovarian cancer. Epidemiology. 2000;11:111–7.
42. Yamada Y, Shigetomi H, Onogi A, Haruta S, Kawaguchi R, Yoshida S, Furukawa N, Nagai A, Tanase Y, Tsunemi T, Oi H, Kobayashi H. New insights into pattern recognition receptors and their ligands in gynecologic pathologies. Hum Immunol. 2011;72:213–8.
43. Yamaguchi K, Mandai M, Toyokuni S, Hamanishi J, Higuchi T, Takakura K, Fujii S. Contents of endometriotic cysts, especially the high concentration of free iron, are a possible cause of carcinogenesis in the cysts through the iron-induced persistent oxidative stress. Clin Cancer Res. 2008;14:32–40.
44. Kobayashi H, Yamada Y, Kanayama S, Furukawa N, Noguchi T, Haruta S, Yoshida S, Sakata M, Sado T, Oi H. The role of hepatocyte nuclear factor-1beta in the pathogenesis of clear cell carcinoma of the ovary. Int J Gynecol Cancer. 2009;19:471–9.
45. Kajihara H, Yamada Y, Kanayama S, Furukawa N, Noguchi T, Haruta S, Yoshida S, Sado T, Oi H, Kobayashi H. Clear cell carcinoma of the ovary: potential pathogenic mechanisms. Oncol Rep. 2010;23:1193–203.
46. Tsuchiya A, Sakamoto M, Yasuda J, Chuma M, Ohta T, Ohki M, Yasugi T, Taketani Y, Hirohashi S. Expression profiling in ovarian clear cell carcinoma: identification of hepatocyte nuclear factor-1 beta as a molecular marker and a possible molecular target for therapy of ovarian clear cell carcinoma. Am J Pathol. 2003;163:2503–12.
47. Kobayashi H, Kajiwara H, Kanayama S, Yamada Y, Furukawa N, Noguchi T, Haruta S, Yoshida S, Sakata M, Sado T, Oi H. Molecular pathogenesis of endometriosis-associated clear cell carcinoma of the ovary. Oncol Rep. 2009;22:233–40.
48. Kato N, Sasou S, Motoyama T. Expression of hepatocyte nuclear factor-1beta (HNF-1beta) in clear cell tumors and endometriosis of the ovary. Mod Pathol. 2006;19:83–9.
49. Zanetta GM, Webb MJ, Li H, Keeney GL. Hyperestrogenism: a relevant risk factor for the development of cancer from endometriosis. Gynecol Oncol. 2000;79:18–22.
50. Tanase Y, Yamada Y, Shigetomi H, Kajihara H, Oonogi A, Yoshizawa Y, Furukawa N, Haruta S, Yoshida S, Sado T, Oi H, Kobayashi H. Modulation of estrogenic action in clear cell carcinoma of the ovary. Exp Ther Med. 2012;3:18–24.
51. Swedenborg E, Power KA, Cai W, Pongratz I, Rüegg J. Regulation of estrogen receptor beta activity and implications in health and disease. Cell Mol Life Sci. 2009;66:3873–94.
52. Suzuki F, Akahira J, Miura I, Suzuki T, Ito K, Hayashi S, Sasano H, Yaegashi N. Loss of estrogen receptor beta isoform expression and its correlation with aberrant DNA methylation of the 5′-untranslated region in human epithelial ovarian carcinoma. Cancer Sci. 2008;99:2365–72.
53. Mandai M, Yamaguchi K, Matsumura N, Baba T, Konishi I. Ovarian cancer in endometriosis: molecular biology, pathology, and clinical management. Int J Clin Oncol. 2009;14:383–91.

Index

T. Harada (ed.), *Endometriosis: Pathogenesis and Treatment*,
DOI 10.1007/978-4-431-54421-0, © Springer Japan 2014

MIX
Papier aus verantwortungsvollen Quellen
Paper from responsible sources
FSC® C105338

If you have any concerns about our products,
you can contact us on
ProductSafety@springernature.com

In case Publisher is established outside the EU,
the EU authorized representative is:
Springer Nature Customer Service Center GmbH
Europaplatz 3, 69115 Heidelberg, Germany

Printed by Libri Plureos GmbH
in Hamburg, Germany